MW01350508

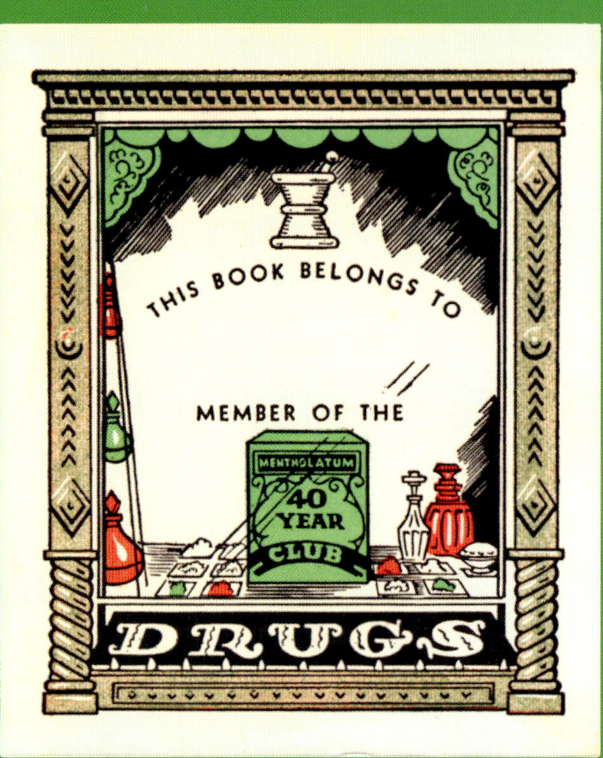
THIS BOOK BELONGS TO
MEMBER OF THE
MENTHOLATUM
40
YEAR
CLUB
DRUGS

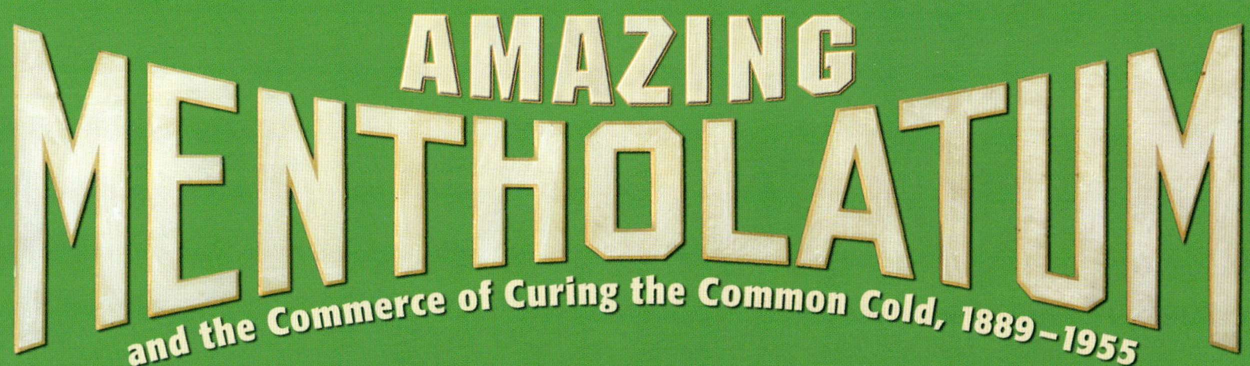

by Alex Taylor

with an introduction by John M. Hyde

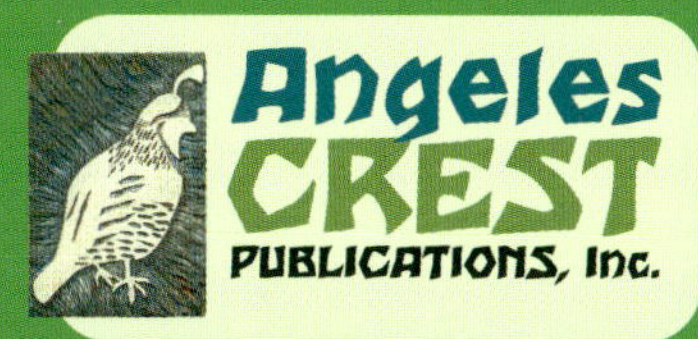

To Vickie, Jane, and Pattie

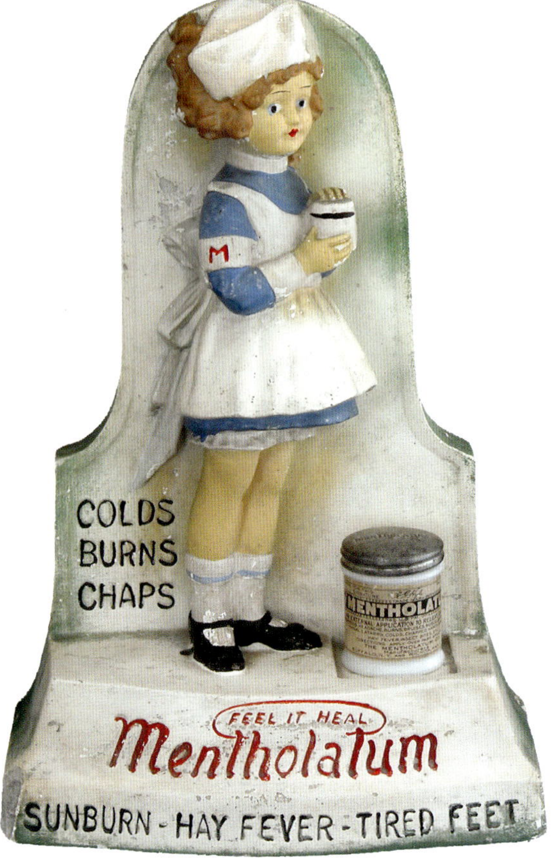

▲ **c. 1917** cast plaster countertop display, 13″H × 8½″W × 4¼″D

Book design and production by Susan H. Hartman
(www.suettcommunications.com)

First Edition

ISBN 0-9786173-0-4 Softbound edition
ISBN 0-9786173-1-2 Hardbound edition

Angeles Crest Publications, Inc.
P. O. Box 1211, La Cañada, CA 91012-5211

SAN: 851-1365

Printed in China

Contents

Catalog of Packaging and Advertising Art CD

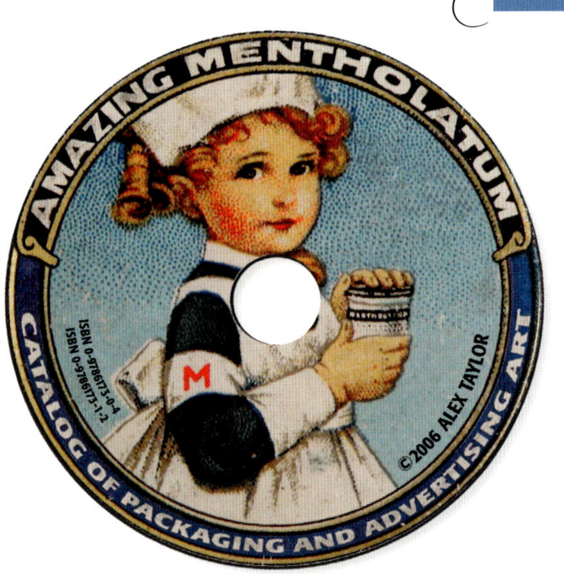

To view the catalog you will need Adobe Reader 3.0 or later. Download it free at www.adobe.com.

Product Packaging

Advertising

Marketing and Sales

Lost and Found

It's remarkable that the history of a business as old and respected as the Mentholatum Company could be lost, but it was. What is more remarkable is how fast it was recovered, with the help of the Internet.

My great-grandfather founded the Mentholatum Company. For as long as I can remember I have studied people's reactions when I mention my relationship to Mentholatum®. There are typically three different responses: blank, effusive, and guarded. The first response generally comes from younger folks who have not heard of the salve or know only of the currently popular Mentholatum Softlips®. The second, and most enjoyable, response begins with a big smile and a sigh, followed by a heartfelt testimonial, which will often go like this: "I remember Mentholatum—my mother always put it on my chest when I had a cold," or "My grandmother loved Mentholatum—she put it on her feet before she went to bed," and the best one, "I love Mentholatum—I use Mentholatum all the time." Then there are the "Vicks VapoRub® people," who try to be polite and not disappoint me, or mistakenly ask, "Didn't Mentholatum become Vicks?"

When I was growing up in the '50s and '60s, it seemed that my world was divided over a handful of popular brands, like the contest between people who drank Coke and the people who preferred Pepsi. My neighborhood was also split between Ford and Chevy owners (although my dad was a Pontiac man). There were many smaller factions, but only a few main tribal allegiances clearly divided us. The division I was particularly sensitive to was between the Mentholatum people and the Vicks people. From my perspective, as a fourth-generation member of the family that manufactured Mentholatum, the Vicks people were not particularly bad, they were just different. I felt pity for them. After all, Mentholatum represented all that was good in America; it was mom and apple pie! It was as plain as day and night that Mentholatum's green jar represented growth and life, while the dark purple Vicks VapoRub jar signaled danger . . . well, you see my youthful logic.

In 1988, a year before the Mentholatum Company's centennial anniversary, the stockholders in my family sold the company to a Japanese buyer, Rohto Pharmaceutical Co., Ltd. Rohto was a fitting choice to acquire the American icon. The Mentholatum Company had nurtured a long and prosperous relationship with the Japanese who, in the early years, provided Mentholatum with its signature ingredient, menthol, a product of the northern island of Hokkaido. Additionally, the company's founder and my great-grandfather, A. A. Hyde, supported the Christian missionary work of the Omi Brotherhood in Omi-Hachiman. After building a new factory there in 1921, he licensed the manufacture and sale of Mentholatum in Japan to the Brotherhood. Japanese consumers have remained loyal to Mentholatum ever since, and today they constitute the brand's largest market worldwide.

It was no fault of Rohto's new management team that when they celebrated Mentholatum's one hundred–year anniversary in 1989, they were unable to tell much of its history. Sometime beyond living memory a great deal of it had been lost. The family mythology told how Grandfather reversed a financial disaster by inventing Mentholatum, then became extremely wealthy, living on 10 percent and tithing 90 percent to people with a greater need than his own. Perhaps it was true in the earliest days that "the product sold itself," but in order for the company to grow, A. A. Hyde had to advertise and market his new salve. The nuts and bolts of how he used advertising and marketing to build the Mentholatum Company into a major international concern rivaled only by Vicks was absent from our simple family tradition.

I first became aware of the problem back in the early 1980s, when I asked my cousin George Hyde, who was then president of the company, for historical information about some old sample tins I found. He told me he could not help me, because it did not exist. So I had to look elsewhere if I was going to find the story. George Irving's *Master of Money: A. A. Hyde of Wichita* (New York: Fleming H. Revell Company, 1936) provided background on A. A. Hyde's spiritual and philanthropic life but offered nothing about the company. John M. Hyde's, "A Balm in Gilead" (*Kansas History: A Journal of the Central Plains*, vol. 9, no. 4, winter 1986/1987: 150–163) provided more information on the company's founding and a framework for the early history, but it also focused largely on A. A. Hyde. Fragments of the marketing story could be gleaned from the company's quarterly "pocket magazine" *Menthology* (1916–1944), but a complete collection was as yet unknown. Old magazine ads were another source, but finding the right issues was like locating a needle in a haystack. As it turned out, the most important clues would come from the containers, packaging, and handouts that I was finding at random in flea markets and thrift shops.

With pestilence, flood, and fire working around the clock, it is a miracle any of these items survived. The lucky few pieces that were not thrown out and remained intact did so because they were neglected in some out-of-the-way place. They were hidden throughout North America in the back of medicine cabinets, inside steamer trunks in attics, in cluttered dresser drawers at estate sales, and in forgotten, dust-covered shipping crates in the basements of old drugstores. It would have taken me a lifetime of searching through rummage sales and auctions to find enough of the surviving pieces to reconstruct the entire Mentholatum puzzle.

My collection expanded a bit faster when a neighbor and fellow collector, Duane Shrader, offered to bring back any Mentholatum artifacts he found from the antique shows that he annually visited in the Midwest and on the East Coast. I was impressed with the wide variety of objects he was able to find. Along the way, Duane also taught me a few tricks of the trade, the most important being not to trust another collector to do your collecting. Duane easily became hooked on Mentholatum, and after that, all I ever saw were his "seconds." He now has quite a nice collection of his own!

Then everything about the way I collected Mentholatum changed. In early September 1999, Jack Melton, the director of the Dorsey Museum in Estes Park, Colorado, gave me a call. Jack and his wife, Lulie, have created a wonderful little history museum on the grounds of the YMCA Conference Center that includes a fine display of Hyde family and Mentholatum artifacts. Jack thought it would be a good idea for me to take a look at eBay. It turned out that on any given day in cyberspace there are an average of one to two dozen Mentholatum-related items up for auction. They include jars, sample tins, blotters, booklets, posters, letters, and artifacts that I had not known existed. They are gathered up not just by the antique dealers who specialize in drugstore collectibles, but by all sorts of people living in many different countries. On-line trading has made everybody a potential dealer and every computer screen a virtual showroom.

A few months later, I was comparing the labels on several new auction jars that had arrived in the mail with the labeled jars in my original collection when I noticed that they could be placed in chronological order. It dawned on me that if I could date the jars this fast, reconstructing Mentholatum's lost history was now within my reach. Seizing the opportunity, with my wife Vickie's enthusiastic and loving support, I dropped all other projects and began acquiring anything and everything that had to do with Mentholatum. I found more than three hundred new items within the first twelve months and close to one thousand by the book's completion. This collection produced the illustrations for the text and the product catalogs that make up the second part of this book—on CD-ROM—that will help dealers and collectors to identify and authenticate what they find.

As my studio was transformed into an oversized curio cabinet, a picture of Mentholatum's first fifty years began to emerge. I was able to create a time line so that advertising and packaging could be identified chronologically. I enlisted the help of my cousin, John Hyde, who is professor emeritus in the history department at Williams College in Williamstown, Massachusetts. John is the keeper of the Hyde family history as well as custodian of a small collection of records from the early years of the Yucca Company. John agreed to help critique my manuscript, and I owe him a huge debt for suffering through many terrible drafts while I struggled to find my voice. I knew I was going to make it when he finally wrote in the margins of one chapter that it was as good as any graduate thesis. John's generosity did not end with his editing and copious notes; he also contributed the introduction that follows this preface.

With my background in art and design I was still going to need professional help creating the picture book I envisioned. Susan Hartman is a graphic designer with a specialty in book design. I got to know Sue and her husband, Ed, as parents at our children's school and became familiar with her work doing joint projects for the school. We found that our design instincts were complementary, and the past several years spent collaborating on the book have been a delight. Though I was involved every step of the way, the overall look of the book was her fault. In addition to supporting Sue, Ed kept my computer up and running so that I could shoot, clean, and cut out the hundreds of digital images that Sue needed for layout. Ed also contributed product photography for the catalog. Sue's longtime associate Dawn Shoemaker expertly edited the final manuscript. Dawn's colleague Sharon Duffy compiled the index.

Additional thanks go to Gayle Thompson for assisting in the organization of the collection; to our mail carrier Paul Anderson for delivering everything I purchased on eBay; to our son, Charles Taylor, for helping me in the beginning with computer trauma; to my sister, Julia Taylor, for curating the family photo archive; to my cousin Kevin Taylor and aunt Carol Taylor; to Jami Frazier Tracy, curator of collections at the Wichita-Sedgwick Historical Museum; to Craig Miner, Willard W. Garvey Distinguished Professor of Business History at Wichita State University, for editing the first chapters for historical content; to Mike Kelly and Mary Nelson at the Wichita State University Libraries, Department of Special Collections; and to Bob Boewe, owner of the Spice Merchant.

A special acknowledgment goes to my old friend Dr. George Caughey, chief of the Pulmonary and Critical Care Medicine Division at the University of California at San Francisco's Veterans Hospital, for editing the manuscript for scientific accuracy. Admiration to Sarah Young for her illustration of *Mentha arvensis*. Thanks go to Janice Kwarta and Jeanine Sortisio at the Mentholatum Company; Yoko Matsumoto at the Omi Brotherhood Company; Richard Foster at the New York Public Library; the staff at the Los Angeles Public Library, Central Library; Kim Mann; Edgar Simon; Duane Bouliew Jr.; Robert E. Newnham; Kathlyn Schoof; Robert Mitchell; Lynn Payne; Ethel Willard (d. 9/18/01); George Jordan (d. 5/26/03); and Albert Taylor Hyde (d. 12/25/03).

A product history would not be complete without a review of the nineteenth-century patent medicine industry out of which Mentholatum emerged. I expanded my search for a sampling of the rivals in the cold-remedy market. Examples of rival brands throughout the book provide a context for evaluating Mentholatum's early success and a clue to what worked in the marketplace and what didn't.

The advertising art produced by the Mentholatum Company is a reflection of its time, providing us with a clue to what attracted our grandparents' attention, what images caught their eyes, and what made them feel good about a product. In the days before antibiotics, it tells us what they knew about illness and the serious efforts they would take to "cure" a cold before it grew into something life-threatening. This is the story of how a handful of patent medicines rose above the crowd, and how one in particular shook off the stigma of quackery and nurtured the transformation of the rural drugstore into the modern pharmacy of today.

In the 1920s, '30s, and '40s, Mentholatum and its archrival, Vicks, were the most recognized cold-remedy brands in the world. They were indeed the Coke and Pepsi of the cold season, and, somewhat as Coke and Pepsi have today, they have entered a secondary collectors' market of vintage packaging and advertising art. A. A. Hyde certainly never dreamed that his healing emollient would survive to enter the marketplace for a second time, to be bought and sold for its utilitarian and artistic value. And now that the first half of Mentholatum's history has been resurrected, a better understanding of the part it played in the lives of our ancestors will perhaps encourage collectors to take better care of these antiques and assure their existence for another hundred years.

Introduction

Mentholatum and A. A. Hyde are names that have become indissolubly linked. The product was developed and named by Hyde, and he presided over more than four decades of its growth as a salve that became known throughout the world. It seemed appropriate, therefore, to introduce this history of Mentholatum with a brief essay on the life of A. A. Hyde, emphasizing the values and ideals that influenced not only his personal life but his business practices and goals as well. A family-owned and -managed company for the first century of its existence, Mentholatum's association with the Hyde family is reflected in this history of its origin and growth, which was compiled and written by Alex Taylor, a great-grandson of A. A. Hyde, and in this introduction, which was written by a grandson, John M. Hyde.*

In 1792, Alvan Hyde, the new young minister of the Congregational Church, "built me an house" and "moved with my wife into it and began to live in family state." More than two hundred years after it was built, the house still stands on a small rise just west of the center of the town of Lee in the Berkshire Hills of western Massachusetts. Later generations added to and renovated the house, but the original structure remains the dominant feature of the building. It was in this house that Albert Alexander Hyde was born in 1848, the second son and fifth child of Alexander Hyde who, in turn, was the youngest son of the Reverend Alvan Hyde. Having inherited the family homestead and the responsibility for caring for his aging mother, Alexander became deacon of his father's church and established a "family boarding school" in the house in order to support himself and his growing family. His son, Albert Alexander (known to the family as Bert), grew up in that environment of church, family, and school in a small New England town whose institutions and traditions inevitably shaped his view of the world. That view was also influenced by the events of the Civil War and their impact on the community, which the young boy recorded in his diary: the reports of life on the battlefront in northern Virginia in letters from Bert's older brother, the losses suffered by neighbors and friends, and the excitement of hearing the church bell ring out to announce great "victories." The end of the war coincided with the end of Bert's high school education, and as did many young men from the small towns of New England, he went west in 1865 to

*The sources quoted in the Introduction are drawn from Dr. Hyde's collection of A. A. Hyde papers and memorabilia, which will ultimately be deposited in the Special Collections of the Ablah Library at Wichita State University.

join his older brother in Leavenworth, Kansas, where he was employed as a bank clerk.

In 1872, he was sent to the newly established community of Wichita to become the cashier of a new bank. A booming frontier town, Wichita had recently become the terminus of the cattle drives up the Chisolm Trail upon the completion of a rail line by the Santa Fe Railroad to carry the cattle to market. The young man soon settled into the life of a growing community, and by 1885 he was an officer of the Kansas National Bank, a member of the Board of Education, a leader of the First Presbyterian Church, and the father of a growing family. A respected member of the community, a "square-toed man of pronounced convictions," he seemed an unlikely prospect to be caught up in the "land boom" of the 1880s, but for reasons that he never fully explained, he resigned from his position with the bank in 1887 and became a "loan broker," a real estate speculator.

He had invested in real estate in prior years, as had many of his business colleagues, and one of his successful ventures left a lasting imprint on the present city of Wichita. Developing and platting a section of land, known as Hyde's Addition, he reserved one square block for a park to provide recreational space for the neighborhood, which came to be called Hyde Park. And he named the streets in the section after the important women in his life including his wife, Ida, her sister, Pattie, and her sister-in-law, Laura. During the "boom" years, he became on paper a wealthy man, buying and selling mortgages in Wichita and surrounding communities. As a sign of his new prosperity, he built a large and imposing home on a hill to the east of the town, which he was confident would anchor a valuable residential area as the city grew. But predictably the "boom" collapsed, and A. A. Hyde was left with a growing family, a heavily mortgaged home, and significant debts. It was this experience of the sudden loss of his wealth that was to have a profound influence on Hyde and on his subsequent conduct of personal and business affairs.

His was a moral and ethical crisis as well as a financial one, for he felt responsible not only for his own losses but also for those of friends and family who had entrusted their money to him. He therefore sought understanding and direction in scripture and in prayer, traditions and ideals in which he had been raised. The familiar words of the Sermon on the Mount, which he had known by heart since he was a boy, suddenly took on new meaning for him in its admonition to "lay up treasures in heaven" rather than on earth "where moth and rust consume, and where thieves break through and steal." His efforts to accumulate earthly wealth had not brought satisfaction "but brought instead anxiety and a distrust of fellow men" and a realization that "accumulated wealth was a source of worry, shortened life, and was deleterious to character; that the time spent worrying over these investments, attending meetings and brooding over reports, might be put to much better advantage for my own satisfaction, good of my family, and for the benefit of the community."

Hyde's first responsibility was to provide for the needs of his growing family. In 1889, he entered into a partnership to form the Yucca Company for the manufacture and sale of a toilet soap made from the oily pulp of the yucca plant. From that partnership ultimately came Mentholatum, and in the chapters to follow, the origins and development of that product will be traced both in text and in illustrations. By 1898, the success of this venture and the dramatic increase in the sale of Mentholatum brought the sudden realization to A. A. Hyde that he was becoming a very rich man. Mindful of the lesson he had learned from his earlier experience with accumulated wealth, he now turned to applying the admonition of the Sermon on the Mount to "lay up for yourselves treasures in heaven" rather than on earth.

Thus began the association of Mentholatum with the philanthropy of A. A. Hyde. Caring for the needs of others was not a responsibility suddenly thrust upon him by financial success. From those institutions of family, school, and church that were his heritage, he had learned to tithe, to give away one-tenth of one's income, and had been a generous supporter of his church and of the YMCA in Wichita. But tithing, Hyde wrote, was for "those without accumulated wealth." Those who had gained surplus wealth, as he was now doing, were responsible for giving away *all* the surplus, rather than only a tenth. A person who died with accumulated wealth, therefore, died disgraced. There was nothing particularly original or profound about this philosophy of giving, which bore a strong resemblance to Andrew Carnegie's "Gospel of Wealth." Hyde never acknowledged any debt to others for his ideas, nor did he associate his good fortune with any particular political or economic theory. His wealth was not a sign of God's favor toward him or the economic system that produced it; it was simply a gift of which he was the trustee or steward. That sense of stewardship provided the incentive for his giving. In doing so, he may have oversimplified life, as his friend and widely known Kansas newspaper editor William Allen White once remarked, but "if he did he erred in the right direction."

Having made this commitment in principle to give away his accumulated wealth, Hyde then faced the practical questions of how it should be done and to whom these funds should be given. Two institutions were of particular interest to him and had already benefited from his tithing—the First Presbyterian Church of Wichita and the YMCA. The minister of the church, the Reverend Charles E. Bradt, had aroused the energy and enthusiasm of his congregation for the work of foreign missions, and in 1898, the members of the First Presbyterian Church resolved to "become and be known as a Missionary Church." To assist in this endeavor, A. A. Hyde had published a booklet of Bible verses, which was distributed with each jar of Mentholatum. It was dedicated to all those who obeyed the words of the "Great Commission" to go into "all the world" and "preach the gospel to every creature." Included in the booklet was a message from the Reverend Charles Bradt endorsing the message of the booklet and certifying that "one-tenth of the profits from the sales of Mentholatum" will be donated "each year to the cause of Missions." The secretary of the Kansas YMCA seconded Bradt's message and urged that the Biblical "texts be applied to the spirits and Mentholatum to the bodies of tens of thousands."

As the sales of Mentholatum increased, so too did Hyde's wealth. To provide a framework for his philanthropy, he set aside a significant block of Mentholatum stock to establish a foundation, the Hyde Benevolent Society, which was to be the vehicle for his philanthropy. As the stock grew in value, Hyde was able to increase the range and number of beneficiaries. From this generosity came many of the apocryphal stories of the origins of Mentholatum and of Mr. Hyde's wealth. The popular evangelist Aimee Semple McPherson accounted for his success by saying that when he was a destitute young man, he had turned to the Bible and "entered into a definite contract with the Lord" who immediately "began to prosper him." Therefore, she concluded, the "Lord prospered him in a wonderful way," and changed him "from a penniless, deeply indebted man to a multi-millionaire." A copy of these remarks was sent to Hyde, who wrote at the end of the article in carefully hand-printed block letters: "All Bosh. A.A.H."

By 1906, Mentholatum had become a patent remedy with nationwide sales and distribution. The volume of business led to the opening of a branch plant in Buffalo, New York, in 1903 and the construction in 1909 of a new factory on Douglas Avenue in Wichita. A new corporate entity named, appropriately, the Mentholatum Company was formed. Like its predecessor, the Yucca Company, the stock in the new company was largely owned by A. A. Hyde and members of his family. With the business prospering and his sons gradually assuming responsibility for the day-to-day affairs of the company, Hyde began to devote more and more of his time to his philanthropy. His objective in giving away his wealth was almost too simple, as White had noted: it was to support any person, organization, or institution which Hyde felt would contribute to the Kingdom of God on earth. What was required of all was a religious, but not necessarily a denominational or even Christian, commitment. With such a broad mandate, the results were predictably eclectic, ranging from the Piney Woods Country Life School for black youths in Mississippi to Oberlin College, from the Gilbert Street Mexican Mission in Wichita to a playground in Athens, Greece, for refugees from the war with Turkey; from the National Anti-Cigarette League to the American Friends Service Committee. He always reserved a special place for foreign missions and the YMCA—the first of his many charitable interests. In 1925, the city of Wichita honored him at a civic banquet at which his neighbor, former governor Henry J. Allen, described Hyde as "the wisest man I've ever known about wealth. . . . He distributes wealth under an unshakeable conviction that he's investing in the happiness of others—and that by this course of action, he contributes to a holy purpose in a better world."

Mindful of his age and health as he approached his eightieth birthday, he decided to dissolve the Hyde Benevolent Society and to sell its stock *for cash* only, which he would then distribute in accordance with his intention of dying without accumulated wealth. By January 1935, he was nearing his eighty-seventh birthday. Still actively engaged in the affairs of the company that he had started almost fifty years earlier, he was asked to say a few words to a group of Mentholatum salesmen who were meeting in Wichita. His message to them was to be his valedictory. It was a reaffirmation of his faith that "we are not here to lay up worldly treasures but to be of service." Six days later he was dead. As he had wished, he did not die disgraced.

John M. Hyde
Williamstown, Massachusetts

Dr. John M. Hyde received his B.A. degree from Williams College, his M.A. from the University of Minnesota, and his Ph.D. from Harvard University. He spent his career teaching history at Williams College, where he served as chairman of the history department and dean of the college.

Everything Goes in Wichita

The founding of the Yucca Company in September 1889 was the genesis of Mentholatum. It was a hopeful venture begun by three Wichita, Kansas, businessmen during an economic depression. Walter R. Binkley, a former partner of the Stallings Palmole Soap Co., saw an opportunity to start his own soap business when D. W. Stallings sold out to investors. Binkley had already developed a method of manufacturing vegetable-based soaps using the indigenous yucca or "soap tree," which grew in abundance on the Kansas prairie. Now all he needed to get started was financing. Binkley met Clayton K. Smith, a pharmacist trained at the Philadelphia College of Pharmacy who had recently arrived in town, and convinced him to join the venture. They capitalized their new company with $600 from Smith's brother-in-law, Albert Alexander Hyde, a local real estate developer and small-business investor. Binkley and Smith set up the Yucca Company on the ground floor of a three-story brick building owned by Hyde on Douglas Avenue, Wichita's main thoroughfare and route of the old Chisholm Trail.[1]

The Empire House

A. A. Hyde (inset) stayed here when he arrived in Wichita in 1872. The hotel also housed the stagecoach ticket office.

A. A. Hyde was one of the young businessmen who helped build Wichita. As a twenty-four-year-old bookkeeper employed by the Leavenworth banking firm Clark and Company, he was sent to Wichita to open a new bank in early July of 1872. To launch the new bank, Sol and Morris Kohn, Wichita merchants and longtime customers of Clark and Company, matched Clark's $20,000 investment. Hyde put down $500, and the rest of the stock was purchased by "a majority of the best business men of the place." With nearly $70,000 of the $100,000 goal on the books, the Wichita Savings Bank elected officers on the 17th of July. The new bank's rival in town was the First National Bank of Wichita, the only other bank Hyde said was "worth speaking of." The Kohn brothers were among a core group of wealthy speculators in their mid- to late twenties who had orchestrated a plan to lure the profitable Texas cattle trade to Wichita. Within two weeks of his arrival, Hyde had become a bit player in the launching of a new cowtown.[2]

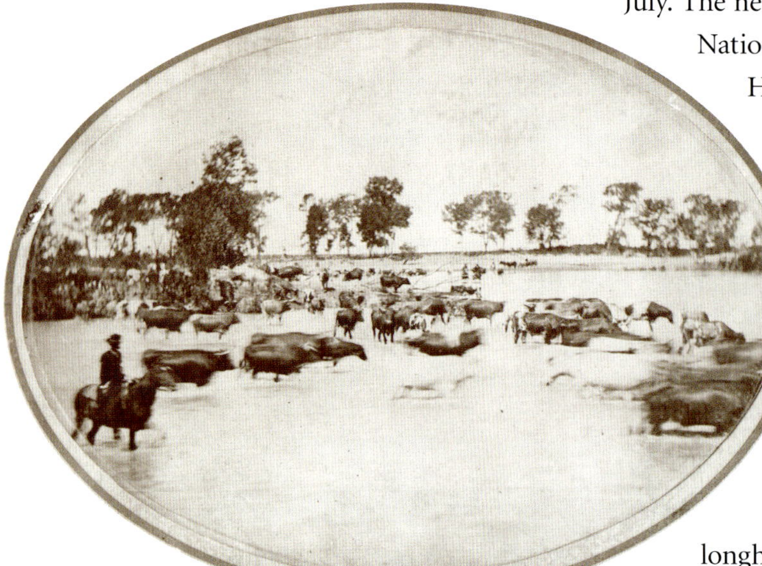

The Best Place to Cross

Crossing rivers could become a dangerous undertaking for Texas cattlemen on the trail to Abilene, like the outfit shown in this 1869 photograph, who chose to safely cross the Arkansas River at the Wichita trading post.

Each summer, Texas cattlemen drove longhorns up the Shawnee Trail to the railroad lines in Kansas City and St. Louis where their herds were loaded onto boxcars and shipped to the beef-hungry eastern markets. In 1868, a shorter route called the Chisholm Trail was surveyed. Drovers left Red River Station in Texas, crossed Indian Territory up into Kansas (where they forded the Arkansas River at a frontier trading post used by the Wichita tribe of Indians), and then crossed rolling grasslands northward to the Union Pacific Railroad at Abilene. But the Abilene terminus was not to last long. After only four years, the local citizens (called "nesters" by the cowboys) became fed up with herds trampling their crops, rowdies tearing up the streets at all hours, and the vice and crime that followed the cattlemen. The *Abilene Chronicle* announced to the cattlemen in February 1872 that the citizens would "no longer submit to the evils of the trade."[3]

Wichita Opens for Business

Other frontier towns immediately stepped up to compete for the profitable cattle business. Speculators at the Wichita settlement were already building a new town that they hoped would become the next cattle terminus and shipping point. They convinced the Atchison, Topeka & Santa Fe railroad to secure a rail extension from the main line at Newton, and the new track was completed in May of 1872. They also hired agents who traveled south to the cattlemen and east to the buyers to spread the news that Wichita

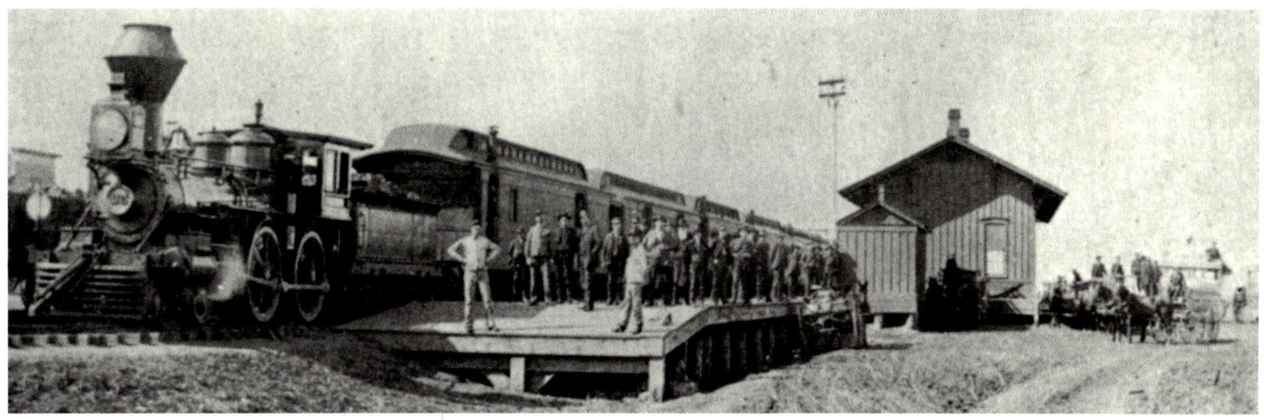

New Terminus of the Chisholm Trail

A spur line brought the Santa Fe Railroad to Wichita, where speculators created an ideal destination for eastern meat packers and Texas ranchers to conduct their business and have a good time.

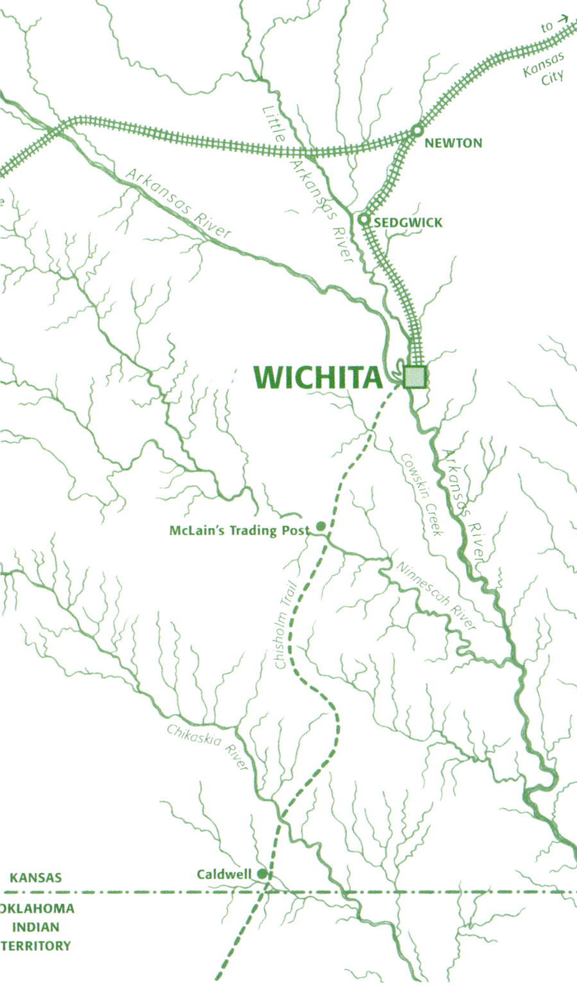

was ready with the necessary banks, hotels, livery stables, stockyards, outfitters, and entertainment for the 1872 driving season.[4]

As the tired drovers approached Wichita, they were greeted by a sign posted at the edge of town that read, "Everything Goes in Wichita," with one exception listed at the bottom: "Leave your revolvers at police headquarters and get a check." The dusty streets and boardwalks were crowded with men on horseback and foot, and endless herds of "beeve critters" passing through to the stockyard east of town. There were bowlegged Texas cowboys, Mexican vaqueros, ex-slaves, Plains Indians, long-haired frontiersmen, immigrant sodbusters, merchants, Eastern adventurers, gamblers, and assorted loose characters. Bert Hyde, as A. A. was known by family and friends, recalled that the gambling houses and saloons, which operated all night and day, outnumbered grocery and outfitting stores. A variety theater, called a "Free and Easy," gave nightly exhibitions of exotic female dancers. A brass band played all afternoon seated on a balcony perched over the sidewalk. Bert wrote in his diary: "So much swearing I never heard before . . . the majority can hardly construct a sentence with out an oath as emphasis." He also observed, "The principal occupation here seems to be loafing. In front of every store the whole length of the street (half a mile) you will see from one to a dozen men occupying themselves whittling, talking or dozing. Whether it is the nature of the country or the nature of the inhabitants I have been unable to discover, possibly both."[5]

In this wild and uproarious setting, Hyde opened the bank up for business in a temporary location: a small wood building on Main Street, which had formerly been a saloon. At night, he pulled a bed up in front of the safe, placed his pistol under the pillow, and tried to sleep through the outside din of drunks and keno gamblers. The room above him was used as a flophouse

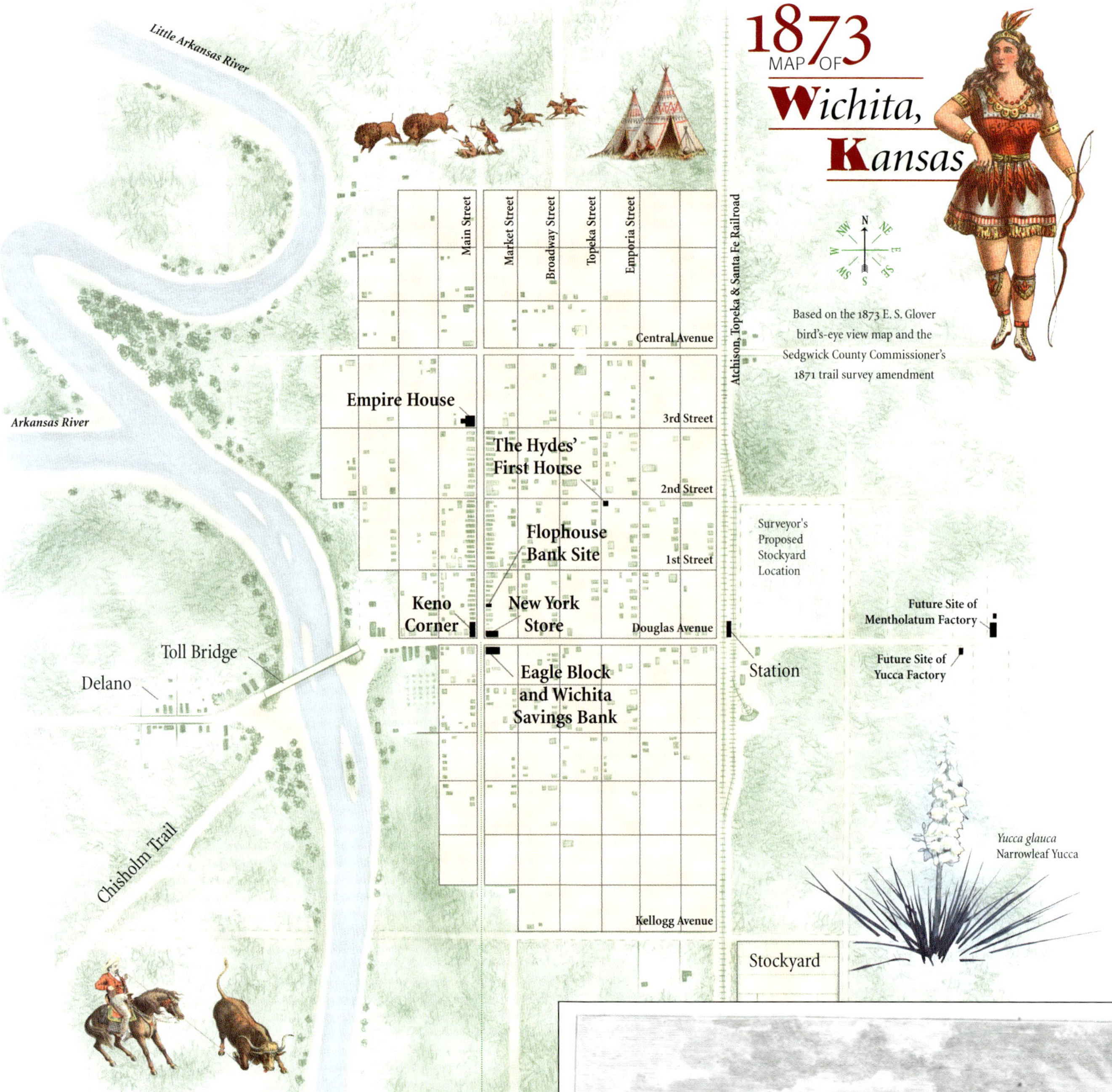

1873 Map of Wichita, Kansas

Based on the 1873 E. S. Glover bird's-eye view map and the Sedgwick County Commissioner's 1871 trail survey amendment

Little Arkansas River
Arkansas River
Main Street
Market Street
Broadway Street
Topeka Street
Emporia Street
Atchison, Topeka & Santa Fe Railroad
Central Avenue
3rd Street
2nd Street
1st Street
Douglas Avenue
Kellogg Avenue
Empire House
The Hydes' First House
Flophouse Bank Site
Keno Corner
New York Store
Eagle Block and Wichita Savings Bank
Toll Bridge
Delano
Chisholm Trail
Station
Surveyor's Proposed Stockyard Location
Future Site of Mentholatum Factory
Future Site of Yucca Factory
Stockyard
N NE E SE S SW W NW
Yucca glauca
Narrowleaf Yucca

Wichita in 1873

The new cowtown at the fork of the Arkansas River already had more than five hundred buildings, a toll bridge, train station, and stockyard. The engraving (right) from *Harper's Weekly* depicts Main Street looking north and shows the predominance of business establishments located there. The artist's view is from atop the Eagle Block on the southeast corner of Douglas and Main. Keno Corner and the balcony where brass bands often played can be seen on the left, the New York Store is on the right, and the Empire House is just visible at the far end of the street.

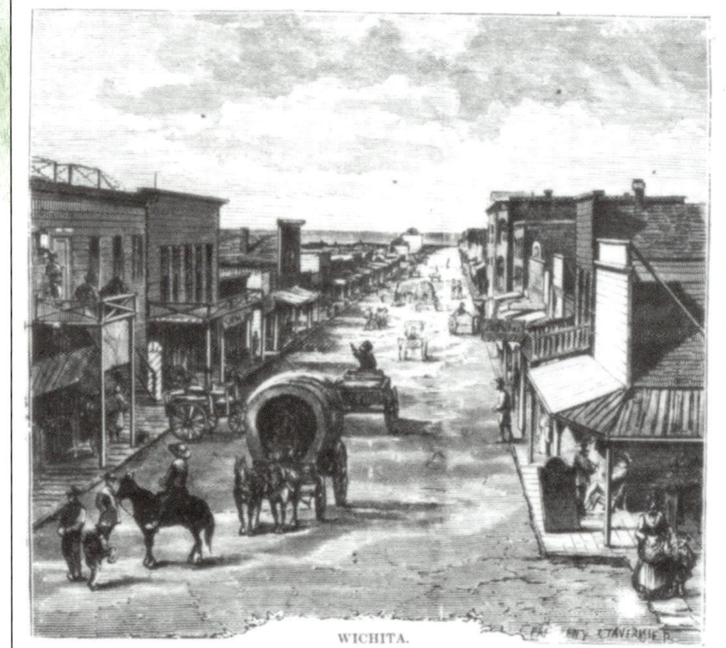

where there happened to be a hole cut in the floorboards just above his bed large enough for a man to drop through. In later years, he characterized this as "a fool arrangement on my part, but in those days horse stealing was the fashionable crime, and hold-ups and bank robbers were almost unknown." Within a few months he moved the operation into the newly completed Eagle Block office building on the southeast corner of Douglas and Main. This intersection was fast becoming the center of Wichita's economic and social life.[6]

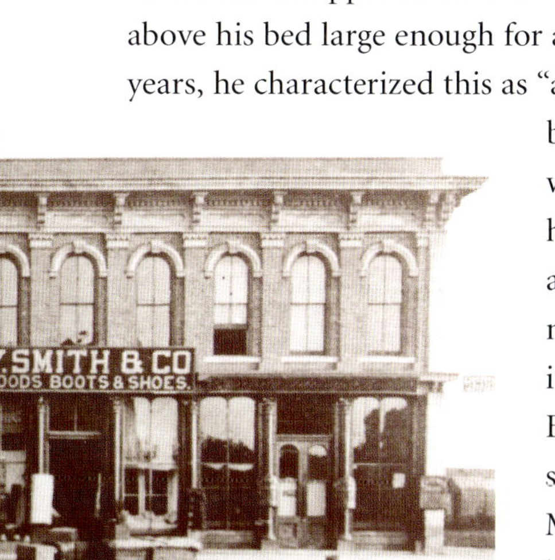

Millions of dollars changed hands during the next few years, and Hyde and his bookkeeper, Johnnie Walters, handled a large portion of it. In addition to the books, Johnnie's chief business was running the big saloon and gambling house called "Keno Corner" located diagonally across the intersection from the bank. Throughout the day, he would run over to the saloon to see how business was doing. For a few years in the early 1870s, Douglas and Main also marked the center of America's Wild West. Here was the proverbial crossroads between anything goes and law and order, a manifestation of that singular contradiction in the American psyche—that we want it both ways. Sometimes the two collided, as for several weeks in 1874 when Wichita was held hostage. The Texas desperado William Martin, known as "Hurricane Bill," and his gang of cattle rustlers shot up the streets and terrorized the residents. To stop them, Marshal Bill Smith hired several new policemen, including the young Wyatt Earp. Because the city did not tax its citizens, Marshal Smith used funds from gambling license fees and prostitution fines to pay his lawmen. Wichita wanted it both ways for most of the next decade. Hyde's conservative neighbors were torn between their disdain for open drinking, gambling, and prostitution on the streets, and their appetite for the tax-free prosperity that the cattle trade brought to their town.[7]

The Eagle Block

This 1872 photograph (above) of Wichita's first stone building, named the Eagle Block, illustrates the wide range of personalities inhabiting the business community. Notice the contrast between the clean sidewalk in front of the corner Wichita Savings Bank (complete with spittoon) and that of the trash-strewn walk in front of the Drygoods & Groceries store. The photo of Wichita Savings Bank below was taken a few years later. It shows a gas lamp over the bank's front door and additional length to the building beyond where the *Wichita Eagle* newspaper offices were located.

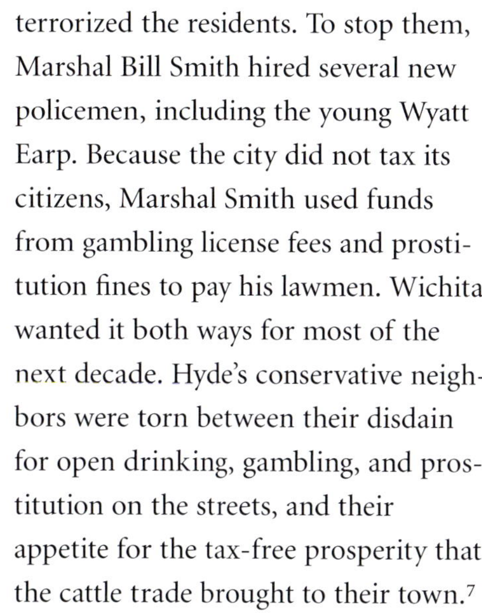

In 1874, merchants were relieved when cattle were no longer allowed to enter at the Douglas Avenue crossing. The new Kellogg Avenue route to the stockyard put an end to longhorns crowding through the business district and kicking up dust.

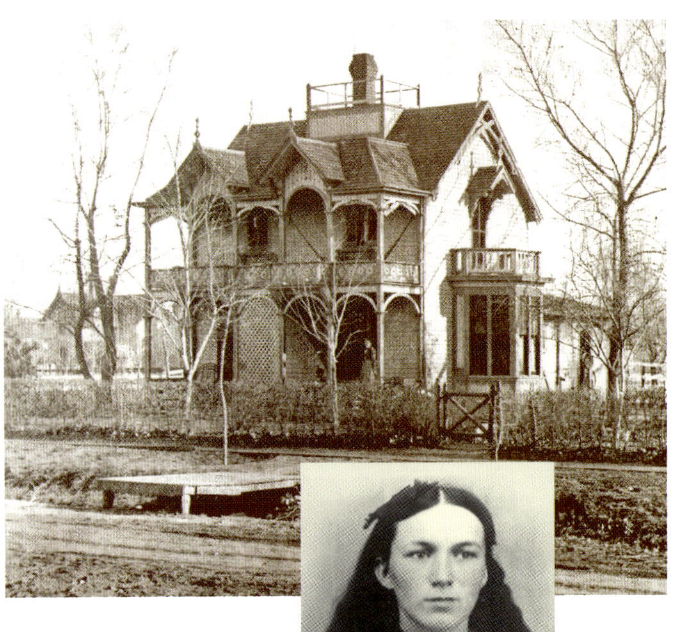

Ida Todd

Ida (inset), a relative of Mary Todd Lincoln, married A. A. Hyde in 1875. The Hydes' first house (above) cost $1,000 and occupied two lots. Within the first year they added a new barn for their horse, Betty; a cistern; and a "hot house" garden. They also planted fruit trees on the open lot and elm and ash trees along the sidewalks.

In 1875, Bert married Ida Todd, the daughter of James H. Todd, a local grocery merchant and a cousin of Mary Todd Lincoln. In a bachelor town where most men had to return east to find a wife, Bert was lucky. Caught geographically in the middle of a popular saying of the time, "There is no Sunday west of Junction City and no God west of Salina," they were married on Tuesday, January 19, in Mr. Todd's home by Rev. McCabe of Topeka. Bert vacated the bank's back room that he had shared with Johnnie Walters and moved with Ida into a house that he purchased a week before on the southeast corner of Second Street and Topeka Avenue. The first of their nine children, Albert Todd Hyde, was born a year later in 1876.[8]

Wichita's cowtown days had been numbered from the very beginning. Texas longhorns carried ticks that could infect domestic cattle with a deadly fever, so the Kansas state legislature had established a quarantine line to keep the two herds apart. As new settlers pushed farther west, the quarantine line had to be adjusted accordingly. In 1876 the line was moved west of Sedgwick County, closing the Chisholm Trail, and Wichita's trade in Texas cattle came to an end. A hard winter wheat called "Turkey Red," which improved prairie farm yields, replaced cattle as Wichita's number one product and changed the town into an agricultural center.[9]

Increased circulation of silver coins through the bank compelled Bert to invent a device to organize them, and in 1877 he applied for and received a patent on the "improved tray to hold silver" (patent number 189,101).[10] He sold the manufacturing rights to William Mann of Philadelphia for a royalty of 50¢ on each tray Mann sold. In 1878, Bert's diary notes, "We have put up the first telephone in town lately between the two banks and it works pretty well when there is not too much noise." Bert continued as cashier for Sol Kohn until August 1879, when he left to join the Farmers and Merchants Bank owned by Col. H. W. Lewis, a real estate investor and staunch fellow prohibitionist.

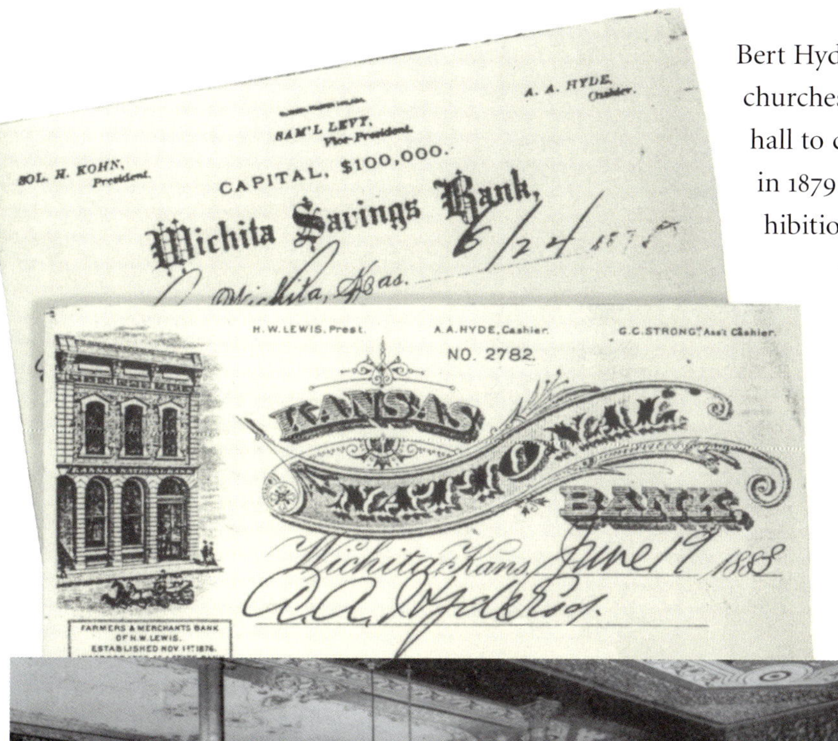

A Period View of a Wichita Bank Interior c. 1887

This is a reflection of the opulence during the boom years in Wichita, and A. A. Hyde's fifteen years as a cashier (i.e., bank manager) in Wichita's financial community.

Bert Hyde and other prohibitionists in Wichita's churches and women's clubs tirelessly pressured city hall to close down prostitution, finally succeeding in 1879. This was followed in 1881 by statewide prohibition. But Wichita's vice industry, which by then had retreated mostly west of the river to Delano, simply went underground and continued in a less conspicuous fashion. When Hyde ran unsuccessfully for mayor in the 1883 city election, the *Wichita Eagle* described him as a "square-toed man of pronounced convictions on the liquor traffic." A protégé of Lewis, Hyde also invested in real estate. By 1885, the year Kansas completely shut its borders to Texas cattle, the thirty-seven-year-old bank manager had become an officer of the renamed Kansas National Bank, a member of the board of education, and a leader in the First Presbyterian Church.[11]

Wichita in 1885 looked much different than it did during its cowtown days. The wooden storefronts that once lined the center of town were replaced with two- and three-story crenelated brick buildings. Mule-drawn trolleys transected the busy intersection of Main and Douglas. New electric lightbulbs were strung up next to older gas lamps. Neighborhoods that once stood starkly against the prairie's flat horizon now were lost among emerging treetops, interrupted by sharply pointed church steeples and distant factory smokestacks. Wichita's twenty-five thousand–resident population was surrounded by prairie that was plowed up for wheat and corn or grazed over by cattle. Greedy ranchers crowded grasslands and depleted the buffalo and grama grasses necessary to support healthy animals. Wichita's industry was strong, corn was now "king," and the real estate market was booming.[12]

In the fall of 1885, as the first snows blanketed the Great Plains, city hall was busy approving preliminary work on a sewer system and considering offers to install electric street lighting. Then came a series of terrible storms that hit harder, longer, and colder than anyone had experienced. After they passed, nearly 85 percent of cattle on the southern plains froze to death. The following winter, storms hit the northern plains, once again killing cattle. Creditors called in loans throughout the prairie states. Bankrupt cattle operations were eventually replaced with sheep herds.[13]

Ecological and economic catastrophes often walk hand-in-hand. The 1880s saw ever-increasing droughts throughout the western states. Geologist John Wesley Powell warned the lawmakers in Washington that the West was too dry to farm, but the government's settlement policy continued unabated. In spite of this evidence, Wichita's economy seemed immune to the hardships of its neighbors. The year 1886 saw ever-increasing property sales as thousands of people flooded in and found work in the city's robust industrial and construction trades. The value of property sold during peak periods was sometimes as much as $1,000,000 a month, much of these dollars coming from Boston, New York, and San Francisco investors. In an 1887 survey of real estate markets by Bradstreets, Wichita ranked number three, behind New York and Kansas City. The population grew 60 percent, and Wichita's boom was the talk of the nation.[14]

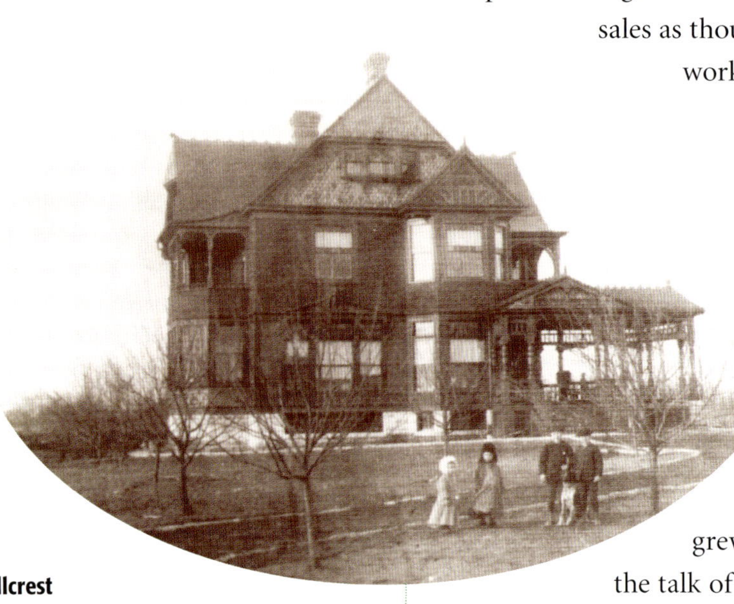

Hillcrest

Located on the top of College Hill, on the northwest corner of Second Street and Roosevelt Avenue, the large, Victorian structure was designed by Proudfoot and Bird Architects and constructed by a prominent local builder named Sullivan. The Hydes moved into Hillcrest in December 1887 and kept it filled with family for the next forty-eight years. Because of the real estate crash of 1888, Hillcrest stood alone for many years without neighbors, to the chagrin of Hyde, who was uncomfortable with any appearance of elitism. The house was torn down following A. A. Hyde's death.

Hyde's land speculations were so successful that he resigned his position with the bank and started his own business as a loan broker. He hired the best architects in town, Willis Proudfoot and George Bird, to design a stately, $10,000 house for his growing family in the newly platted district that came to be called College Hill. He was now a successful thirty-nine-year-old man with an estimated worth of $100,000.[15]

The Bubble Bursts

Hard times eventually caught up with Wichita, and the boom went bust. There followed several years of drought and depression, which inflicted great hardship on the farmers. The exodus of people calling it quits over the next decade depleted some Western counties of as much as half of their population. Wichita lost 30 percent from an estimated 1888 peak of forty thousand residents. Two of the three banks in which Hyde owned stock

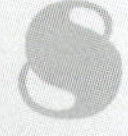

closed their doors, and he lost everything. The third bank, his former employer Kansas National Bank, fell in value to 37¢ on the dollar. His mortgage business became too dangerous to continue, and a stationery store that he had financed and where he kept his office had to be sold, netting only $7,000 for his $40,000 investment. Now all that stood between him and financial ruin was a partnership in the Maple Grove Cemetery and his $600 capital investment in Binkley and Smith's Yucca Company. Prospects of starting over were not pleasant for the forty-one-year-old breadwinner with a wife, seven children, and a spinster sister and aunt living at home. He and the rest of Wichita were going to have to pull themselves up by their own bootstraps.[16]

During its first year of operation in 1889, the Yucca Company introduced several yucca-based soaps to the Kansas, Indian Territory (Oklahoma), and Colorado market, including a sandalwood-scented soap, eczema soap, and shaving soap, as well as a "tooth soap." Specialty items included sticky fly paper, Quick Corn Cure, and silver polish. Hyde took over the bookkeeping and front office while his four older boys pressed and packed soap in the factory after school. The Yucca Company was one of hundreds of small-town operations to take advantage of the relatively simple "stove top" technology of the toiletries industry. Catalogs from wholesale distributors in Kansas City, Chicago, and elsewhere supplied necessary ingredients such as essential oils, perfumes, and packaging materials: glass bottles and jars, tin lids, corks, and paper boxes. Once considered exotic and rare ingredients, essential or volatile oils were becoming commonly available as new steel-hulled ships powered by steam turbines were doubling the tonnage and cutting the time to foreign markets in half. The infrastructure was in place to support a cottage industry almost anywhere in North America. The Yucca Company turned a slim profit at the close of its first year in operation.

Clayton Smith's understanding of medical remedies influenced the company's development of the eczema soap, Corn Cure, and a new cough syrup that was based on a formula that

* * *

A Good Joke.

Will Russell cut from a newspaper the other day an advertisement of this popular Vegetable Yucca soap and stuck it on his window and then stood inside and smiled as he caught the eyes of those who stopped and read it carefully through supposing it to be a 'literary gem' The Yucca company also appreciated the joke and sent Will around a box of their best white Yucca Toilet Soap.

The old joke of a man not starving in the desert "because of the sand-which-is-there," reminds us that considerable wealth is now-a-days being found in desert places. The Yucca plant from which this Vegetable Yucca Soap is made is a desert plant, and the soap made from it is surely the purest and finest toilet soap to be had anywhere. Ask for "Yucca" made only by Yucca Co., Wichita.

Modern Shakespear.

He who steals my purse steals trash, but he who filches our good name (Yucca) steals that of the best toilet soap made. Try "Yucca" and you will be convinced of the truth of the above. Beware of imitations. See that all boxes and cakes are stamped "Yucca Company Wichita." For sale at leading stores.

The Poet of the Plains.

Some people are fat;
Some people are lean,
Some people are dirty,
Some people are clean.
Some people are lively,
Some people mope,
All but the foolish
Use "Yucca Soap."

Truth compels us to say that while this poem took only second prize at the Royal Academy exhibition in London last year, "Yucca Soap" came out way ahead.

Shaving Made Easy,

By lathering with "Yucca Shaving Soap." It holds lather longer, leaves the skin softer, and is altogether the most desirable shaving soap made. Ask your dealer for "Yucca Shaving Soap." It is as much better than other shaving soaps as the "Yucca Toilet Soaps are than the common article.

Who Pays the Fiddler?

Some millions of dollars worth of Pears Soap are sold annually in the United States. The profits go to England. London grease makes no such soap as as our own Yucca plant, and the people are finding it out. If you want pure, healthful soaps at a reasonable price, which will clean the skin and leave it smooth and soft, ask for those make by the Yucca Company. No chapped hands where "Yucca" is used. Though only a few years before the public, "Yucca Soap" is already being imitated. See that every cake and box is stamped "Yucca Company, Wichita, Kansas," and you will get soap fit for a queen. For sale at leading stores.

GOOD AND BAD.

Both good and bad, in life we find,
Together often mingle,
We need to discipline the mind,
The good from bad to single.
To love the good and hate the mean,
And ever live in hope,
Keep hands and face forever clean
By using Yucca Soap.

—Wheeler. Autograph of the author given away with each 25c box of Yucca Soap.

Truth.

It is a well known truth that if you want to know the faults of any article, ask a competing manufacturer. So when other soap factories imitate the name of the well known "Yucca" toilet soap, they virtually say "Yucca is the best soap made." The people agree with them. Do not be deceived. Take only soaps made by the Yucca Company and so stamped on each cake and box. Pure, Cleansing, Healing.

The Poet of the Plains

The Yucca Company could afford to advertise its soap only by printing small stickers on gummed paper that were then cut apart and posted all over town. These examples, found in A.A.'s scrapbook, include some lighthearted jokes, poetry, and product claims.

the family doctor from his hometown in Aiken, South Carolina, had prescribed. This recipe used a crystalline peppermint extract from Japan called menthol. Menthol was known for its penetrating odor and mild anesthetic effect. Hyde gave a bottle of the aromatic tonic to his minister at church for testing. Duly convinced, the clergyman passed it on to the other divines in Wichita, who in turn were impressed. They found that just a few drops on the tongue distracted a coughing fit and one swallow cured "preacher's throat." The partners decided to package the potent syrup (which contained 35 percent alcohol) in a small bottle to fit in a man's vest pocket for easy access in time of distress. They named it "Vest Pocket Cough Specific."

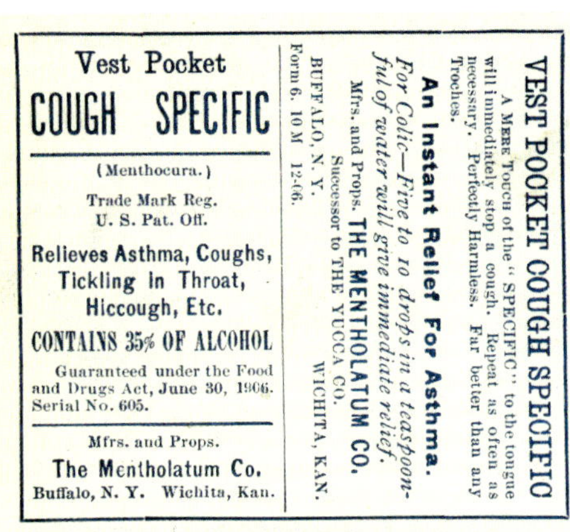

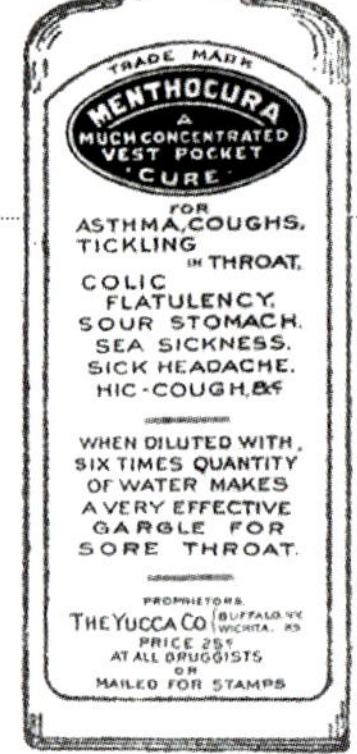

Vest Pocket Cough Specific

Clayton Smith's cough syrup was later renamed Menthocura, and this 1906 label (top) and earlier bottle illustration (below) are the only examples of what the first 1890 packaging may have looked like. See also page 53.

Despite modest success the first year, it became clear that the little company could not provide incomes for three families. In May 1890, Hyde bought out his two partners, replacing them with a schoolteacher from New York named Dewey Wheeler, who went on the road to sell their goods. Wheeler and Hyde each drew $10 per week from the business. Over the next few years, Hyde expanded the product line to include shoe polish, face powder, and sewing machine oil. With little money to spend on newspaper advertising, he printed product claims and whimsical verses on gummed paper and stuck them around town on "posts, seats, old windows &c. mostly at night." He incorporated the company in 1892, naming himself; his wife, Ida; Dewey Wheeler; T. I. Humble (his old partner in the stationery store); and A. C. Jobes (a well-known banker) as the incorporators.[17]

The national panic of 1893 caused Wichita's already weak economy to hit bottom again. With no way to go but up, income for the Yucca Company steadily increased as it did for other Wichita businesses. But from the time he bought out Binkley and Smith, Hyde knew that hard work was not going to be enough. Even with increasing income, it was evident that he needed a product that would be more profitable than common soap. His limited success with Vest Pocket Cough Specific pointed him in the direction of menthol and the other volatile oils, and by 1893 he was completing tests on a new menthol-based salve, or as he called it, "healing emollient."[18]

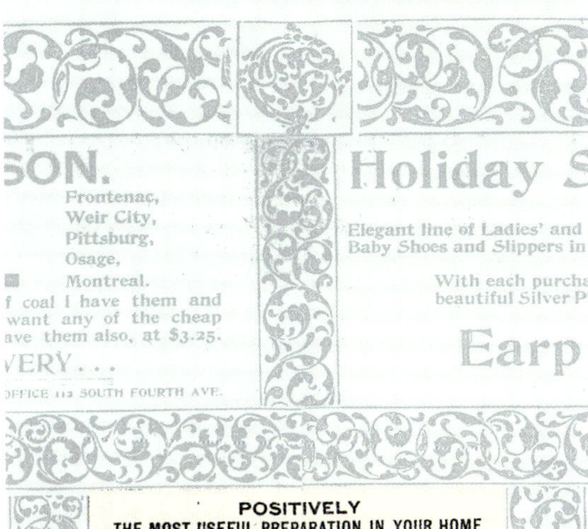

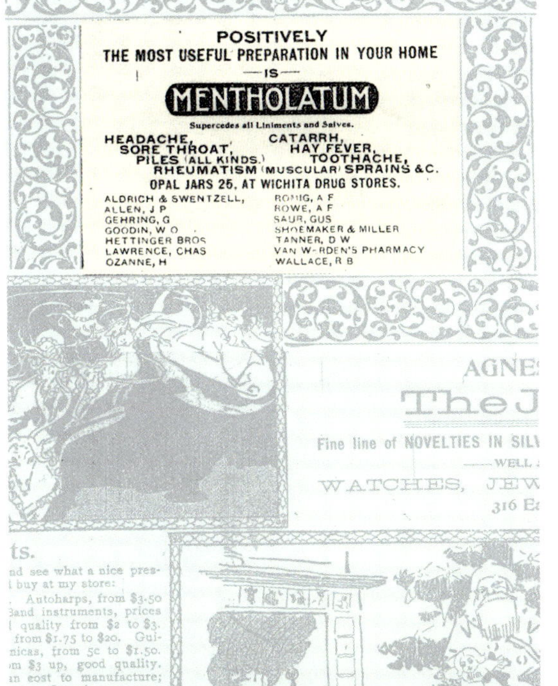

A Brand Is Born

This modest advertisement in the *Wichita Daily Eagle* marked the close of Mentholatum's freshman year and the beginning of a marketing phenom.

MEN·THO·LA·TUM

"The excellent name, a compound of its chief ingredients, Menthol and Petrolatum, came to [me] as a happy inspiration from Above. [I] well remember the occasion, walking home from the factory one evening after closing and just east of Hydraulic Avenue, this euphonious and slightly descriptive name flashed in my mind."

—A. A. Hyde

The earliest known advertisement for Mentholatum appeared on a decorative full-page Christmas layout for local merchants in the *Wichita Daily Eagle*, Sunday morning, December 22, 1895. The ad read Mentholatum "Supercedes [*sic*] all Liniments and Salves" for "Headache, Sore Throat, Piles (All Kinds), Rheumatism (Muscular), Catarrh, Hay Fever, Toothache, Sprains &c." Then, it listed the fourteen Wichita drugstores where "opal jars" could be purchased. How Mentholatum came into being was not by some fortunate accident or discovery, as so many innovations sometimes are. Rather, it was the result of a deliberate and systematic effort.

Based on his experience with Vest Pocket Specific, A. A. Hyde had become intrigued with the medicinal qualities of peppermint oil and the other volatile oils such as eucalyptus, camphor, and pine. He had learned about the innovative new process that was being used to transform distilled mint oil into a concentrated crystalline form, reducing large barrels of oil into small boxes of menthol crystals that demonstrated powerful healing abilities. The Yucca Company already used a variety of aromatic oils to create its scented soaps, and their effect on the olfactory nerves was not lost on Hyde. But it was the anesthetic quality of menthol crystals that excited his and everyone else's interest. The small amount of menthol used in Clayton Smith's Vest Pocket Specific worked well to dull a sore throat, but in syrup form it was not a practical way to treat the other symptoms of a cold such as sinus congestion (inflammation of the mucous membranes) and sore muscles. A small number of "cures" had already become available on the market, each capitalizing on the volatile nature of menthol. They used various methods such as inhalers, snuff, smoke, steam vapor, and douche to reach the sinus cavities within the upper respiratory passage. Traditional methods used to administer the healing oils and ease sore muscles included rubbing a liniment into the skin or applying a sticky poultice. But like Vest Pocket Specific, each of these techniques could treat only one symptom.[1]

Hyde had surely experienced during his boyhood the smelly and often painful mustard plaster. If so, his mother would have mixed a warm poultice of mustard powder, flour, and water then spread it on a cloth that would hold it in place over a swollen, bruised, or otherwise sore muscle. Another standard treatment for colds was camphor oil and turpentine (distilled from pine oil). Druggists mixed the two into a clear jelly-like

Imported Menthol and Camphor

Labels from K. Kobayashi in Yokohama, Japan (above) and the Nippon Camphor Company in Kobe, Japan (right) were found in A. A. Hyde's scrapbook. The companies were likely the first suppliers of Mentholatum's two most important ingredients. The menthol crystals in the tall apothecary jar are as clear as glass.

substance called white petrolatum to create a balm. This undiluted mixture must have been an intense experience when rubbed onto the neck and chest! Hyde could see that if the different oils were blended like a perfume, the result would be a dramatic and desirable improvement.

The petrolatum base that the druggist used to hold the oils was a derivative of petroleum "crude oil." Petrolatum is a thicker form of kerosene and a softer form of paraffin, which are derivatives of petroleum. In 1859, an enterprising kerosene salesman from Brooklyn, New York, named Robert Chesebrough discovered that petrolatum applied to a small cut helped it heal faster, so he packaged and sold it to druggists under the brand name Vaseline®. It became a common practice for druggists to buy Vaseline in bulk containers and repackage it in smaller sizes with the pharmacy label. Based on Yucca Company records, Hyde was doing the same thing. Hyde saw that petrolatum was an ideal base for his "emollient." It was thicker than a liniment, not as messy as a poultice, yet sticky enough to hold the volatile oils against the skin long enough to be absorbed into the muscles or vaporized into the sinuses. It was also odorless and therefore would not compete with the stimulating smell of the menthol and camphor additives. After all, a pleasing fragrance would be the proverbial sugar that helps the medicine go down.[2]

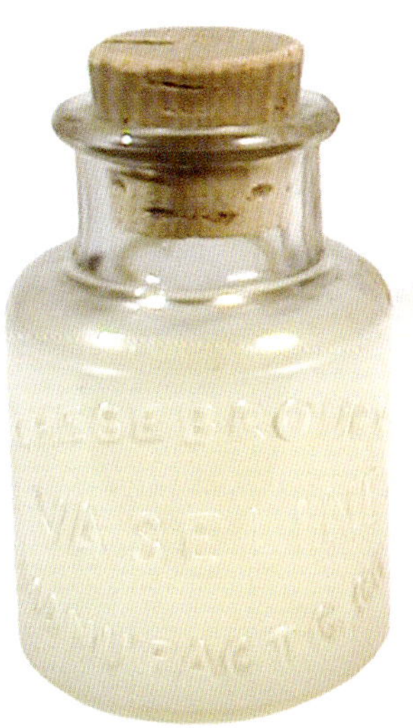

Vaseline,
Paraffin, and Eucalyptol

This antique three-ounce Vaseline jar represents the petrolatum base A. A. Hyde used in early batches of Mentholatum. If he wanted to stiffen the base he could add paraffin. Eucalyptus, birch, pine, and wintergreen oils were added to create the sweet smell of success.

The Yucca Company kept Hyde busy and limited the time he could experiment with the emollient. When he did find time, bookkeeping skills from the bank days served him well in the task of recording each test batch. Hyde mixed countless blends of different volatile oils to find the right quality of smell and potency—sweet, but not too strong to harm the eyes nor too weak to penetrate to sore muscles. We know from early labels that Hyde was working with blends of menthol, camphor, sweet birch oil, pine oil, eucalyptus oil, and "Oil of Gaultheria" (or wintergreen). Whenever he created a promising batch, employees, family, neighbors, and even the innocent passersby on Douglas Street were roped into trying it out. He sought the advice of local doctors and chemists who no doubt stressed the importance of adding boric acid into the mix to act as an added preservative and antiseptic. Today, there are eighty-year-old jars of Mentholatum that still contain ointment and smell as strong as the day they were manufactured!

The story of Mentholatum's invention has reached mythic proportions over the years, but pragmatically, there was nothing revolutionary about its creation. The spotlight must shine instead on Hyde's pleasing blend of ingredients and his ability to coin such a fine-sounding name. Trade-mark names fall into two categories: they can either be a real or descriptive name, or they can be an invented or fictitious name. When considering a real or descriptive name, the ex-banker ruled out using his own name, as was popular with the nostrum makers, because he was not a doctor. There were other descriptive brand names on the market that had already exploited the word *menthol.* For example, the Chicago-based wholesale druggists Lord, Owen & Co. listed two menthol products in their 1885 price catalog: "Menthol Plaster" and "Menthated Camphor." Menthol Plaster was manufactured in Lowell, Massachusetts, by the National Plaster Company, and it claimed its product was "The Most Wonderful Plaster Made for Relieving Pain at Once." Another product being advertised was Japanese Oil, manufactured in New York by the National Remedy Company (established in 1888), which boldly exploited the Japanese connection to menthol.[3]

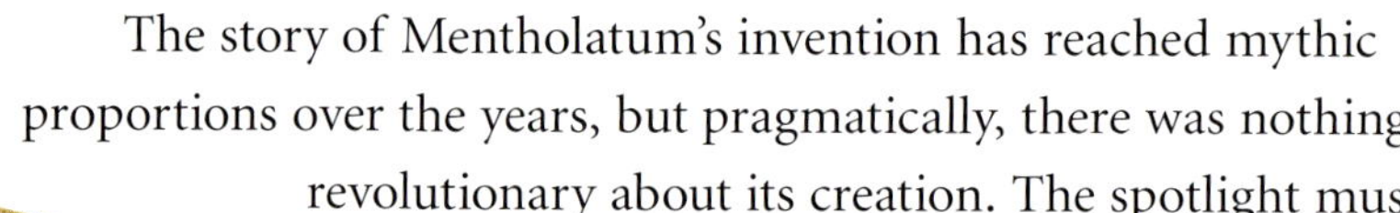

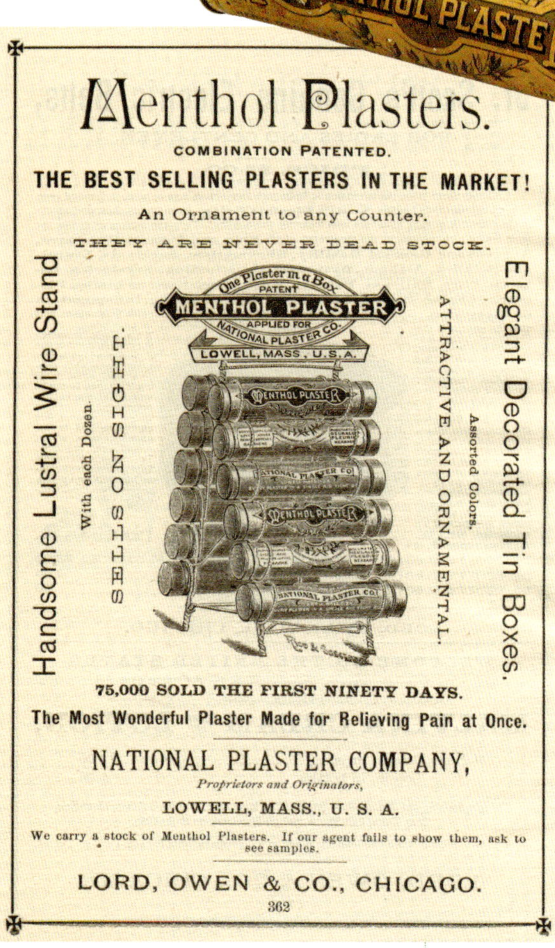

Menthol's Popularity

This advertisement from an 1885 wholesale druggist catalog provides evidence that the new ingredient, menthol, was sought after and sold well. The cylinder-shaped tin "boxes" came in an assortment of colors, and the twisted wire display stand must have looked very modern in its day. Note: this form of plaster is not to be confused with plaster of Paris.

The remaining option was to invent a fictitious name. Hyde felt it should be descriptive of the product, either of its function or its contents. But the new ointment was hard to categorize by function because it was multifunctional—it could be vaporized, stick like a plaster, and be rubbed in like a liniment. Happily, by combining the names of two of its ingredients, **menth**ol with petr**olatum**, he found an honest and effective solution. Lord, Owen & Co.'s Menthated Camphor (mentholated is the proper adjective) was actually more descriptive of Hyde's recipe, Mentholatum's primary additive being 9 percent camphor, compared to only 1.3 percent menthol. But menthol was the wonder ingredient that commanded the public's attention.

By the time Hyde introduced his new salve at the 1896 Kansas State Fair, he was immersed in the competitive and controversial world of patent medicines. Other manufacturers were flooding the market with thousands of brands of elixirs, bitters, pills, salves, and other remedies each competing for the few dollars American families had to spend on their health. This proliferation of brands was possible because the industry had a low barrier to entry, and there were absolutely no limitations imposed by federal or state governments as there are today. Anyone could blend a concoction in his or her kitchen, put it in a bottle, slap on a label, and call it a cure. Additionally, there was a welcome market for sweet-tasting nostrums. For a majority of nineteenth-century Americans, a visit to the doctor was too expensive or too remote for all but the direst emergencies. Treatments that came in a bottle packaged with the testimonials of customers who had been cured were an easy sell to someone looking for relief.

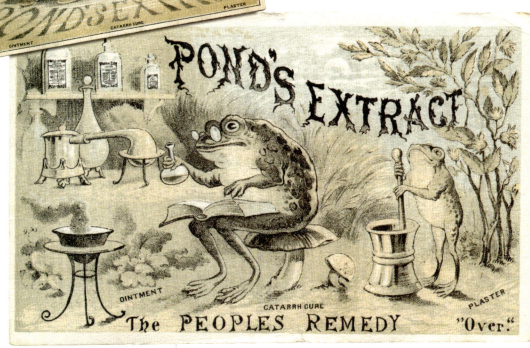

Fanciful Victorian Trade Card?

Or a rare glimpse into a toadstool millionaire's laboratory? A popular brand imported from Great Britain, Pond's used images of ponds and swamps in its advertising with surprisingly successful results.

The Age of Nostrums

The word *patent* in *patent medicine* was nothing more than a trademark registration and did nothing to protect the propriety of a nostrum's formulation. James Harvey Young's landmark book *The Toadstool Millionaires* is a remarkable account of the history of patent medicines in the United States. Young tells of a competitive patent medicine industry several hundred years ago in England whose products were marketed throughout the British Empire. Merchants in Colonial America imported English patent medicines such as Daffy's Elixir, Anderson's Pills, Bateman's Drops, and Turlington's Balsam of Life. The first American to receive a British patent for a proprietary medicine was Mrs. Sybilla Masters in 1715. She sold a consumption (tuberculosis) cure called "Tuscarora Rice," which she manufactured from milled Indian corn. Later, in 1731, Benjamin Franklin's mother-in-law advertised one-ounce "gallypots [*sic*]" of her "well known Ointment for the ITCH" in the *Pennsylvania Gazette.* After the Revolution in 1793, the fledgling Congress enacted the first U.S. patent law, to "promote the Progress of Science and the useful Arts." The first patent to be registered for medicine under this act was issued in 1796 to Samuel Lee Jr. of Windham, Connecticut, for his "Bilious Pills."[4]

Doctors were a rare commodity during the Colonial period, and their knowledge of disease was rudimentary. They might have had some schooling and possessed a few books, but they were not much better prepared to treat illness than was the neighborhood midwife, folk healer, or Indian medicine man. It has been estimated that only one in nine eighteenth-century American medical practitioners went abroad to medical school.[5] Also in short supply were the apothecaries that were typically located in large population centers such as Charleston, Philadelphia, and Boston. Rural practitioners were kept busy collecting their own supply of herbs and mixing their own prescriptions by dissolving dried herbs with water to make a tea or with alcohol to make a tincture. Of necessity, they were physician, surgeon, apothecary, and midwife, all in one, as exemplified by the famous pioneer surgeon Ephraim McDowell (1771–1830). McDowell first apprenticed for several years under Dr. Alexander Humphreys in Staunton, Virginia, before traveling to Scotland to study for two years at the Royal College of Physicians at the University of Edinburgh. Upon his return he set up practice in Danville, Kentucky, where he also kept an apothecary shop at the side of his house supported by a large herb garden in the backyard.[6]

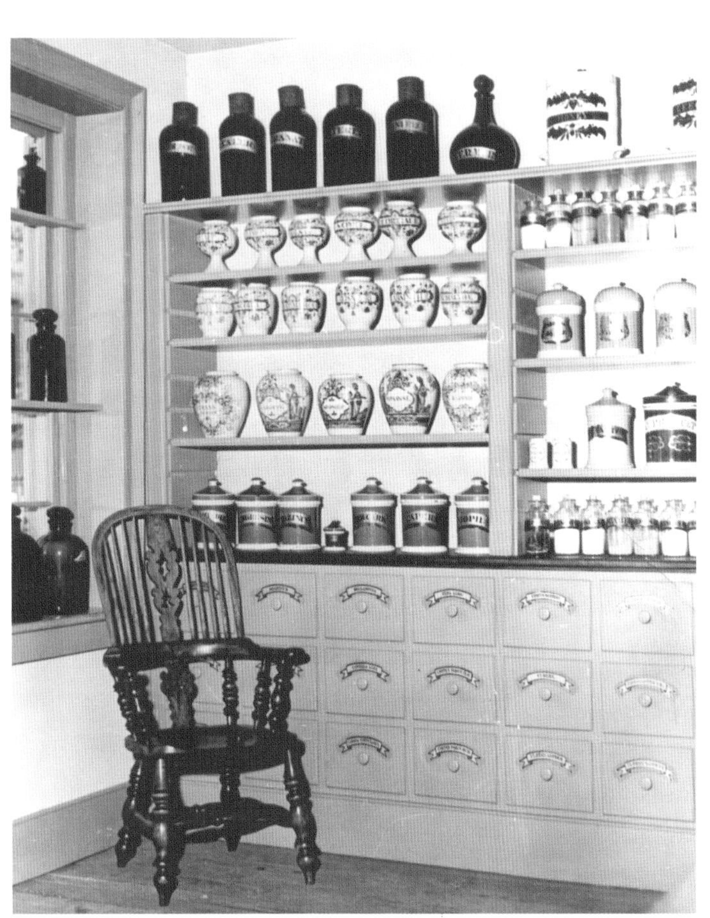

Dr. McDowell's Apothecary Shop

Considered to be the first "drugstore" west of the Allegheny Mountains, Ephraim McDowell's apothecary shop is part of the McDowell House Museum in Danville, Kentucky, and houses this rare collection of eighteenth- and nineteenth-century pharmacy equipment, glassware, and ceramic jars.

While physicians today might enjoy gardening like Dr. McDowell, they would consider mixing their own prescriptions an unreasonable burden if not a totally illegal act. A pioneer in the attempt to separate pharmacy from the practice of medicine

Gallipot

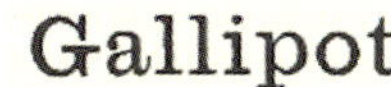

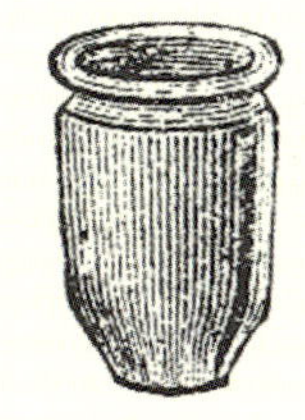

Benjamin Franklin's mother-in-law sold her "Ointment for the Itch" in this type of small, glazed earthenware jar or pot. The design of a gallipot is similar to the amphora and is of ancient origin: the base was sized to seat tightly into the mouth of another pot; that way many same-sized pots could be stacked one on top of another in the hull of a ship or in a storage room. The lip around the mouth of the pot allowed for a cover to be stretched over the top and tied around the neck with cord like the head of a drum. This formed a gasket when the base of another pot was seated on top. There was no need to stack the tiny one-ounce-sized gallipots, so they were probably covered with a colorful patch of cloth and tied with a ribbon.

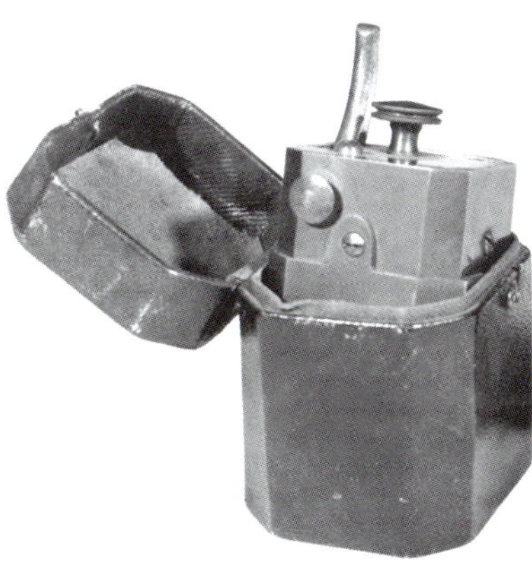

The Dreaded Scarificator

This brass instrument holds six spring-loaded steel lancets. Scarificators were developed to aid physicians in bleeding their patients, which was thought to be an essential treatment during the eighteenth and nineteenth centuries. However, bleeding was not only harmful to patients but helped turn them away from physicians and toward alternative care.

was John Morgan, who in 1765 helped found the first medical school in America. Dr. Morgan believed that the three branches of medicine—pharmacy, surgery, and doctoring—employed different talents and would improve only if practiced individually. When his idea was criticized, Morgan replied:

> *After visiting the sick, do not [the doctor's] apprentices make up their prescriptions? I should ask, is not an apothecary acquainted with the art of compounding and making up medicines as skillful in it as an apprentice? Is not a man educated in the profession to be trusted in preference to one who is only learning the business?*

Morgan became the first teacher of pharmacy, pharmaceutical chemistry, and materia medica at the College of Philadelphia (later the University of Pennsylvania), and during the Revolution, he replaced the eminent Benjamin Church as Director-General and Chief Physician in the Continental Army.[7]

Morgan's successor at the college, Benjamin Rush (c. 1746–1813), is credited with ushering in the "heroic" age of American medicine. Rush advised a generation of young medical students to bleed patients to unconsciousness and administer large doses of mercury-laden calomel, which could cause their teeth to fall out and lead to premature death. It is no wonder that sick people came to dread the trained doctor's lancet and mercury treatment and to welcome the sweet-tasting nostrums that promised to cure without the violence and pain. After the War of Independence came a period of great national pride and optimism and a feeling that all areas of life could be improved now that America was free of England's social and institutional controls. At the dawn of the nineteenth century, almost eighty American-based nostrum proprietors were already cutting into the profits of imported English brands.[8]

At the same time, the healing community was being split irretrievably into two branches: scientific and commercial—those who prescribed mineral-based emetics and diuretics vs. those who prescribed vegetable-based nostrums. Unfortunately for the first group, who mistakenly considered themselves scientists, Rush had steered them in the wrong direction. On the other side, botanical practitioners capitalized on the public's fear of violent doctors by posing as the guardians of public health, and so they came to dominate the market for the next century. The word *quack* was worn ragged by both sides in mutual attempts at discreditation.[9]

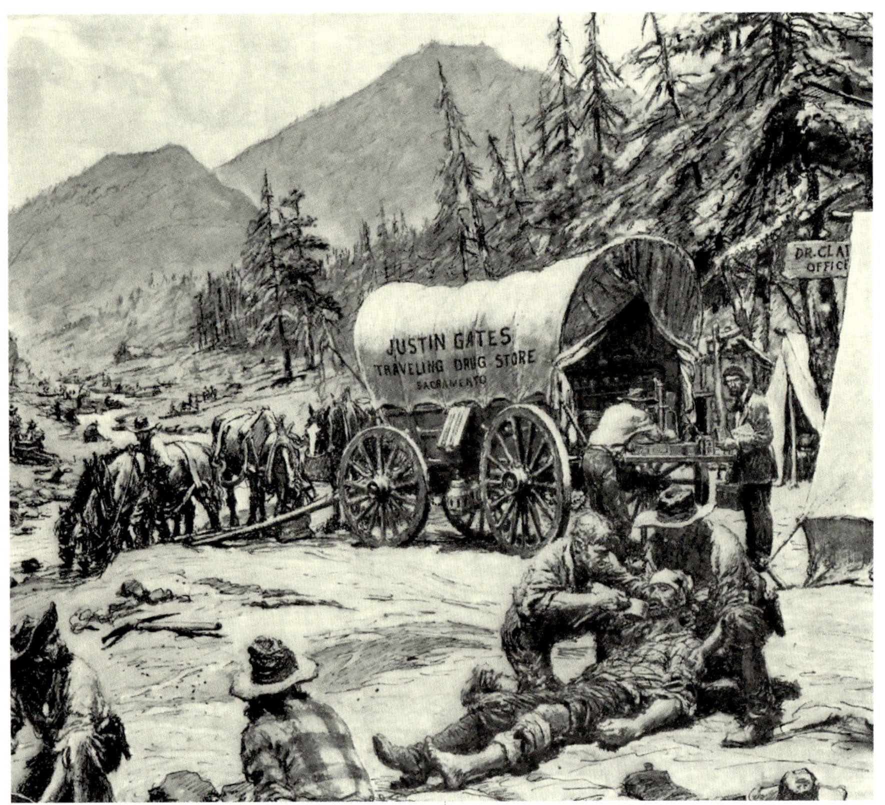

Portable Remedies

A Sacramento druggist named Justin Gates outfitted a pharmacy on wheels so that he could reach remote mining camps in the California gold country. It is likely that patent medicines constituted a significant portion of his inventory.

By the mid-nineteenth century and throughout the Civil War, physicians were abandoning the bloodletting and mineral medications out of economic necessity. But the bloody stigma was only one of the challenges they had to overcome. During the great Western expansion, doctors were few and far between, leaving a majority of Americans beyond their reach. Patent medicines, on the other hand, were portable and traveled easily via horseback and covered wagon to wherever people settled. Complicating this was the fact that many nostrums contained narcotics that deadened pain and could convey a false sense of recovery, thus delaying a call to the doctor until it was too late. And finally, doctors could not ignore the fact that sick people wanted to hear something hopeful rather than the truth about their condition. On that score, nostrum copywriters were the experts.[10]

The nostrum makers were notable for their tendency to put more effort into elixir packaging than into science and manufacture. Secret formulas added an air of mystery and were an effective sales device. The manufacturers tended to be lax in controlling the quality and proportions of ingredients. But their worst offenses were fraudulent claims. Labels were crowded with long lists of ailments they claimed to cure. Advertisements listed so many general symptoms that a perfectly healthy person might be persuaded into taking unneeded medications, and thus run the risk of becoming addicted to the narcotics that many products contained.[11]

In Mentholatum, A. A. Hyde had found a product that would eventually be more profitable than manufacturing specialty soaps. But for that to happen he first had to learn the ropes of the patent medicine industry. Although he would eventually rewrite the rules, his new product started out looking and behaving just like all the other packaged remedies for sale. The earliest surviving jar labels contain the slogan "The Great Japanese Salve"

A Handy Corkscrew

"Cactus Bloom Catarrh Cure
Cures Catarrh
Compliments of
The Arnold Distributing And Mfg. Co.
Omaha, Nebraska.
Sole Agents"

above the trademark scroll and "An External Application for Cure of All Imflammations [*sic*]" written below. Each year the number of uses for Mentholatum grew, as did the use of the word *cure*. Mentholatum was found to be a "Speedy Cure" for catarrh and hay fever. "For Piles" was marked in bold letters. Hyde, who was an avid fisherman and loved outdoor activities, soon added "Insect Bites, Sunburn, Poison Vine Swellings, &c." to the list. Druggists were asked to test Mentholatum on croup and pneumonia during one upcoming winter season, presumably to see if their claim that "It Saves Lives" could be substantiated. "We positively guarantee Mentholatum to stop Spasmodic Croup in five minutes, cure Sore Throat in one night, and give prompt relief for Pneumonia." Hyde was a natural nostrum copywriter with lines like: "Unequivocally Guaranteed" . . . "To cure or relieve" . . . "To cure promptly" . . . "The best cure" . . . "An instant relief," etc. By 1903, the "Great Japanese Salve" circular that the druggist wrapped around each jar of Mentholatum, listed almost two dozen ills that it cured, including "Brain Fag."[12]

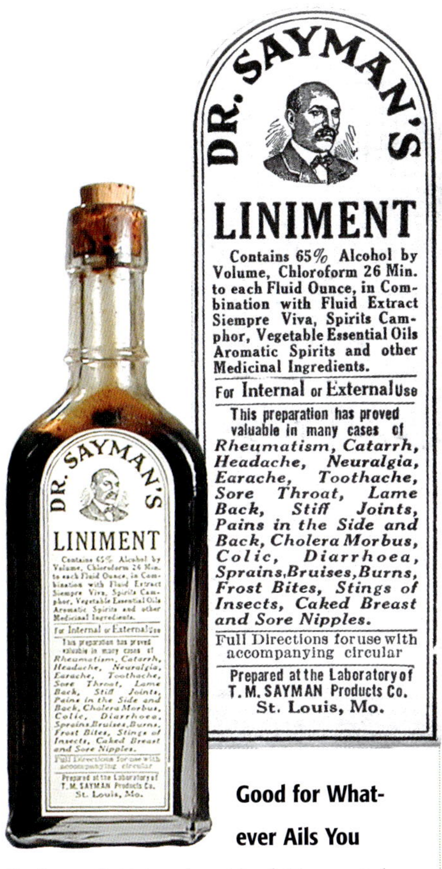
DR. SAYMAN'S
LINIMENT
Contains 65% Alcohol by Volume, Chloroform 26 Min. to each Fluid Ounce, in Combination with Fluid Extract Siempre Viva, Spirits Camphor, Vegetable Essential Oils Aromatic Spirits and other Medicinal Ingredients.
For Internal or External Use
This preparation has proved valuable in many cases of Rheumatism, Catarrh, Headache, Neuralgia, Earache, Toothache, Sore Throat, Lame Back, Stiff Joints, Pains in the Side and Back, Cholera Morbus, Colic, Diarrhoea, Sprains, Bruises, Burns, Frost Bites, Stings of Insects, Caked Breast and Sore Nipples.
Full Directions for use with accompanying circular
Prepared at the Laboratory of T. M. SAYMAN Products Co. St. Louis, Mo.

Good for Whatever Ails You

Dr. Sayman's Liniment contained 65 percent alcohol, and its label was covered with a list of twenty ailments for which it "has proved valuable."

Hyde would eventually break the conventions of nostrum packaging and criticize the trade's often deceptive advertising and marketing practices. The demand for packaged cures was high, and the competition to supply them was fierce, yet he would refuse to play by Madison Avenue's rules. With estimates of twenty-eight thousand to fifty thousand patent medicines in the United States during the final decades of the nineteenth century,

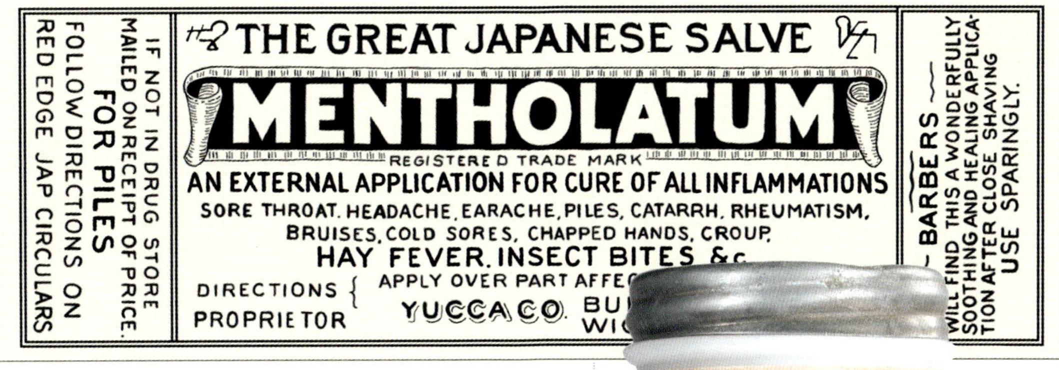

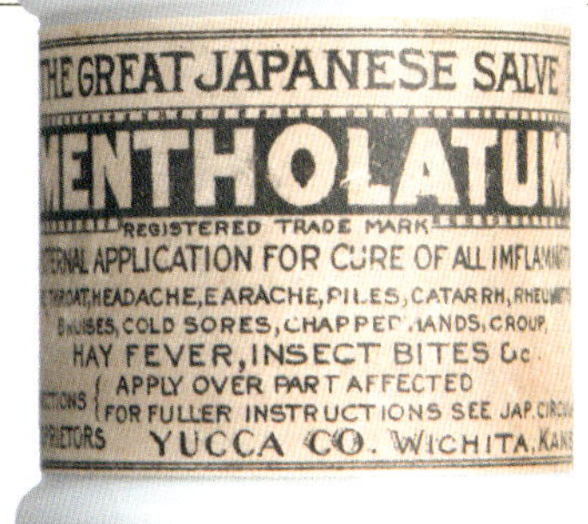

Early Mentholatum Label and Jar

When Mentholatum was first introduced, its hand-drawn label gave top billing to the exotic new ingredient from Japan. This rare jar was found in a drugstore in Sheldon, Iowa.

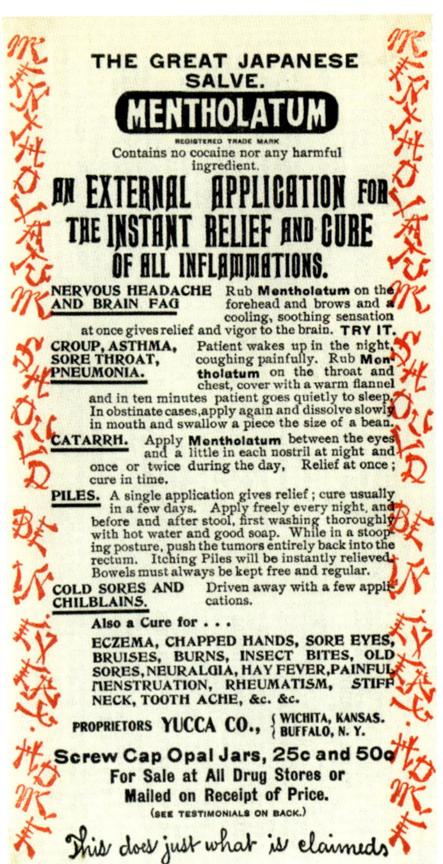

Mentholatum Cures All

Like other remedy makers of the time, A. A. Hyde initially touted a long list of ailments that Mentholatum could cure. Take a closer look at the Japanese-like letters that decorate the sides of this circular for some subliminal fun.

Mentholatum rose above them all to become one of a handful of beloved household brands. At the time, it was estimated that no more than fifty proprietors of patent medicines ever made more than $100,000 annually, and perhaps only a dozen became millionaires. Remarkably, Hyde would soon be joining their ranks.[13]

Nationwide, more money was spent on nostrum advertising than on any other sector. Advertising costs alone could exceed $50,000 just to create demand for a new product. A manufacturer might spend as much as $250,000 before sales of a new product began to cover the cost of bottles and packaging. In fact, advertising costs were responsible for bankruptcies among entrepreneurs and experienced manufacturers alike. Many ad agencies became the owners of nostrum patents as a result of foreclosure for failure to pay their rates. The high cost of advertising also hurt druggists. Hyde warned the druggists:

> *Do you know that newspaper advertising has done more than anything else to hurt the drug business and the medical profession? First. —It has beguiled the people into purchasing worthless and even harmful preparations, until many sensible folks reject all medicines and say: "They do more evil than good." Second. —It compels druggists to sell these largely advertised mixtures at an unreasonably small profit to themselves and an enormous profit to the manufacturer.*[14]

The physicians were determined to increase their portion of the retail prescription business. Starting soon after its founding in 1847, the American Medical Association (AMA) began a campaign to "enlighten" the public to the dangers of quack remedies. Eventually the beseiged leaders of the patent medicine industry formed the Proprietary Medicine Manufacturers and Dealers Association in 1881 to consolidate their lobbying power in Washington. Known as the the Proprietary Association, it also helped its members fight counterfeiting and copyright infringement, which was egged on by the AMA and pernicious medical journals that periodically revealed industry formulas in their print. Despite the high cost of advertising and pressures imposed by competitors and detractors alike, one druggist complained that the number of nostrums in the United States had become "epidemic." But the tide was about to turn.[15]

DO YOU KNOW that newspaper advertising has done more than anything else to hurt the drug business and the medical profession?

FIRST.— It has beguiled the people into purchasing worthless and even harmful preparations, until many sensible folks reject all medicines and say: "They do more evil than good."

SECOND.— It compels druggists to sell these largely advertised mixtures at an unreasonably small profit to themselves and an enormous profit to the manufacturer. Now when an excellent thing like this MENTHOLATUM is put on the market, which absolutely does what is claimed; which is expensive to put up; which sells at a reasonable price and a fair profit; it makes a sensible man tired to hear a dealer say: "Have no calls for it; can't sell it; you must advertise."

Where is your pride in your profession, man? A clerk that would talk like that would not be worth his salt, and you would justly fire him out of your store. Mentholatum does what we claim, as you can see by testimony of druggists enclosed.

It is needed in every family! SELL IT!!

WE GUARANTEE EVERY JAR. YUCCA CO., WICHITA, KANSAS.

Hyde Speaks Out

On this card, inserted with regular business correspondence, A. A. Hyde took a stand against the common practice of manufacturers promoting remedies in newspapers at the expense of druggists' profits.

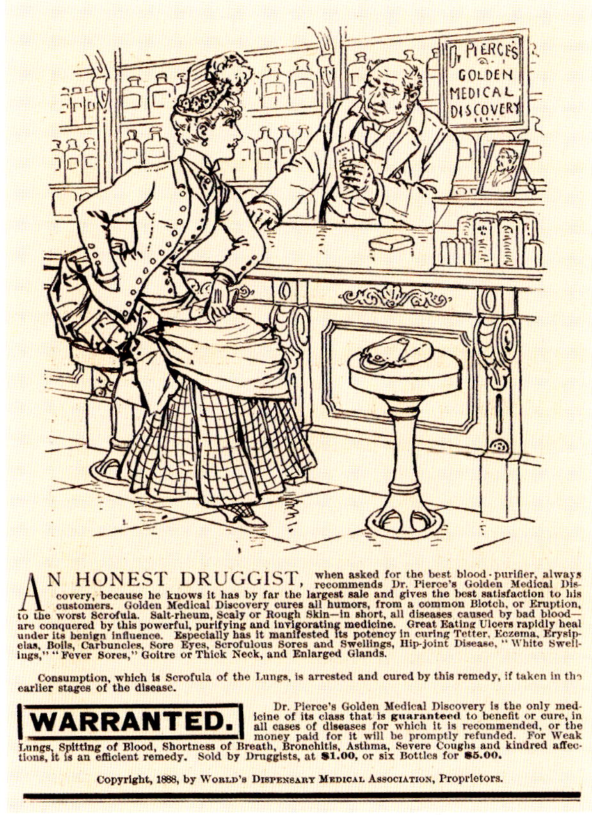

An Honest Druggist or Bartender?

In this 1889 magazine advertisement, Dr. Pierce not only wanted the reader to believe that the druggist preferred to sell his Golden Medical Discovery because it was the best medicine, it appears he also wanted independent-minded women of the day to know that the druggist's counter was the only publicly acceptable place for her to obtain alcohol in the guise of his tonic.

Along the way, the physicians' camp was steadily strengthened by chemists and pharmacists who had once been caught in the middle. At the start of the nineteenth century, apothecaries began their struggle to break free from the control of medical practitioners. The founding of the Philadelphia College of Pharmacy in 1821 was the first step toward professional independence. By 1864, they chartered seven more schools and founded the American Pharmaceutical Association (1852) to nationalize the standards and ethics that had originated in Philadelphia. While the "A.Ph.A." represented the professional and scientific interests of pharmacists, the National Association of Retail Druggists was founded in 1898 to represent their business and economic interests. But recognition came slowly from the doctors, many of whom guarded their right to dispense medicines from their offices (a practice that was continued by some well into the 1930s). By the end of the nineteenth century, though, enough respect had accumulated for them to form an alliance against the pseudoscience of the nostrum pushers.[16]

Chemists were also steadily improving their art and techniques. Progressive state governments began to hire agricultural chemists to help look after the health of their citizens. By 1884 these state chemists had formed the Association of Official Agricultural Chemists. As the chemists pursued their investigations of tainted food products, they could not help but uncover fraud in the patent medicine industry.[17]

A Chicago druggist on the floor of the 1893 American Pharmaceutical Association convention appealed to the membership to stop selling nostrums, claiming it siphoned away millions of dollars that "rightly" belonged to the prescription druggist. At the 1905 convention, another druggist asked:

> *How stupid can pharmacists be? They give away valuable window display space to show goods which are making their sworn enemies rich; they hang the pictures and tack signs of their biggest rivals . . . to the end that a quack living in a distant city, a doctor who is too sick to practice, or a "retired missionary" who is too strong to work, may wax opulent.*

As men of science, the druggists knew it was wrong to sell ineffective and possibly dangerous packaged medicines, but as

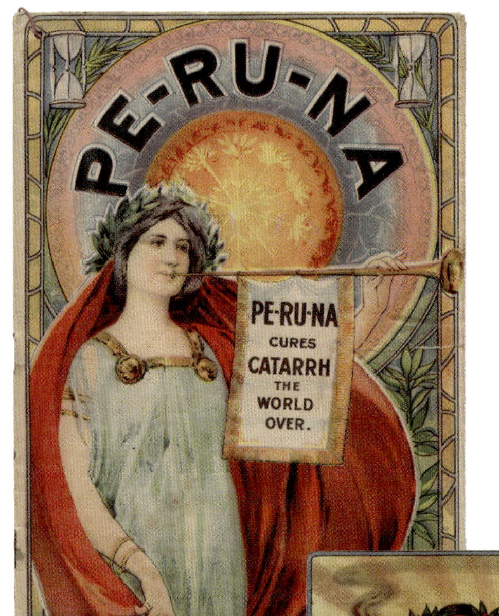

merchants, they knew proprietaries improved profit margins. Many rationalized that there were good and bad patent medicines, and if they stuck with the good they could sleep at night. Others said flat out that if they didn't sell the quack stuff in their shop, the grocer down the street certainly would, so they continued to sell nostrums as usual.[18]

The nostrum makers' ascendancy began to reverse in the fall of 1905, when *Collier's* published a series of articles by Samuel Hopkins Adams, entitled "The Great American Fraud." The magazine also printed a muckraking article by the Harvard-trained journalist Mark Sullivan, entitled, "The Patent Medicine Conspiracy Against the Freedom of the Press." Attempts to enact national food and drug regulations, which had begun back in 1879, looked promising when a bill was finally passed by the Senate in 1906. The Proprietary Association was confident the bill would die in the House, where one representative gibed, "Peruna seems to be the favorite Congressional drink." What happened next was totally unexpected. Upton Sinclair published his book *The Jungle*, exposing filth and contamination in Chicago's meatpacking industry, and the public outcry demanding government regulation decided the final outcome. The bill passed on June 23, and Theodore Roosevelt signed the Pure Food and Drugs Act into law on June 30, 1906.[19]

The historic law required manufacturers to print the truth on their labels. Dangerous drugs were to be listed, while the other ingredients would remain optional. No longer could the word *cure* be used unless it was proved to be true. People continued to drink or swallow whatever they pleased, but after 1906, they were given a fair warning of the risks.[20]

Remedy for the Cure

The 1906 Pure Food and Drugs Act was the first federal law to regulate claims made by proprietary medicine manufacturers. The cover of this 1902 Pe-ru-na testimonial booklet (above) claimed it "cures catarrh," while another cover printed sometime after 1906 (right) could only claim it was a "catarrh remedy." The label on this little sample bottle (left) revealed Pe-ru-na's top-secret formula. It is no real surprise that it contained 18 percent alcohol. Of its ten dubious ingredients, cubeb was the only catarrh fighter. How effective was swallowing cubeb as a tonic when the catarrh was in the nose and sinuses?

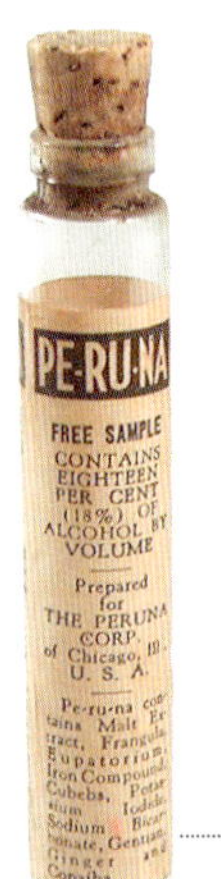

King Catarrh
The Perfect Disease

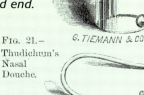

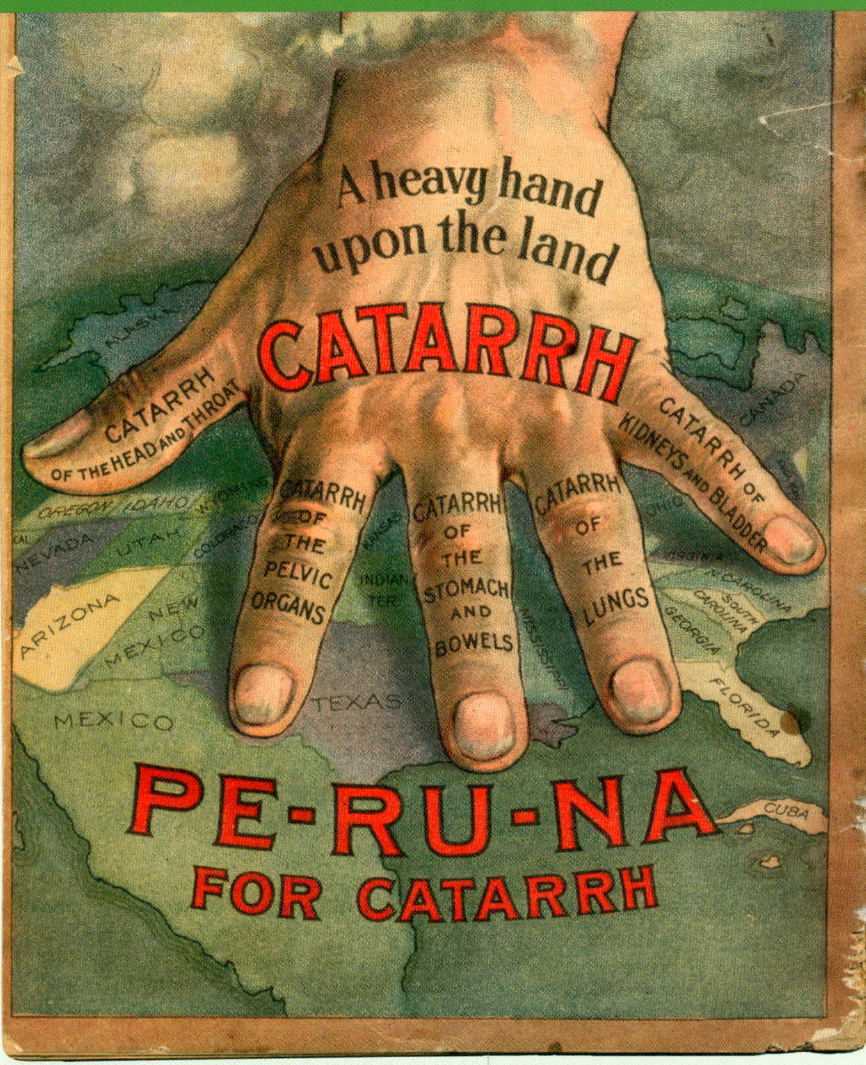

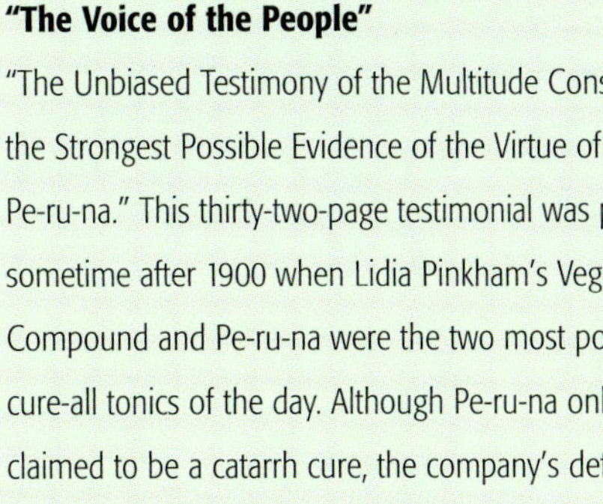

"The Voice of the People"

"The Unbiased Testimony of the Multitude Constitutes the Strongest Possible Evidence of the Virtue of Pe-ru-na." This thirty-two-page testimonial was printed sometime after 1900 when Lidia Pinkham's Vegetable Compound and Pe-ru-na were the two most popular cure-all tonics of the day. Although Pe-ru-na only claimed to be a catarrh cure, the company's definition of catarrh included everything from consumption to female complaints.

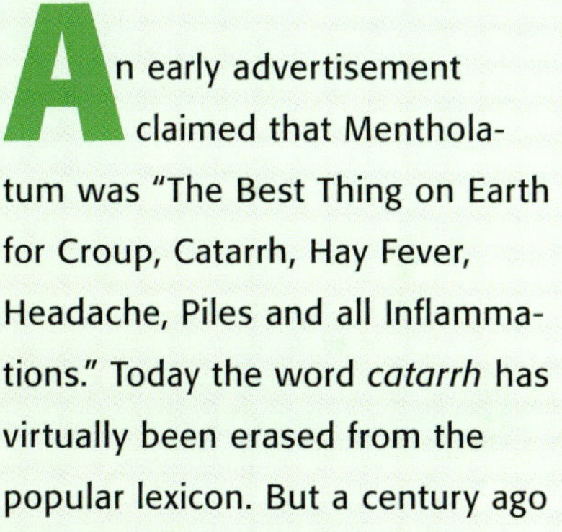

An early advertisement claimed that Mentholatum was "The Best Thing on Earth for Croup, Catarrh, Hay Fever, Headache, Piles and all Inflammations." Today the word *catarrh* has virtually been erased from the popular lexicon. But a century ago it was universally known as the common cold. The dictionary's first definition of catarrh is the "inflammation of mucous membranes, especially of the nose and throat." In 800 A.D., the School of Salernum, the earliest school of medicine in Christian Europe, defined catarrh in the following remedy for a cold:

Fast well and watch. Eat hot your daily fare.
Work some, and breathe a warm and humid air;
Of drink be spare; your breath at times suspend,
These things observe if you your cold would end.
A cold whose ill effects extend as far
As in the chest, is known as catarrh.
Bronchitis, if into the throat it flows—
Coryza, if it reach alone the nose.[1]

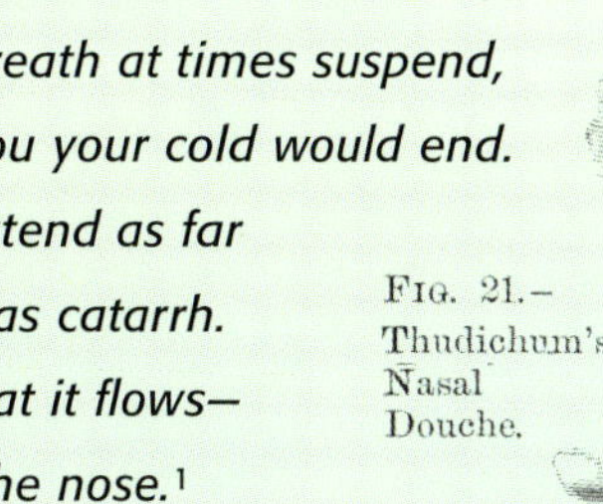

Fig. 21.– Thudichum's Nasal Douche.

SPRAY
DOUCHE
ATOMIZER
VAPORIZER
INHALER
POWDER-BLOWER

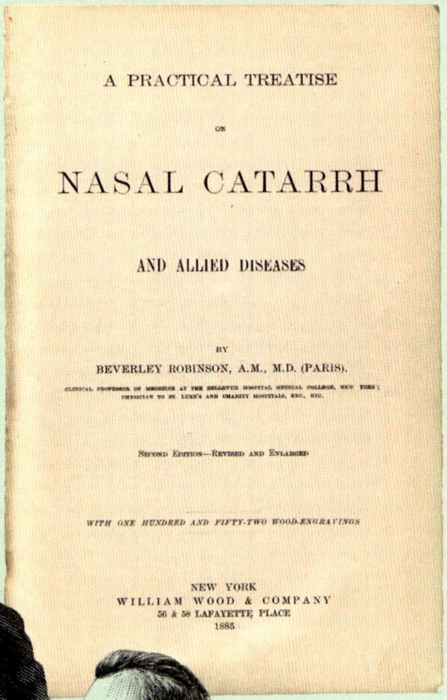

A PRACTICAL TREATISE
ON
NASAL CATARRH
AND ALLIED DISEASES
BY
BEVERLEY ROBINSON, A.M., M.D. (PARIS).
CLINICAL PROFESSOR OF MEDICINE AT THE BELLEVUE HOSPITAL MEDICAL COLLEGE, NEW YORK;
PHYSICIAN TO ST. LUKE'S AND CHARITY HOSPITALS, ETC., ETC.
SECOND EDITION—REVISED AND ENLARGED
WITH ONE HUNDRED AND FIFTY-TWO WOOD-ENGRAVINGS
NEW YORK
WILLIAM WOOD & COMPANY
56 & 58 LAFAYETTE PLACE
1885

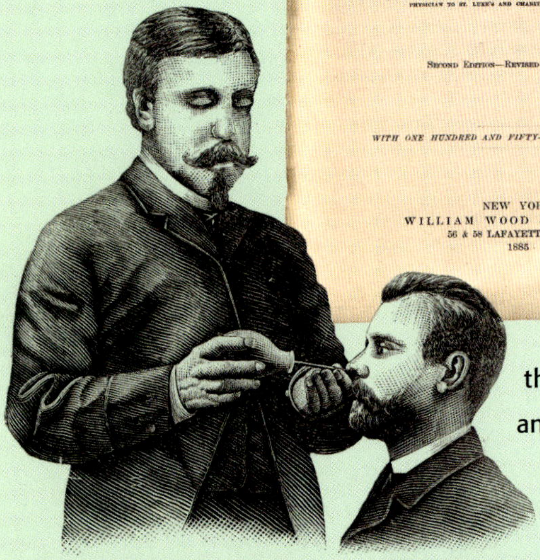

FIG. 91.—The Eustachian Catheter in Position (Roosa).

FIG. 44.—Hard-rubber Powder-blower with Ball.

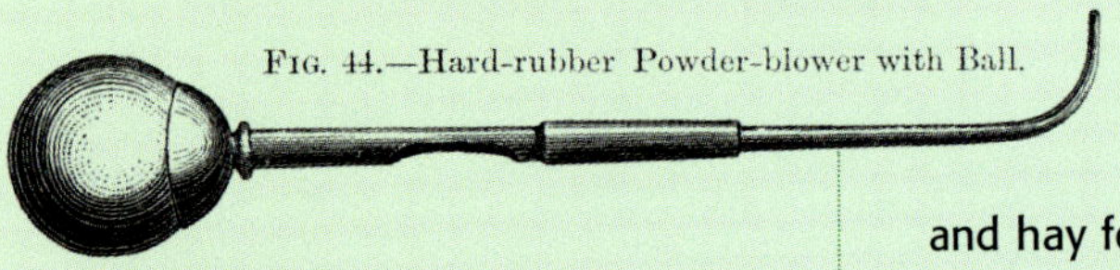

Treatment Systems

Dr. Beverley Robinson's book contained 152 wood engravings that illustrated the tools used by doctors in 1885 to treat nasal catarrh. In addition to many serious looking examination and surgical tools, there were a number of devices used for treatment of the nasal cavities. They included spray, douche, atomizer, vaporizer, inhaler, and powder-blower.

The patriot physician Benjamin Rush published a specific treatment for catarrh in his 1787 *Directions for the Cure of Sundry Common Diseases Suited to Country Gentlemen in the United States*. He instructed:

> *Bleed occasionally, if the pulse is hard or full. Abstain from eating meat and butter. Drink freely of bran or flaxseed hysop [sic] teas. Take ten grains of niter [saltpeter] three or four times a day. When cough attends and is troublesome, take thirty or forty drops of laudanum [a tincture of opium] every night at bedtime. Keep bowels open with the pills made of aloes and soap.*

Published in 1819 and again in 1828, the English physician John Bostock coined "Catarrhus Æstivus," and "Summer Catarrh" to name the symptoms of a "periodical affection of the eyes and chest" (hay fever). In 1826 a paper in the medical journal *Lancet* used "catarrhal ophthalmia" to name the inflammation of the mucous membrane that lines the surface of the eye. The scope of catarrhal inflammation had expanded from the chest to include eyes.[2]

In addition to inflammation, doctors knew that colds and hay fever also shared the dictionary's second definition of catarrh, "a flowing down" of mucus. So when they treated the symptoms of colds, hay fever, and asthma, they were basically treating catarrhal inflammation and flowing mucus. If the treatment was going to be the same for all three diseases, then it became academic which one of the three the patient actually had, and more practical to call it by its common denominator, "catarrh."

George Beard, in his 1876 treatise on hay fever, wrote about the early history of catarrh and associated it with hay fever or "hay-asthma," which some observers thought was brought on by "vegetable matter of the atmosphere." Beard cited a Professor Phoebus at the University of Giesson who wrote in 1859 that hay fever was an Anglo-Saxon disease more common in England than in the rest of Europe. Charles Blackley, a surgeon in Manchester, England, was more specific. He said the cause was pollen and suggested it be called "pollen catarrh." Dr. Blackley believed that the reason cats, rabbits, and guinea pigs "excited asthmatic symptoms" was due to their fur collecting pollen "while roaming amid the hay."[3]

"The healthful and beneficial influence of the summer climate here in cases of weak or diseased lungs is recognized by the best physicians, and total exemption from hay fever, asthma and catarrh is usual."

—Ned A. Lindsey
May 1, 1886

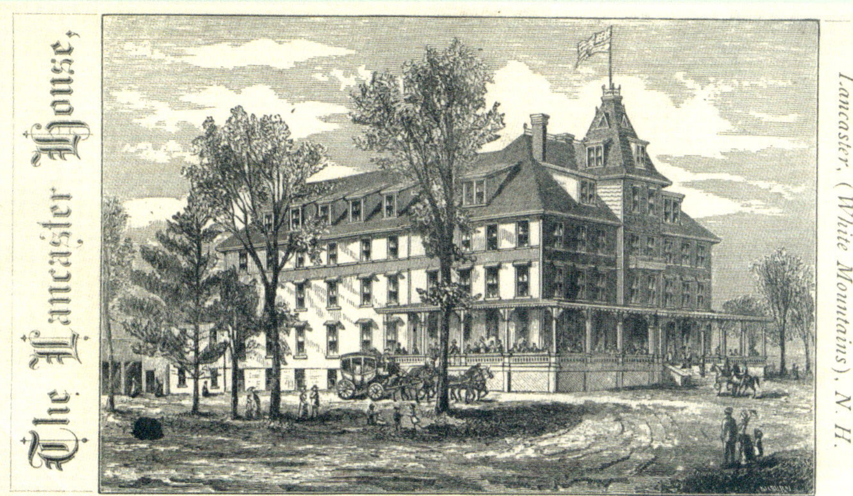

A Fashionable Affliction

In America, the word *catarrh* began to circulate among the East Coast intelligentsia—the university professors and doctors who frequented the vacation resorts in the White Mountains of New Hampshire. Catarrh's broader usage had piqued their interest. The more they began to write about it, the more important it became, advancing catarrh's status from a mere symptom to a full-fledged disease. They made it as complex as they could, devising theories, performing tests, and then calling in the press. Only when news of catarrh's arrival at the forefront of medical research reached the yacht clubs and boardrooms of the industrial elite did it achieve star power. The publishing houses, advertising agencies, and patent medicine moguls made sure catarrh became a household name.

(Text continues on page 27.)

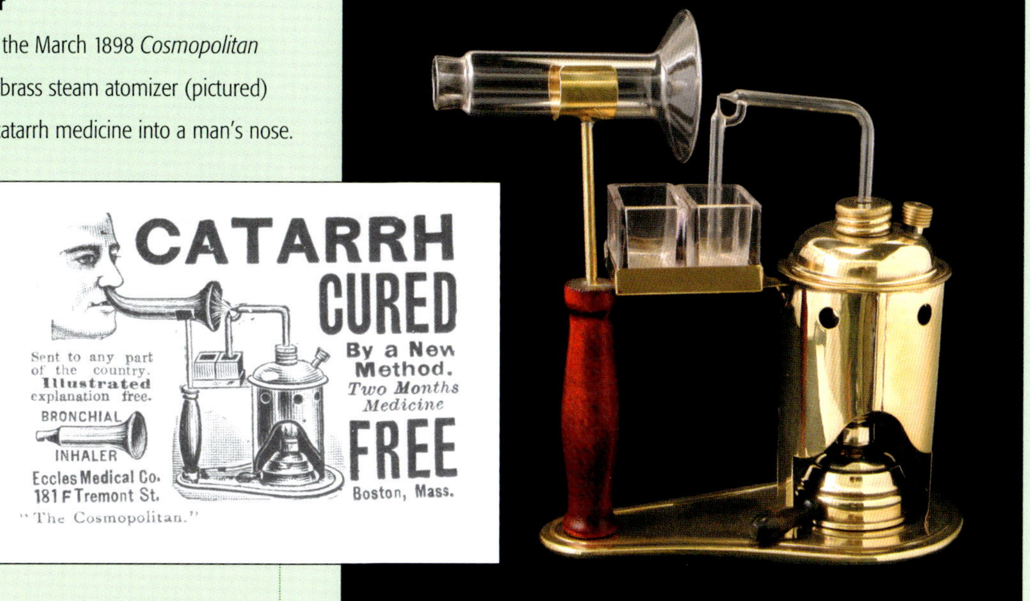

Eccles Bronchial Inhaler

This small ad (inset) from the March 1898 *Cosmopolitan* magazine shows how the brass steam atomizer (pictured) was used to spray Eccles catarrh medicine into a man's nose. A range of hot to cold inhalations could be achieved by adjusting the length of the glass inhaler tube; a short tube produced a hot mist, and a long tube produced a cold mist. See page 35 for more on steam atomizers.

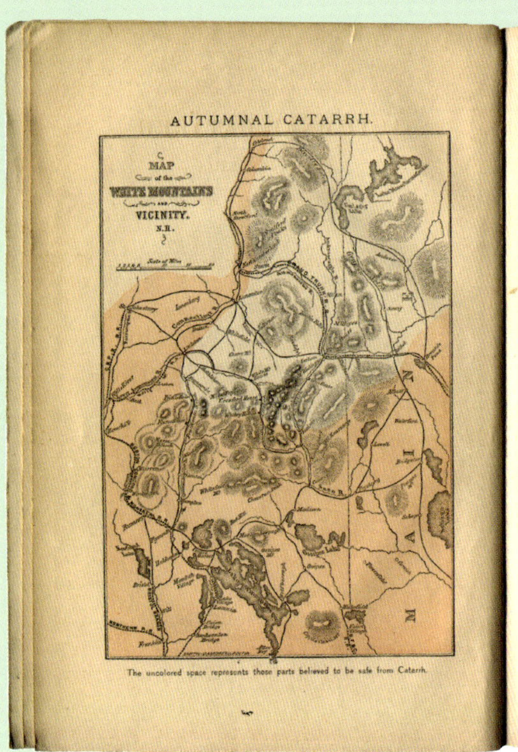

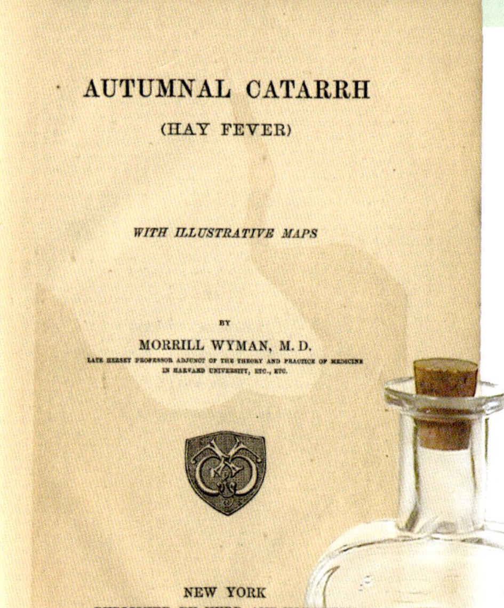

Dr. Wyman's Autumnal Catarrh

Dr. Morrill Wyman was a Cambridge physician and adjunct professor at Harvard University, "etc., etc.," who suffered cold-like symptoms at the close of every summer since his graduation from Harvard in 1834. In the late summer of 1865 he was visiting the White Mountain region of New Hampshire and discovered that he had skipped his annual cold. Dr. Wyman had unwittingly joined the legions of hay fever sufferers who escaped there each year to avoid getting sick. His discovery was reason for celebration and provided new material for a scientific paper.

According to Dr. Wyman's thesis, there were two forms of annually recurring catarrh; the first and most common form afflicted people throughout the month of June and was called "June Cold" or "Rose Cold," and the second, less understood form, struck sufferers during the month of September, which he named "Catarrhus Autumnalis" or "Autumnal Catarrh" (a salute to Bostock) before the Massachusetts Medical Society in 1866. Over the next decade, Wyman collected one hundred case histories that became the foundation for his book titled *Autumnal Catarrh: (Hay Fever)* published by the Riverside Press in 1876 (the same year Beard's book was published). In addition to a thorough description of symptoms, an added feature of Wyman's book were four maps marking areas in the eastern United States where Autumnal Catarrh was known to occur and highlighting the locations of catarrh-free zones.

Case No. 2: Rev. Henry Ward Beecher

Brooklyn, September 25, 1868.

Henry Ward Beecher (1813–1887), Protestant clergyman, editor, abolitionist leader, and brother of Harriet Beecher Stowe (1811–1896) [author of Uncle Tom's Cabin], was an Autumnal Catarrh sufferer since the age of thirty-six. His hay fever returned, with the exception of two years, so punctually that he came to admire nature's regularity. Beecher wrote that the Catskill Mountains, Adirondacks, Lake Superior region, and even the ocean coast of Long Island were good places for fugitives from hay fever to hide. He preferred to retreat to Peekskill, forty miles above New York on the Hudson River during July, August, and September. "A sister is a sufferer, and a brother's son. No others of our family have been attacked. Many gentlemen in New York arrange their business so as to make an August voyage to Europe, thus escaping the inception." As to a medical treatment, he had not found one—yet. Sometime after 1880 and before his death in 1887, he must have been impressed with Dr. M. M. Townsend's new remedy because he allowed the Maryland manufacturer to use his name as an endorsement on the specific's label (above).

Case No. 8: Hon. Daniel Webster

Taken from personal correspondence.

Daniel Webster (1782–1852), statesman, administrator, and diplomat suffered his first attack at the age of fifty while living in Boston. Each year thereafter "my incurable catarrh" caused Webster to loose weight and become depressed. Some years it lasted longer than a month. No matter if he was in Washington, New York, Boston, or at his seaside home in Marshfield, Massachusetts, it affected him so severely that he considered resigning his office as Secretary of State in the Fillmore administration. Ironically, Webster once visited the White Mountain region during late August and early September and noticed that his annual catarrh was late, but unfortunately he failed to make any connection.

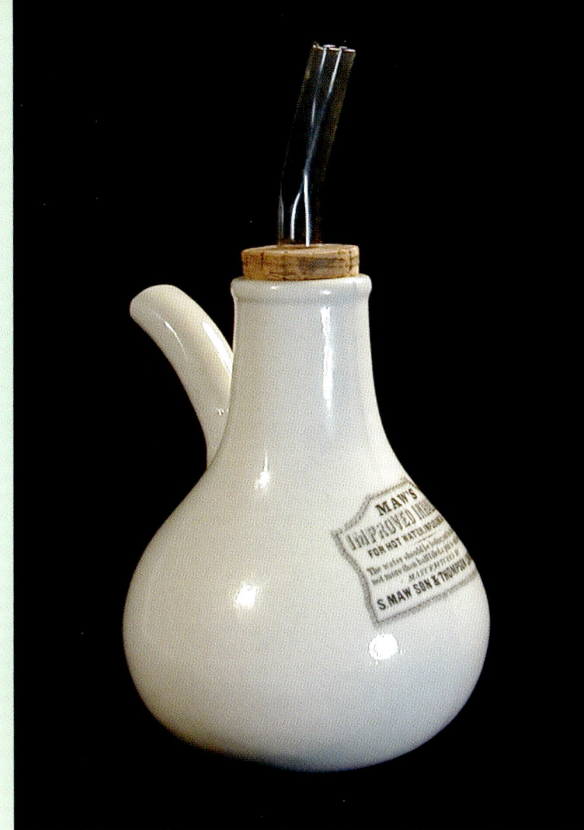

The U.S. Hay-Fever Association was organized in Bethlehem, New Hampshire, in 1874 to promote research and to comfort its many sufferers. The once trifling aggravation was now being called a "disease of the fashionable and the thoughtful—the price of wealth and culture, a part of the penalty of a fine organization and an in-door life."[4]

Catarrh was soon "discovered" to have seasonal phases such as "Rose Cold," "Peach Cold," or "June Cold" in the spring, followed by "Summer Catarrh" and "Autumnal Catarrh." It was classified a "Nervous Disease" because it afflicted only people with a "nervous susceptibility" to the "enervating" influences of heat, dust, and "vegetable matter of the atmosphere." The experts also found catarrhal symptoms manifest throughout the body. There was catarrh of the stomach, bowels, lungs, kidneys, bladder, head, and throat. Doctors were advised to prescribe treatments that included sea voyages, mountain retreats, Turkish and Russian baths, as well as doses of arsenic, whisky, galvanic electricity, strychnine, cod-liver oil, opiates, cold powders (camphor), belladonna, digitalis, caffeine, ether, and chloroform, to name a few.[5]

Merck's 1899 *Manual of the Materia Medica* expanded treatments to include the inhalations of diluted carbolic acid, "sulphurous [*sic*] acid," ammonia, formaldehyde, camphor, menthol, and arsenic as cigarettes; opium (as Dover's powder); and even a "hot foot bath." George Beard offered general advice on diet, exercise, and proper clothing. He spoke to the "laity" and the "sufferers" advising they get plenty of sleep during an attack of catarrh and, most important, abstain from shaving as "a hygienic measure of great value."[6]

Vapor Infusions

In 1885, Dr. Robinson found the Maw's Inhaler (above) to be the "most recommendable" form of hot water vaporizer. To use, mix "active ingredients" with one pint of boiling water and place into the earthenware vessel, cork it, place the glass straw up one or the other nostril and breath until your nose is clear, or five minutes. The hot water vaporizer pictured is the plain institutional variety; others were ornately decorated, and these have become highly collectable. Reproductions of Victorian earthenware like this were made for the tourist trade and are quite common on Internet auctions.

Dr. Robinson considered Dr. Morell Mackenzie's "eclectic" inhaler the most "perfect instrument" for inhaling vapors.

FIG. 35.—Mackenzie's Steam Inhaler.

Capitalist Dream

The patent medicine industry wasted no time exploiting catarrh. It was the capitalist's dream, the perfect illness. Catarrh would not kill off their customer base, and as a bonus, it recurred with the seasons, which guaranteed repeat business, year after year after year. It took top billing on many national brand labels. And, because their success relied on the "threat-reassurance" model—threaten with imminent death, then reassure with a sure cure—they demonized catarrh with the standard adjectives: *systemic*, *acute*, *chronic*, and *epidemic*.

(Text continues on page 30.)

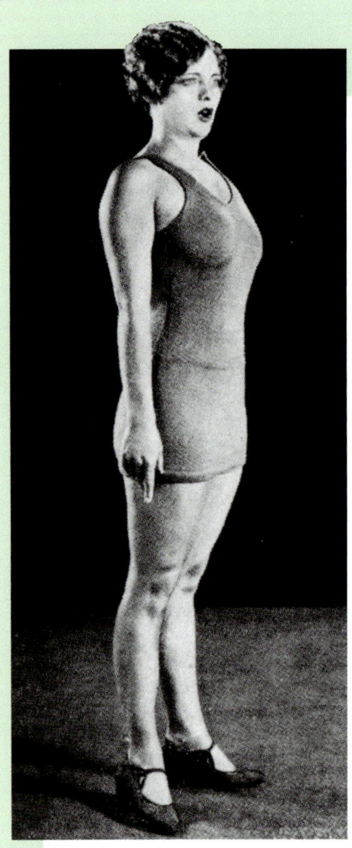

Deep Breathing Exercise

Macfadden on Catarrh

"Rational Living" was to the Golden Age what the holistic life movement is to us today. It was a lifestyle movement that influenced a generation to question all things artificial and to search for natural and rational alternatives in their foods, medicines, and physical well-being. Early followers shunned wearing corsets and tight-fitting clothes, taking pills, and consuming processed foods. They sought out massage, chiropractic, and colonic therapies. And, they slept with the windows open, ate fresh food in small portions, and advocated physical exercise for both men and *women*—scandalous!

"Hay Fever is a disease arising from putrefaction within the intestinal canal and reflected throughout the circulatory system."

—Elmer Lee, M. D., editor, *Health Culture*[8]

The magazine *Health Culture* (est. 1894), "A Monthly Journal of Practical Hygiene," was at the forefront of the movement, and its editors published what they called "rational cures for everyday disorders, without drugs." The cover article for February 1912 was titled: "Chronic Nasal Catarrh; Its Cause and Radical Cure" by Dr. George H. Patchen. The doctor wrote that during a case of chronic nasal catarrh it was desirable to let the mucus flow because that was how "impurities" were discharged from the blood. He explained that the cause of impurities in the blood was the "defective digestion and assimilation of food." The cure? "Purify the blood and invigorate and fortify the entire system." Catarrh "cannot exist in any one who possesses good digestion and assimilation of food, whose skin, liver and kidneys are normally active and whose blood is rich and pure and in a good state of circulation."[7]

In addition to health and diet, Rational Living practitioners took a new look at their own physique. Men were inspired to try out strength training by strongmen like the Great Sandow who staged muscle displays to show the world what an ideal man's body should look like. Another such strongman was an ambitious heavyweight boxer from St Louis, Missouri, named Bernarr Macfadden. While performing his muscle show in New York he evolved a philosophy that combined body building with the principals of Rational Living and called himself "the greatest living authority on physical culture." A natural exhibitionist and tireless egomaniac, Macfadden collected a large following, and in 1899 he launched his own magazine, *Physical Culture*. In addition to its primary focus of creating the perfect human body, *Physical Culture* also challenged the medical establishment or what Macfadden coined the "pill-pushers." During his long and controversial

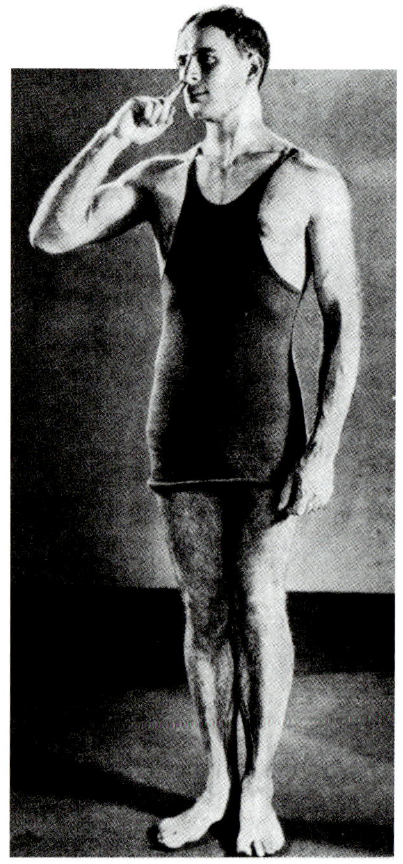

Resistive Breathing Exercise

life, Macfadden wrote an estimated 150 health books that codified the doctrine first established by Drs. Latson, Lee, Patchen and the other luminaries of the Rational Living movement.[9]

Macfadden's 214-page *Colds, Coughs and Catarrh* was published in 1926. In the book he repeated what Patchen had written more than a decade earlier and added some of his own eccentric procedures. He updated it a little by acknowledging that germs had "become very popular of late" as the "supposed cause of colds." But he was not impressed with the germ theory and stubbornly maintained the old line that germs were "more of a symptom." He went on to describe many of the "actual causes," and the following list is a collection from throughout the book: improper diet; lack of fresh air; too little exercise, bathing, and sleep; overclothing; overheating of houses; destructive emotions or thoughts; bad habits of any kind (which included coffee, tea, candy, alcohol, and tobacco); vaccination and inoculation; the medicine habit (he warned his readers against using the 25¢ cough cures advertised in the drugstore window); gossiping and the bargain sales habit; and mental sexual abuse which may "predispose to a cold and other worse conditions. . . ."[10]

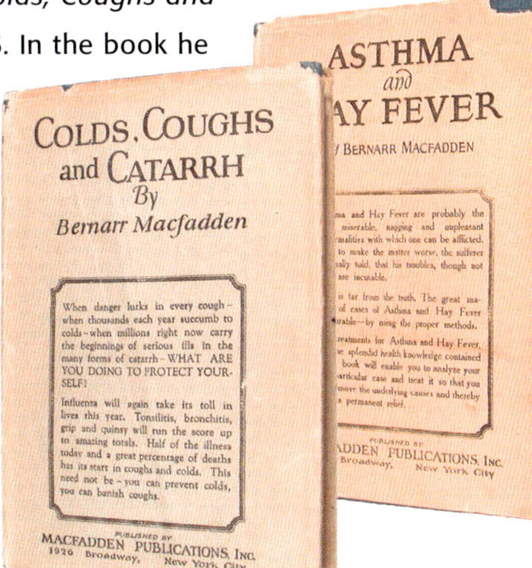

The treatment for catarrh? Daily: a diet of six oranges, hot bath, enema, lots of sleep, fresh air bath with dry-friction rub, nude sun bath followed by a cold bath, wool wraps, walking, and rhythmic breathing. After a few days when the symptoms have subsided, the orange diet is replaced with fresh raw milk, twelve glasses a day, and more enemas, for two to four weeks "or longer if desired." Macfadden demonized drugstore medicines but made an exception for cough drops, throat atomizers—"use oils of eucalyptus, menthol, pine, etc.," and nasal douches—which he said "are excellent." Ironically, that constituted most of the 25¢ catarrh and cold "medicines" found in the drugstores at the time. Tragically, after Macfadden's eldest son became seriously ill and died, it was learned that the millionaire publisher had refused to summon a doctor because he believed the boy's body would heal itself with plenty of fresh air, fasting, and "right living."[11]

"The treatment of nasal catarrh has afforded a rich field for quacks, and has been a source of almost infinite annoyance to physicians."

—J. H. Kellogg, M.D.,
inventor of corn flakes,
director of the
Battle Creek Sanitarium,
author of *Man the Masterpiece*[12]

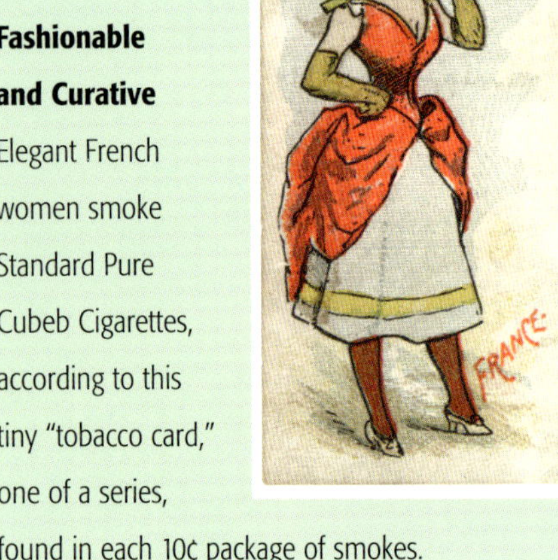

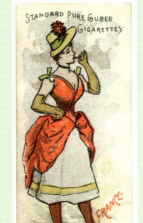

Fashionable and Curative
Elegant French women smoke Standard Pure Cubeb Cigarettes, according to this tiny "tobacco card," one of a series, found in each 10¢ package of smokes. L. W. Warner & Co., Incp'd. Sole Proprietors. 69 Murray St., New York.

■ Sanford's Radical Cure for Catarrh "instantly relieves and permanently cures acute, chronic and ulcerative catarrh."[13]

■ Piso's Remedy for Catarrh "gives immediate relief—the Catarrhal virus is soon expelled from the system, and the diseased action of the mucous membrane replaced by healthy secretions."[14]

■ Wei DeMeyer's Catarrh Cure announced, "Catarrh Poison—No other such obstinate and offensive disease, afflicts mankind, as Catarrh. One-fifth of our Children die of diseases it fosters, and fully one-fourth of living men and women, have but miserable existences from the same cause. A Malignant Virus nursed in the System from Infancy until Death. Putridity, Deafness, Bronchitis, Scrofula and undetermined Constitutions."[15]

■ Marshall's Cubeb Cigarettes described the symptoms of catarrh: "profuse discharges of mucous or purulent matter—there is more or less dropping of mucus from the head into the throat; and a hawking up of toughened or inspissated mucus, often in the shape of scales or crusts—or the profluvia is so great as to necessitate constant spitting of glairy mucus."[16]

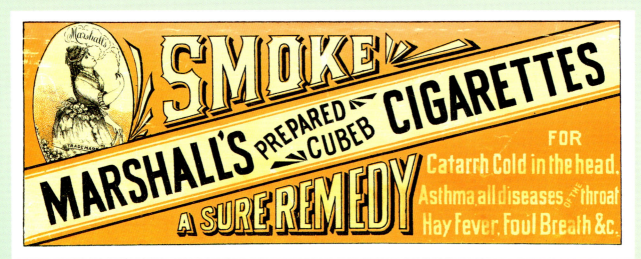

Smoke—A Sure Remedy
Smoke was another form of delivery—nothing like inhaling hot smoke when you have a sore throat! Smoking dried cubeb berries was a traditional catarrh cure in southeastern Asia.

Catarrh was worked overtime at the famous Invalids' Hotel and Surgical Institute in Buffalo, New York. The Invalids' Hotel was founded in 1871 by Dr. Ray V. Pierce as a front for his quack nostrum manufacturing enterprise and his star tonic Pierce's Golden Medical Discovery. Pierce also published *The People's Common Sense Medical Adviser in Plain English; or, Medicine Simplified*. In this 1,008-page "doorstop," Pierce described a new "ulcerous or more aggravated stage of the disease" called ozaena. Ozaena was "so acrid, unhealthy, and poisonous" that it produced an "excessively fetid" discharge that required "the frequent use of the handkerchief" and rendered the "poor sufferer disagreeable to both himself and those with whom he associates." Pierce also wrote:

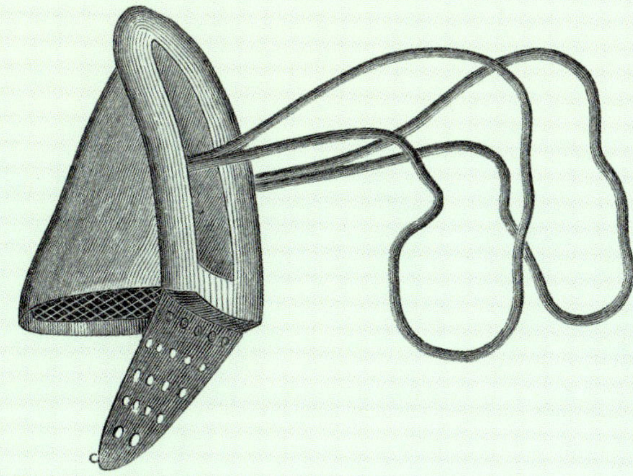

Fig. 55.—Nasal Respirator.

Portions of cartilage and bone, or even entire bones, often die, slough away, and are discharged, either in large flakes, or blackened, half-decayed, and crumbly pieces; or, as is much more commonly the case, in the form of numerous minute particles, that escape with the discharge and are unobserved. It is painfully unpleasant to witness the ravages of this terrible disease, and observe the extent to which it sometimes progresses. Holes are eaten through the roof of the mouth, and great cavities excavated into the solid bones of the face; in such cases only the best and most through [sic] treatment will check the progress and fatal termination of the disease.[17]

Symptoms of catarrh to look out for included, "inflamed eyes, ringing in the ears, deafness, hawking and coughing, ulcerations, death and decay of bones, nasal twang, offensive breath, dizziness, mental depression, nausea, tickling cough, difficulty in speaking plainly, general debility, idiocy, and insanity." Pierce and his associates left nothing to the poor reader's imagination while exhausting their own. However, they debunked the notion that catarrh came in different varieties, such as "Rose Cold" or "Autumnal Catarrh," separating hay fever out as another disease more closely related to "coryza, or cold in the head." To the "skilled eye of the practical and experienced physician," catarrh was caused by an "enfeebled, impure, or otherwise faulty condition of the system—weakened or deranged with bad humors." Hay fever was caused by pollen and "odors" from grasses, flowers, and feather beds and affected people with an "over sensitiveness of the nervous system."[18]

Treatment included two of Pierce's products: the Golden Medical Discovery as the natural helpmate of Dr. Sage's Catarrh Remedy, followed ironically by a special warning not to be influenced by "Unprincipled quacks and charlatans." Profits from the

A Practical Remedy

When a federal tax was levied on the sale of goods during the 1898 Spanish American War, Dr. Pierce printed a tax revenue stamp (above) that doubled as a package closure. Also shown is Dr. Sage's Catarrh Remedy bottle with its paper wrapper and regular gummed stamp closure.

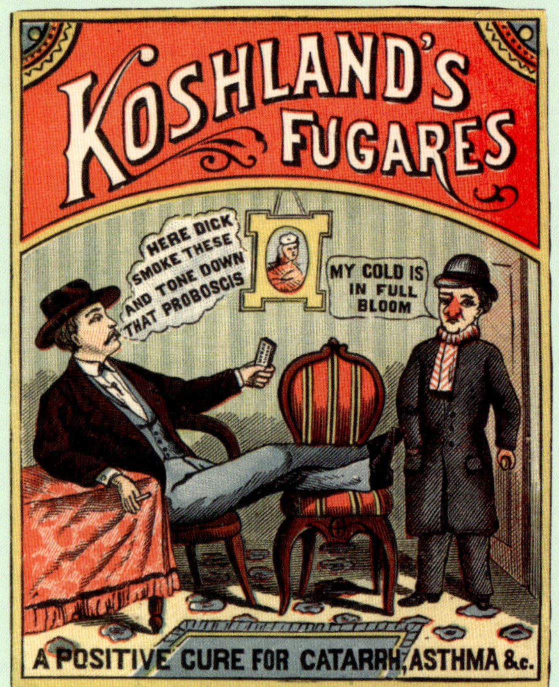

nostrums, clinic, and publications eventually supported speculative ventures in the West, a pleasure island off the coast of Florida, and other capitalist investments, making Ray Pierce a very wealthy man.[19] (See more about Pierce on page 49.)

Sometime after 1922, the Mentholatum Company dropped its use of the word *catarrh* from packaging and advertising. The 1906 Food and Drugs Act was a wake-up call to the industry. The constant hounding by watchdog groups like the Council of Pharmacy and Chemistry of the American Medical Association kept at bay giants like Pe-ru-na, who claimed only to cure catarrh. And, although the word *catarrh* continued in common usage, its meaning among men of science returned to its origin, as a simple "flowing down" of mucus.

In 1925, Dr. R. L. Alsaker, a writer of self-help health books, published *Curing Catarrh Coughs and Colds,* one of the last books on catarrh. Alsaker perpetuated the theory that catarrh was caused by a weak constitution, but he associated it only with colds, no longer with hay fever. He debunked ozaena as simply undrained mucus that caused bad breath. Alsaker said, "The mucus is an albuminous fluid [albumin is a water-soluble protein found in blood plasma] and when it is discharged as catarrhal waste it weakens the body." This discharge removes "impurities" from the blood, but when the mucus dries into crusts he observed that the membrane is unable to keep itself clean. Alsaker warned that "most of the children who have the disgusting habit of picking their nose are suffering from catarrh" and blamed the parents for feeding them improperly. "If catarrh is allowed to remain long the mucous membrane is forced into degeneration—[and] becomes an ideal site for many different kinds of diseases." He claimed that it was "one of the most prolific causes of consumption," which he thought killed "more than fifteen out of every hundred individuals." Alsaker concluded that a weakened constitution was the result of improper eating and that "sickness [was] a bad habit, not a necessity." *Catarrh* was eventually dropped by advertisers completely, and the word became lost among the childhood memories of those born before the Second World War.[20]

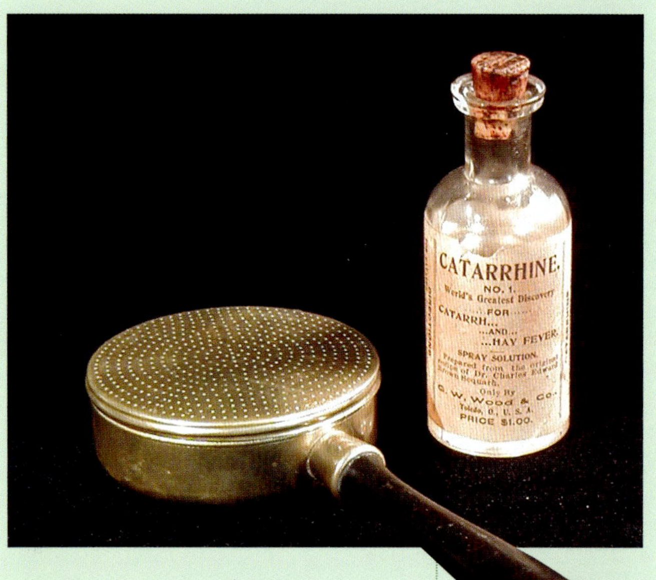

Catarrhine and Brass Inhaler Pan

Simple evaporation was the principle behind the design of this inhaler. A small amount of liquid remedy was poured onto an asbestos fiber mat inside the pan and allowed to evaporate at room temperature. The sufferer would hold the pan under the chin and inhale the escaping fumes. This design was used for a broad range of medical inhalations.

Science on Catarrh

Where were the "real" doctors and scientists, one might ask, when all these wild theories about catarrh were being published? The twentieth century's leading authority on colds, the eminent virologist, Sir Christopher Andrewes (1896–1989), wrote that "the history of serious research into the causes of colds need not go further back than 1860–70 when Pasteur did the first great work on the causative relation of bacteria to infectious disease."[21]

The next "serious" step would then be the 1914 experiments of Dr. W. Kruse of the Hygienic Institute at the University of Leipzig. In January, Kruse collected nasal discharge from his cold-suffering assistant, Dr. Hilger, put it in solution, filtered out all the bacteria, then placed drops up the noses of twelve of his staff causing four of them to develop colds. In June, Hilger arrived at work with another cold, and Kruse used this second

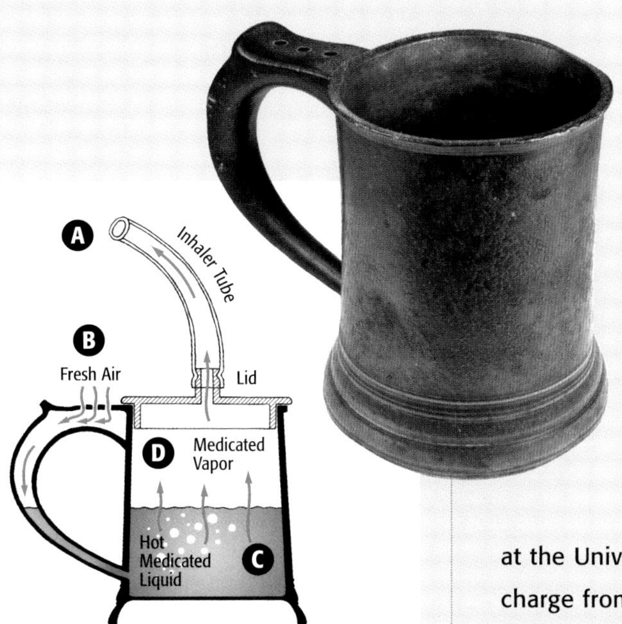

Vapor Inhalers: Pewter Tankard Inhaler

Inhaling spirits from a pewter tankard at the corner pub was nothing new to an Englishman in 1850, but inhaling Friar's Balsam vapors from a tankard in the hospital ward certainly might have been! Sometime in the early to mid-nineteenth century, a closed system was devised to ensure that all of the valuable medicated vapors went into the patient's respiratory system and not out to the rest of the room. This is how it worked: holding the tankard with the thumb on top of the handle (**B**), the patient sucked on the rubber inhaler tube (**A**) to create a vacuum inside the lidded tankard (**D**). When the thumb was released, air rushed through the three holes in the top of the hollow handle to equalize the pressure. As the air passed through the liquid inside the handle and down through a hole at the bottom of the handle, it entered the tankard and mixed with the volatile molecules of the hot balsam tea (**C**) and vaporized at the surface (**D**), where it was inhaled through the tube by the patient. The length of the tube and the temperature of the balsam tea determined if it was going to be a cold, warm, or hot inhalation.

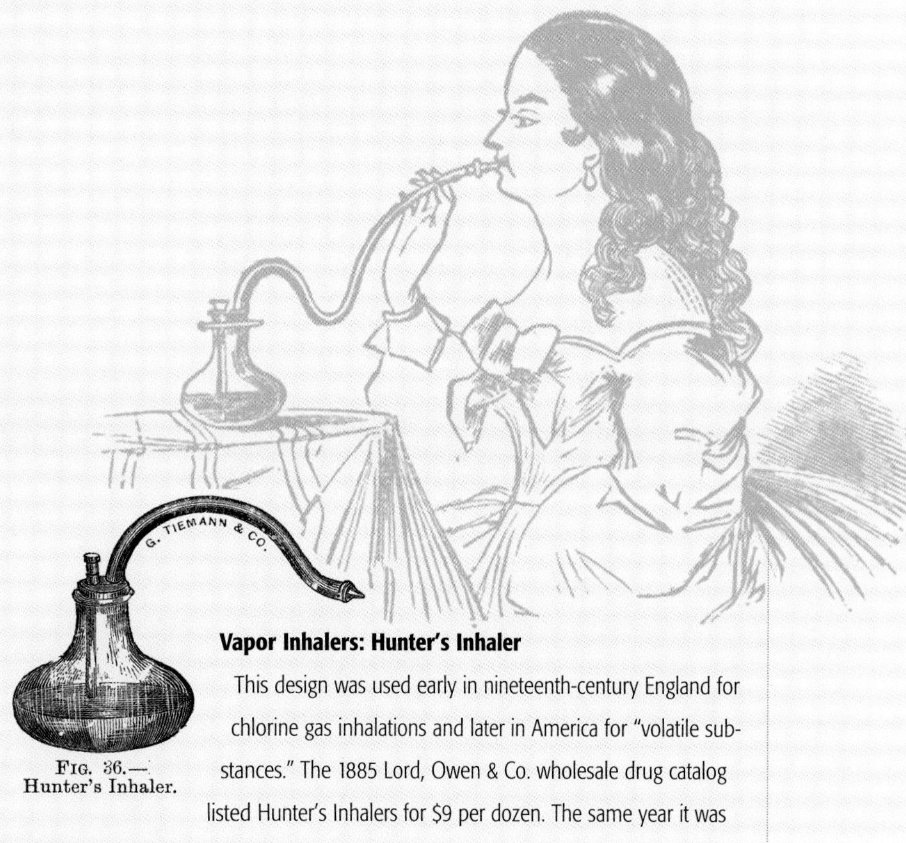

FIG. 36.—Hunter's Inhaler.

Vapor Inhalers: Hunter's Inhaler

This design was used early in nineteenth-century England for chlorine gas inhalations and later in America for "volatile substances." The 1885 Lord, Owen & Co. wholesale drug catalog listed Hunter's Inhalers for $9 per dozen. The same year it was included in Dr. Robinson's book on nasal catarrh, where he described it as inexpensive and simple. That was a good reason why Hunter's Inhaler remained a viable commodity for more than fifty years. It operated on the same principles as the pewter tankard and was more attractive and efficient. Its stopper produced a tighter seal, and thus a better vacuum could be achieved.

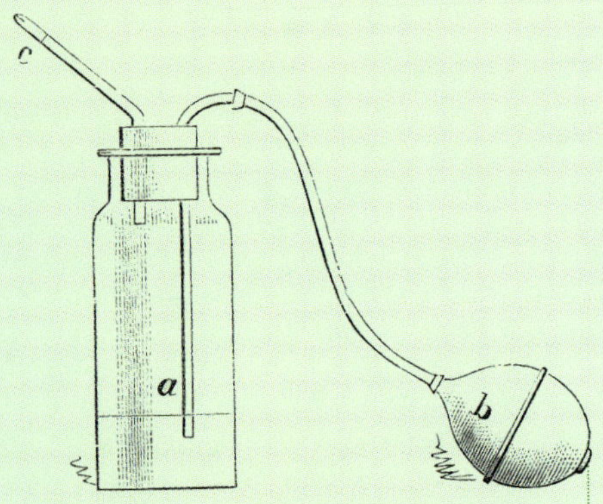

Fig. 38.—Apparatus for Injecting Vapor into the Nasal Passages (Smith).

Vapor Inhalers: Cold Vapor Spray Inhaler

Based on the same principles as Hunter's closed system vaporizer, and credited to A. H. Smith, the vapor spray inhaler utilized a rubber bulb to pressurize the chamber, and a long metal inhalation tube that allowed the exit spray to be placed inside the nasal cavity or throat. This was the forerunner of later-day atomizers and nebulizers.

opportunity to inoculate his class of thirty-six bacteriology students. Fifteen promptly became infected with Hilger's cold. The professor suspected there must have been an invisible, poisonous agent, or "virus," involved in the transmission of the disease. He managed to publish a report of his findings just weeks before the start of World War I, which, unfortunately, put an end to his investigation.[22]

Evidence that catarrh is contagious was recorded back in Pasteur's day when explorers in Greenland observed epidemics of colds rage through the Eskimo populations of isolated villages whenever a foreign ship arrived. However, this was not widely known. Remarkably, for the next half century, doctors continued to believe that colds were unique to each individual, were caused by a chill or bad blood, and were not contagious. The surgeon on Sir Ernest Shackleton's 1907–08 expedition to the Antarctic, Dr. Eric Marshall, reported that there had been no sickness among the crew until a bale of new clothing was opened and the men were "seized with acute nasal catarrh." Based on Blackley's theories of the day, it was not unreasonable to suspect that hitchhiking pollen had caused this hay fever attack. But, as it turned out, investigators who later read Dr. Marshall's account misinterpreted catarrh to mean "cold," and the fast recovery of the explorers naturally threw doubt on the credibility of the twenty-eight-year-old doctor's report.[23]

(Text continues on page 36.)

ONE or MORE of these Cards Mailed to any one on request.

TABLE OF ERUPTIVE FEVERS

W-WEEKS D-DAYS

NAME	INCUBATION	RASH APRS.	ERUP. LASTS	DIS'SE LASTS
Chicken Pox...	4 to 14 D	2d or 3d D	4 to 8 D	1 to 2 W
Erysipelas......	1 to 5 D	1st to 3d D	4 to 8 D	1 to 3 W
Measles	10 to 12 D	4th D	3 to 5 D	10 to 14 D
" German	7 to 17 D	1st or 2d D	1 to 3 D	4 to 7 D
Scarlatina	1 to 8 D	2d D	4 to 10 D	2 to 3 W
Small Pox......	8 to 14 D	3d or 4th D	16 to 25 D	3 to 5 W
Typhoid........	10 to 21 D	7th to 10th		3 to 4 W

In all eruptions (and for Piles) MENTHOLATUM will give instant relief from itching and is remarkably soothing, cooling and healing. MENTHOLATUM CO. BUFFALO, N. Y. WICHITA, KS.

Form 4.-35-M-11-07. H.W. OVER.

1907 Free Handout

This wallet-size card provided sobering information at a time in our history when there was no defense against these deadly diseases. Mentholatum was a staple in the sick room helping caregivers provide relief from the pain and suffering of their loved ones.

Atomizer 101

Dr. Horatio C. Wood Jr., professor of materia medica at the Philadelphia College of Pharmacy and Science, wrote in the July 1932 issue of *American Druggist* that Dr. Bergsen of Berlin invented the first steam atomizer in 1860. The atomizer requires steam under pressure, and at its heart is the siphon (above). The siphon's "operation is based on the principle that a current of air passing at right angles over a tube creates a partial vacuum in that tube." The vacuum draws liquid medicine up the venturi tube 1, which then intermixes with the steam in tube 2.[24]

The example above right was manufactured by Codman & Shurtleff of Boston under three U.S. patents dated 1868, 1869, and 1886, and though it is well over 110 years old, its delicate blown glass siphon is still intact. The atomizer below right is a later model using an Eccles siphon (inset above) which was clearly a massive improvement over glass—it is unbreakable, easy to clean, and has a spring-loaded gasket connection to the boiler. Another steam atomizer is shown on page 25.

Anatomy of a Steam Atomizer

A small oil burner (**A**) heats the water inside a spherical boiler (**B**), releasing a head of steam that escapes through a special glass siphon tube (**C**), which draws liquid medication up from the glass container (**D**) and intermixes it with the steam inside the inhaler tube (**E**). The atomized steam and medication cools enough inside the glass tube so as not to scald, and excess vapor that is not inhaled condenses and drips back into the second container (**F**).

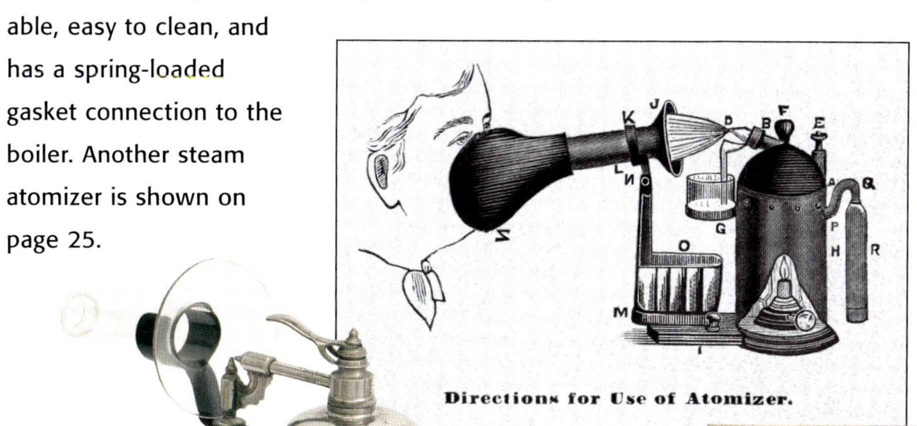

Directions for Use of Atomizer.

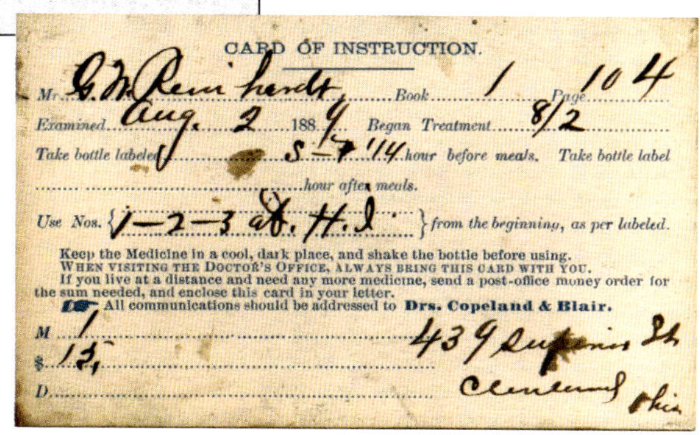

CARD OF INSTRUCTION.

Mr. G. W. Reinhardt .... Book 1 .... Page 104

Examined Aug. 2 188 9 Began Treatment 8/2

Take bottle labeled .... hour before meals. Take bottle label .... hour after meals.

Use Nos. {1—2—3 ....} from the beginning, as per labeled.

Keep the Medicine in a cool, dark place, and shake the bottle before using.
WHEN VISITING THE DOCTOR'S OFFICE, ALWAYS BRING THIS CARD WITH YOU.
If you live at a distance and need any more medicine, send a post-office money order for the sum needed, and enclose this card in your letter.
☞ All communications should be addressed to **Drs. Copeland & Blair.**

M 1 ....
$ 15 ....
D ....

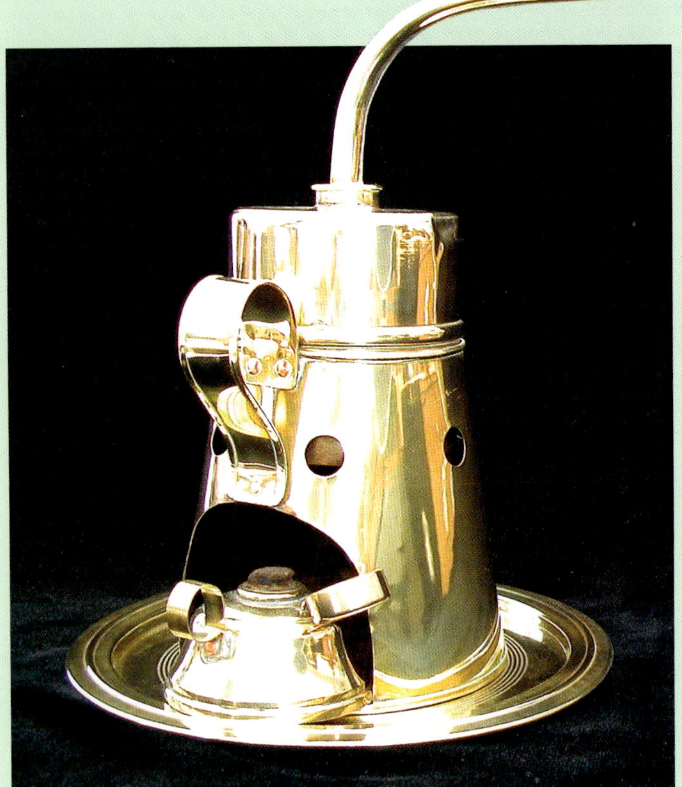

Cool Vapor

This vaporizer of undetermined make is from Utrecht, the Netherlands.

Solving the mysteries of simple catarrhal disease was turning out to be extremely frustrating. In 1916, George B. Foster Jr., a Harvard professor of preventive medicine and hygiene, surveyed the state of medical knowledge on the cause of "catarrhal affections." He wrote that there were some who believed it had a complex etiology; "wet and cold, drafts, irritating vapors, overheated rooms, worry, fatigue, sexual excess, dietetic errors, alcohol, and what not. . . ." Another group, he reported, believed that "chilling, sudden changes in temperature, and fatigue . . . act as predisposing factors by lowering resistance, and thus pave the way for infection by micro-organisms commonly believed to be present normally in the nasal cavities." Foster concluded: "In short, present knowledge of the etiology of the common cold is in a most chaotic state." In 1919, researchers at Washington University Medical School in St. Louis, Missouri, took on one of the more obvious questions, does cold weather play a part in the etiology of head colds? They chilled their student volunteers, tested the collected mucous cultures, and discovered that cold air caused only vasoconstriction inside the nose. Their logical conclusion—cold air was good for combating colds, and not for causing them.[25]

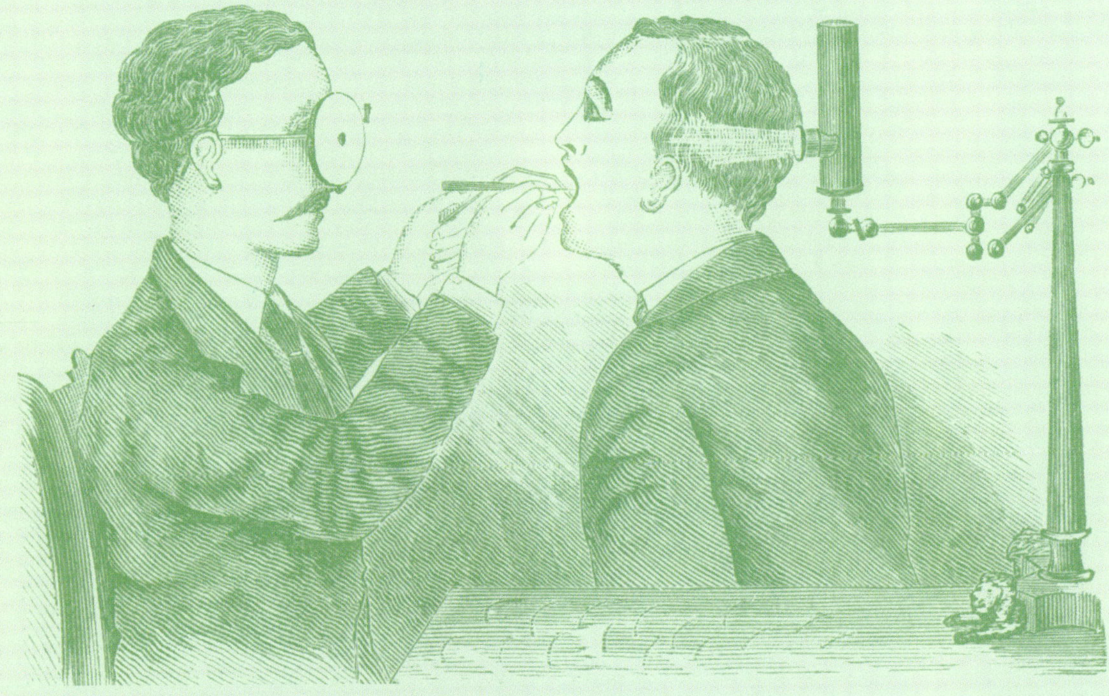

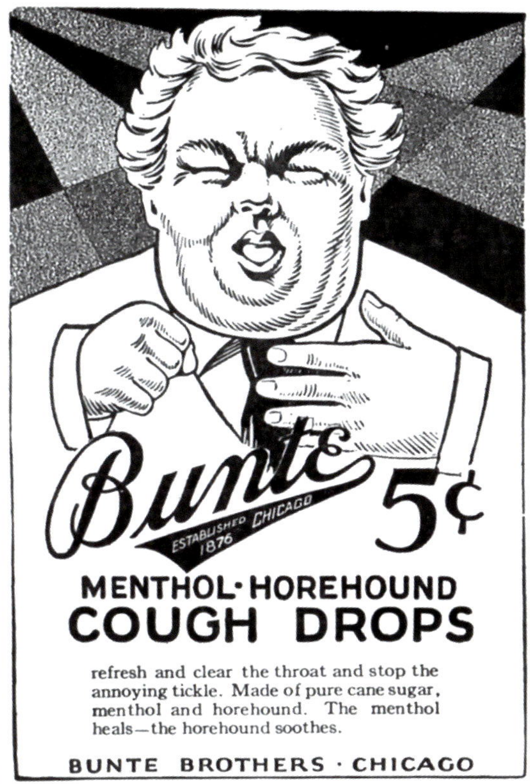

1924 Bunte Ad

This ad appeared in *Popular Mechanics*, February 1924. "The menthol heals–the horehound soothes."

The decade of the '30s marked the ascendancy of scientific thought that now informs our modern understanding of colds. However, the issue of virus vs. bacterium was by no means settled. As an example, the important work of Dr. Alphonse Dochez at Columbia University in 1931, confirming the existence of Kruse's cold virus, was contested in 1932 by Drs. David and Robert Thomson in their 700-page book *The Common Cold*, which advocated a bacterial cause. Dr. Andrewes helped isolate the first human influenza virus in 1933 and went on to pursue the cold virus for the rest of his career. Nevertheless, Andrewes generously recommended the Thomsons' book to be a "very useful review on the common cold."[26]

Starting in 1860 with Pasteur, as Dr. Andrewes suggested, and ending seventy years later with the confirmation of a cold virus by Dochez, hundreds of dedicated and intelligent investigators in association with universities, hospitals, chemical laboratories, and, yes, the proprietary and drug manufacturers, searched for the cure of the common cold. Theirs was an age of great exploration and invention. They tried out everything looking for cause, remedy, and cure. Indeed, some of their theories seem absurd by present standards, but someone had to chart the dead ends on the road map. To say they failed because they couldn't find the etiology within just seventy years would be petty. After all, we have not found a cure during seventy years of modern research since the discovery of a flu virus in 1933! The "nostrum" makers' legacy is their remedies to relieve symptoms. On this front the war against catarrh was most successful. Fueled by competition, the industry isolated the compounds that had the greatest effect and designed the most efficient delivery mechanisms, many of which are still being used today. Labeling them as quacks and dismissing their chapter in medical history as humorous would be intellectual snobbery. While Dr. Andrewes and his colleagues helped to bring us closer to a cure for the common cold, the only remedy he used for himself and would recommend to others to help clear the nasal passages was steam with eucalyptus and menthol. . . .[27]

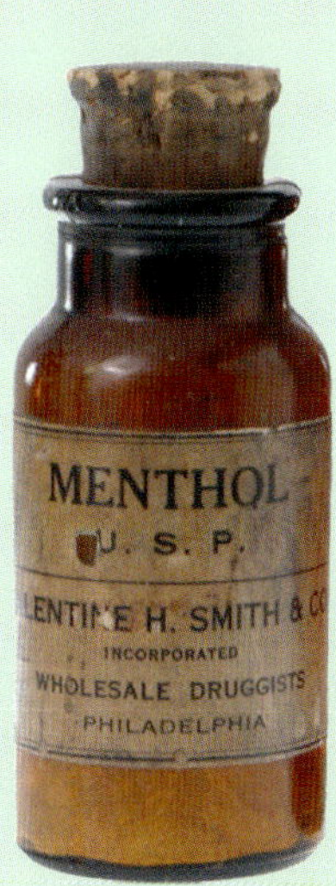

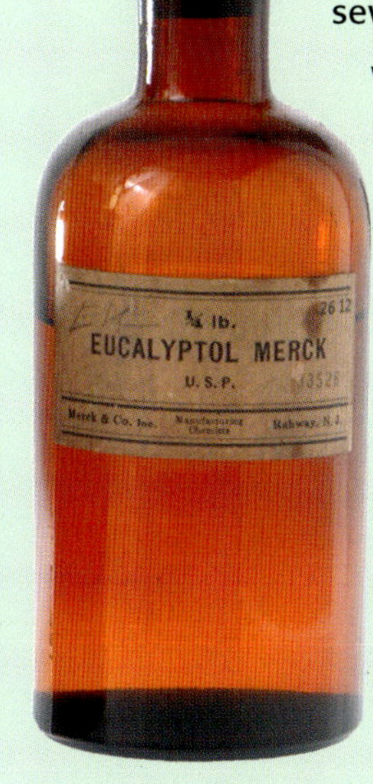

The Friendly Salve

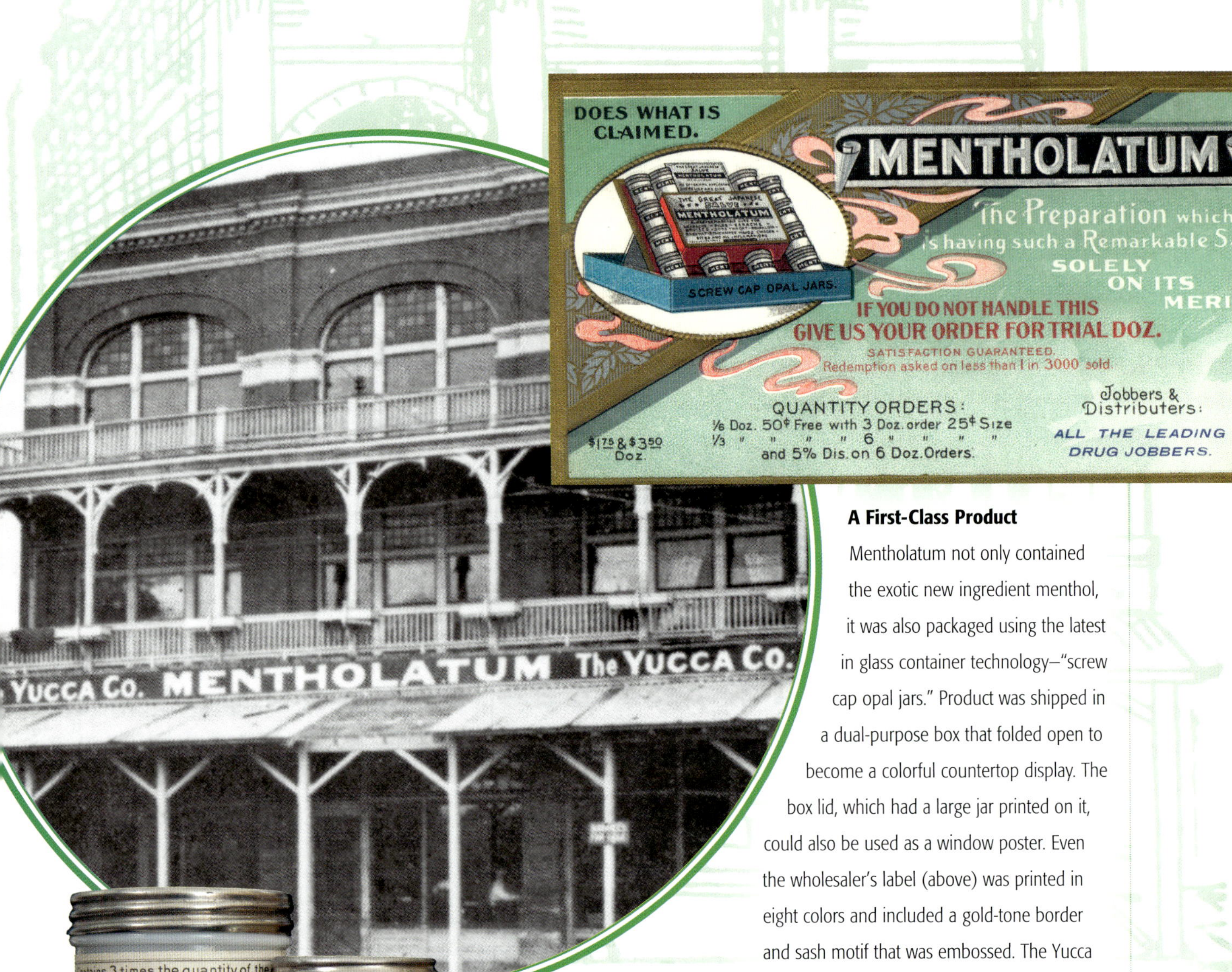

A First-Class Product

Mentholatum not only contained the exotic new ingredient menthol, it was also packaged using the latest in glass container technology—"screw cap opal jars." Product was shipped in a dual-purpose box that folded open to become a colorful countertop display. The box lid, which had a large jar printed on it, could also be used as a window poster. Even the wholesaler's label (above) was printed in eight colors and included a gold-tone border and sash motif that was embossed. The Yucca Company would soon outgrow its factory, which occupied the first floor of this modest building located at 1213 East Douglas Avenue.

SAMPLES MENTHOLATUM

Give circular for Directions with each Sample

☞ **Mentholatum Samples HANDED OUT BY DEALERS WITH PERSONAL WORD OF COMMENDATION make SURE CUSTOMERS.**

What is worth doing is worth doing well.

Pattee Park Pharmacy
JOHN W. KOCH, PROP.
Citizens Tel. 304. 1121 S. Tenth St.

St. Joseph, Mo.
Jan. 30, 1899

YUCCA Co.,
Wichita, Kan.

--Am having the best sale on Mentholatum of anything I ever sold. Your plan of introducing Mentholatum has always been my plan. When I hand a customer a sample and tell him of its merits and ask him to try it faithfully, ''I've got him'' better than all the full page ads and posters in the city will do.

Respectfully,

J. W. Koch.

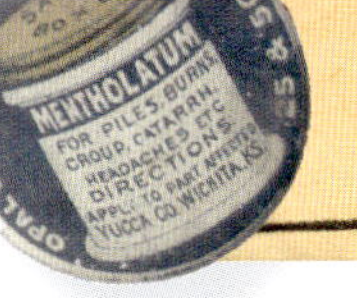

Priming the Pump

Much of the income from early Mentholatum sales went back into the distribution of free samples packaged in little one-inch-diameter tin "boxes." This particular design was in use between 1898 and 1903 and was manufactured by the American Can Company, plant 73-A, run by Norton Bros., Maywood (Chicago), Illinois.

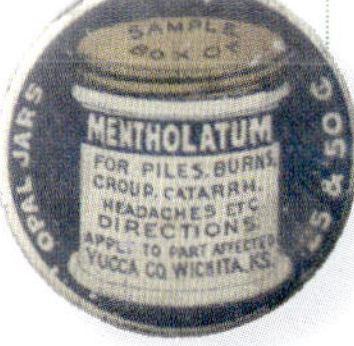

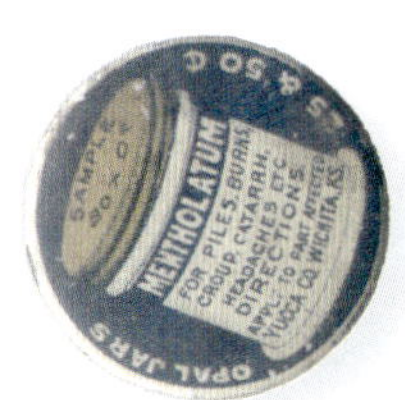

"Mentholatum Salve . . . Does its own advertising."

Commerce in the nineteenth century was dominated by advertising, as it is today, and advertising was very expensive. Then and now, the manufacturer of a new product first had to establish brand recognition and customer demand, then find a way to distribute it to end users. Barring the path to market, there were two gatekeepers: advertisers and the distributors. These institutions governed the market terrain and extracted a high price for entry. The Yucca Company already conformed to the distribution status quo by selling its soap only to wholesale supply houses and "jobbers." These middlemen produced a catalog of the brands they represented and sent it to the businesses within their territory. They handled all the resulting orders and arranged for shipping the Yucca Company's soaps and toiletry articles to their commercial hotel and laundry accounts, as well as to retail drugstores. Hyde planned to market Mentholatum the same way, which explains why there was no mention of the Yucca Company in the 1895 Christmas newspaper ad (see page 11)—he didn't want people coming down to the factory to buy Mentholatum.

Advertising was another matter. Hyde was convinced that brand recognition and demand would be generated by the product itself. As the *Wichita Daily Eagle* reported after observing the Yucca Company exhibit at the 1896 Kansas State Fair, "Mentholatum salve . . . does its own advertising." The druggist at Miller's Pharmacy in Topeka told the company, "Every jar of Mentholatum we sell, sells another." What had started out as just the latest specialty item in the small soap manufacturers' growing product line was rapidly moving to the top of the list.

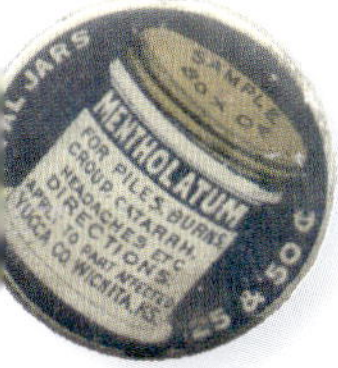

Hyde witnessed the effect his new emollient had on people when first tested and correctly reasoned that all he had to do was introduce the product and Mentholatum would do the rest. A druggist in Charleston, West Virginia, drove home the point when he said Mentholatum "makes friends wherever it goes." The Yucca Company therefore began a grassroots campaign of introduction that circumvented the advertising gatekeepers.

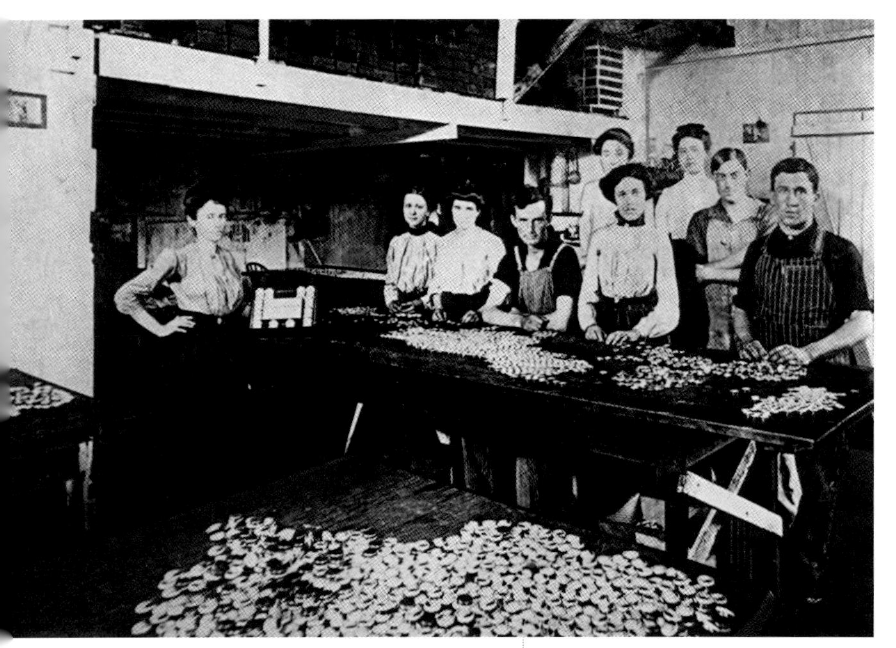

Yucca Company Employees

This early photograph shows the workers gathered around a table covered with what look like sample tins. Notice the woman on the left holding up a counter display for one-ounce jars like the one on page 38.

A proper introduction required a personal endorsement and a free sample. Samples of the friendly salve were provided to the retailer with the suggestion that he pass them on to his customers with a personal commendation. Hyde knew that if Mentholatum was first recommended by a trusted member of the community rather than by a testimonial printed in a newspaper ad, then it would surely become "the best seller in the house." Social scientists today have identified six basic tendencies of human behavior that will affect a customer's decision to buy a product; they are reciprocation, authority, consistency, liking, social validation, and scarcity. Hyde's approach satisfied five of them. Reciprocation was achieved when a gift sample was given, and the receiver felt obliged to reciprocate later by purchasing a jar. Authority was demonstrated when the customer purchased a jar after a trusted druggist or doctor recommended the product. Consistency was evident when the Yucca Company made a public commitment not to raise prices or change the formula, which then secured the future buying actions of its customers. Liking and social validation were satisfied when the pleasant smell and attractive packaging first made a positive personal impression, and they were further reinforced when the customer saw that his friends also liked the product. A group social bonding took place that supported brand loyalty over several generations. Scarcity was probably not a significant factor in Hyde's case.[1]

The first "traveling agent" for Mentholatum was a forty-five-year-old woman named Ella B. Veazie. Beginning in 1896, Veazie ranged the windy prairie states of Kansas, Missouri, and Nebraska, mostly by railroad, stagecoach, and on occasion by

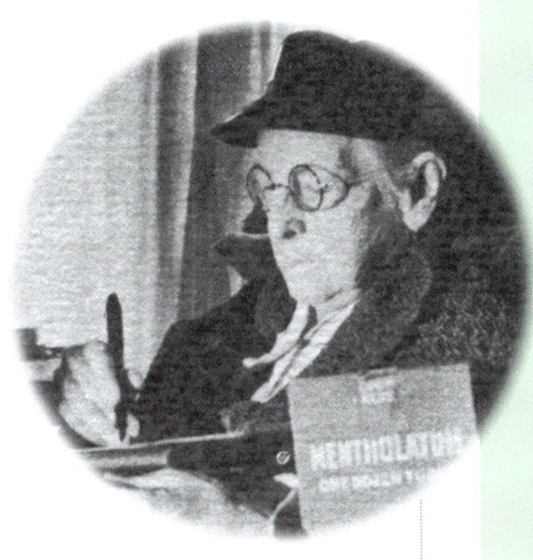

Dr. Ella B. Veazie

Mentholatum's first traveling agent as she appeared in 1939, almost eighty-eight years old and still "pushing" the product. In an early endorsement, she claimed that she had successfully used Mentholatum to cure her own case of deafness.

E. B. Veazie's Mentholatum treatment for deafness:

"The Catarrh that usually causes deafness affects the throat and Eustachian tubes. Air must pass from the inner ear out else we do not hear, hence the inflamed condition must be reduced in the throat and Eustachian tubes. Therefore treat for deafness same as for Catarrh i.e., use in nostrils and outside, on forehead and then in throat on tonsils with gentle massage, using finger anointed with Mentholatum. Use also on the outside of throat well up under the jaw bone, back of ears, well up into roots of hair as the nerve center at base of brain is strengthened thereby. Also apply over the fifth pair of nerves just above ears. In short, a thorough anointing of nostrils and throat inside and out with Mentholatum at least twice a day. Keep out of the ears unless there is soreness there. Trouble is seldom in outer ear. Use persistently and you will get relief."

—from the Hyde Collection, *Some Remarkable Uses for Mentholatum*, c. 1901–1903

horse and buggy, personally introducing the product to druggists, doctors, dentists, and nurses. In 1900, her territory expanded to include Washington, Oregon, and California. She left the company for a few years after the turn of the century to earn a degree at the American School of Osteopathy under Dr. Andrew Taylor Still, followed by a brief practice in Kansas City. But she missed the life of a traveling "man." Dr. Veazie returned to work for the company and traveled from coast to coast as its "Little Emissary of Mentholatum."[2]

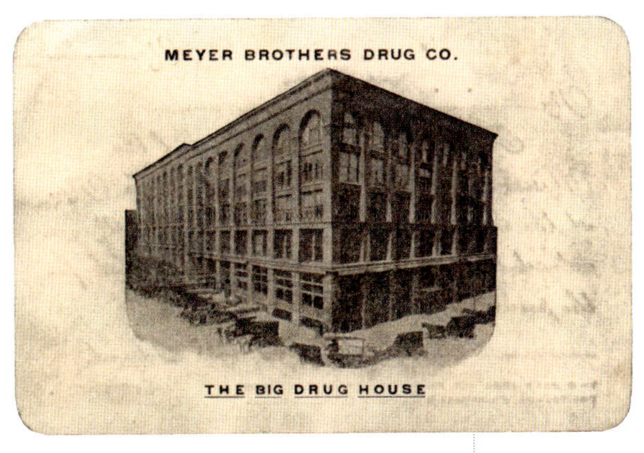

Meyer Brothers

The company was described as "The Largest Drug House in the World."

Her boundless energy and enthusiasm for the product warmed the heart of even the toughest old drugstore proprietor, wary of greedy nostrum salesmen and their overpriced goods. She spread the word that Mr. Hyde promised to make it as easy and profitable as possible to introduce Mentholatum to their customers. And, while other nostrum and remedy manufacturers continued to pay huge sums for print advertising, Hyde invested his advertising budget in free sample "boxes" and in larger profit margins for the druggists. The St. Louis wholesaler, Meyer Brothers Drug Company, recognized his unique approach when it wrote, "We compliment you on the remarkable increase we are having in the sale of Mentholatum. Not being backed with printers' ink, we feel as if merit alone is advertising and creating demand." This policy would stay in effect through the turn of the century, as evidenced by a 1904 flyer that proclaimed, "We Pay MEN Instead of BILL BOARDS."

The Mentholatum trademark, registered under the Trademark Act of 1881, was issued in 1895. The application stated that the product name had been in use since December 1894 and that the product was also produced in commercial quantities since 1894. But later statements made by the company indicate that the product was actually being sold as early as 1893. Interestingly, the application also stated that the product would be for use "in commerce between the United States and foreign nations or Indian tribes, and particularly with the Caddo and Wichita tribes of Indians. . . ." Mentholatum was registered International Class 5 (pharmaceuticals) and U.S. Class 6 (chemicals and chemical compositions).[3]

Shipping Mentholatum

Freight was loaded from the front of the Yucca Company building and not the back as would be the case today. The wagon was parked alongside the porch, and the horse and front wheels were turned out into the street to steady it for loading.

MENTHOLATUM.
A MOST REMARKABLE CURE FOR
—HEADACHE—PILES—EARACHE—
—BRUISES—SORE THROAT—NEURALGIA—
—RHEUMATISM—CHAPPED HANDS—CHIGGER BITES—
AND ALL INFLAMMATIONS
SEE TESTIMONIALS ON CIRCULAR
GUARANTEED
PRICE 25¢
LARGER SIZE 3 TIMES QUANTITY 50¢

A one-ounce jar of Mentholatum sold retail for 25¢. In 1895, that was equivalent to the cost of ten pounds of flour, or a little less than the cost of one gallon of milk delivered. The price became a problem for Hyde's partner, Dewey Wheeler, who felt that they should sell at a minimum profit. Hyde was diametrically opposed to this and said he could not see "much business progress or a broad and liberal standard of life built up on such a basis." Remarkably, Wheeler sold his stock to Hyde for $200 and left the company just as Mentholatum was about to take off. The cost to manufacture a one-ounce jar was 4.2¢. The wholesale price to druggists was $1.75 per dozen, or 14.6¢ per jar. In 1898, they introduced a three-ounce jar that sold for 50¢ retail; one dozen were $3.50 or 29¢ each wholesale and cost 7¢ each to manufacture. Income for the Yucca Company between 1894 and 1898 was averaging about $10,000 annually. It would seem that Mentholatum was making little or no increase over traditional soap sales, when in all probability, income from the product was going straight into promotion, and they were breaking even on their manufacturing costs. Then, in 1899 income doubled! The books show the dramatic results.[4]

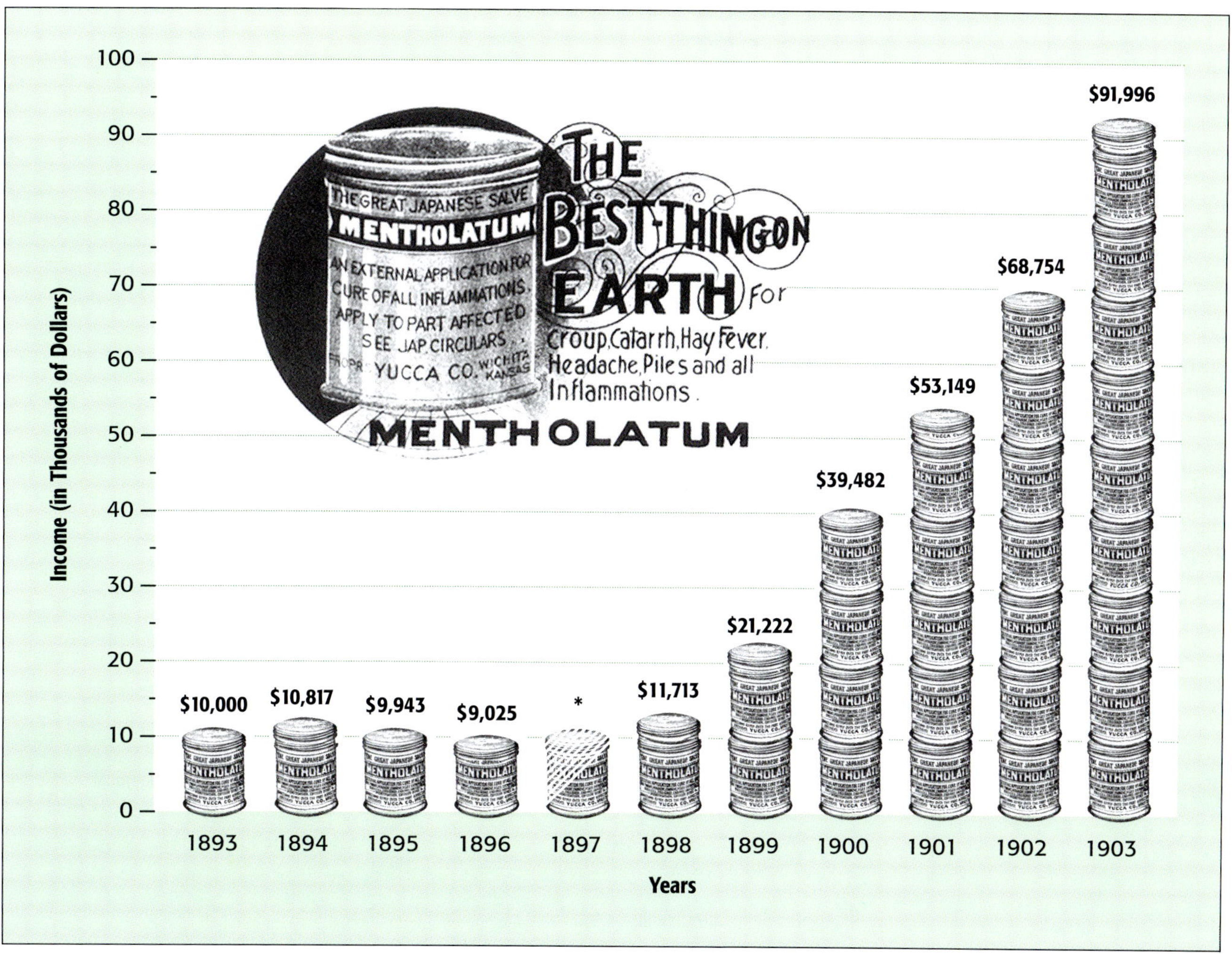

Mentholatum's First Decade of Earnings

The Yucca Company's ledger book recorded combined income from all of its soap and toiletry products, yet it is still easy to see the impact Mentholatum had on the bottom line. Starting in 1893, the year of the National Panic, Wichita businesses were already struggling to recover from what Col. Lewis called the "awful sweat." Earnings understandably remained flat for several more years.

*In 1897, figures for only the first five months were recorded in the ledger. However, there was an increase of $170 from the same five-month period in 1896, so it is safe to assume that the year ended without much difference from the previous year. Then in 1899, income almost doubled, and it did so again in 1900! Sales averaged a phenomenal 33 percent increase annually thereafter. The nineteenth century's Golden Age produced many industries with similar growth rates, and Mentholatum was not alone in its meteoric success. Unfortunately, financial records from the company after 1903 have been lost.

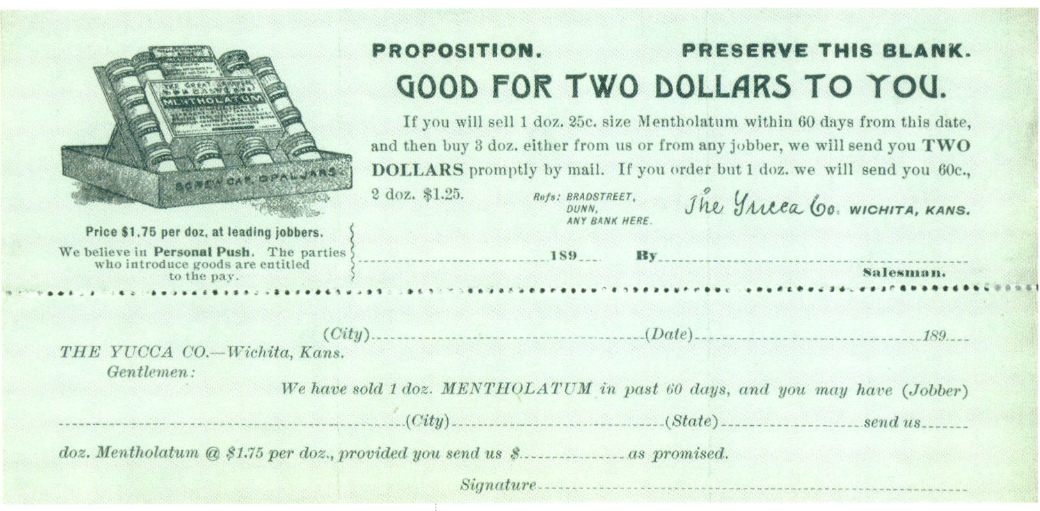

PROPOSITION. PRESERVE THIS BLANK.

GOOD FOR TWO DOLLARS TO YOU.

If you will sell 1 doz. 25c. size Mentholatum within 60 days from this date, and then buy 3 doz. either from us or from any jobber, we will send you **TWO DOLLARS** promptly by mail. If you order but 1 doz. we will send you 60c., 2 doz. $1.25.

Refs: BRADSTREET, DUNN, ANY BANK HERE. The Yucca Co. WICHITA, KANS.

Price $1.75 per doz. at leading jobbers.

We believe in **Personal Push**. The parties who introduce goods are entitled to the pay.

................189.... By................................ Salesman.

(City)................................(Date)................................189....

THE YUCCA CO.—Wichita, Kans.

Gentlemen:

We have sold 1 doz. MENTHOLATUM in past 60 days, and you may have (Jobber)

..............................(City)..............................(State)..................send us.......

doz. Mentholatum @ $1.75 per doz., provided you send us $..................as promised.

Signature..

Cash Back for Sales

Druggists used this form in the late 1890s to take advantage of a Mentholatum sales campaign.

The company sent literature to druggists stressing the importance of a personal endorsement by the clerk before handing out a sample. It offered cash inducements to push Mentholatum over rival brands by selling an introductory quantity within a specified period of time. It also offered additional jars of Mentholatum in return for a listing of names "to whom sold."

WRAP A CIRCULAR FOR DIRECTIONS WITH EACH JAR SOLD.

Please set up card in box as shown above and DISPLAY ON COUNTER OR SHOW CASE.

The BIG JAR pictures on cover make good Window Signs.

The Dealers who SHOW Goods SELL them.

WHEN LOW ORDER THROUGH JOBBER.

Display Instructions

Instructions came with each shipping/display box for its proper setup. Prior to the use of individual boxes, druggists were asked to wrap a circular with each one-ounce jar sold.

Druggists could claim premiums such as a Parker "14k Gold Fountain Pen" (continued past 1906), a "3 Line Rubber Stamp," an ink pad, or a leather wallet (to about 1915). Cardboard favors like the "medicine time indicator" and "Mentholatum Horse" puzzle were also provided for the druggist to hand out to customers. A druggist in Holden, Missouri, wrote to the company on April 7, 1900, to say, "Gentlemen—Made a nice window display of Mentholatum today and pushed it personally. Result, sold 73 jars in a few hours and now have the people talking Mentholatum to their friends. It is O.K. and any wide awake druggist can sell Mentholatum if he has a mind to. Yours for more business, M. L. Golladay."

Mentholatum was first sold in a one-ounce jar. Generic glass jars called "ointment pots" were obtained from a wholesale supplier. The white colored "opal" or "milk glass" jars (created when tin or zinc is added to the molten glass) were capped by a plain tin lid and marked with a simple black-and-white paper label. Jars were shipped by the dozen in a pasteboard carton that folded open to become a shelf display and was still in use by 1903. Jars were not individually boxed until 1898, when the three-ounce jar was introduced. That same year, a small Bible tract titled "Seed to the Sower and Bread to the Eater" was given

Incentives Pay Off

When Not in Use, Keep

MEDICINE

TIME INDICATOR

In This Envelope so as not to Soil.

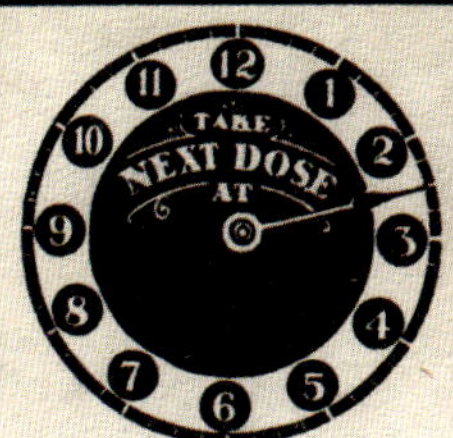

IF NOT AT YOUR DRUGGISTS

These "Indicators" may be had together with a Sample Box of Mentholatum by sending 6c in stamps to

YUCCA CO.

BUFFALO, N. Y.

WICHI

MENTHOLATUM

IS NEEDED IN EVERY FAMILY

IT RELIEVES SUFFERING

IT CURES

CROUP
CATARRH
CHILBLAINS

BUR
PILE
OLD

At Your Druggists, 25c and 50c.

&c. &c.

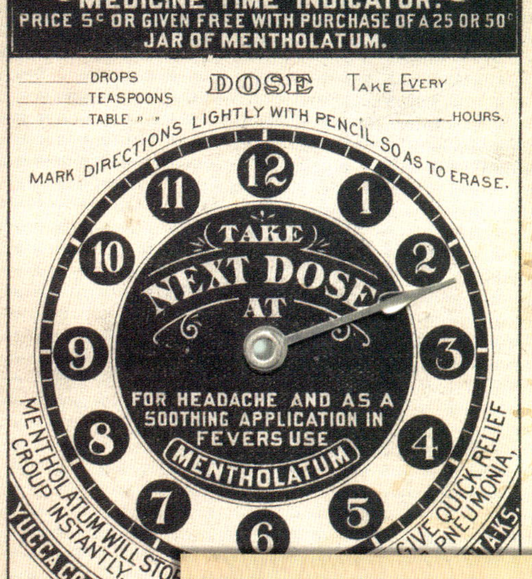

Medicine Time Indicator and Protective Envelope This was one of several cardboard favors supplied druggists to hand out to their customers.

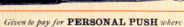

Private Mailing Card

AUTHORIZED BY ACT OF CONGRESS OF MAY 19 1898

PLACE A ONE CENT STAMP HERE

Agent for "Mentholatum,"

THIS

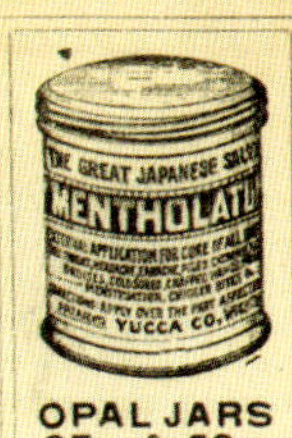

OPAL JARS 25c & 50c.

To Mentholatum Agent: Please bring me a (25c.) (50c.) jar of Mentholatum, and oblige:

(Write Plain.) *(Name)* ....

No .... *Street* ....

"Mentholatum gives the **best satisfaction for Sore Eyes, Headache and Catarrh, and is the best Pile remedy I ever sold.**
W. S. PELHAM,
Druggist,
Kirkville, Iowa.

"**Mentholatum** is the best thing I have ever tried for **Catarrh, Cuts, Burns, Etc.** I cannot be without it."
THOS. N. BARGER,
Pub. of Morning Call, Normal, Ill.

"For **Piles** and for **Catarrh** I think **Mentholatum** has no equal."
C. A. KNAPPENBURGER,
Druggist, La Harpe, Ill.

"My mother was afflicted with **Asthma** for several years **but two small jars of Mentholatum completely cured her.**
MRS. G. H. LOHMAN,
(Formerly Miss Olive Mathis,) Coronado, Cal.
(Kansas City.)

"Your **Mentholatum** has healed an **open sore** of 18 years standing in the palm of my right hand, and I take pleasure in recommending it."
WM. D. MCHENRY,
Riverside, Cal.

"My wife has for years been troubled with ulcerated **Varicose Veins:** your **Mentholatum** removed the pain, healed the ulcers and reduced the swelling. It has also cured my daughter of **Nasal Catarrh** and **Inflamed Eye Lids.** We keep a supply constantly on hand."
C. WIMPERIS,
445 E. Ninth St., Riverside, Cal.

"We find an application of **Mentholatum** relieves the children's **Earache** and stops **Croup** almost instantly."
MRS. JACKSON,
Matron Children's Home, Wichita.

"**Mentholatum does what is claimed. It should be in every home.**"
M. H. MERRIMAN,
Ex. Pres. Y. M. C. A., Los Angeles, Cal.

Return Postcard This was worth one introductory jar of Mentholatum if returned with name and address.

GOLD FOUNTAIN PEN OFFER

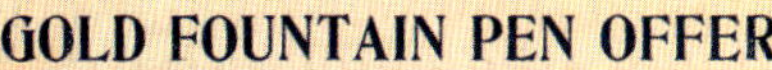

Given to pay for **PERSONAL PUSH** *where Mentholatum is not selling well.*

We Pay MEN Instead of BILL BOARDS

Yucca Co.,
Wichita, Kansas.

Gentlemen:—As soon as

Mr ....

of this town sends you this Report Blank showing names of 20 People to whom he has sold Mentholatum after this date, SEND HIM ONE OF YOUR BEST 14 K. GOLD FOUNTAIN PENS, EXCHANGEABLE and GUARANTEED BY MFR.

Date ....

.... Salesman for Yucca Co.

Town ....

I hereby certify that since I received above offer I have sold Mentholatum to the 20 people whose names and addresses are shown on opposite side of this blank. Send me best Gold fountain pen as promised.

Name ....

Address ....

WRITE PLAINLY

This offer will be redeemed by us promptly when this report is sent in and names given as indicated.

THE YUCCA CO.
BY A. A. HYDE, PRES.

WICHITA, KAN.

Parker Fountain Pen This was awarded for the names of twenty new customers.

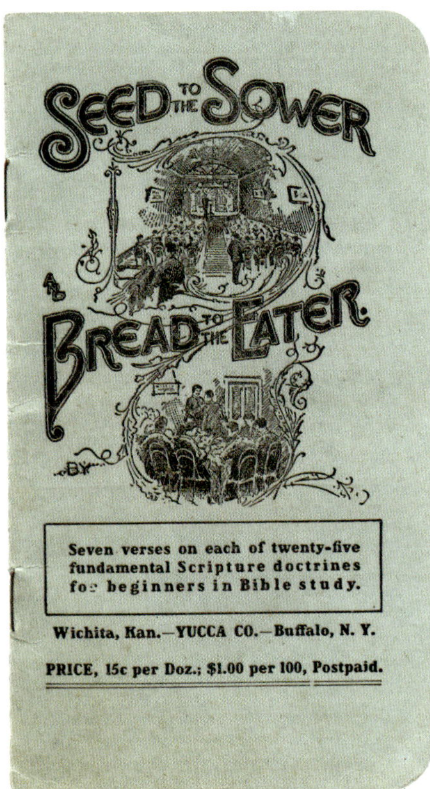

Spreading the Word

"Seed to the Sower" was handed out with each jar sold if the customer wanted one. It was called the "text book" in company promotional literature and inventory lists. It cost less than a penny to print, and additional copies were available for sale at "15¢ per Doz.; $1.00 per 100, Postpaid." There were two variations printed, one for Mentholatum and another for Menthocura (formerly Vest Pocket Specific).

out with the sale of each jar. This sixteen-page booklet contained endorsements inside the front cover by Charles Bradt, the pastor of Wichita's First Presbyterian Church, and by the church's missionary pastor in China, Hunter Corbett. Bradt's introduction reveals the company's unique policy of tithing. He wrote: "I know further that the Yucca Co. have given bond to donate one-tenth of the profits from sales of Mentholatum each year to the causes of missions," and concluded, "we see no reason why it should not bring quite a revenue to the Missionary Boards." This was certainly not the typical business profile of a nostrum manufacturer.

In early 1902, the company printed a list of testimonials by six northwestern jobbers and eleven retail druggists. C. F. Weller, president of the Richardson Drug Company in Omaha,

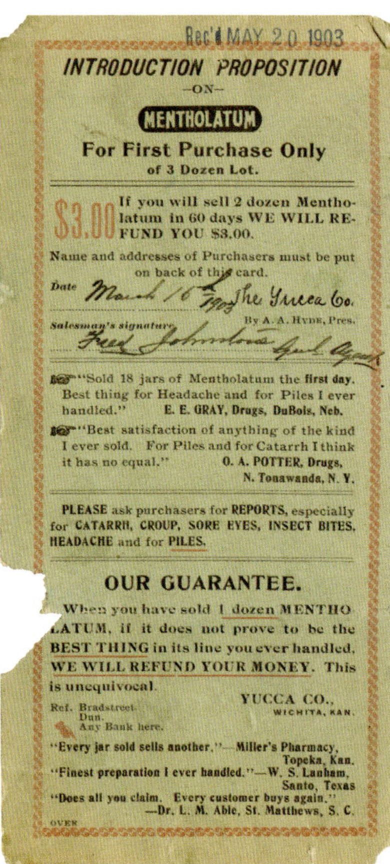

Rec'd MAY 20 1903

INTRODUCTION PROPOSITION
—ON—
MENTHOLATUM
For First Purchase Only
of 3 Dozen Lot.

$3.00 If you will sell 2 dozen Mentholatum in 60 days WE WILL REFUND YOU $3.00.

Name and addresses of Purchasers must be put on back of this card.

Date March 16 1903 The Yucca Co.
By A. A. Hyde, Pres.

Salesman's signature Fred Johnston Genl. Agent

"Sold 18 jars of Mentholatum the first day. Best thing for Headache and for Piles I ever handled." E. E. GRAY, Drugs, DuBois, Neb.

"Best satisfaction of anything of the kind I ever sold. For Piles and for Catarrh I think it has no equal." O. A. POTTER, Drugs, N. Tonawanda, N. Y.

PLEASE ask purchasers for REPORTS, especially for CATARRH, CROUP, SORE EYES, INSECT BITES, HEADACHE and for PILES.

OUR GUARANTEE.

When you have sold 1 dozen MENTHOLATUM, if it does not prove to be the BEST THING in its line you ever handled, WE WILL REFUND YOUR MONEY. This is unequivocal.

YUCCA CO.,
WICHITA, KAN.

Ref. Bradstreet.
Dun.
Any Bank here.

"Every jar sold sells another."—Miller's Pharmacy, Topeka, Kan.
"Finest preparation I ever handled."—W. S. Lanham, Santo, Texas
"Does all you claim. Every customer buys again."
—Dr. L. M. Able, St. Matthews, S. C.

OVER

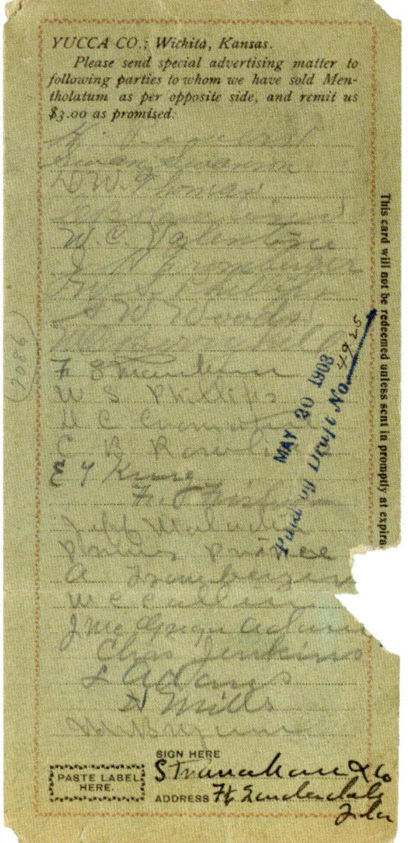

YUCCA CO.; Wichita, Kansas.
Please send special advertising matter to following parties to whom we have sold Mentholatum as per opposite side, and remit us $3.00 as promised.

This card will not be redeemed unless sent in promptly at expira

MAY 20 1903

PASTE LABEL HERE.

SIGN HERE

ADDRESS

Write Plain

This is an actual refund slip that was given to a Fort Lauderdale, Florida, druggist on March 16, 1903, by Mentholatum's sales agent there. The druggist collected the signatures of two dozen customers and returned it to the company on May 20, 1903. Draft No. 4925 was cut for $3 and sent to the druggist as promised. Deciphering the handwriting on these slips became the bane of front-office workers for many years to come.

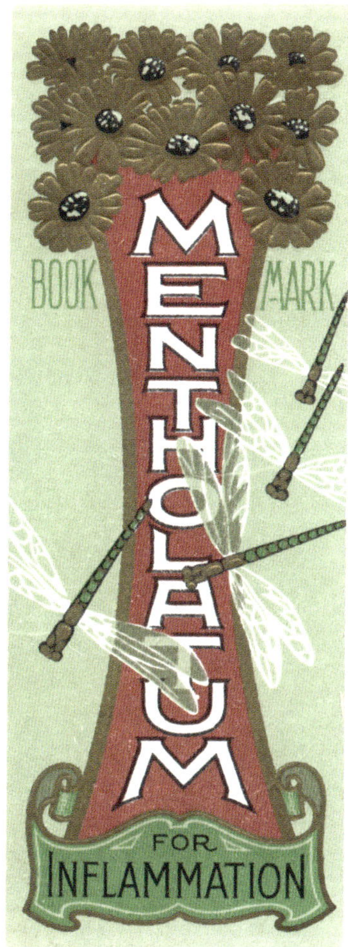

Mentholatum Nouveau

This six-color chromolithographic bookmark was printed by Stecher Lithographic Co., Rochester, New York, sometime around 1910.

Nebraska, wrote, "We have handled Mentholatum for several years and consider it one of the most meritorious articles on the market. The Yucca Co. are people who do as they agree every time." The Des Moines Drug Company, Wholesale Druggists and Stationers, said, "We are glad to add our endorsement to your methods of doing business." Harle-Haas Drug Company in Council Bluffs, Iowa, claimed, "Mentholatum talks for itself if you give it a chance." And E. E. Bruce & Co. in Omaha, Nebraska, announced, "We have never dealt with a manufacturer who was more attentive to his agreements." The retail druggist Kirkwood Pharmacy at 406 Walnut Street in Des Moines, Iowa, exclaimed, "In regard to Mentholatum, it is the best seller we have. Always gives satisfaction and makes friends wherever introduced. We consider it the greatest remedy on the market today for all the ailments it claims to cure."[5]

"He Is a Liar"

If imitation is the highest form of flattery, then A. A. Hyde was the wrong man to flatter. A number of similar menthol- and camphor-based salves came onto the market soon after Mentholatum demonstrated profit potential. After the turn of the century, franchise brands like Rexall, Watkins, and Rawleigh's jumped onto the bandwagon. Small regional proprietors did their best to eat away at Mentholatum's customer base. One in particular got under Hyde's skin. In a warning the Yucca Company sent to the druggists, Hyde wrote under the heading, "He Is a Liar":

> *There is a slick salesman pushing a so-called "improvement on Mentholatum" imitating not only the* Style of our package *but* also our manner of introduction.
>
> *The only originality about him seems to be his faculty of lying about the Yucca Co. and Mentholatum. If he calls on you* please *get him to* put his stories down on paper and sign them. *We want to nail him. Double postage returned.*
>
> *From the* lying imitator *"Good Lord deliver us."*
> *YUCCA CO., Wichita, Kansas*[6]

By 1917, the company claimed that more than thirty imitators existed.[7]

MENTHOLEUM
MENTHOLINE, The Japanese Headache Cure
VICTOR MENTHOLENE
JAPANESE MENTHODINE
MENTHO VAPO
MENTHENE
MENTHOLYPTUS

Free sample tins became a liability in some areas of the country where Mentholatum had become well known. Druggists complained that people returned to their stores to ask for another sample rather than buying a new jar. In those cases, samples were no longer included in stock shipments. By 1903, salesmen were being asked to evaluate whether or not druggists they called upon would "use judiciously a special package of samples and advertising matter." They were admonished on their daily sales reports to be certain that samples were really wanted "as it means quite an expense for goods and express charges, which we have to pay."[8]

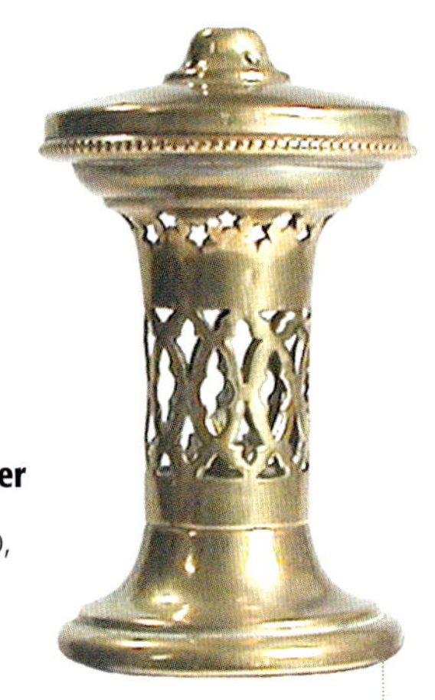

Travel-Size Vaporizer
On the cars to Buffalo, this classy little six-inch-tall brass vaporizer fit snugly on the shelf beside a Pullman bunk. The small oil lamp in the base projected a soft, glowing pattern upon the drawn and darkened curtains. The gently tapered lid ensured that jolts upon the track would not cause splashes of sizzling inhalant, while at the same time tiny holes on top vented the sweet and comforting menthol vapors.

Buffalo, New York

As Mentholatum's commercial field extended further across the United States, the little Yucca Company factory began to strain under the demand for more product. Hyde began searching for an additional location from which to manufacture and distribute product to Eastern markets. His New York sales agent, George Buckner, suggested he look at Buffalo, so in 1901, the same year Buffalo hosted the Pan-American Exposition, Hyde took the long train ride east. An important consideration in Buffalo's favor was proximity to Canada, which he felt was his next "commercial field." Hyde was familiar with Buffalo, which he had passed

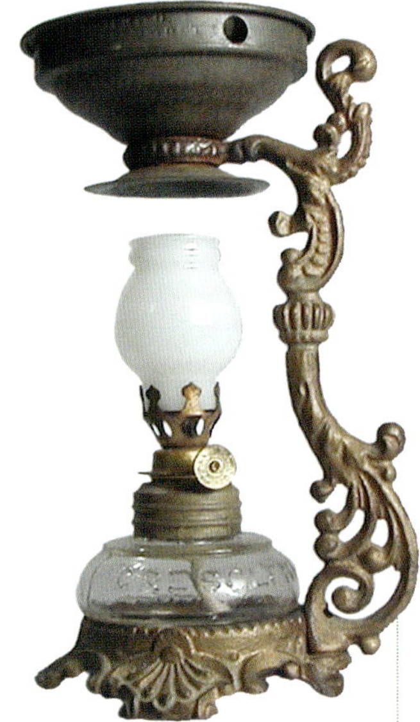

Bedside Vaporizer
This gaudy, six-inch-tall, cast-iron, oil lamp vaporizer was mass-produced by the Vapo-Cresolene Company. Although it was created to vaporize poisonous cresol tar as a sick-room disinfectant, there was no reason why it couldn't also be used to vaporize safe menthol, eucalyptus, and camphor inhalants.

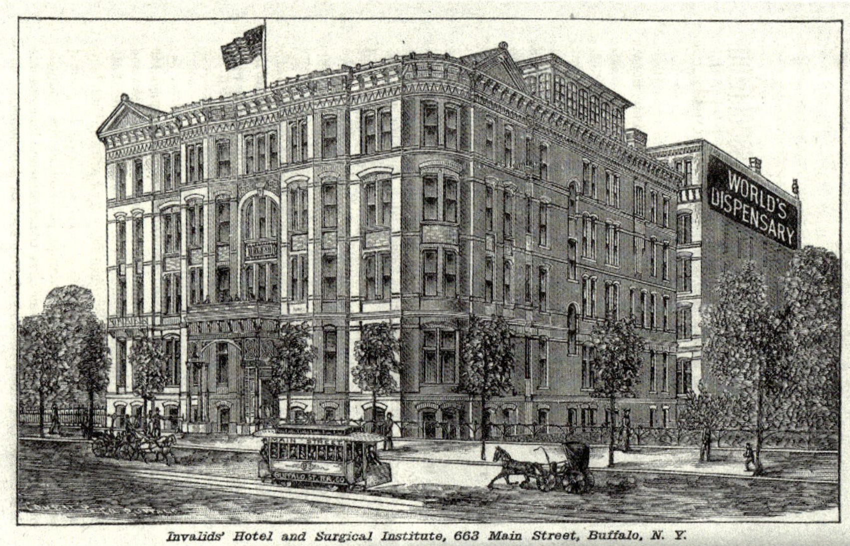

"A Spa for the Nervous & Careworn"
Dr. Pierce first built the lavish Palace Hotel that was destroyed by fire in 1881. He replaced it with the smaller Invalids' Hotel, which stood until 1941. Its full name was the "Invalids' Hotel and Surgical Institute," and it was located at 663 Main Street in Buffalo.

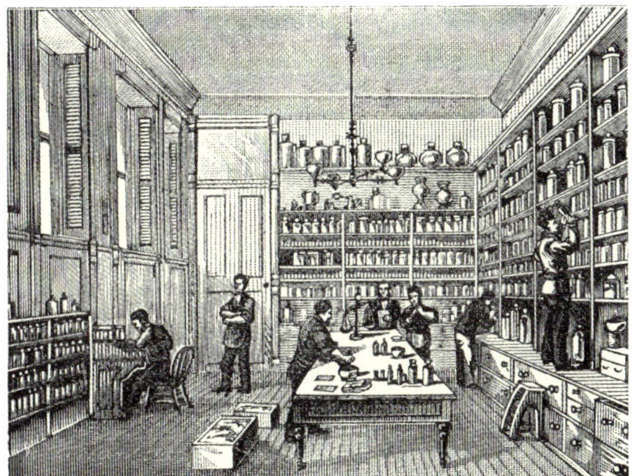

Prescription Department—Invalids' Hotel and Surgical Institute.

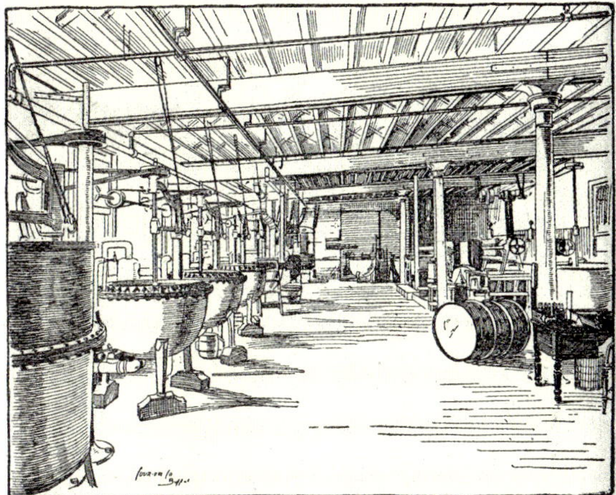

Section of Chemical Laboratory.—World's Dispensary.

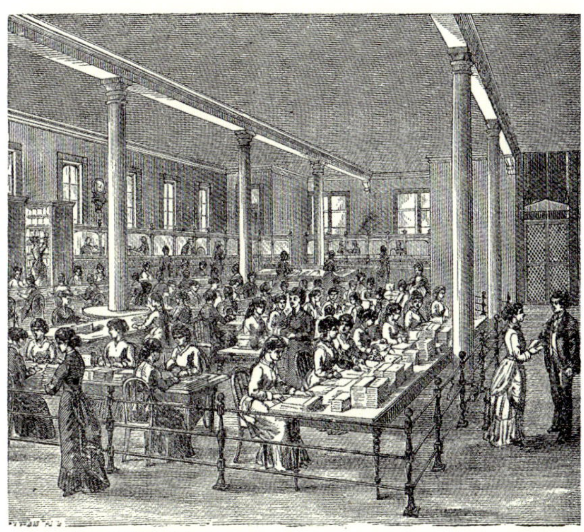

Postal Advertising Department, Wrapping and Mailing-room.

World's Dispensary Medical Association

Three important aspects of Dr. Pierce's business operation are shown above.

through as a young man during various train trips between Leavenworth (and later Wichita) and his hometown of Lee, Massachusetts. On one trip in July 1871, he and his friends stopped over at Buffalo and "took a hack to see the City." He recalled in his diary: "In the evening we attended the fire works which had been postponed there from the 4th on account of bad weather. We had a fine position on top of a hotel and enjoyed them very much as they were well gotten up and looked beautifully." The next day, the party packed a lunch and set out to explore Niagara Falls.[9]

Buffalo was a key east/west transshipping center between the Great Lakes and the overland route through the Mohawk Valley to the Hudson River and port of New York. During the first of America's three westerings, the Mohawk Trail funneled a steady flow of pioneers through Buffalo on their way to Ohio and Indiana. The Erie Canal opening in 1825 improved transport of people and goods until replaced by railroads during the 1850s. Buffalo also became a major port of entry between Canada and the United States. Heavy industries, such as iron and steel works, brick plants, and glass factories located there to take advantage of shipping and rail lines. However, it was Buffalo's health industry that probably did more to put the city on the map and made it a likely setting for Mentholatum's new factory.[10]

After the Civil War, Niagara Falls became an ever more popular tourist attraction as passenger train service improved. Travelers transferred cars at the Buffalo Station and often took overnight lodging in local hotels before visiting the Falls. Niagara Falls's reputation for healing energy made it a mecca for the ill and troubled, who in turn attracted a number of charlatans and healers. The most notable of the late nineteenth-century quacks was Dr. Ray Vaughn Pierce. The inventor of "Dr. Pierce's Alterative Extract or Golden Medical Discovery GMD," Dr. Pierce was a tireless promoter of Buffalo, his "World's Dispensary Medical Association," and his "Invalids' Hotel and Surgical Institute." Pierce's sales literature for the Invalids' Hotel stressed the "Extreme Healthfulness of Buffalo," due in part to the "zephyrs" that blew in from Lake Erie.[11]

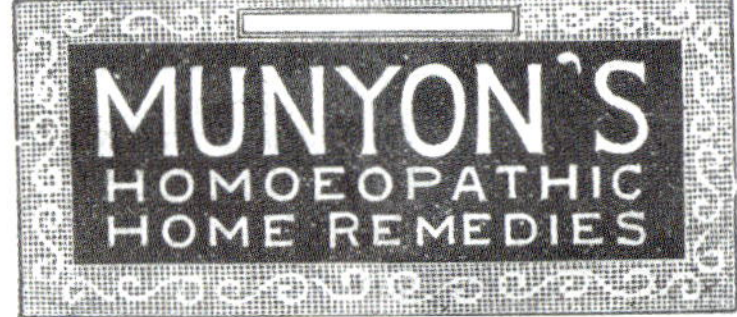

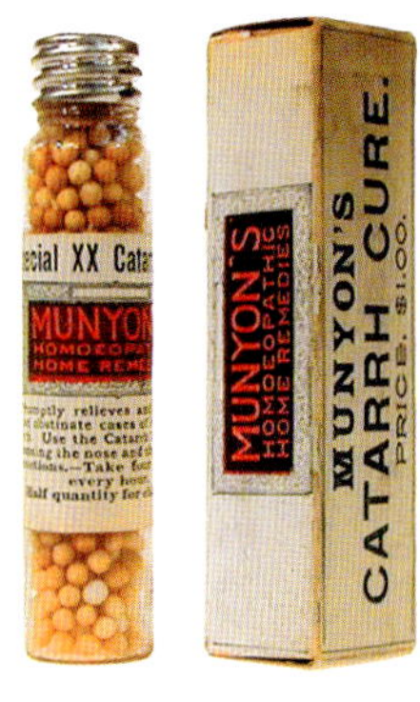

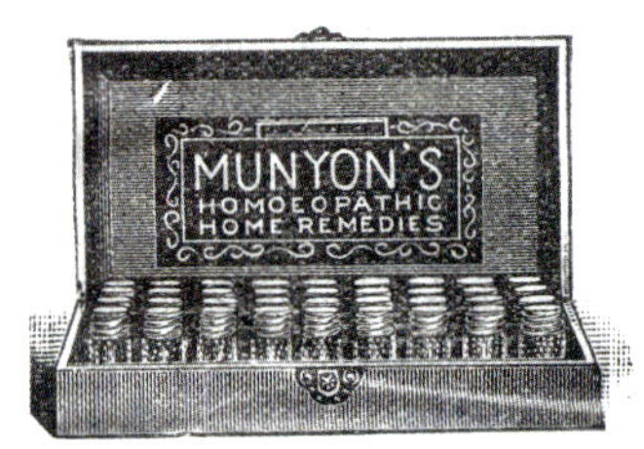

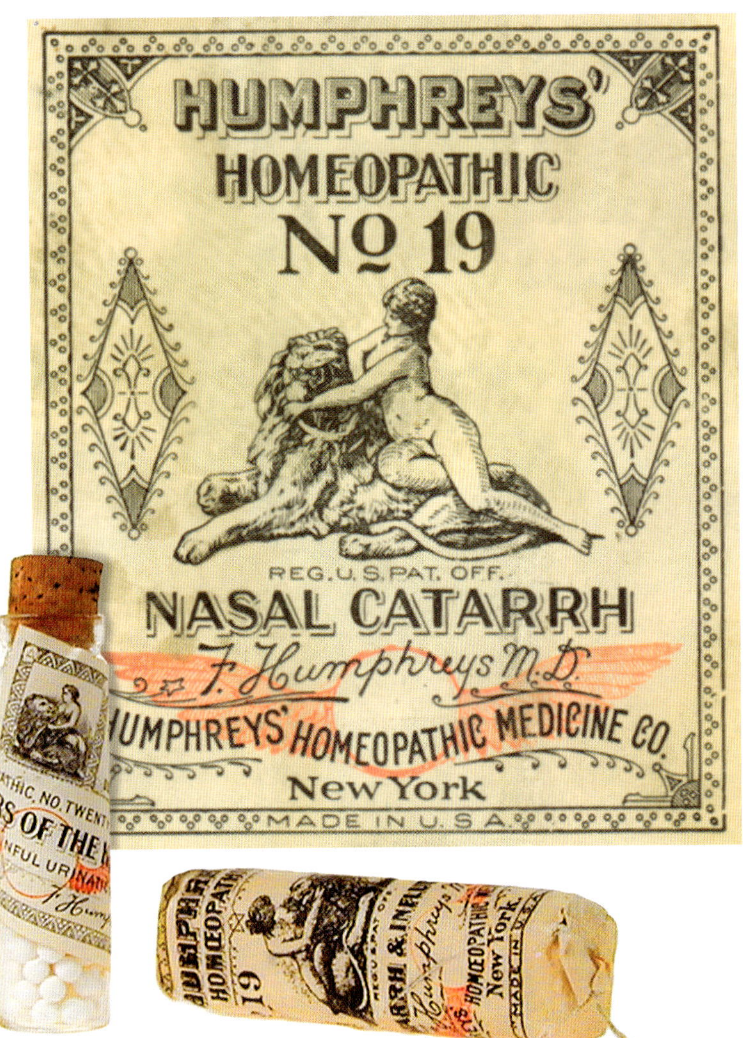

Homeopathic Catarrh Cures

Here are two of the largest brands in the country, Munyon's from Philadelphia (top), and Humphreys' from New York. Humphreys' erotic logo of the maiden and lion (three variations are shown) probably had more healing influence than the sugar and starch pellets found inside each corked glass vial.

A lively competition existed in Buffalo among a variety of health practitioners. In addition to midwives and assorted fringe sects, one of the larger groups was the homeopathic physicians, followers of the German physician Samuel Hahnemann. Homeopaths were recognized and licensed by New York state to practice medicine in 1857. Their association opened a homeopathic hospital in 1872; a homeopathic college was teaching students by 1880. "Regular" doctors were rivals who themselves were divided over the causes of disease and how to treat them. They founded a medical school in 1846, which later became the University of Buffalo. One of the school's founders, Austin Flint, helped shape the "conservative" school of medical practice, which opposed the mainstream "heroic" method of bloodletting and purging, which had been practiced since the days of Benjamin Rush. Dr. Flint's approach to the treatment of tuberculosis, for instance, was to take "plenty of fresh air, and whiskey in quantity." Finally, there was Ray Pierce, who believed in the *business* of medicine.[12]

Dr. Pierce was the champion of free enterprise and mail-order nostrums. Between 1867 and 1880 his ventures earned him almost half a million dollars a year. His factory shipped out nearly a million bottles of remedies annually. And his printing press published *The People's Common Sense Medical Adviser*,

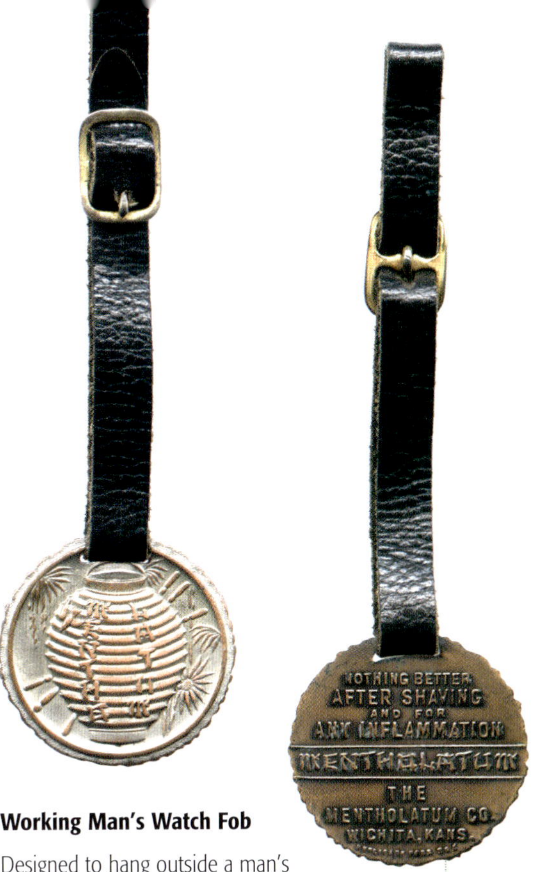

Working Man's Watch Fob

Designed to hang outside a man's blue jean watch pocket. This was a promotional gift sometime soon after 1906.

which went through one hundred editions and remained in print for sixty years (1875–1935). At the time, Pierce was one of Buffalo's two most famous citizens (William G. Fargo of Wells Fargo fame being the other) and was admired by sickly enervated people throughout the country who read his book and swallowed his cures. Buffalo elected Pierce to the New York State Senate and in 1878 to the U.S. Congress, where he served for only two years before resigning his seat due to ill health.[13]

A. A. Hyde decided that Buffalo was the best site for his operations. In 1903 his second son, Edward K. Hyde (1878–1974), relocated there with "authority" to set up business. Edward started out in November by renting a large storeroom at 137 Prospect Avenue, near the post office, and by 1906 he had purchased an old three-story building at 146 Seneca Street. (The 1912 *Cosmopolitan* and 1913 *Modern Priscilla* ads gave a different address—"136 Seneca Street.") As a teenager, Edward had spent several years working for the Potts Drug Company, where he gained valuable training and business experience.[14]

The Yucca Company filed for additional trademark protection for its label copy on April 17, 1905, and received registration number 47783 on November 21, 1905. The copy read:

> *A Salve for External Application in the Treatment of Inflammations and Eruptions of the Skin and Mucous Membrane and in the Treatment of Croup, Asthma, Sore Throat, Pneumonia, Catarrh, and Like Afflictions Involving or Resulting from Congestion.*[15]

This is curious because the label that was in use between 1903 and 1906 read, "An External Application for Cure of All Inflammations." The label used in 1906 read, "An External Application for Relief of Inflammation," in compliance with the 1906 Pure Food and Drugs Act. And the label that followed 1915 read, "An External Application to Relieve or Soothe. . . ." The actual wording of the trademark copy appears to have never been used.[16]

Key Ring

Three railroad switch keys were found on this promotional key ring. The bottom key belonged to the Union Pacific, and the top two were from the Northern Pacific Railroad.

The Great Flood of 1904

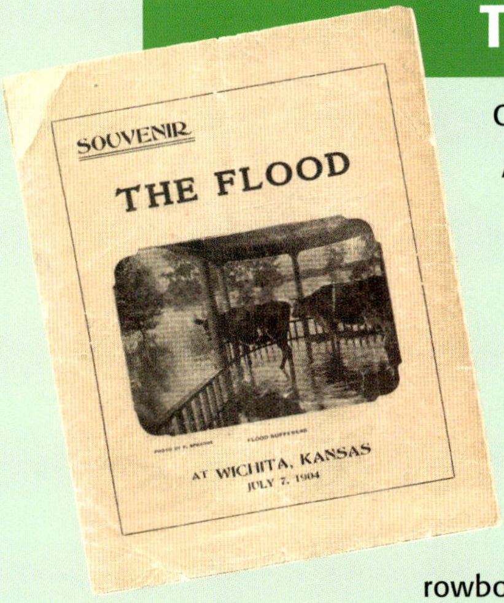

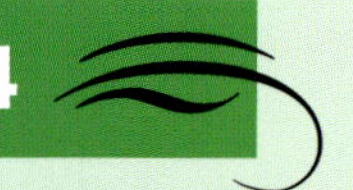

On July 6, 1904, heavy rains caused the Arkansas River to crest at the Douglas Avenue bridge seven feet above the high-water mark. By the 7th, temporary dikes had broken and the city was flooded, causing an estimated $200,000 in damage. The Wichita Engraving Co. quickly got out a souvenir booklet with the photographs of F. Sprague recording the event. Among the pictures were two cows stranded high and dry on a residential porch, some boys swimming in a downtown intersection, and the Yucca Company building with water at its doorstep. In this faded old lithograph, the employees can be seen still standing on the flooded porch where they are watching a rowboat go up the middle of Douglas Avenue. The little factory where Mentholatum was manufactured was already a Wichita landmark.

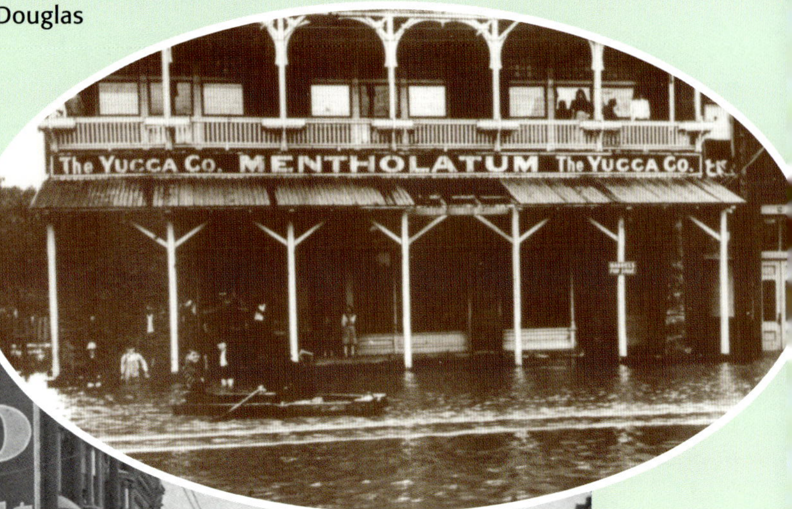

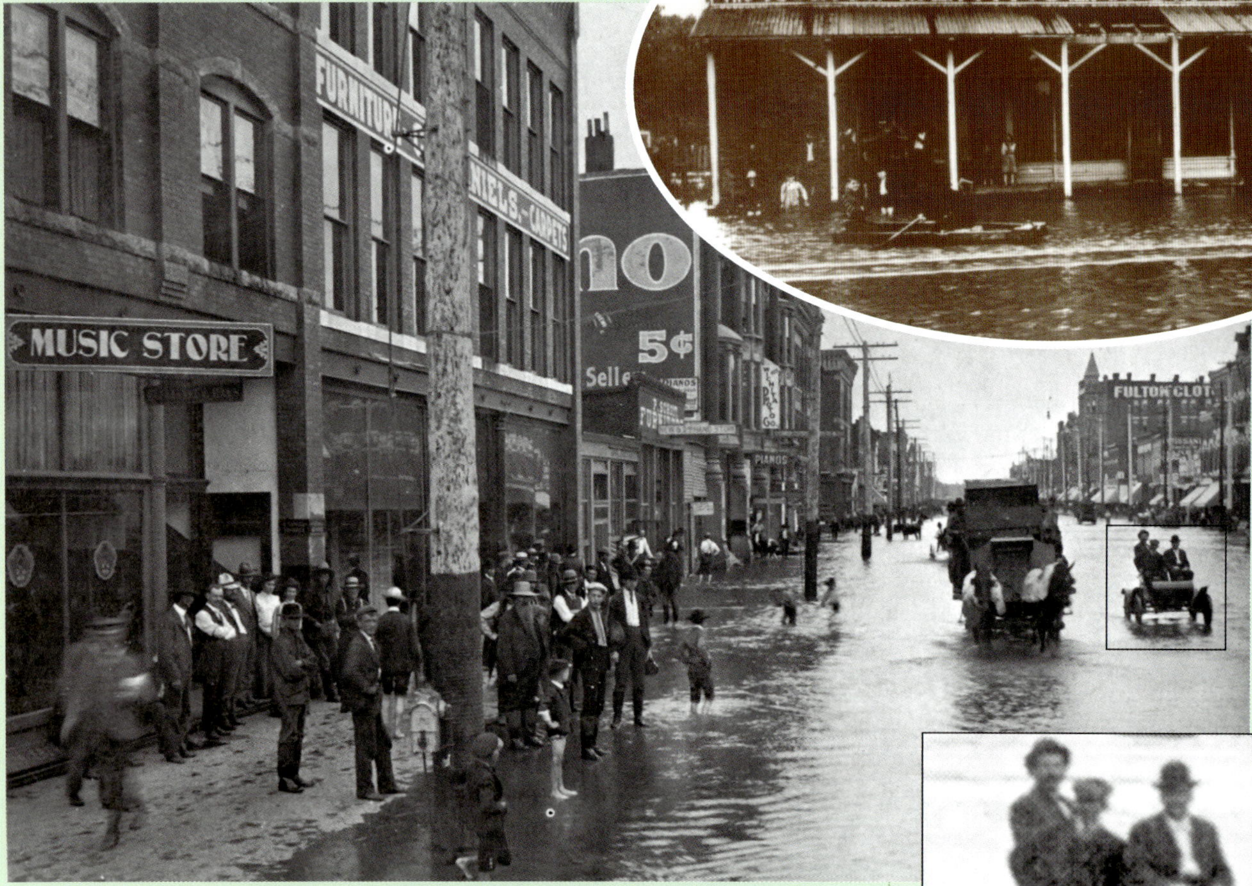

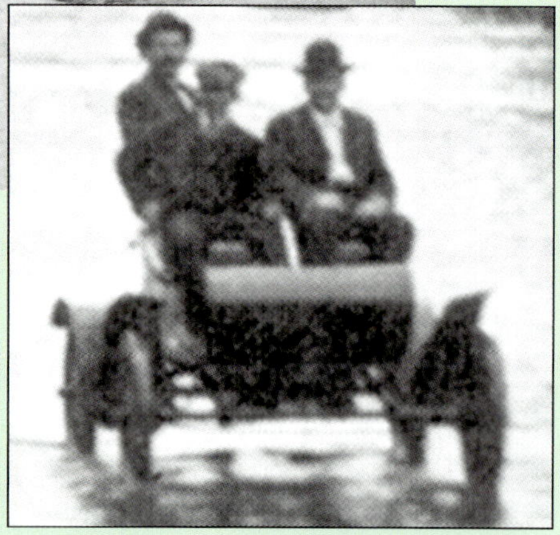

Touring the 1904 Wichita Flood

While work had come to a standstill at the factory (inset above), A. A. Hyde decided to tour the flood damage. His driver and mechanic, Billy Mitchell, brought thc Oldsmobile Runabout around and they set off down Douglas Avenue where a photographer caught this image. In the enlarged view, Billy is the dapper young black man in the sports cap with his hand on the tiller, the fifty-six-year-old Hyde is characteristically planted with his hands in his lap, and the man in the back has not been identified.

By 1906 the Yucca Company was distributing Mentholatum throughout the United States and Canada. Few of the soap company's original products were still in production, and Vest Pocket Specific had been renamed "Menthocura." In November, four months after the Pure Food and Drugs Act was passed, the Yucca Company was dissolved and the Mentholatum Company was incorporated as a family-owned operation. Edward and Alex were the only two Hyde boys working for the company at the time, and they each received a 10 percent share of the stock. By 1909, Charles had joined them to complete the management structure: A. A. Hyde was president; Edward Hyde, vice president and manager of the Buffalo plant; Charles Hyde, secretary; and Alex Hyde, treasurer.

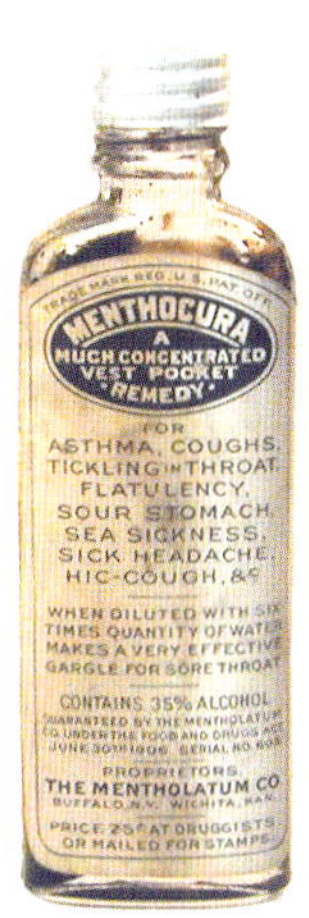

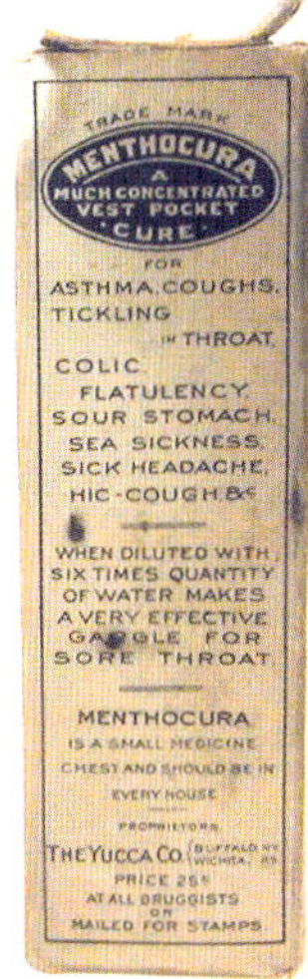

Rare Menthocura Bottle and Box

This is a 1906 "remedy" bottle with its older "cure" box.

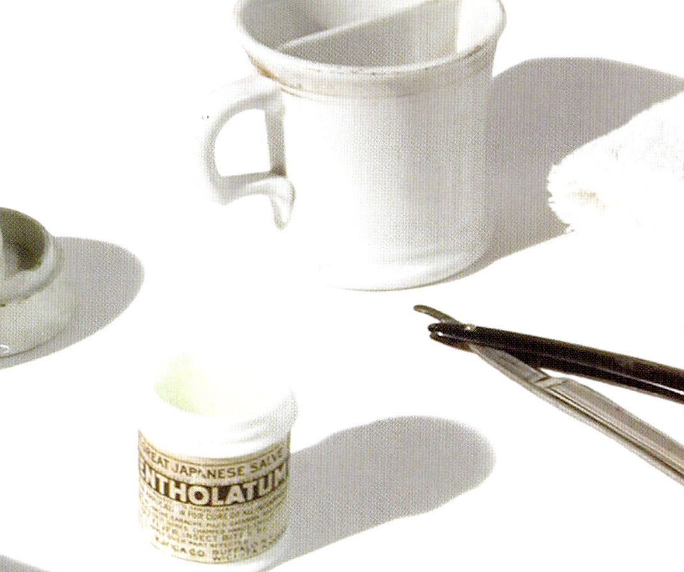

After Shaving

The "healing and soothing" use of Mentholatum for sore and tender skin revealed a new application as an aftershave, and it was quickly marketed to barbers. Labels were printed "For Piles" at one end and "Barbers" at the other.

Directions For Use of

MENTHOLATUM

AFTER SHAVING

TAKE a small portion the size of a pea and rub between the hands until dissolved. Then massage the face lightly with the hands—apply a hot towel to remove the surplus oil, and the skin will feel delightfully cool and soft.

Mentholatum is the most healing and soothing application known for all skin and scalp diseases.

READ WHAT BARBER SAYS

OPAL JARS 25c

ALL DRUG STORES

50c Size Three Times as Large

RED CROSS BARBER SHOP

Dixon, Illinois, July 12, 1900.

YUCCA CO., WICHITA, KS. "I have been in the barber business for over twenty years and have used all kinds of skin remedies, but for sore and tender skin, ingrowing hair, pimples and sunburn, Mentholatum beats them all, and it will cure in from one to five applications. No barber shop is complete without it." Yours respectfully,

HARRY O. WHEELER, 106 First St.

AFTER SHAVING MENTHOLATUM COOLING REFRESHING

MENTHOLATUM RELIEVES HEADACHE AND CATARRH ALL DRUGGISTS

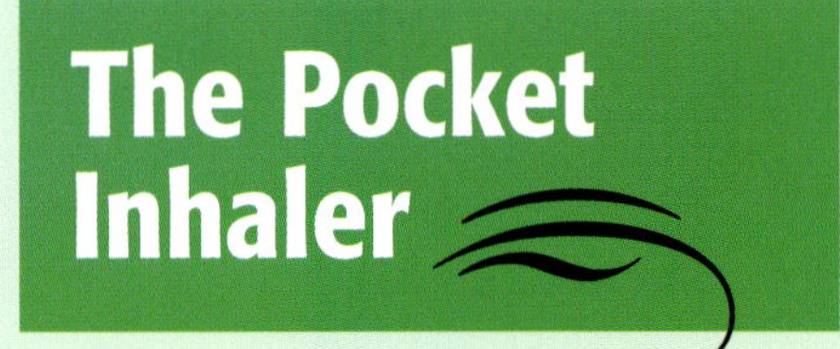

The Pocket Inhaler

In the Victorian age, steam inhalers and nasal douches were standard mechanisms for delivering medicine to the sinuses. These treatments required the support of a bathroom or kitchen and were typically carried out in the privacy of the home. So, how did sufferers find relief when they were away from home?

1875

PORTABLE. In 1875, an enterprising doctor named N. B. Wolfe self-published a seventy-two-page paperback book he titled *Inhalation, How to Cure Consumption, Asthma, and Catarrh*. In his book Wolfe used historical references to convince the reader of the merits of inhalation as therapy. He wrote that long ago the Greek physician, Hippocrates, recommended injecting into the lungs of a person who suffered with pneumonia "fumigations of hyssop, cilicia, sulphur, and asphalt, to bring away phlegm." Wolfe added that the Roman scholar, Pliny, praised the "resinous woods for their healing odors, [which were] more beneficial to the consumptive than a voyage to Egypt, or a course of milk in the mountains." Dr. Wolfe searched through the English literature on catarrh and hay asthma all the way back to Sir John Floyer's 1698 *Treatise of the Asthma* and concluded that not one of the experts had discovered a reliable pathology or treatment that would lead to a cure.

So, in 1848 Dr. Wolfe set out to do what no one else in recorded history had been able to do. He spent the next twenty-five years treating diseases of the nose, throat, and lungs with his own inhaled patent remedies. At last he invented **Wolfe's Inhaler** and with it "succeeded in curing Consumption, Asthma, and Bronchitis, after all hope of human relief [had] been abandoned."

Of his invention, Wolfe wrote, "The instrument is simple, portable, and inexpensive. It can not easily get out of order or broken; and may be carried about the person, and used at any time or place, at home or abroad, sitting or standing, in the house or the open field, without discomfort or inconvenience to the most feeble."

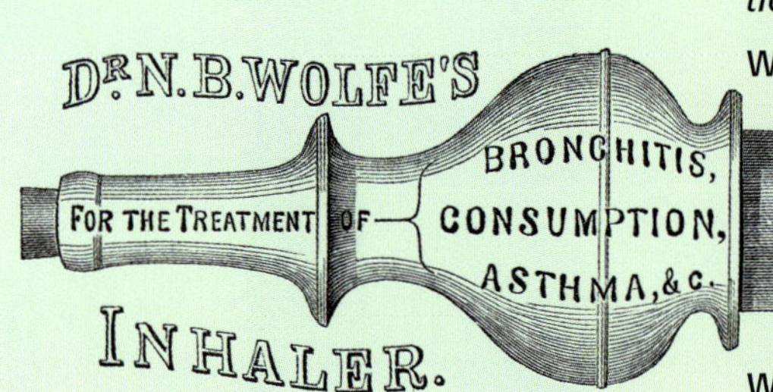

Dr. Wolfe Was Cool on Hot Vapors

N. B. Wolfe agreed with other early nineteenth-century pioneers in the field of inhalation treatment that "hot vapors enfeebled the pulmonary structure, and broke down its organic power." It may not have been the temperature as much as the chemical additives that were causing the "organic" breakdown. It's a wonder how much damage these self-styled visionaries of scientific research were causing! To offer a consumption cure for sale when none existed was criminal.

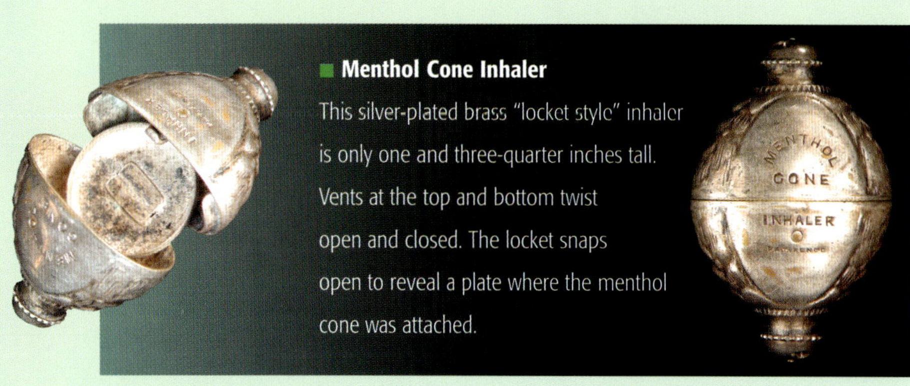

Menthol Cone Inhaler

This silver-plated brass "locket style" inhaler is only one and three-quarter inches tall. Vents at the top and bottom twist open and closed. The locket snaps open to reveal a plate where the menthol cone was attached.

1885 **MENTHOLATED.** In the 1885 Lord, Owen & Co. catalog of druggists' supplies, another delivery device was listed that had the advantage of being portable and allowing for easy and discrete use. The illustration of **Cutler's Pocket Inhaler** in this catalog showed a glass tube with stoppers tied on string leashes that were used to plug each end to keep the medicine (carbolate of iodine) fresh. When the medicine in a glass inhaler of this design was used up, the entire device was thrown away and replaced with a new one. The glass tube or "pipe" became the standard shape for menthol pocket inhalers that were marketed under many different name brands well into the next century.

■ **The Electric Inhaler** Abbotts Menthol Plaster Co., Worchester, Massachusetts

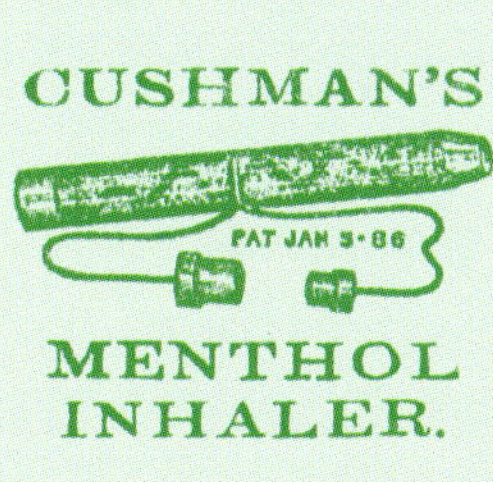

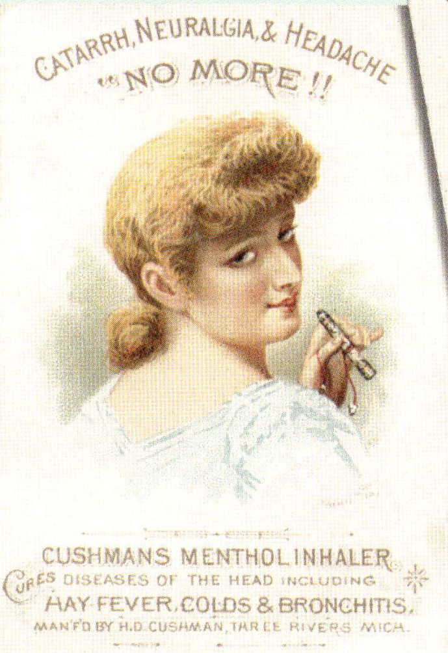

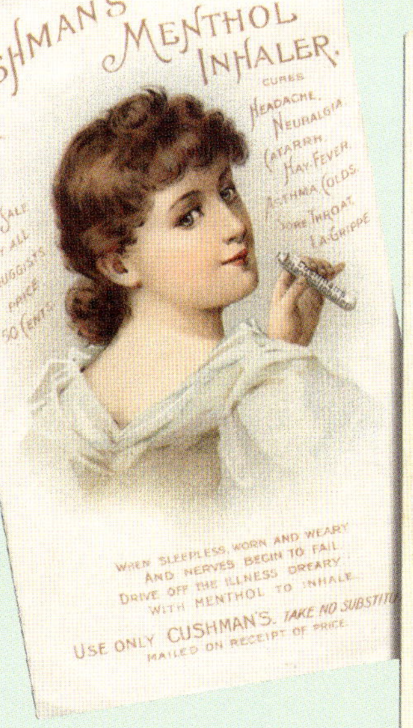

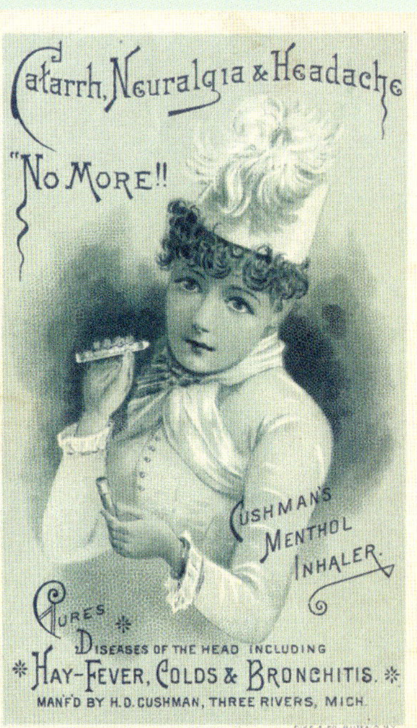

■ **Cushman's Menthol Inhaler (patented 1886)** The first inhaler (above) started out with stoppers at each end, but Cushman soon improved on this method with an airtight plated brass canister (below) to maintain freshness when the glass inhaler was not in use.

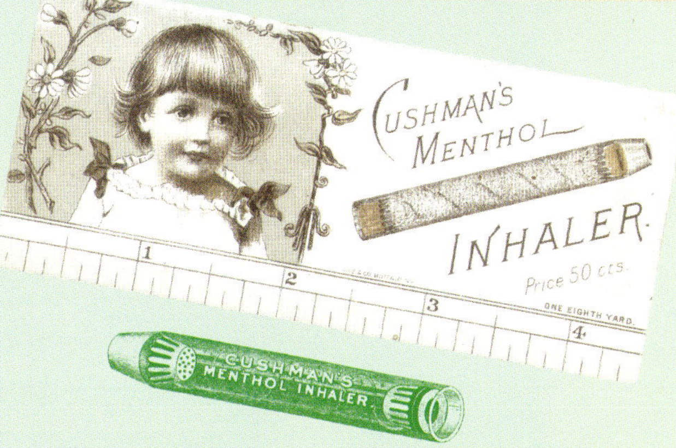

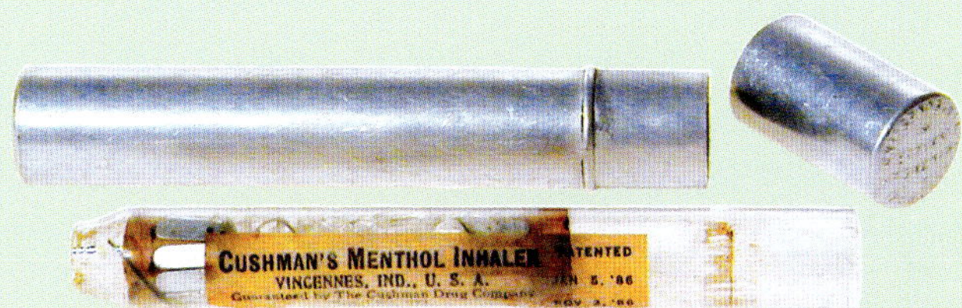

1900

REFILLABLE. While these early portable puffers were mostly disposable commodities, the next generation were made more durable. Predicated on the need to be refilled when the menthol ran out, inhaler designs became more inventive, and some sturdier materials were used. Glass was often replaced with vulcanite (hardened rubber) and later with Bakelite (a phenolic resin patented by Dr. Leo Baekeland in 1910). These durable inhalers typically came boxed with a bottle of refill solution, instructions, and any necessary tools and replacement gauze that was needed.

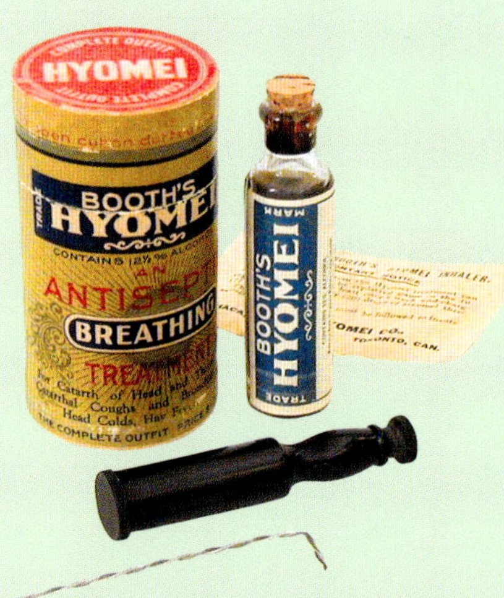

■ **Booth's Hyomei Dry-Air Cure (c. mid-1890s)** One of the first and most successful examples of the self-loading systems, the Hyomei "Pocket Inhaler Outfit" functioned like the glass tube inhaler but was made of vulcanite, followed later by Bakelite. Instead of corks to seal each end, it had threaded end caps. A bottle of eucalyptus-based "antiseptic" provided the drops that rehydrated the cotton gauze inside the curvilinear plastic tube.

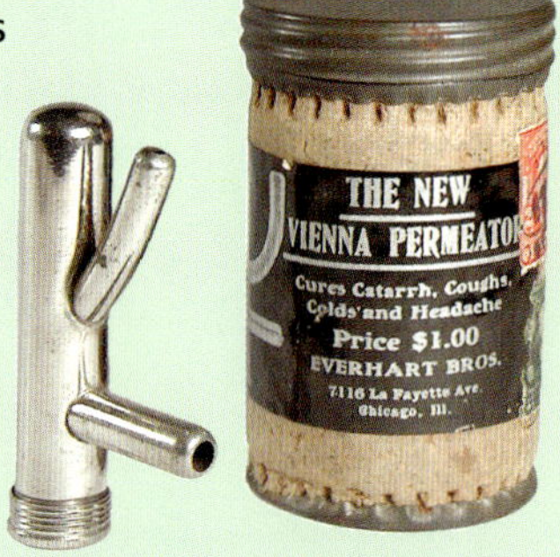

■ **Vienna Permeator (c. 1902)** Absorbent material in the main cylinder chamber was saturated with solution. The curved arm was placed up one nostril and the straight arm into the mouth to blow vapors into the sinus cavities.

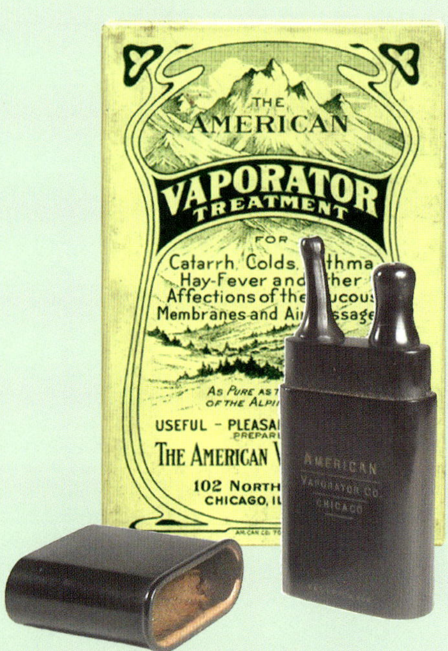

■ **The American Vaporator Treatment (c. 1915 and earlier)** The Vaporator was a Bakelite flask with a lid covering two nozzles, one for the nostrils and the other for the mouth to blow on. Both nozzles unscrewed to refill the reservoir below.

■ **Maxim's Inhaler (patented 1909)** The inventor, Sir Hiram Maxim (1840–1916), was also the inventor of the machine gun. Maxim suffered from catarrh and was not happy with treatments then on the market. He studied the problem and decided that pine oil and menthol were the two best ingredients. He then designed two elongated glass pipes that delivered "the vapours at exactly the right spot" in the back of the throat. The "Pipe of Peace" delivered the pine "essence," and the Maxim Inhaler delivered menthol's "soothing influence." "The little pocket appliance which I call the 'Maxim Inhaler' never leaves my person day or night. At the first sign of trouble, it is brought into play." The pinched section of each pipe was for the teeth to rest. The wadding in the bulb was used to hold and reload the menthol crystals.

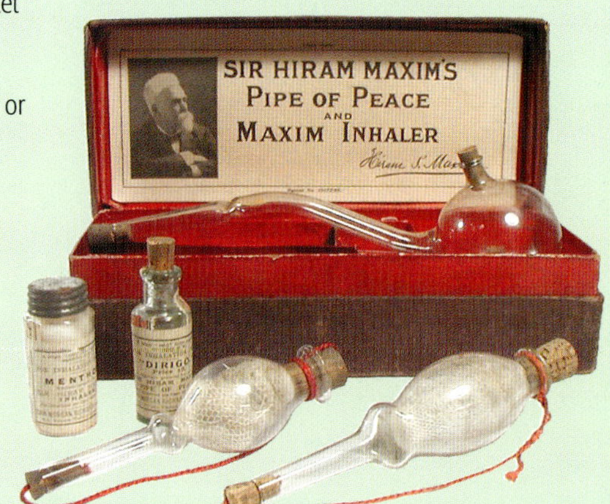

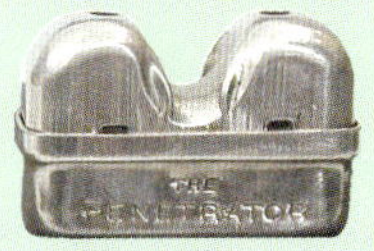

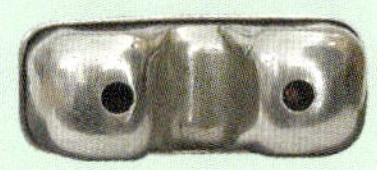

The Penetrator (patented August 27, 1918) This "Menthol Inhaler-Pencil" said, "For use as pencil remove cover." Instead of crystals or solution, this tiny sniffer contained a menthol stick that was mentholated paraffin or wax. This example must be missing a cover.

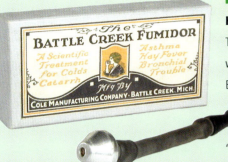

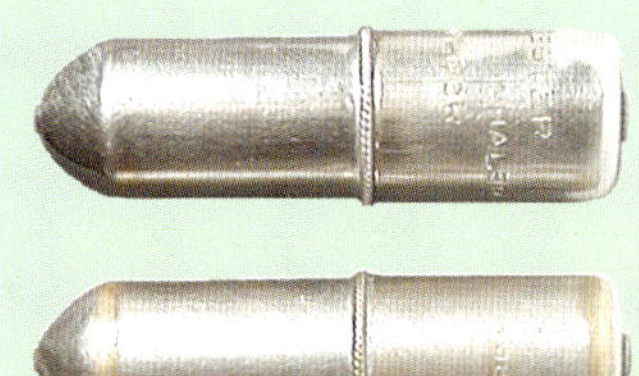

Winchester Menthol Inhaler (top); **Sharp & Dohme Menthol Cone Inhaler** "PAT APL FOR" (dates unknown). This smart little plated brass device was probably too expensive to manufacture on a mass scale. The bullet shape slid up into the nostril. With a simple twist of the base, a plunger dropped and the air passage through the center of the bullet opened, allowing the menthol vapors inside to be inhaled. Another twist and the plunger closed airtight.

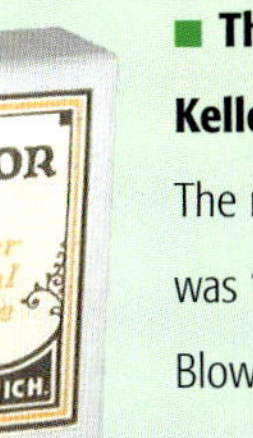

The Battle Creek Fumidor (from Dr. Kellogg's famous sanatorium, c. 1920s) The nozzle chamber, containing sterilized gauze, was "Charged" with five drops of "solution." Blowing on the Bakelite mouthpiece through the flexible rubber tube into the aluminum nozzle placed against alternating nostrils forced "the vapor back into the otherwise inaccessible nasal passages."

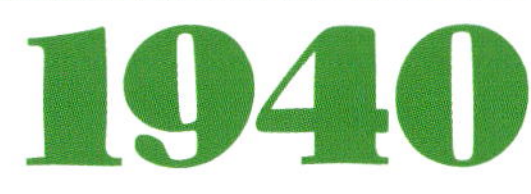

DISPOSABLE. As manufacturing technology improved toward midcentury, allowing complicated shapes to be mass-produced in strong, yet lightweight materials, pocket inhalers became disposable again. The torpedo-shaped aluminum inhalers developed by Penetro and Vicks were, and still are, by far the best menthol pocket inhalers ever produced. Eventually the aluminum parts were replaced with plastic parts, as was the fate of almost everything else during the 1950s and '60s. Remarkably, with new medications making the need for pocket puffers obsolete, this design is still being marketed sixty-plus years later!

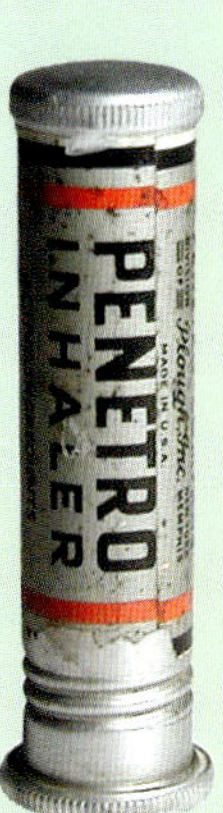

Penetro Inhaler (c. 1939) The first modern menthol inhaler, this was first listed in the company's 1939 Trademark Registration application. After removing the aluminum cap, the torpedo-shaped aluminum tube was inserted into one nostril at a time, while holding the other nostril closed. Upon inhaling, air entered the tube through intake holes located next to the twist grip and collected vapors from a menthol stick inside the tube, exiting through a hole in the top into the nasal cavity. The cap screwed down tight against a rubber gasket inside the twist grip to seal in the vapors when not being used.

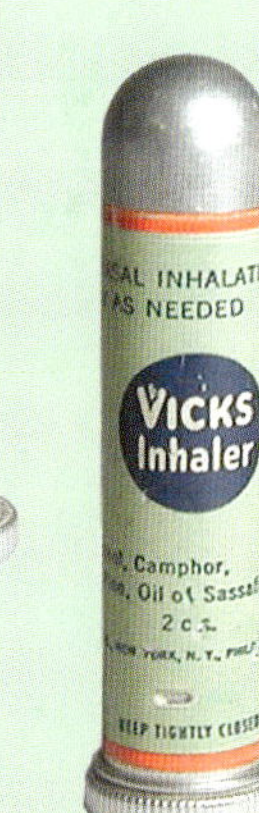

Vicks Inhaler (1940) Smith Richardson wrote in his 1975 book, *The Early History and Management Philosophy of Richardson-Merrell*, "Then in 1940, we developed, successfully test-marketed and nationally introduced the *Vicks Inhaler*, which rapidly attained multimillion dollar sales and has continued to be a leader in its field." There are very few differences between the Vicks and Penetro designs.

Live Druggists Are the Best

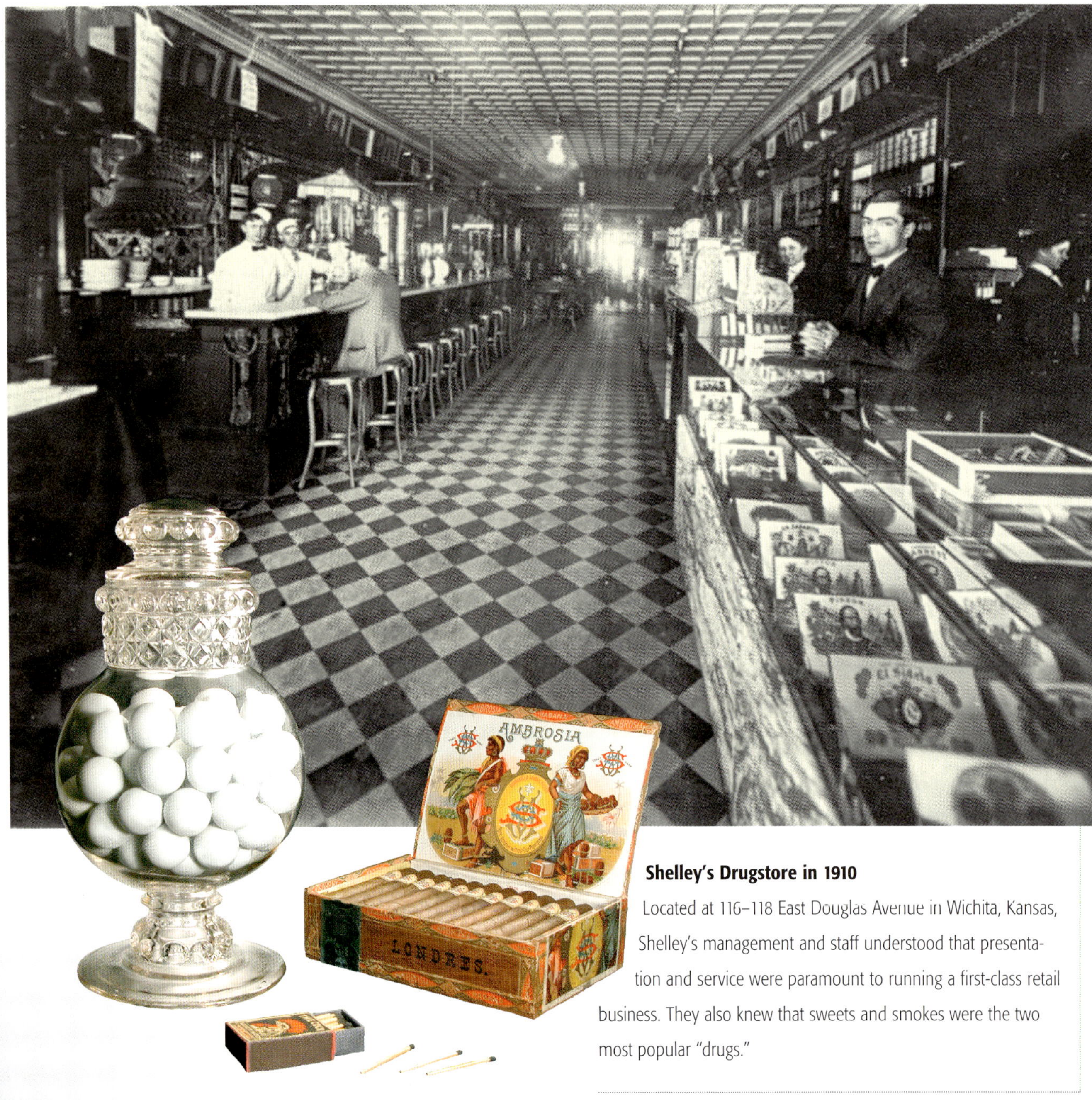

Shelley's Drugstore in 1910

Located at 116–118 East Douglas Avenue in Wichita, Kansas, Shelley's management and staff understood that presentation and service were paramount to running a first-class retail business. They also knew that sweets and smokes were the two most popular "drugs."

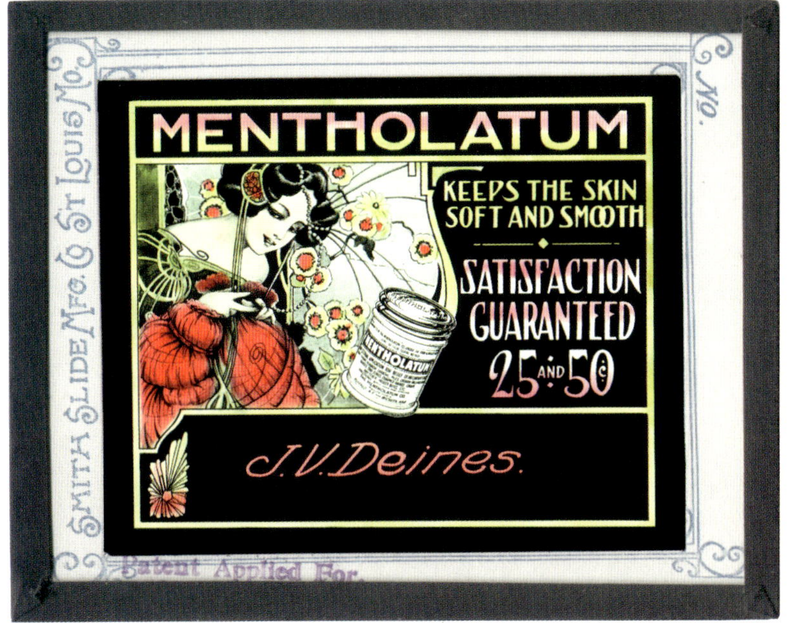

Lantern Slides

The Mentholatum Company took advantage of the advertising opportunities offered by the emerging motion picture industry. Images from these hand-tinted, glass lantern slides were projected onto the screen before the featured attraction was shown. Space at the bottom was customized with the name of the local druggist.

"We prefer to pay Druggists for advertising rather than Newspapers. Have tried both. Live druggists are the best."

Form 41-5M-10-08

A main street American institution, drugstores were where the pulse of the community was measured. Unlike the hardware and feed stores where men gathered or the grocery where women shopped, the drugstore was where everyone congregated. Women with small children dropped in throughout the day, businessmen lined up at lunch break, and teenagers crowded in after school let out. A typical drugstore had a soda fountain on one side and a merchandise counter on the other. In the back of the long room was the pharmacy. If it was wide enough, there were small, round tables and chairs set out in the middle for the customers to use while they ate and visited. Unlike stores today, the merchandise was kept on shelves and cabinets behind the counter and produced by the druggist or his clerk upon request.

In a counter cabinet that could be seen through the window from the street, fancy cut-glass jars packed with colorful penny candy were set at eye level for children. A wooden rack by the door held newspapers and the latest national magazines like *McCall's*, *Woman's World*, *Red Book*, *Farmer's Wife*, and *Delineator* (the latter contained the latest and much anticipated Butterick sewing patterns). The glass cabinet in front of the checkout displayed ornately printed cigar boxes. Further down the counter there were popular dime novels

Match Strike

This perforated tin sign was useful for sparking a sulfur match as well as an advertising pun.

and books. There were boxes of aromatic toilet soaps, a brightly colored display of Diamond fabric dyes, a decoratively scrolled cabinet of Willimantic sewing threads, and stacks of stationery and school supplies. Razors, brushes, mirrors, creams, and perfumes were displayed inside other glass-front cases.

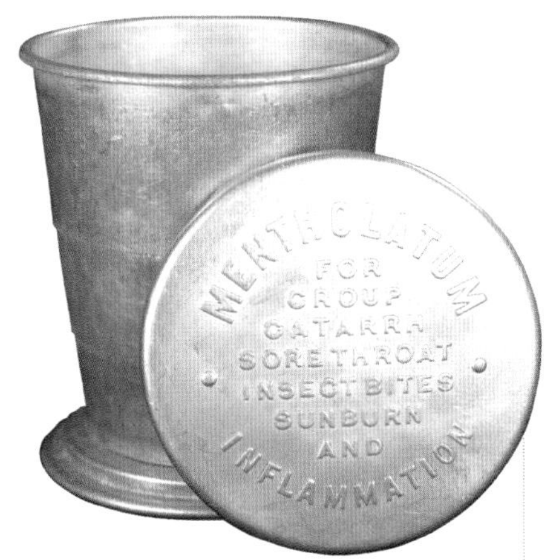

Telescoping Aluminum Drinking Cup

This camp cup with lid was given as a premium to all who responded to a 1912 advertisement in *Good Housekeeping* magazine. (See ad on page 73.)

In the back of the store was the pharmacist's counter. Behind the counter was a wall covered with matching apothecary jars labeled in incomprehensible Latin. The pharmacist poured and measured liquids and powders; he dispensed cascara, sulfur, soda pot ash, powdered charcoal, and quinine from a spice drawer cabinet. He poured calomel, mercury, Black Draught, iodine, pine oil, glycerin, alcohol, digitalis, and a dozen more from dark brown bottles. Shelves were stacked with packages of Castoria, Pe-ru-na, Hall's, Piso's, Bromo Seltzer, and Pond's Extract. On the counter sat boxed jars of Mentholatum and perhaps a few rival brands like Musterole, Saratoga Ointment, or Dr. Sayman's Healing Salve. He always had a new remedy to show to the customer.

When a family came in from the farm for supplies, the drugstore would be their first stop. Before Dad went over to the hardware store, he would start a tab with the clerk and grab a few cigars and a box of matches. The children made a beeline to the soda fountain and scrambled up the tall stools to sit at the shiny marble counter. They ordered chocolate ice cream sodas and banana splits. While waiting, they spied their

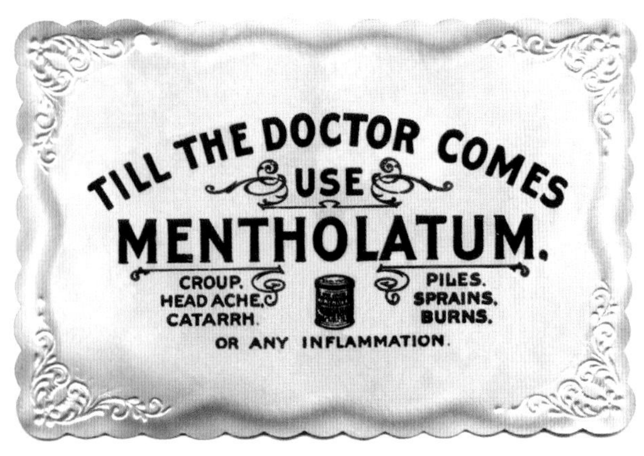

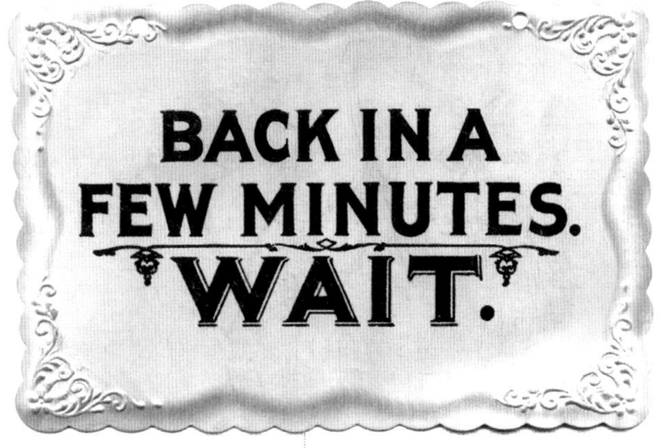

Aluminum Novelty

Mentholatum salesmen left these little, two-sided signs with doctors after each sales call. Prior to 1900, they were printed on cardboard. Then, from 1900 to 1908, the signs were printed on shiny, decoratively embossed and die-cut aluminum plates. This was made possible by technological advances in the 1890s that brought down the price of manufacturing the exotic alloy and increased experimentation and discovery of new commercial applications. One example was the Wright brothers' novel use of aluminum to build a lightweight engine for their 1903 *Flyer*, which helped make their flight at Kitty Hawk, North Carolina, possible. To own a piece of aluminum during the first decade of the twentieth century was analogous to holding the future in your hands.

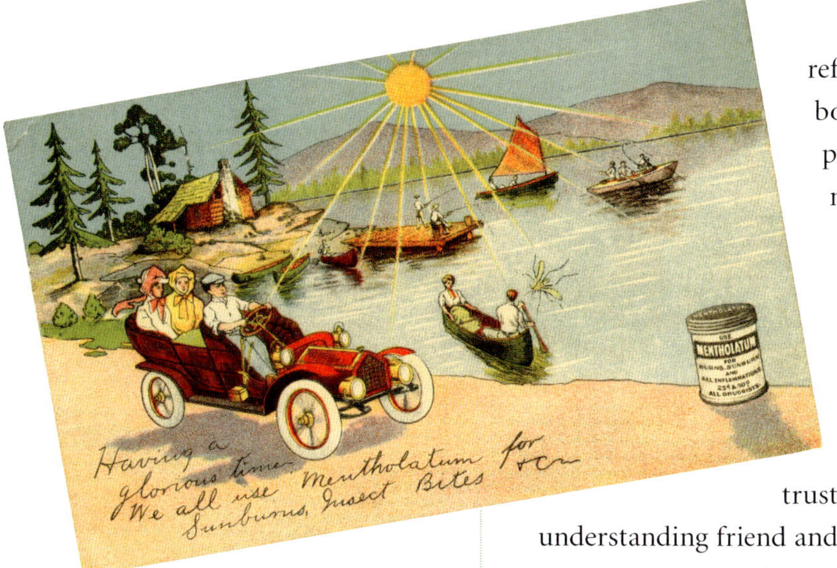

First Advertising Postcard

The activities depicted on this 1910 postcard represented everything that made A. A. Hyde happy, e.g., a sunny day at the lake, fishing, boating, and motoring. Notice that the artist captured a likeness of Billy Mitchell behind the wheel of the motor car.

reflections between and through colored bottles of lime, root beer, vanilla, sarsaparilla, and cherry syrups that lined the mirrored wall and watched the soda clerk (later called "jerk") assemble their treats. Mom consulted in back with the druggist and caught up on the town's gossip.

The druggist was a respected neighbor, a church member, and a trusted community leader. He could be an understanding friend and always knew the names of his customers. He was easily approached for health tips and for his opinion about goings-on in the community. Besides the front-door trade, the druggist also conducted business out of the back door. In the South, Jim Crow laws forced black customers to wait outside the back door for access to the pharmacy. Despite this insulting segregation, they were still paying customers, and the druggist would be there to fill their orders. In most cases, he was their only link to medical care, as he was for just as many in the poor white community. All too often there was no money to pay and he took trade goods or services in exchange.

MENTHOLATUM IS USEFUL EVERY DAY IN THE YEAR

CATARRH, SORE THROAT, BURNS

SORE EYES, PILES, ECZEMA, ETC.

CROUP, CHAPPED HANDS,

MEMORANDUM

(ERASE WITH DAMP CLOTH)

MEN - THO - LA - TUM

FOR INFLAMMATION

Aluminum Calender/Memo Pad

Aluminum pocket calenders were also handed out in the early 1900s. The flip side of the metallic card was labeled "Memorandum" and was left blank so that notes could be written in pencil and then erased with a damp cloth.

For those people without means to consult a doctor until their illness became serious, a knowledge of packaged and home remedies was very important. Jane Baker remembered that around 1915 her mother collected and dried sweet flag root and catnip leaves to store until she needed to make tea for a sore stomach. When Jane caught a cold, her mother would rub Mentholatum on her chest and wrap her up in warm flannel. To loosen the phlegm in her throat, her mother would make a towel tent over her head and a pot of steaming water. The water contained a dab of Mentholatum, and she inhaled its vapors.

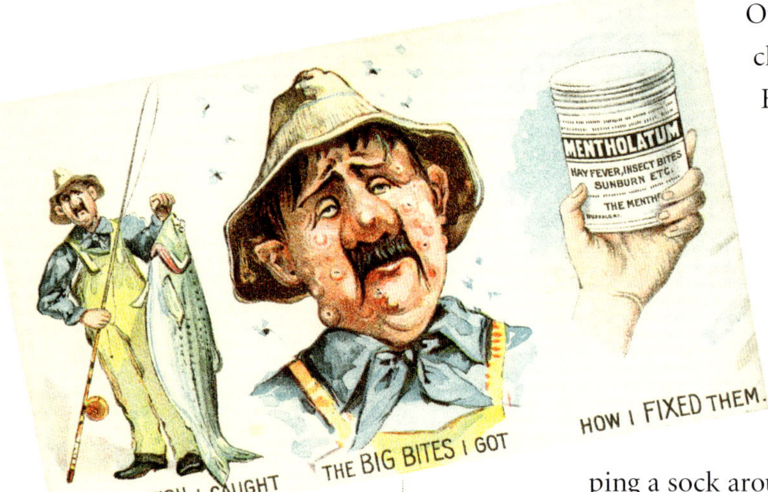

1912 Postcard

There is little doubt who inspired the creation of this comical character. A.A. always enjoyed a good joke on himself, particularly if it involved his favorite pastime and documented an award-winning catch!

Other basics in her mother's medicine chest were castor oil, ipecac, and Epsom salts.[1]

Helmuth Huber, whose German/Russian parents immigrated to America and homesteaded outside Ashley, North Dakota, said his family was never without Mentholatum. For sore throat, his mother heated it as an inhalant and rubbed it on his neck, wrapping a sock around it. He remembered it got hot and made him feel good.[2]

Joyce Gibson Roach, from Horned Toad, Texas, reported her grandmother didn't bother with camphorated oil and turpentine for the flu, because, she said, "Mentholatum was her personal choice for nose and chest. But then she also treated cuts, scrapes, callus, bunions and sores with Mentholatum—anything short of brain surgery." Mrs. D. C. Gibson of Buffalo, New York, wrote to the company, "I call Mentholatum the Little Doctor." For good reason, the company used the slogan "The World's Medicine Chest" for many years.[3]

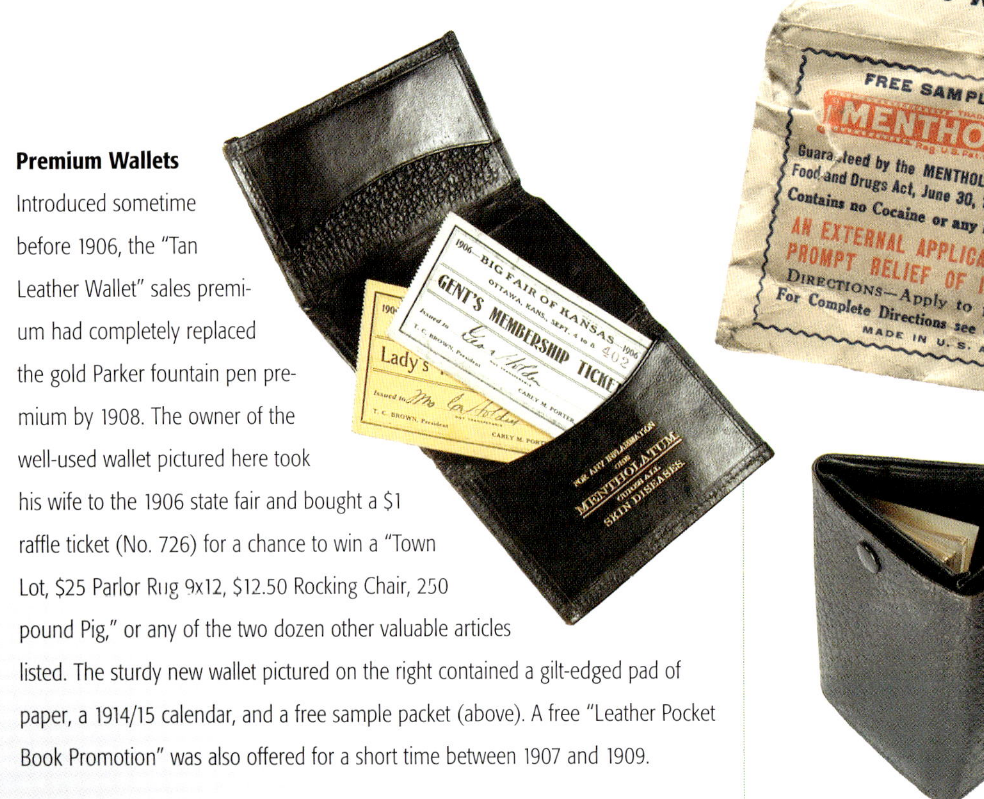

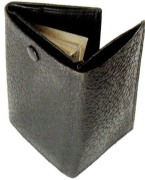

Premium Wallets

Introduced sometime before 1906, the "Tan Leather Wallet" sales premium had completely replaced the gold Parker fountain pen premium by 1908. The owner of the well-used wallet pictured here took his wife to the 1906 state fair and bought a $1 raffle ticket (No. 726) for a chance to win a "Town Lot, $25 Parlor Rug 9x12, $12.50 Rocking Chair, 250 pound Pig," or any of the two dozen other valuable articles listed. The sturdy new wallet pictured on the right contained a gilt-edged pad of paper, a 1914/15 calendar, and a free sample packet (above). A free "Leather Pocket Book Promotion" was also offered for a short time between 1907 and 1909.

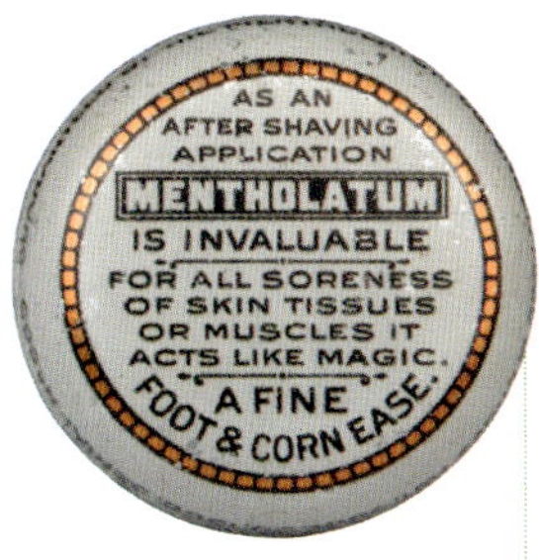

"Acts Like Magic" Trial Box

This rare tin is dated 1906.

American industry boomed during the first decade of the century and employed all who wanted to work, yet denied labor its fair share of the prosperity. Farming, like factory work and mining, was an unregulated and dangerous occupation, and like other workers, farmers labored long hours for extremely low wages. The men in charge hid behind syndicates and trusts, monopolizing wealth and flouting America's democratic values. President Teddy Roosevelt tried unsuccessfully to regulate the trusts before his term ended in 1908. His successor, William Howard Taft, had no better luck with antitrust suits. Not until the presidency of Woodrow Wilson (1913–1921) would the Federal Reserve Act (1913) and the Clayton Antitrust Act (1914) be passed, which would lead to an increasingly open economy and more equitable distribution of wealth.[4]

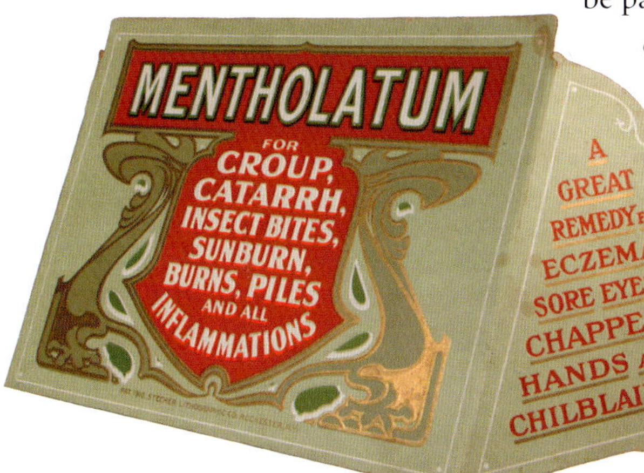

Art Nouveau Counter Card

This 1910 countertop display claims seventeen remedies.

But until then, cash was scarce in working-class and rural communities, and druggists routinely kept a tab book for customers who wanted to pay at the end of the month. One such book, surviving from a drugstore in Willard, Ohio, then called "Chicago Junction," gives us an eight-month window into the buying habits of its patrons between December 10, 1907, and August 10, 1908. The most common purchases were cigars, pencils, magazines, books, and stationery. The druggist received a surprisingly small number of doctors' prescriptions but filled more orders for measured quantities of camphor oil, cascara (a laxative), cough syrup, and turpentine. One citizen went home with quinine, castor oil, and whiskey, while another took home

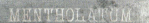

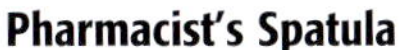

Pharmacist's Spatula

A useful and appreciated gift from the Mentholatum Company, this simple advertising spatula had no markings or paper trail that could be used to reveal its maker or date. Two variations have been found with different brand name type styles (boxed and serif) etched on the blades. The Piso Company gave out a similar spatula.

DRUGS & MEDICINES

Favorite Remedies

Willard, Ohio's favorite packaged remedies in 1908

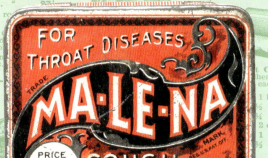

CHAMBERLAIN'S
REG. U.S. PAT. OFF.
COLIC REMEDY

FOR FLATULENT OR WIND COLIC

Each Fluidounce Contains
Chloroform . . . 20 mins.
Ether . . . . . 64 mins.
Camphor . . . . .81 gr.
Capsicum . . . .81 gr.
Alcohol 45%

FOR PRODUCING A WARMING, SOOTHING SENSATION TO STOMACH AND INTESTINES

Dose: Adults: 1 teaspoonful diluted with 10 parts of water. Repeat in 15 minutes if necessary, then every hour until 4 doses are taken. Children: 4 to 6 years, 15 drops—6 to 8 years, 20 drops—8 to 14 years, 30 drops—diluted with 10 parts of water.

Contents ¾ Fl. Oz.

CHAMBERLAIN MEDICINE CO., INC.
NEW YORK ST LOUIS

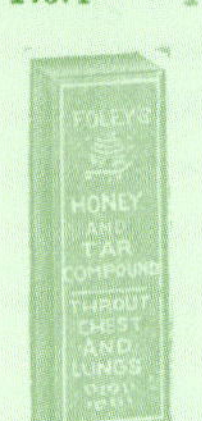

Y7374

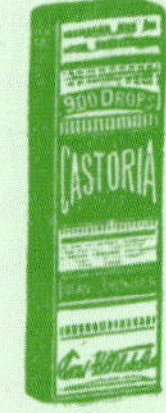

Y7376

Sloan's Family Liniment—25c size.
Y7374—1 doz. in box. Doz. **$1.98**

California Syrup of Figs and Elixir of Senna—
Y7376—½ doz. in box. Doz. **$4.75**

Y7375 Y7371

Foley's Honey and Tar—Small size.
Y7375—1 doz. in carton. Doz. **$1.95**

Fletcher's Castoria—The genuine.
Y7371—1 doz. in box...Doz. **$2.95**

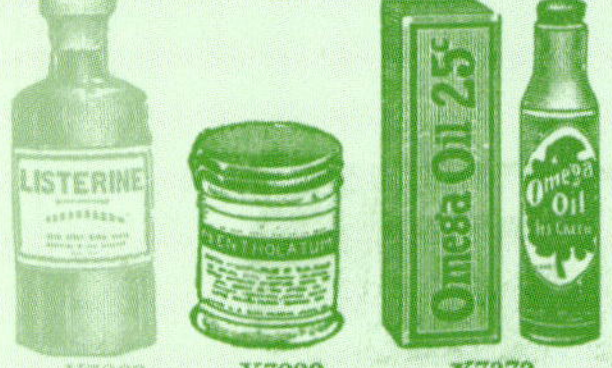

Y7203 Y7229 Y7373

Listerine — 3-oz. size well-known antiseptic.
Y7203—1 doz. in carton. Doz. **$2.20**

Mentholatum—25c size. Relieves catarrh, hayfever, cold sores, skin irritation, etc.
Y7229—1 doz. jars in carton. Doz. jars, **$1.75**

Omega Oil—35c size.
Y7373—1 doz. in box..Doz. **$2.80**

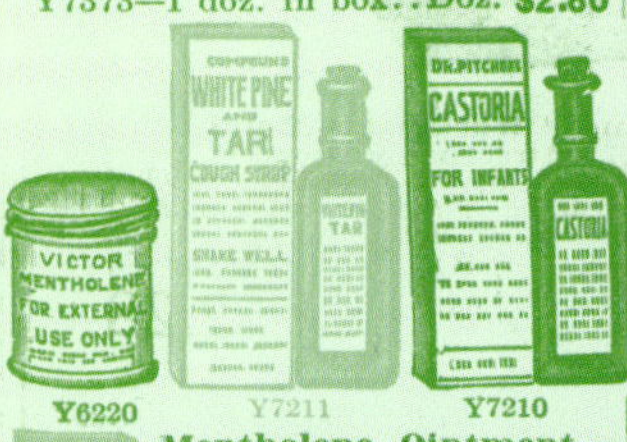

Y6220 Y7211 Y7210

Y7212

Mentholene Ointment—1 oz. opal jar, relieves catarrh, hay fever, fever, piles, sores, etc.
Y6220—1 doz. in box. Doz. **$1.10**

White Pine and Tar Cough Syrup—No. 2 panel bottle. Excellent cough remedy. Each in carton.
Y7211—1 doz. in box. Doz. **$1.35**

Dr. Pitcher's Castoria—No. 4 bottle. Guaranteed, prepared according to original formula, each in carton.
Y7210—1 doz. in box...Doz. **$1.35**

Laxative Fig Syrup—No. 2 panel bottle, pure, each in carton.
Y7212—1 doz. in box. Doz. **$1.35**

Y7288—½ oz. ....Doz. **$0.45**

Senna Leaves—1½ oz.
Y7383—1 doz. in box.

Gum Camphor—43 oz. to make spirits of Camphor in 10 oz. Alco…
Y7362—2 doz. cakes in box.........Doz.

DRUG SPECIAL…

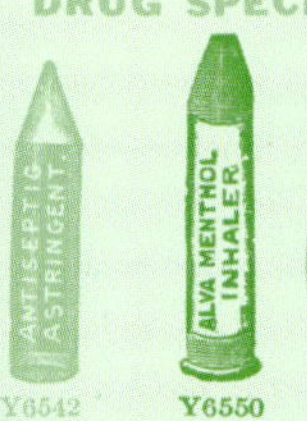

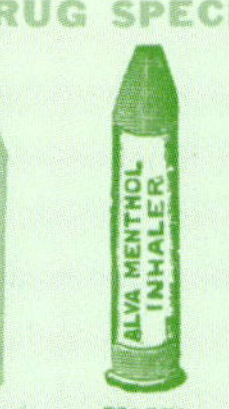

Y6542 Y6550

"Stop-O-Styptic" Penci… tic, astringent, stops flow…
Y6542—1 doz. on card...

Menthol Inhaler—3½ in. glass tube, extra strong for catarrh, cold in head, etc. On display card.
Y6550—1 doz. in box....Doz. **60c**

Carbolic Salve—Large litho tin box in carton.
Y7208—1 doz. in box....Doz. **80c**

Y7242—100 tablets in bottle. 1 in carton..............Each, **88c**

HORLICK'S MALTED MILK

Widely advertised strengthening food for infants, invalids and aged. Free adv. helps included if requested with order. Each bottle in carton. Doz.
Y7200—50c size.. **$4.50**
Y7201—$1.00 size. Each, **75c**
Y7209 — Hospital or family size. Each, **$3.00**

CUBEB CIGARETTES

Y6541—10c size. Quick relief for catarrh, 12 in pkg. with show card. 1 doz. pkgs. in box. Doz. pkgs. **67c**

ABSORBENT COTTON

Y6459 — Full 1 lb. rolls, white U. S. P. hospital cotton........Lb. **45c**
In 10 roll lots or more...Lb. **43c**

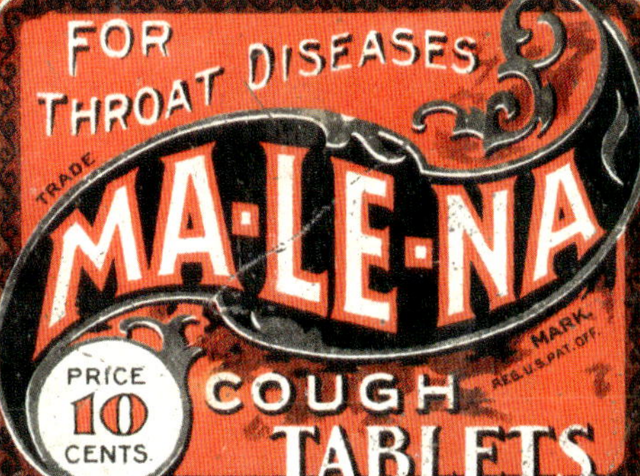

Strengthening Plas…
Y7424—2 doz. in bo… (Total $2.00)

Bella Donna Poro… 5x7½ in.
Y7420—2 doz. in bo… (Total $3.00)

Linton Gauze Banda… in sealed cylinder. …ders in carton.
Y7430—1 in. wide.
Y7431—2 in. wide...
Y7432—3 in. wide...

Y7043—Silk, black, fl… pieces in envelope.

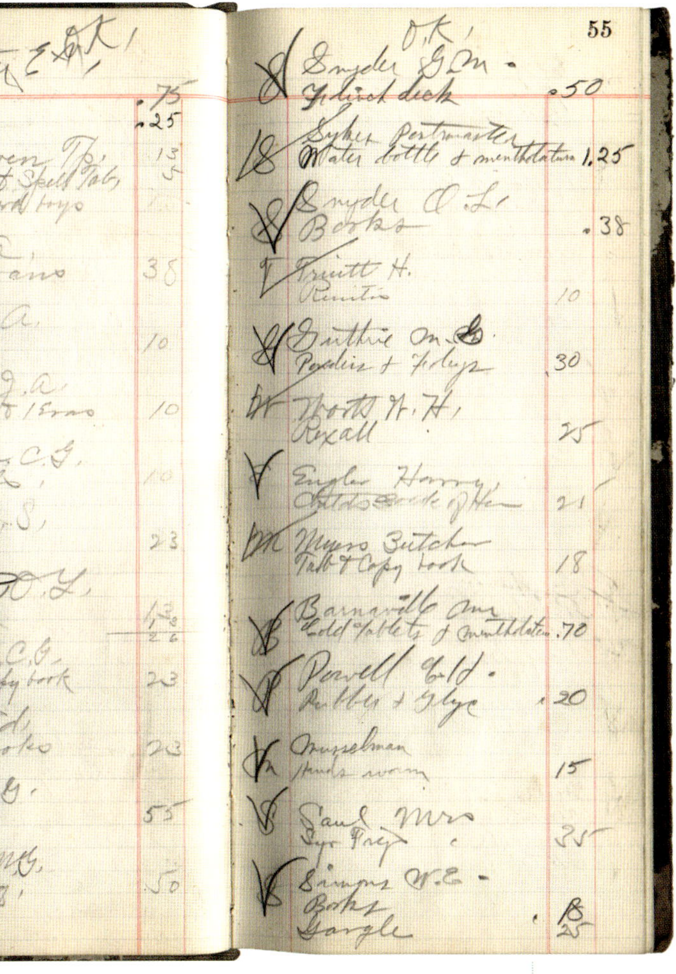

camphor, turpentine, blue bark, and cough syrup. The top-ten-selling packaged remedies were:

1. Doan's pills (sixteen packages of various cures)
2. Chamberlain's (fifteen bottles of various cures)
3. Castoria (fourteen 35¢ bottles)
4. Mentholatum (twelve 25¢ jars)
5. Nervine (ten $1 bottles)
6. Hyomei (eight 50¢ bottles)
7. Vaseline (seven, various prices charged according to the amount taken from a bulk container)
8. Pe-ru-na (seven $1 bottles)
9. Ma-le-na (three 10¢ tins)
10. Omega Oil (two 50¢ bottles)

The top two brands, Doan's and Chamberlain's, could be expected to head the list because they packaged a range of remedies for colds, constipation,

Put It on My Tab, Doc!

This tab book from a drugstore in central Ohio represents a sample of the buying habits of a small rural town in 1908. The second entry on page 55 indicates that Postmaster Sykes took home a water bottle and a jar of Mentholatum and left a tab for $1.25. Further down the page, Mr. Barnaville took cold tablets and a jar of Mentholatum home and left a tab for 70¢. The entries in this book also provide an informal measure of which brands were the most popular.

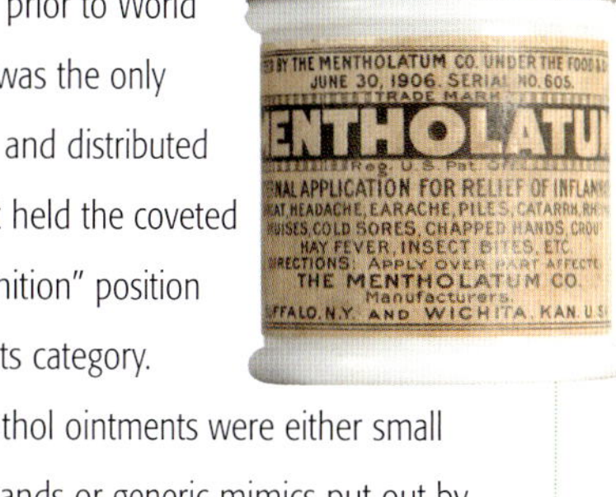

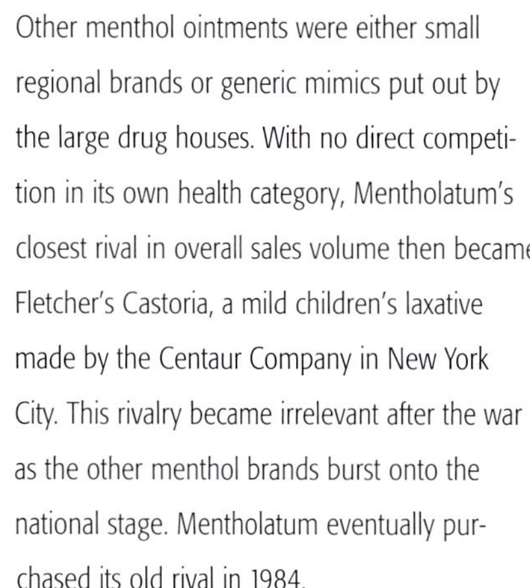

The Contenders

Through the decade prior to World War I, Mentholatum was the only nationally advertised and distributed menthol ointment. It held the coveted "household recognition" position all alone in its category. Other menthol ointments were either small regional brands or generic mimics put out by the large drug houses. With no direct competition in its own health category, Mentholatum's closest rival in overall sales volume then became Fletcher's Castoria, a mild children's laxative made by the Centaur Company in New York City. This rivalry became irrelevant after the war as the other menthol brands burst onto the national stage. Mentholatum eventually purchased its old rival in 1984.

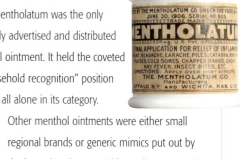

nerves, etc. The book did not detail the kind purchased. Castoria (a laxative) and Mentholatum were specialized products. Mentholatum topped the cold and catarrh remedy list, ahead of Pe-ru-na and Ma-le-na. Because the book was used exclusively for tab accounts, it can provide only a sampling of brand popularity. In 1915, Mentholatum and Castoria topped a more comprehensive survey by a regional sales agent for Mentholatum. He surveyed total sales by the jobbers he knew in four western states, and the top sellers were Mentholatum and Castoria: the former in Montana, Washington, and South Dakota, and the latter in Minnesota.[5]

The American West Was Mentholatum Country!

In 1910, Mentholatum's customer base lived on small family farms and large ranches, at remote mining and logging camps, and in thousands of small towns scattered over the wide prairies and among the high mountain valleys. There were fifty million rural Americans, compared to forty-two million urban residents. Rural populations in aggregate were much larger in the western and southern states than they were in the industrialized northeast. Overall, the nation had nine thousand towns with populations of less than a thousand, and only three cities with populations of more than a million.[6]

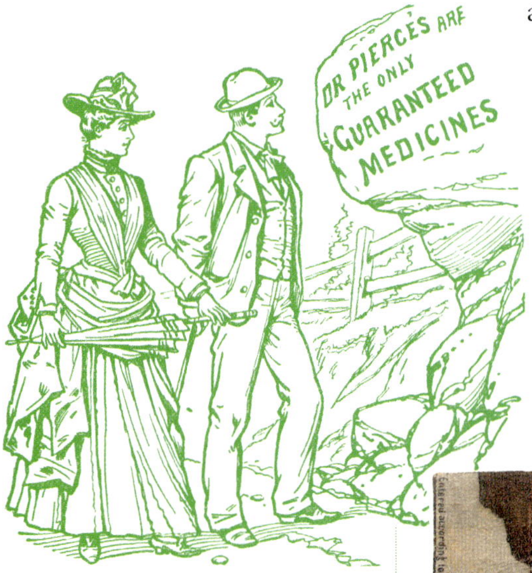

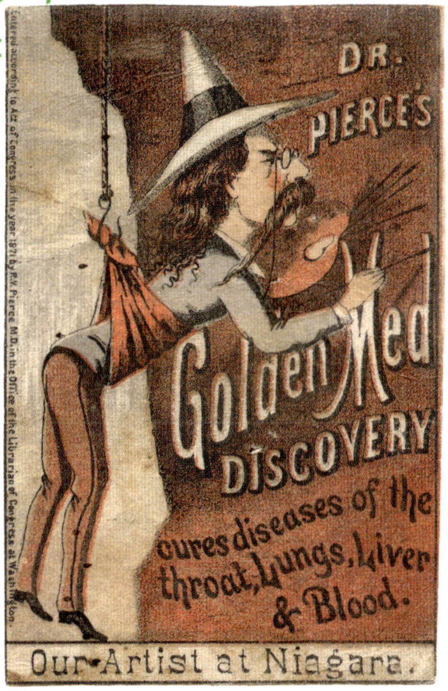

Advertising Had No Limits

Dr. Pierce's disregard for natural rock formations was typical of sign painters during the Victorian age.

No matter how remote, rural families were never completely isolated from the world. They read the newspapers and discussed current events with their neighbors at church socials and the local drugstore. Like their city cousins, country folk were assaulted everywhere they looked with advertisements. Remarkably, by the turn of the century America's remote and empty expanses were covered with ads. Signs were painted on farm buildings and even on roadside rocks; they were nailed

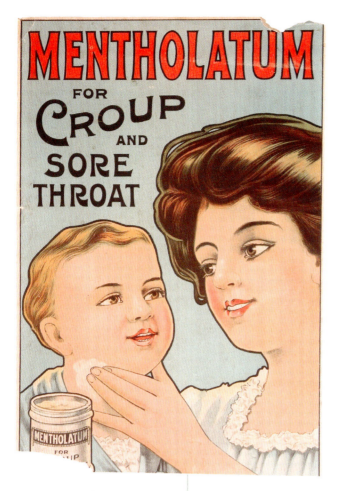

A Nurturing Influence

This early poster introduced the mother and child motif that would go on to play an important role in the company's future advertising imagery. (See Catalog page C142.)

to trees and utility poles. They reached into the humblest homes with Sears, Roebuck and Co. and Montgomery Ward catalogs. They filled up monthly subscription magazines such as *Ladies Home Journal, Woman's Home Companion*, and *Cosmopolitan*. Children poured over their colorful rotogravure illustrations and steel plate engravings, memorizing every detail in drawings of pretty ladies, modern gadgets, furniture, and automobiles.

A distant relative of A. A. Hyde was one such child. Growing up in Duncan, Oklahoma, Harold T. Hyde (1910–1993) remembered when he and the other boys would cut out a magazine coupon and send it in with a nickel postage for a free sample "box" of Mentholatum. Sometimes they were given a tin by their teacher, which they carried in the bib pocket of their overalls. When the salve was gone, it might be replaced with a lucky bird claw or coin. The tins wore a characteristic circular imprint on the outside of the bib, as did the Rooster Snuff tin placed in their hip pocket.[7]

The drugstore in Duncan, Oklahoma, recalled by eighty-two-year-old Harold Hyde was typical of stores in the center of a block. The front was twenty or thirty feet wide with a central door flanked by display windows. If it was a corner drugstore, there was room for more display windows along the side street. Keeping the windows dressed was a big concern for druggists. To help them out, colorfully lithographed, die-cut display boards were provided gratis by the Mentholatum Company. There were also oversized Mentholatum boxes to use as props. For inside the store, the company provided point-of-purchase easel-back display cards for the counter. Harold Hyde recalled that Mentholatum jars were displayed on a cardboard "step-up."[8]

The earliest Mentholatum window displays seem to have been used year-round and might have served for several years in a row. The earliest mention of an "easel card display" appeared on a 1903 sales offer to druggists. Another was printed on a return postcard, "If you want one of our Baby Head Signs, . . ." c. 1903–1905. One 1907 notice to druggists regarding the discontinuation of automatically packed free samples simply said, "special window display." "Display Poster Herewith" was printed on a "Special 4th of July Proposition" sent out in 1909. In 1912, the "Don't Cry Mentholatum Will Fix It" easel back appeared. On a 1915 postcard order form, the company asked if the druggist needed more samples and a "window display." And in 1919 there were boxes to check if you wanted a "Special Barber Offer, Shop Signs," or "Jap Hang." The Japanese Hang was a brightly colored scroll poster depicting three domestic scenes with Japanese families using Mentholatum. The scenes were framed with red, yellow, and blue flowers and topped with an umbrella that proclaimed, "The World's Medicine Chest Mentholatum." Sometime in the mid-

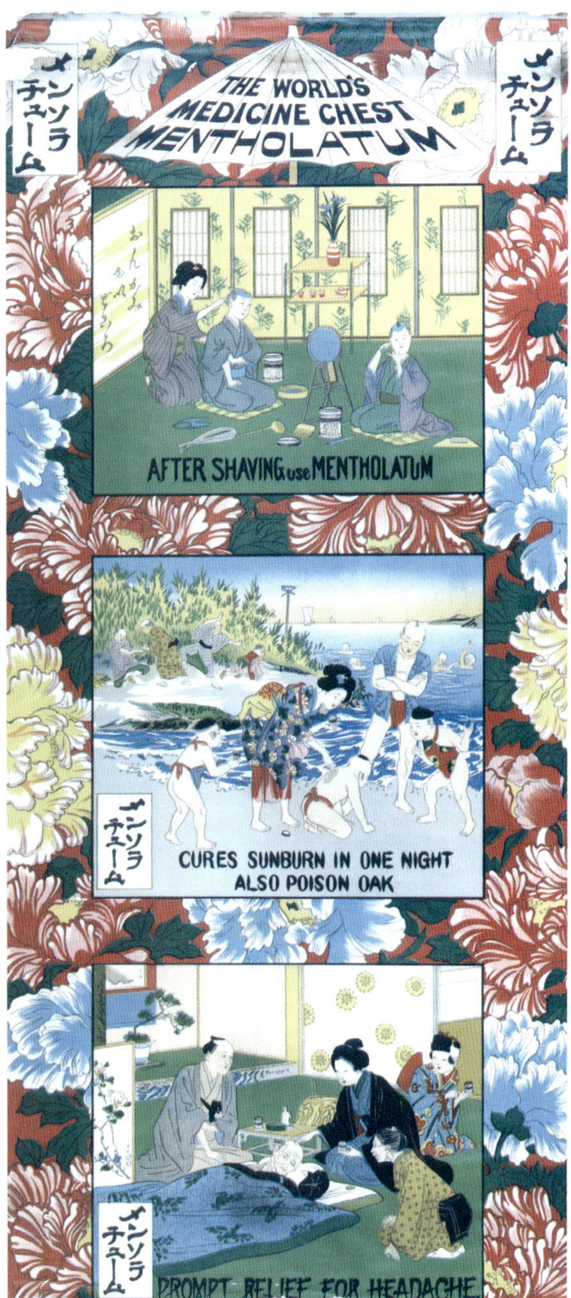

Japanese "Hang" (c. 1919)

Thin metal rods at both top and bottom held the paper poster so that it rolled up like a scroll. It was hung from a string that was tied to holes at both ends of the top rod. (See Catalog page C143.)

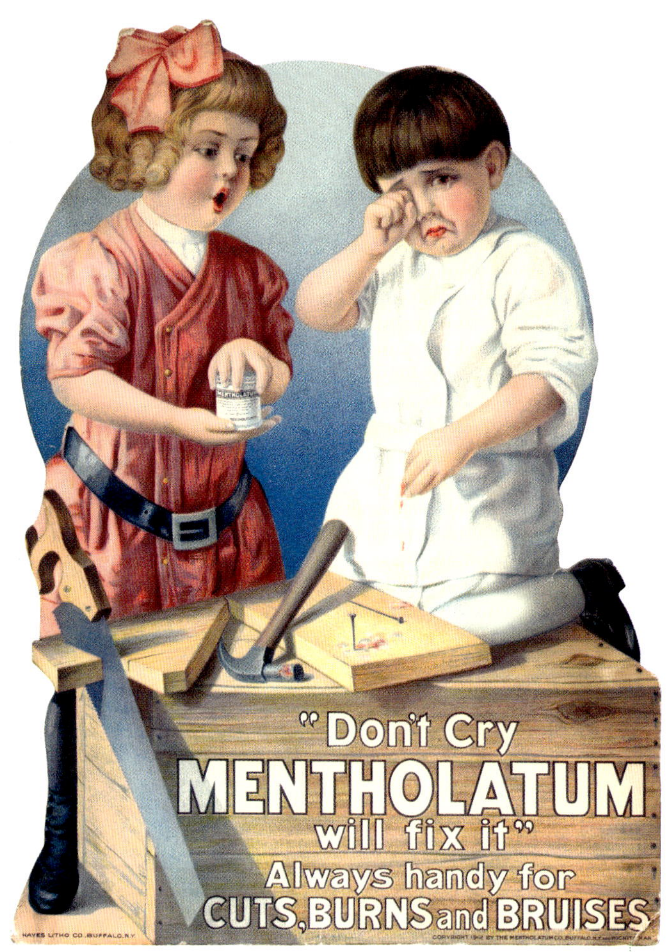

Mother's Little Helper

This 1912 countertop display might have been the inspiration for Little Nurse, which was introduced in a national campaign five years later.

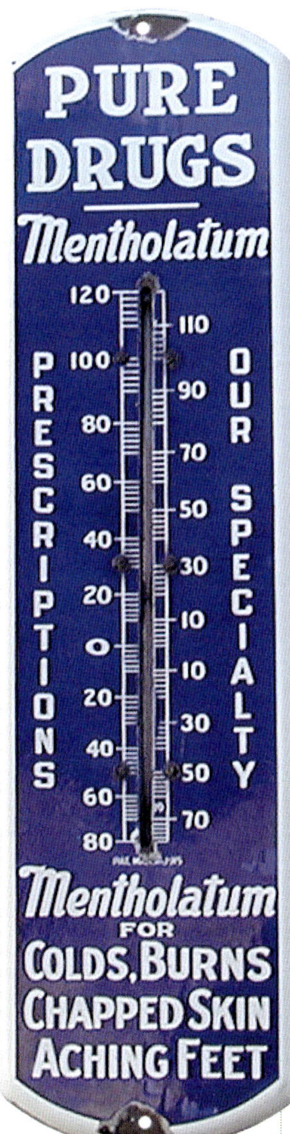

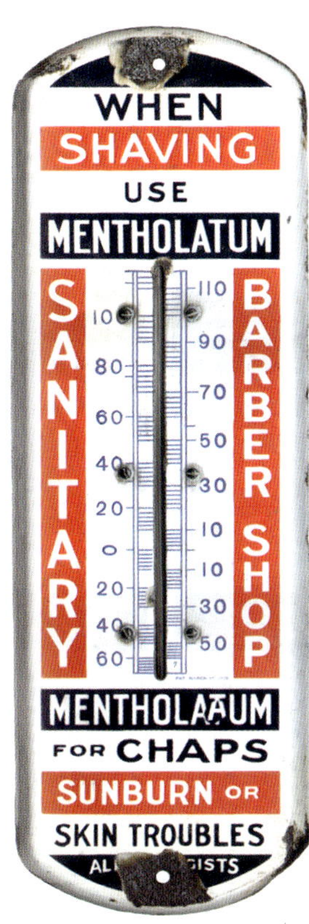

Temperature Signaled the Cold and Hay Fever Seasons

Based on the Mentholatum logo style, the Pure Drugs thermometer was produced sometime after 1916. Both porcelain enamel thermometers have a patent date of "March 16, 1915" printed at the bottom of the temperature scale.

1920s, two new displays were produced each year, one for the summer and the other for the winter sales season. Customized porcelain signs with the Mentholatum logo and the customer's name were produced, as were porcelain thermometers sometime after 1915.

A new product introduced in 1906 was Mentholatum Plaster, which was touted to be "A Prompt Relief for Backache, Chest Colds, Sciatica, Pleurisy, Pneumonia, Neuralgia, Lumbago and All Aches and Pains." The trademark was registered in the U.S. Patent Office and labeling recorded at the Bureau of Chemistry under the Pure Food and Drugs Act. Little else is known about it, other than the four-page illustrated insert with directions in seven different languages. An order card printed in November of that year listed:

Doz. Menthocura @ \$1.75
Doz. Mentho. Plasters @ \$1.75
Doz. Mentholatum @ \$1.75.

But another card printed a month later replaced "Mentho. Plasters" with "Mentho. Corn Oil Soap."[9]

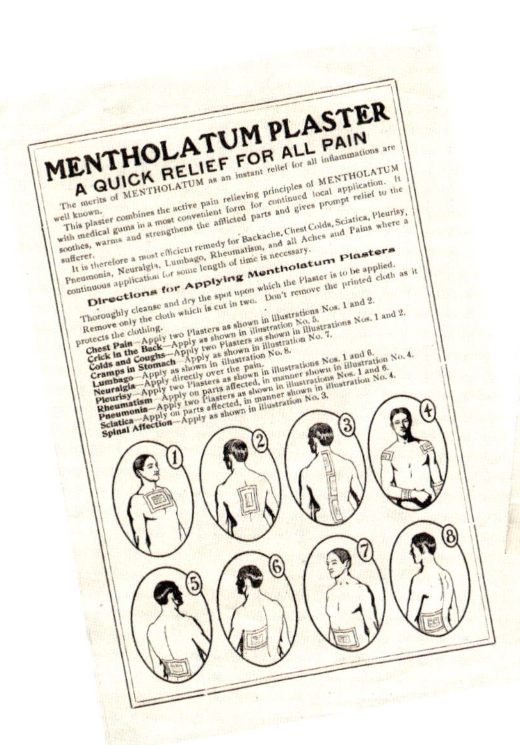

MENTHOLATUM PLASTER
A QUICK RELIEF FOR ALL PAIN

The merits of MENTHOLATUM as an instant relief for all inflammations are well known.

This plaster combines the active pain relieving principles of MENTHOLATUM with medical gums in a most convenient form for continued local application. It soothes, warms and strengthens the afflicted parts and gives prompt relief to the sufferer.

It is therefore a most efficient remedy for Backache, Chest Colds, Sciatica, Pleurisy, Pneumonia, Neuralgia, Lumbago, Rheumatism, and all Aches and Pains where a continuous application for some length of time is necessary.

Directions for Applying Mentholatum Plasters

Thoroughly cleanse and dry the spot upon which the Plaster is to be applied. Remove only the cloth which is cut in two. Don't remove the printed cloth as it protects the clothing.

Chest Pain—Apply two Plasters as shown in illustrations Nos. 1 and 2.
Crick in the Back—Apply as shown in illustration No. 5.
Colds and Coughs—Apply two Plasters as shown in illustrations Nos. 1 and 2.
Cramps in Stomach—Apply as shown in illustration No. 7.
Lumbago—Apply as shown in illustration No. 8.
Neuralgia—Apply directly over the pain.
Pleurisy—Apply two Plasters as shown in illustrations Nos. 1 and 6.
Rheumatism—Apply on parts affected, in manner shown in illustration No. 4.
Pneumonia—Apply two Plasters as shown in illustrations Nos. 1 and 6.
Sciatica—Apply on parts affected, in manner shown in illustration No. 4.
Spinal Affection—Apply as shown in illustration No. 3.

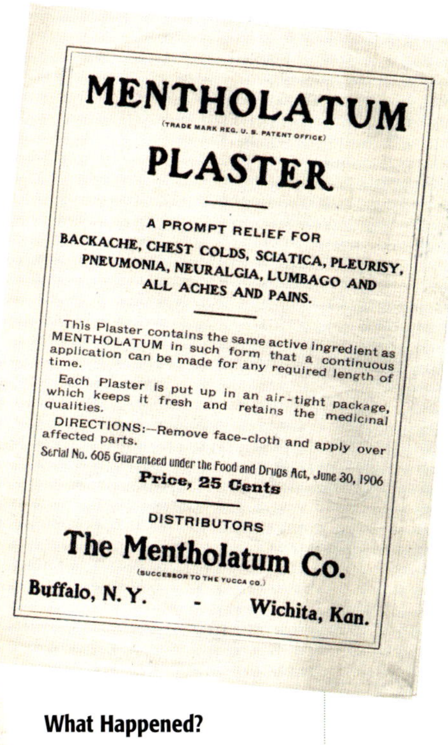

MENTHOLATUM
(TRADE MARK REG. U. S. PATENT OFFICE)
PLASTER

A PROMPT RELIEF FOR
BACKACHE, CHEST COLDS, SCIATICA, PLEURISY, PNEUMONIA, NEURALGIA, LUMBAGO AND ALL ACHES AND PAINS.

This Plaster contains the same active ingredient as MENTHOLATUM in such form that a continuous application can be made for any required length of time.

Each Plaster is put up in an air-tight package, which keeps it fresh and retains the medicinal qualities.

DIRECTIONS:—Remove face-cloth and apply over affected parts.

Serial No. 605 Guaranteed under the Food and Drugs Act, June 30, 1906

Price, 25 Cents

DISTRIBUTORS
The Mentholatum Co.
(SUCCESSOR TO THE YUCCA CO.)
Buffalo, N. Y. - Wichita, Kan.

What Happened?

Mentho Plasters were ready for market and then vanished . . .

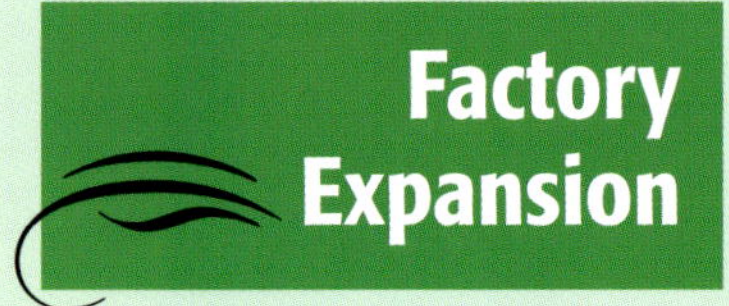

Factory Expansion

In 1906, Charles H. Hyde (1884–1970), A. A. Hyde's fifth child, opened a Canadian subsidiary called Mentholatum Inter-American Inc. Mentholatum's business approach was well suited to serve Canada's frontier market. The subsidiary initially distributed product that was manufactured at the Buffalo plant and imported into Canada. Later, in 1914, "Charlie" oversaw the construction of a new ten-thousand-square-foot, two-story factory on Lewis Street in Bridgeburg, Ontario, and began manufacturing product locally. The building sat on the bank of the Niagara River immediately south of the International Railway Bridge (built in 1870), which crossed the river into Buffalo. The factory was in the township of Bridgeburg, which by 1932 was renamed Fort Erie. Charlie Hyde remained general manager of the plant until 1933, when he was succeeded by G. H. Stratton Sr., who was later followed by his son, G. H. Stratton Jr. The factory was in operation for almost eighty years before being closed in March 2004 due to consolidation in the U.S. facility.[10]

Back in Wichita, construction began in 1908 on a new eight-thousand-square-foot factory on the northeast corner of Cleveland and Douglas, one block east of the old building. Designed by U. G. Charles, the building was the first reinforced-

Fort Erie started out as a French trading post and stockade in 1750 and became a British fort in 1764, after the French and Indian War. The area around the fort was later settled by Royalists who were deported at the end of the American Revolution. During the War of 1812, Yankee militiamen captured and burned the already battered old fortification. It remained a ruin until the 1930s, when it was resurrected and turned into a history museum and symbol of national pride. On August 7, 1927, a new 4,900-foot-long steel and concrete bridge was opened connecting Fort Erie with Buffalo or, more important, Canada with the United States. It was named the "Peace Bridge" to commemorate one hundred years of peace between the two countries. For more than eighty years Mentholatum has been represented in all twelve provinces with "Made in Canada" on the label.[11]

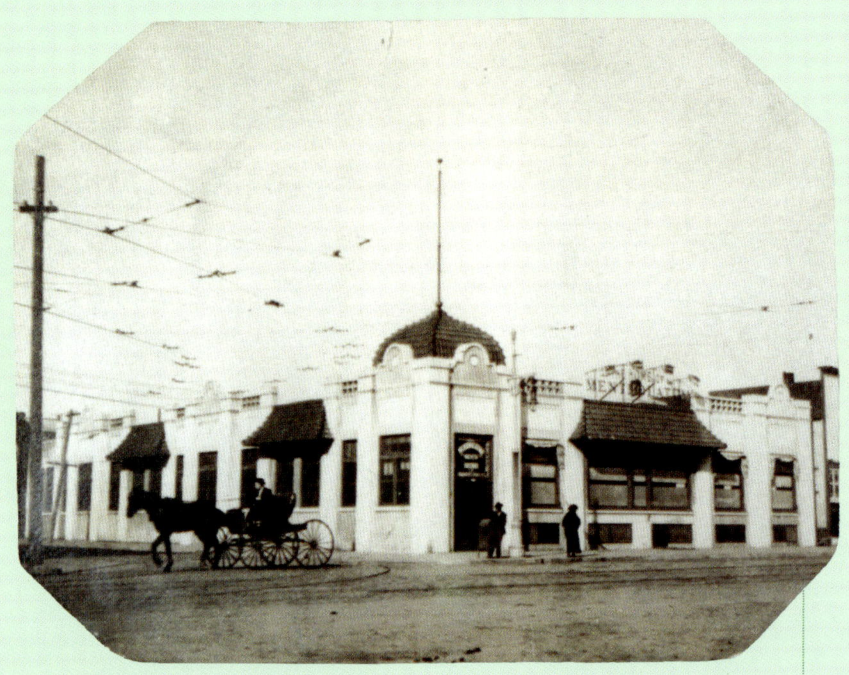

Early View

This photograph showed the Wichita factory with its original exterior colors, white with mint green trim. The "UFOs" in the sky were actually cable spacers for the electric trolley cars.

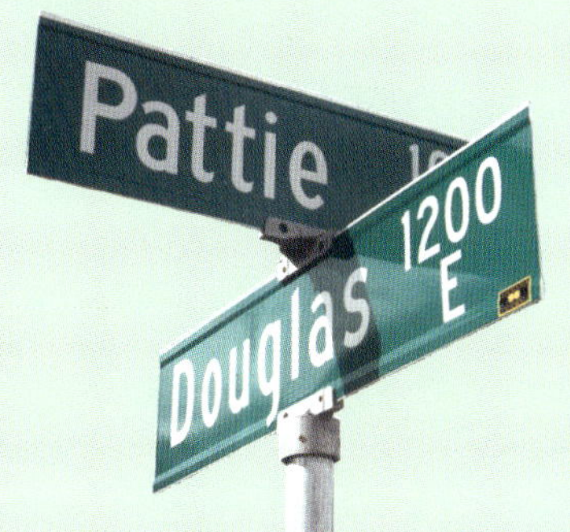

concrete structure to be erected in Wichita. It contained a skylight over the packing floor, a steam heating plant, and an evaporative cooling system. When it opened in 1909, a large sign on the roof read "The Home of Mentholatum." The exterior was painted white and mint green. The dome over the corner entrance was tiled with terra cotta, as were the three large awning structures. The packing floor in the center of the building constituted more than half the square footage, and two raised floors, fore and aft, made up the rest. (See floor plan on page 109.) An additional 1,700 square feet were added in the rear sometime later. Today, the building looks the same, minus the mint green paint, the electric sign, and the three tiled awnings. The original Yucca Company building on the south side of Douglas and Pattie is still standing, but now without its distinctive two-tiered wood balcony and awning.[12]

Souvenir Postcard c. 1917

This five-color picture postcard shows that the annex at the back of the building had already been completed by the time the photograph was taken. It also shows a new street lamp had replaced the old telephone pole on the street corner. The printers at E. C. Kropp Company in Milwaukee, Wisconsin, also made a few fictional improvements of their own when they covered the trolley cables with a painted sky, added a flag, and placed an automobile in the foreground. This traditional view is taken from across Douglas, standing under the Pattie street sign.

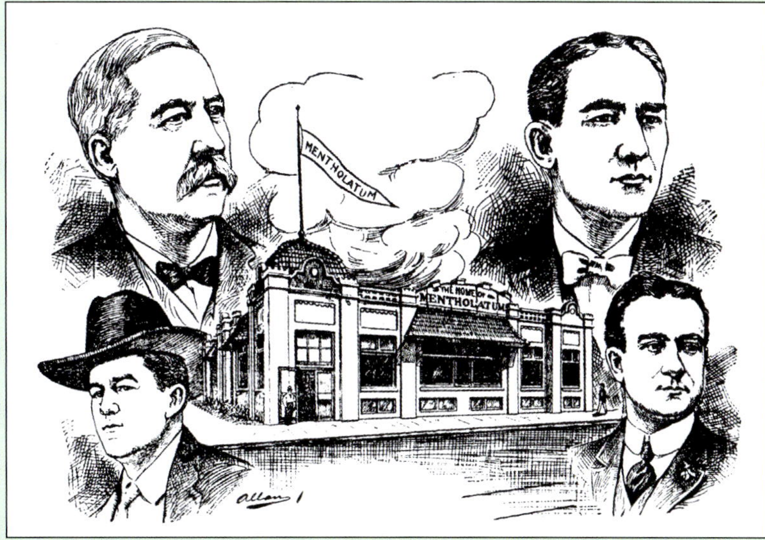

"The Quartet of Hydes"

Published in the *Wichita Eagle*, c. 1909, this drawing pictures A. A. Hyde, founder and president, at upper left. Also shown (clockwise) are Edward K. Hyde, vice president of the company and manager of the Buffalo plant; Charles H. Hyde, company secretary; and Alexander Hyde, company treasurer.

For Sunburn and Windburn

The Cooling, Soothing, Healing Cream for Daily Use

MENTHOLATUM

Accept No Substitute

Mail Coupon now for Free Sample or Jap Pocketbox

TRADE MARK
MENTHOLATUM
Reg. U.S. Pat. Off.

Small Size 25¢
Regular Size 50¢
Family Size $1.00

At All Druggists

Coupon for Free Sample or a Jap Pocketbox

Cut this out and mail to
**The Mentholatum Company,
Dept. A. 7, Wichita, Kansas**

Please send me handsome Jap Box containing a liberal sample of Mentholatum, convenient for handbag or vanity case. I am enclosing 10c to cover postage and packing.

Name ....

Address ....

City and State ....

(If you want free sample only send coupon without 10c)

Milestone Ad Was Aimed at a Female Demographic

This advertisement in the July 1916 *Delineator* is the first full-page color Mentholatum ad. At the time, Mentholatum had achieved household brand recognition in markets influenced by magazines such as *Modern Priscilla* and *Cosmopolitan*. Now it would be recognized in every market within *Delineator*'s infinite reach. (See Butterick Trio, page 82.) Throughout the decade, Mentholatum had been not only the first but the only nationally advertised menthol salve, leading an estimated thirty local and regional competitors.

The ad captured the spirit of the car-crazy nation. The banner threatened "Sunburn and Windburn," a woman's first concern when she was faced with the consequences of motoring around the countryside all day. "Cooling, Soothing, Healing Cream," all qualities that Mentholatum provided, reassured her that she could survive a Sunday drive with "Daily Use." (The "threat-reassurance" model was, and still is, an advertising winner.) Women continued to be Mentholatum's primary consumer demographic.

This ad also introduced the $1 Family Size jar nationwide. The best feature of the layout was the coupon for a free sample of Mentholatum for "handbag or vanity case." The "Jap Pocketbox" is arguably one of the most beautiful sample tins ever produced by an American proprietary.

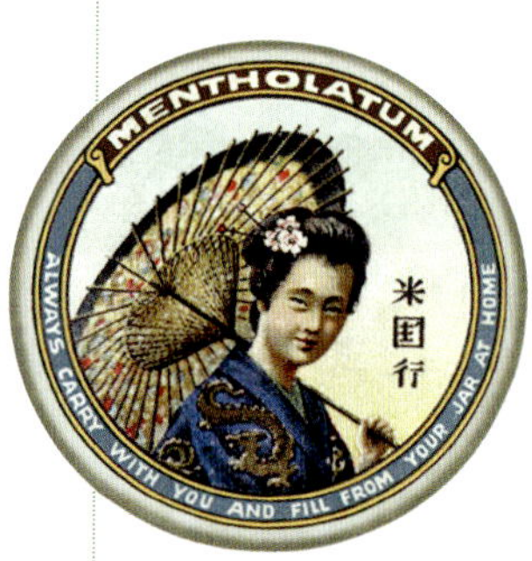

A. A. Hyde's aversion to print advertising softened as Mentholatum's market matured. One of the early magazine ads was in the September 1912 edition of *Cosmopolitan*. The ad depicted a fisherman applying Mentholatum to ward off mosquitoes. Another ad was found in the March 1913 edition of *The Modern Priscilla*. This ad depicted a young girl using a wooden snow shovel, and below the Mentholatum logo was an offer for free samples. Both ads gave the Buffalo, New York, address, which might indicate they were targeting the East Coast market where print advertising was possibly more influential and a more practical form of introduction. Mentholatum's first color advertisement was a full page in the July 1916 issue of *The Delineator*. The illustration was painted in the muted colors of the prairie and depicted a young couple joyriding in their roadster down a country road. The company said the purpose of the color ad was to draw attention to Mentholatum's "seasonable uses." With a few exceptions, magazine advertising from then on was limited to January and February for the cold season and July and August for the hay fever/bug bite/sunburn season.[13]

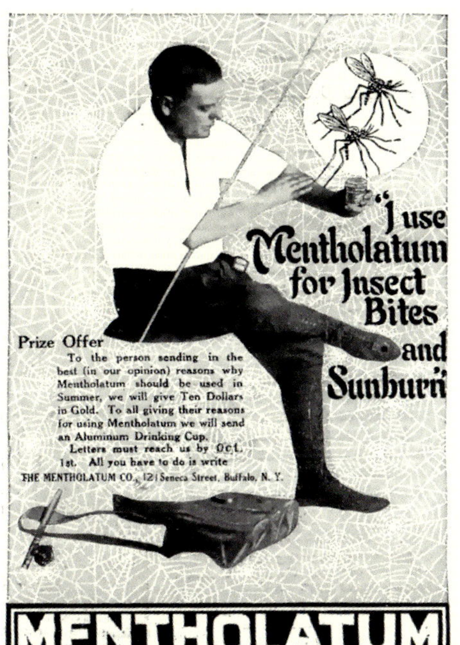

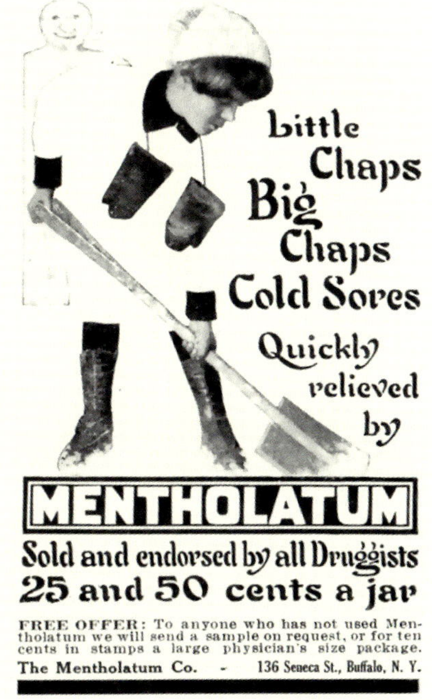

Early Magazine Ads

This advertisement (above) in the August 1912 *Good Housekeeping* magazine is one of the earliest yet found. It, and the March 1913 ad in *The Modern Priscilla* (right), represent a campaign that was characterized by the "fadeaway" illustration style of Coles Phillips, a popular artist of the day. The campaign ran from 1912 to 1914 and was managed through the Buffalo office. Launching a national advertising campaign at this time meant that the company was now prepared to meet the demands that would come from new sales from within each magazine's wide circulation. It also assured Mentholatum's promotion to a nationally recognized brand-name status.

On the evening of Thursday, April 22, 1915, a reporter from the *Wichita Eagle* called Hyde at his home to ask for his response to the recent charges filed against the company by the U.S. District Attorney, Fred Robertson. Hyde told the reporter, "This is the first I have heard and I do not care to say anything now." The suit filed in federal court contained oaths from Barclay C. Winslow, Charles M. Spring, Edward C. Merrill, and Francis P. Morgan charging that the Mentholatum Company made false claims on its labels in violation of the Pure Food and Drugs Act as amended in 1912. In October of 1912, Inspector Winslow of the Bureau of Chemistry purchased a sample of Mentholatum in Joplin, Missouri, from the C. M. Spring Drug Company and sent it to Merrill for analysis at the Bureau in Washington. Dr. Morgan, a physician in the Medico-chemical Analysis Division of the Bureau, analyzed the sample and found, according to his opinion, that it did not contain ingredients or medical agents

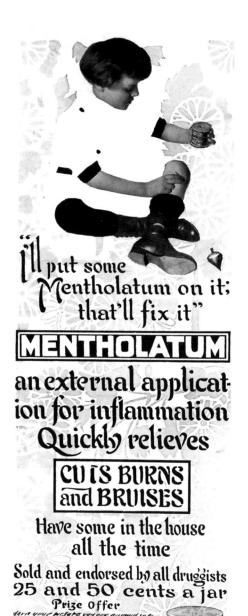

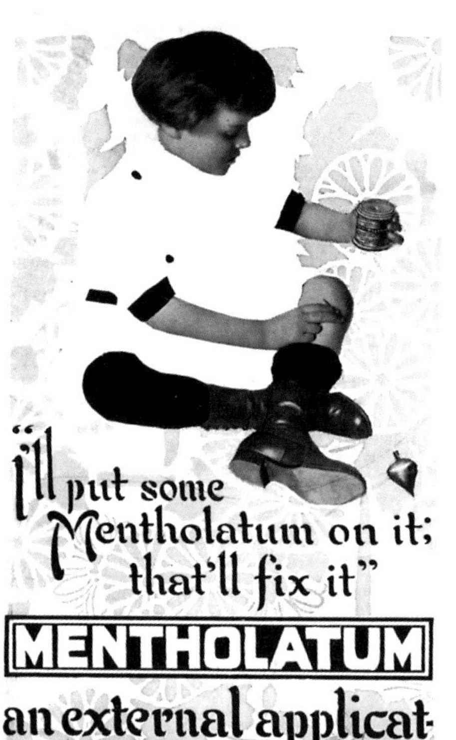

Ad Comp

An (as yet unknown) advertising agency used this comp to show management at Mentholatum what the ad might look like when printed in a magazine. Notice the scribble text at the bottom where a prize offer was being suggested. A variation of the ad ran in the October 1912 *Woman's Home Companion*. The comp was found at an estate sale in the vicinity of Hornell, New York, which is about seventy miles southeast of Buffalo.

effective as a remedy for piles, eczema, skin and scalp diseases, and pneumonia, as claimed on the label.

Attorney Robertson told the *Wichita Eagle*, "It was understood that A. A. Hyde is a man of very good standing in Wichita, and it was decided to bring the action against the corporation." The newspaper said the penalty for the violation was one year in jail and a $500 fine in the case of an individual or an officer of a company, and that corporations could only be fined. The *Wichita Eagle* came to Mentholatum's defense claiming it was "probably the best salve on the market, and its reputation has never been assailed. It has curative powers and the discussion brought up about it by the government relates only to certain alleged curative claims." The article concluded with a résumé of Hyde's philanthropies and called him a "pioneer and the head of a favorably known and excellent family."[14]

On September 27, 1915, the *Wichita Eagle* again reported:

> *The government's action against the Mentholatum Company for alleged mislabeling the Company's products was stopped by District Attorney Robertson. "The violation charged was a technical one under the Shirley [sic] amendment to the pure food and drug act and I came to the conclusion after investigation that the violation was unintentional," said the district attorney after the dismissal. "The company revised its printed matter to comply with the law soon after its passage and is now believed to be fully complying therewith."*[15]

To understand how this happened requires a closer look at the 1906 Pure Food and Drugs Act, and the fact it was regulated by three government agencies: Agriculture, Commerce, and the Treasury. The three agencies assigned enforcement of the law to the Bureau of Chemistry, which was run by scientists who were not familiar with law enforcement. There was confusion over the vague wording of the Act, and the Bureau was quickly overwhelmed with questions from the thousands of nostrum makers who were trying to comply with the law. To sort out who was compliant and who was not, the Bureau decided to issue serial numbers to each brand that passed a necessarily brief inspection of its label. The serial number was to be printed on new labels to indicate compliance and help alert druggists to the difference between legal and illegal packages on their shelves. Though the serial number was never meant as an endorsement or guarantee by the Bureau, many manufacturers nevertheless put "Guaranteed by the 1906 Pure Food and Drugs Act" on their labels. The Men-

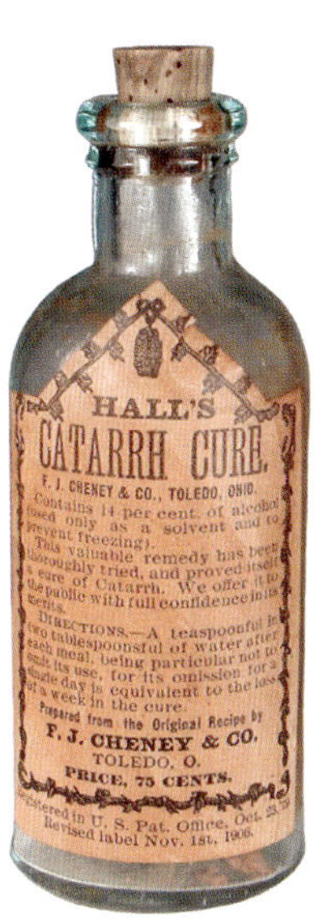

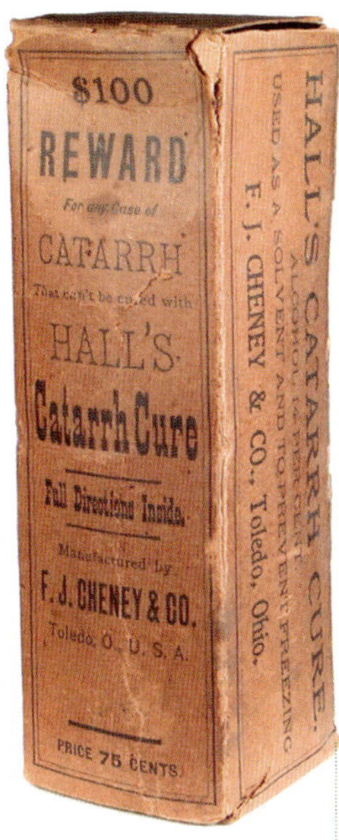

Hall's Wanted It Both Ways

When Congress passed the 1906 Pure Food and Drugs Act, it spelled the end to proprietary claims of cure on packaging and labels. Here the F. J. Cheney Company complied with the new law by revealing the content of 14 percent alcohol, yet it stubbornly refused to drop the word *cure* from the label, which would have put an end to its $100 challenge that had been running since 1886 (for twenty years). The Feds won in the end, and Cheney renamed its product Hall's Catarrh Medicine.

tholatum Company was no exception. Mentholatum's serial number was 605, and it was placed on new labeling in compliance with the law. Confusion also existed over the use of the word *cure*. After all, who could judge if something was a cure or not at a time when science knew very little about the pathologies of disease and the effects of drugs on them? This remained a bone of contention to manufacturers for years to come.[16]

Most of the large national brands came into compliance and dropped the word *cure* from their labels, as did Mentholatum. "Piso's Cure for Consumption," for instance, became "Piso's Remedy, A Medicine for Coughs and Colds." The Bureau took many smaller companies to court that failed to conform, but it found that the penalties levied by most judges amounted to a slap on the wrist. It quickly became evident throughout the industry that it was easier to plead guilty and pay a $50 fine than it was to go to court. The Bureau's inept enforcement tactics were failing, and the scientists' frustration was growing. Eventually, one proprietor chose to fight the law and in 1911 took it all the way to the Supreme Court and won, effectively crippling the 1906 Act. President Taft urged the Congress to fix it, and Congressman Swagar Sherley from Kentucky introduced a bill, which was passed with little fanfare on August 23, 1912. The Sherley Amendment honored the Bureau of Chemistry's wish to push restrictions beyond labeling to include all printed material. A brand was now considered misbranded "if its package or label shall bear or contain any statement, design, or device regarding the curative or therapeutic effect of such article or any of the ingredients or substances contained therein, which is false and fraudulent."[17]

(Text continues on page 78.)

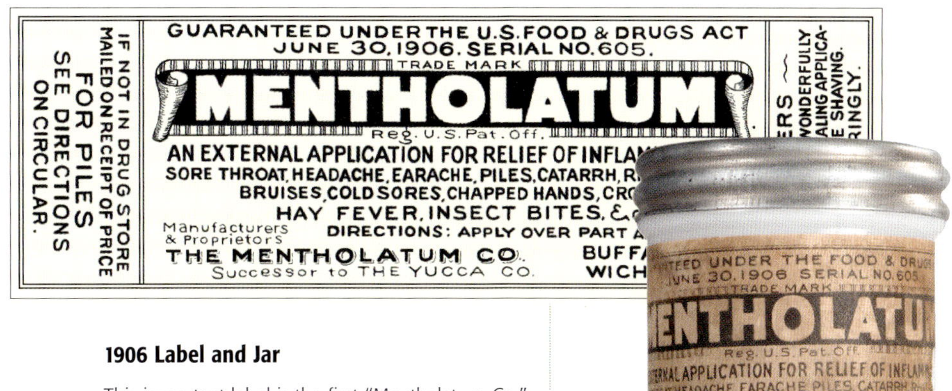

1906 Label and Jar

This important label is the first "Mentholatum Co." label and the first to comply with the 1906 Pure Food and Drugs Act. (See **J4** Catalog page C5.)

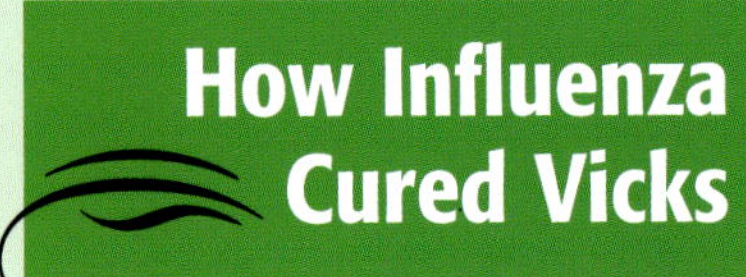

First Vicks Sample Tin

It was 1915, in St. Louis, Missouri, that the first sample tins were introduced. Before that, Vicks salesmen placed newspaper ads that offered free jars "as long as supplies last" to attract new customers into participating drugstores.

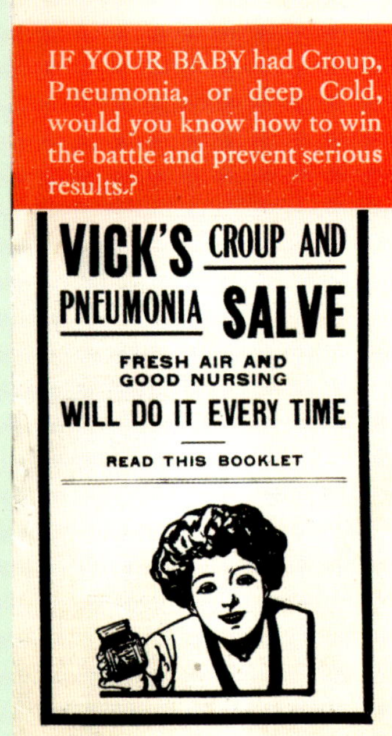

Vicks Was a Salve on a Mission

As they claimed in this 1912 handout, the makers of Vicks VapoRub truly believed that their salve was the best thing for croup and pneumonia! In spite of what some scientist or bureaucrat thought, they continued to boldly say so on their labels and circulars until Congress told them to remove the claim in 1935.

The Rise of Mentholatum's Nemesis

In 1913 a southern regional salve manufacturer began an ambitious marketing campaign to bring its product, Vicks VapoRub, north of the Mason-Dixon Line. By 1916 its salesmen had visited every Midwestern drugstore they could find that was willing to sign up with Vicks. Each new drugstore was given a limited number of free jars to hand out to the first customers who responded to a newspaper ad that the salesmen had placed the day before. However, this approach didn't reach many customers, so in 1917, they entered the New England states with a new campaign to distribute a free sample tin directly to every doorstep with a notice attached giving the name of the local druggist that carried their product. Vicks salesmen hired boys to deliver the tins house to house. This process took four years to complete. The success of the New England model inspired the solution to the problem of reaching new customers in their next campaign, the vast western territory. Vicks mailed thirty-one million, or eight freight-car loads of sample tins through the newly completed rural free-delivery system during a fifty-day period.[18]

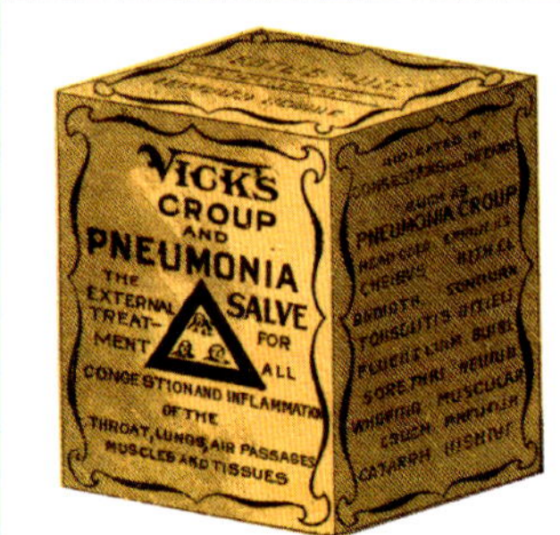

On March 11, 1918, while war raged in Europe, a sturdy farm boy recruited to fight in the war came down with a case of bird or swine flu. Within days his influenza had spread throughout the army's training camp at Fort Riley, Kansas, and began spreading like wildfire throughout the army and adjacent civilian contacts all the way to the Western Front. Erroneously named the Spanish Flu, it became the first of three pandemic waves that would circle the earth during the coming year. The second and most virulent phase began in August and would peak in October. When the third and final phase ended in February of 1919, an estimated twenty million people had died in India alone. In the United States half a million perished, with some parts of Alaska and the Pacific Islands losing more than half of their populations. On the Western Front, forty-three thousand or 80 percent of America's total battle deaths were credited to the influenza, as was the eventual failure of the German offensive that brought an end to the war in November.

The disruption in American community life brought cities almost to a standstill. An estimated twenty-five million clinical cases of influenza were observed during the second-phase pandemic alone—one out of every four U.S. citizens. Philadelphia saw 4,600 deaths in October even though its public meeting places were closed. Hospitals were overflowing and unable to help the victims who clamored for medicine. Unfortunately, the reality in 1918 was that there were no true medicines for viral pneumonia and there was little that caregivers could do but provide prayer and comfort for the afflicted. Healthy adults would sicken and die within twenty-four hours. Entire families were stricken with no one to care for them.[19]

Americans celebrated the end of the war with white cotton masks on. They celebrated New Year's with them off. Then the third-phase pandemic hit—this time with less force and fewer deaths. Pandemic influenza is the most virulent form of influenza virus and is the most likely to result in pneumonia. Coincidentally, the Vick Chemical Company was in the midst of its aggressive sales campaign for their "Croup, Cold and Pneumonia Salve" when the pandemics struck. A panicked public grabbed every jar they could get their hands on. The company called in their salesmen to help man the factory, which ran twenty-four hours a day in an attempt to meet the demand. Sales jumped from $613,000 in 1917 to $2,940,000 in 1919. The epidemic money put Vicks VapoRub into a position overnight to compete head-to-head with Mentholatum.

Pictorial Review for January, 1921

A Gift From Dixie

GREENSBORO, N.C., has a famous drug store where O. Henry, America's greatest story writer, was a clerk, and where Vicks VapoRub was invented by Lunsford Richardson.

Believing that colds should be treated by inhalation and absorption, rather than through the stomach, Druggist Richardson worked out a salve combining the penetrating and vaporizing virtues of Camphor, Menthol, Turpentine, Eucalyptus, Thyme, Cedar, Juniper Tar, Wintergreen and other essential oils.

For hours after Vicks is applied, its volatile ingredients, released as vapors by the body heat, are breathed right into the affected air passages.

Vicks in a few years became Dixie's favorite treatment for all cold troubles. It was just being introduced in the North when influenza broke out. Everybody wanted Vicks. The laboratory was swamped with orders. Ingredients were bought by tons. Production was speeded up. Over 250,000 jars were made in one day. Since then Vicks, from coast to coast, has been the standby in millions of homes for cold troubles, skin eruptions, cuts, burns, bruises, sores, stings, and other inflammations of skin or tissues.

Get a jar of Vicks. Melt a little in a spoon and inhale the vapors. You'll know at once how valuable it is. You'll want Vicks with you always. Write to Vick Chemical Co., Box 9190, Greensboro, N. C. A generous trial tin will be sent.

By Ships That Sail The Seven Seas

Through Vicks, the far ends of the earth supply to American mothers the best of Nature's remedies for colds of head, throat or chest, for skin hurts or itchings and for various bodily aches and pains.

In Vicks there is—Camphor from Formosa—Oil of Eucalyptus from Australia—Menthol from Japan—Oil of Juniper Tar from Northern Africa—Oil of Thyme from the South of France—Oil of Nutmeg from the Dutch East Indies—Oil of Turpentine from our own Southern states—and certain other aromatic, volatile oils.

These valuable ingredients are combined in salve form by the exclusive Vick process.

To be had wherever medicines are sold

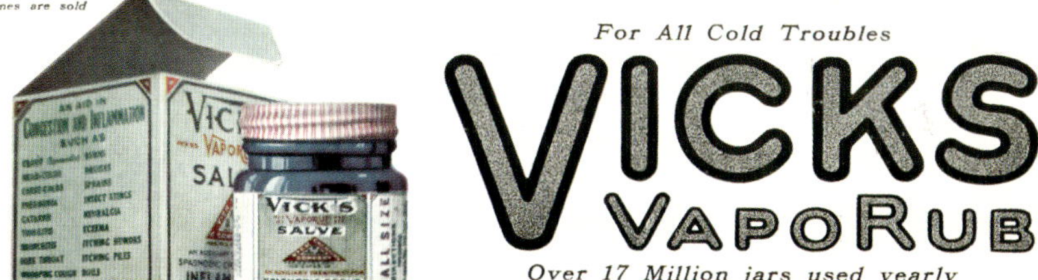

Bragging Rights

Proud of the role Vicks played during the influenza pandemic, and now able to afford to advertise in national magazines, Smith Richardson first composed his company's mythology in this full-page color ad.

It would take another decade before scientists would discover the viral cause of influenza, and all the while Vicks continued to list pneumonia on its list of remedies. Smith Richardson, the son of the founder and at that time the president of the company, when faced by the new scientific evidence, added the modifier "incipient" pneumonia. It would take a visit to the House Subcommittee investigating the Food and Drugs law in 1935 before he would testify that the wording would be removed. (See "The Competition," page 184.)

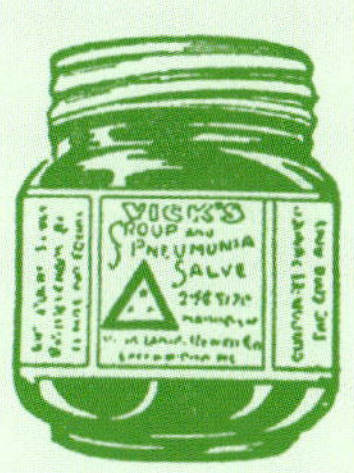

The amendment's passage inspired the press to renew its scrutiny of nostrum makers. Their old adversary, Samuel Hopkins Adams, again wrote a series of critical articles that were published by *Collier's* between 1912 and 1913. (Adams also wrote a novel, *The Clarion*, critical of the industry.) The Bureau's inspectors were back in business with a vengeance. It's not known exactly which "labels and booklets" were collected by Inspector Winslow on October 24, 1912, but the fact that he did it only three months after the passage of the amendment makes it possible that the one gross (144) jars shipped from Wichita to the Spring Drug Company were from old stock. Because the words *eczema*, *skin and scalp diseases*, and *pneumonia* are clearly not on any labels that have been found to date, it would indicate that the "booklet" (or folded circular that came packed with each jar) must have been the culprit. Curiously, the word *piles* (hemorrhoids) was continued on jar labels after 1912. The 1916 booklet titled "Effective Uses of Mentholatum" was printed in eight languages and retained the word *eczema*. The only changes the company made to the new 1915 jar labels were the replacement of "For Relief of Inflammations" with "To Relieve or Soothe," and they added "Look for This Signature on Each Package" with a facsimile of A. A. Hyde's signature above the trademark scroll.[20]

The signature was obviously a big concession for Hyde, who shunned the limelight and insisted that he was only a steward of the wealth his salve had earned. A.A.'s sons were aware of the fact that while Mentholatum's brand recognition had grown, public awareness of A. A. Hyde's largesse had grown concurrently. After

A. A. Hyde's Formal Signature

When seventeen-year-old Bert Hyde first arrived in Leavenworth to assist his brother George at the bank, he was advised to hire a tutor to improve his poor penmanship or lose the position. Although he improved enough to keep legible books, Hyde's hand never was very good. His letters to family were rounded and sloppy, and his formal writing was sharp, self-conscious, and extremely inconsistent in style.

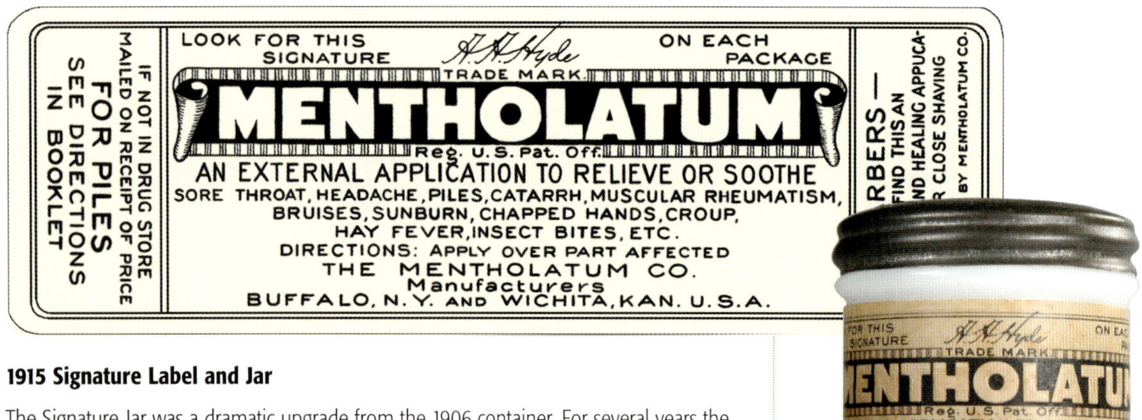

1915 Signature Label and Jar

The Signature Jar was a dramatic upgrade from the 1906 container. For several years the traditional embossing on the side had been removed and placed on the bottom of the jar. A new embossed tin lid had replaced the earlier plain lid. The paper label was die-cut with rounded corners, and the banner lettering was embossed. (See J10 Catalog page C6.)

the events of 1915, it become clear that the two had merged in the public mind. Hyde was frequently listed with the top philanthropists of his day, like John D. Rockefeller and Cyrus McCormick. His support of Christian missionary work, the YMCA's International Committee, and John R. Mott's World's Student Christian Federation had spread his name worldwide. Hyde's celebrity helped introduce Mentholatum to distant markets, which in turn boosted sales and increased the number of beneficiaries.[21]

With the introduction of a new eight-ounce jar, the "Collapsible Tube," and *Menthology*, 1916 was a big year for the company. The large size jar was called the "Family or Hospital Size" and was priced at $1. It proved hard to sell, though, and after an eleven-year run it was discontinued in 1927. The war in Europe caused a shortage of tin that delayed the introduction of the new tube until the end of the year. Tubes were filled and packaged at the Buffalo plant. The publication in January of a new "house organ," or newsletter, launched a twenty-eight-year run that produced 103 issues before ending in 1944. The first issue was named *Mentholatum Magazine*, and it announced a contest to find a better name. Ten druggists shared the $100 prize money for suggesting *Menthology* out of several thousand entries.[22]

Trial Box

(See S7 Catalog page C38.)

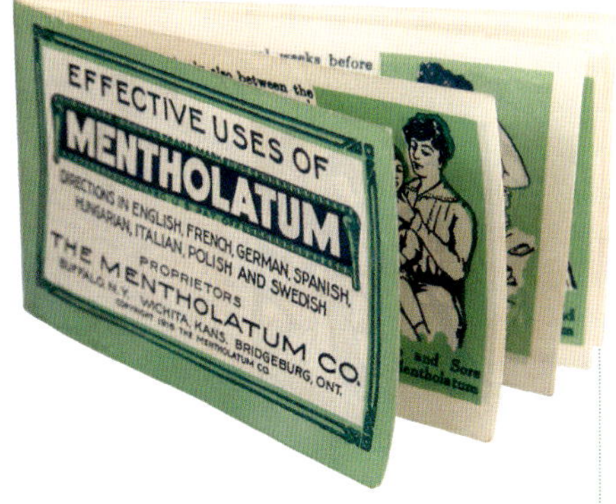

Effective Uses

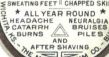

In 1916, a twenty-three-page booklet replaced the folded circular that accompanied jars and tubes of Mentholatum.

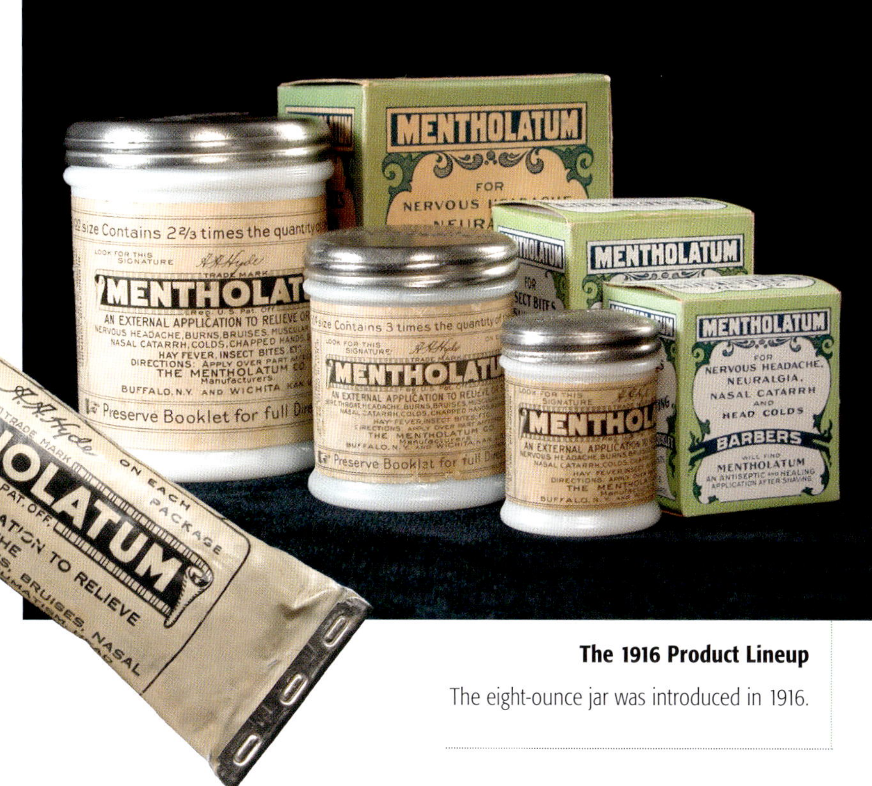

New Collapsible One-Ounce Tube and Sample Tube

(See T1 Catalog page C26.)

The 1916 Product Lineup

The eight-ounce jar was introduced in 1916.

Menthology

A neutral nonexplosive pocket Magazine of Ammunition for the Druggist & Clerk. Advertising Suggestions, Sales Helps, Wit & Humor.

Menthology's first editor was A. A. Hyde's third son, Alex Hyde (1880–1962), who produced the first forty-six issues before he left in 1927. His tenure was characterized by smart and witty commentary, whimsical illustrations, and contributions from many talented artists and writers. McCormick-Armstrong Press in Wichita was the printer. Walt Mason, "the poetic philosopher," and humorist H. E. Gonder made regular contributions to the early issues.[23] (For more see Catalog pages C178–C189.)

Alex Hyde Trick Shot

Alex Hyde's legacy includes positions as corporate officer and treasurer, founding editor of *Menthology*, and, as one employee remembered, the only other Hyde besides A.A. who regularly attended employee dinners and functions. "He was the life of the party" recalled ninety-four-year-old George Jordan (1908–2003), who was a printer's assistant in the Wichita plant from 1927 to 1929. Alex always wore a western-style hat and liked to show off his skills with a six-shooter. He could hit a nickel that was thrown into the air, and George swore that he actually saw Alex do it!

Highlights from the First Issue

Seven million jars sold last year [1915]. An amusing story told: "A Missouri druggist tells us he has the best Mentholatum customer in the world—uses it for everything and devotes his spare time to manufacturing new uses. The other day this Booster made his will . . . after completing the document he added a codicil as follows: 'After you think I am dead rub my forehead, nose, throat, and chest well with Mentholatum. If I don't show signs of life in fifteen minutes, I'm sure dead and you can bury me.'" Offer of $100 to name the magazine.

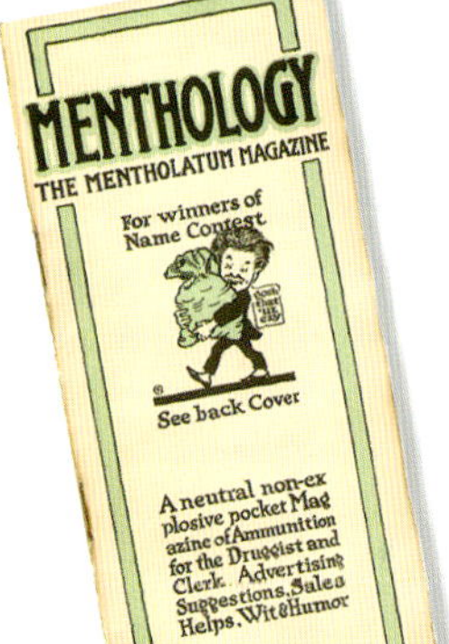

From the Second Issue

The ten name winners were each sent checks for $10. It was announced that plans were in the works for the company's first national magazine ad campaign—to use full pages in color starting in July. Thousands of letters and cards were received from druggists after launching the first edition. January sales of Mentholatum ran 150,000 jars ahead of any previous month. Prize money was offered for new window display designs. The collapsible tube's introduction was delayed.

THE DREAMER

Written for *Menthology*

by Walt Mason

The clerk was mixing up some powders, which were prescribed by Dr. Chowders, for the relief of old Dad Swankles, who had gout in both his ankles. And as the clerk went on compounding, his thoughts roamed far from things surrounding. He thought about the blooming Carrie—the girl that he intends to marry, with eyes like stars and hair so curly, and angel smile and molars pearly. He thought of presents he would buy her, when his small salary went higher. He thought of rivals who were scheming to end his pleasant hopes and dreaming. His thoughts all topics were pursuing—except the work that he was doing.

Old Swankles took the pale white powders that were prescribed by Dr. Chowders, and then he hollered Bloody Murder, and from his cottage kicked a girder, and then he crawled beneath the stable, and died as fast as he was able. The absent-minded clerk had killed him, and now a monument we built him.

Oh, keep your mind on what you're doing, whate'er the task you are pursuing! The idle head that dreams and wonders, a garden is of fatal blunders.

Uncle Walt

Vol. 1, spring edition 1916, no. 2

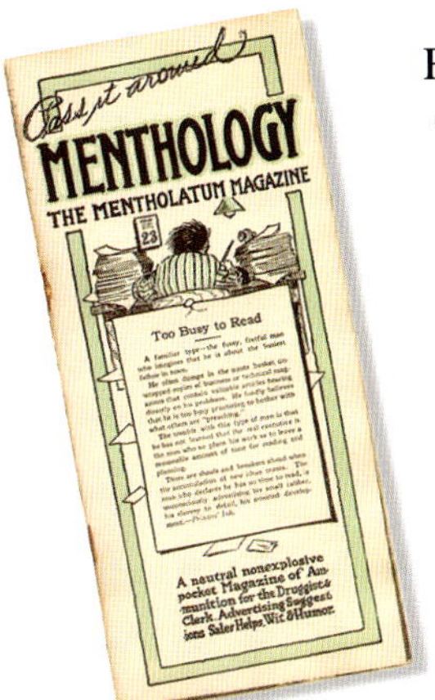

From the Third Issue

The most prominent uses for Mentholatum are: "tired and aching feet, sunburn, windburn, insect bites, after shaving." July 1916—"Mentholatum is now put up in $1.00 size opal jar, called family or hospital size. Just as we are going to press, we learn that our Buffalo House succeeded in getting a few collapsible tubes. Long before our next issue we hope to have the new tube on the market." A new lantern slide was also introduced.

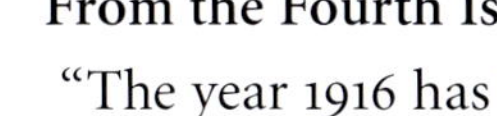

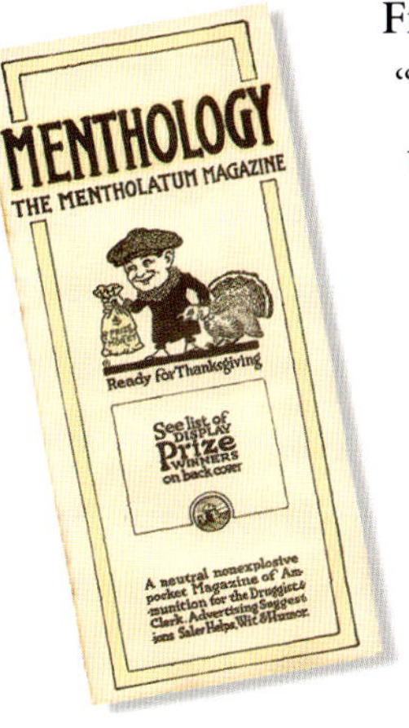

From the Fourth Issue

"The year 1916 has been, in nearly all lines, the most prosperous in history, and this Thanksgiving will find the druggist with many things to be thankful for." Collapsible tube is now obtainable from jobbers. New fire insurance provision announced—if stock is ruined by fire a starter assortment will be sent. "As we grow older we realize that the greatest pleasures of life come from what we do for others. In this connection it may interest you to know that some years ago 40% of the stock of the Mentholatum Company was given to a chartered Benevolent Association [A. A. Hyde's philanthropy]. Thus over one-third of the profits on Mentholatum go constantly to worthy benevolence."

The editor concluded the first year of *Menthology* by requesting a vote whether the magazine should be continued or not, and he received a thumbs-up from the druggists. Letters continued to arrive with sales suggestions and ideas for new uses. In the spring 1917 edition, J. C. Scott, a druggist in Bethel, Ohio, suggested Mentholatum could be used in a "De Vilbiss Nebulizer, No. 49" and explained in detail how to do this. Walter J. Moffitt, the druggist in Cortez, Colorado, reported he sold Mentholatum to cowboys who complained of dyspepsia caused by a diet of baking powder biscuits and strong coffee. Moffitt connected a doctor's prescription for an intestinal antiseptic tablet that contained menthol and thymol with the ingredients in Mentholatum and recommended a small spoonful be mixed into a cup of hot

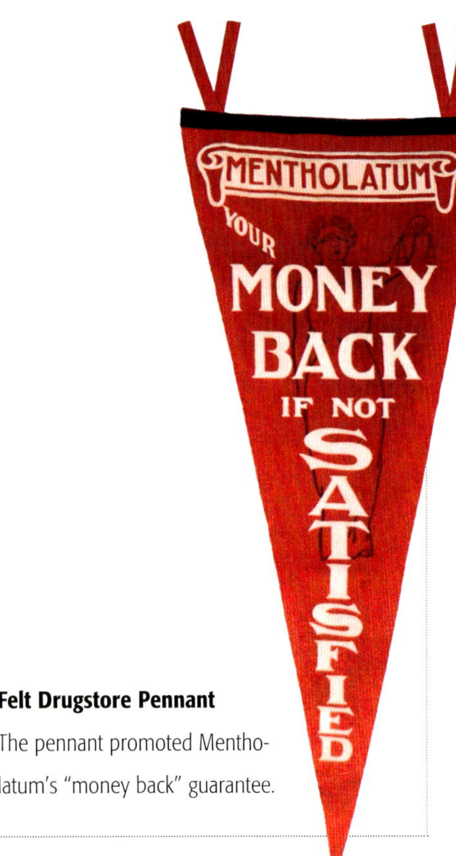

Felt Drugstore Pennant

The pennant promoted Mentholatum's "money back" guarantee.

coffee for relief. The company consulted a doctor who concluded it "certainly ought to give relief to the stomach and it couldn't hurt the cowboy." The editor reminded his readers of the company's "absolute guarantee of satisfaction . . . to make refund cheerfully without question." The Mentholatum Company refunded the full retail price to the druggist whenever a jar was returned and claimed that in the past year "the returns were about one jar in each million sold, or about eight jars in the twelve months—certainly a most pleasing record." Eight million jars were sold in 1917.[24]

With war raging in Europe, Mentholatum began stockpiling supplies. On January 31, 1917, Germany launched unrestricted submarine warfare, and shipping lanes throughout the world were virtually closed down. The company continued to manufacture with no change to its price schedule. But by July, it had exhausted its stockpile and was forced to buy at inflated war prices. Determined to keep the retail price fixed, the company announced in *Menthology* that it could no longer provide free incentives to the druggists. More belt tightening was required in the summer of 1918, when notice was reluctantly given that the wholesale price would be raised beginning on September 1. Cost of raw materials had risen as much as 100 percent, it said. It is known that the company was forced at times during the war to make substitutions when raw materials became scarce, and this might explain why jars from this period show up with plain aluminum lids instead of the typical embossed tin lids.[25]

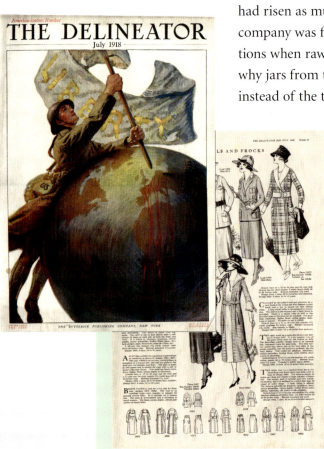

Butterick Trio

Ebeneezer Butterick created the first graded sewing pattern in 1863 and published several magazines to advertise his patterns. These included *Ladies Quarterly of Broadway Fashions* (est. 1867), *Metropolitan* (est. 1868), and *Delineator* (est. 1873). By the turn of the century, *Delineator* was considered the top women's service and fashion magazine, and it became Mentholatum's preferred advertising venue. Butterick operated the largest commercial publishing operation in the United States, next only to the government printing office in Washington, D.C.[26]

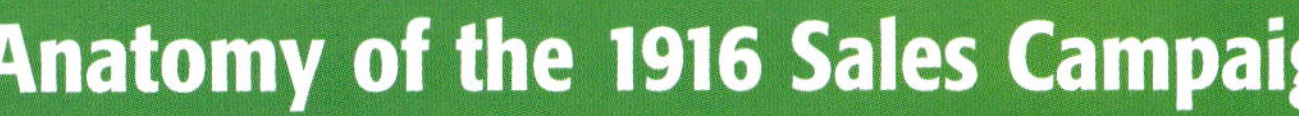

Anatomy of the 1916 Sales Campaign

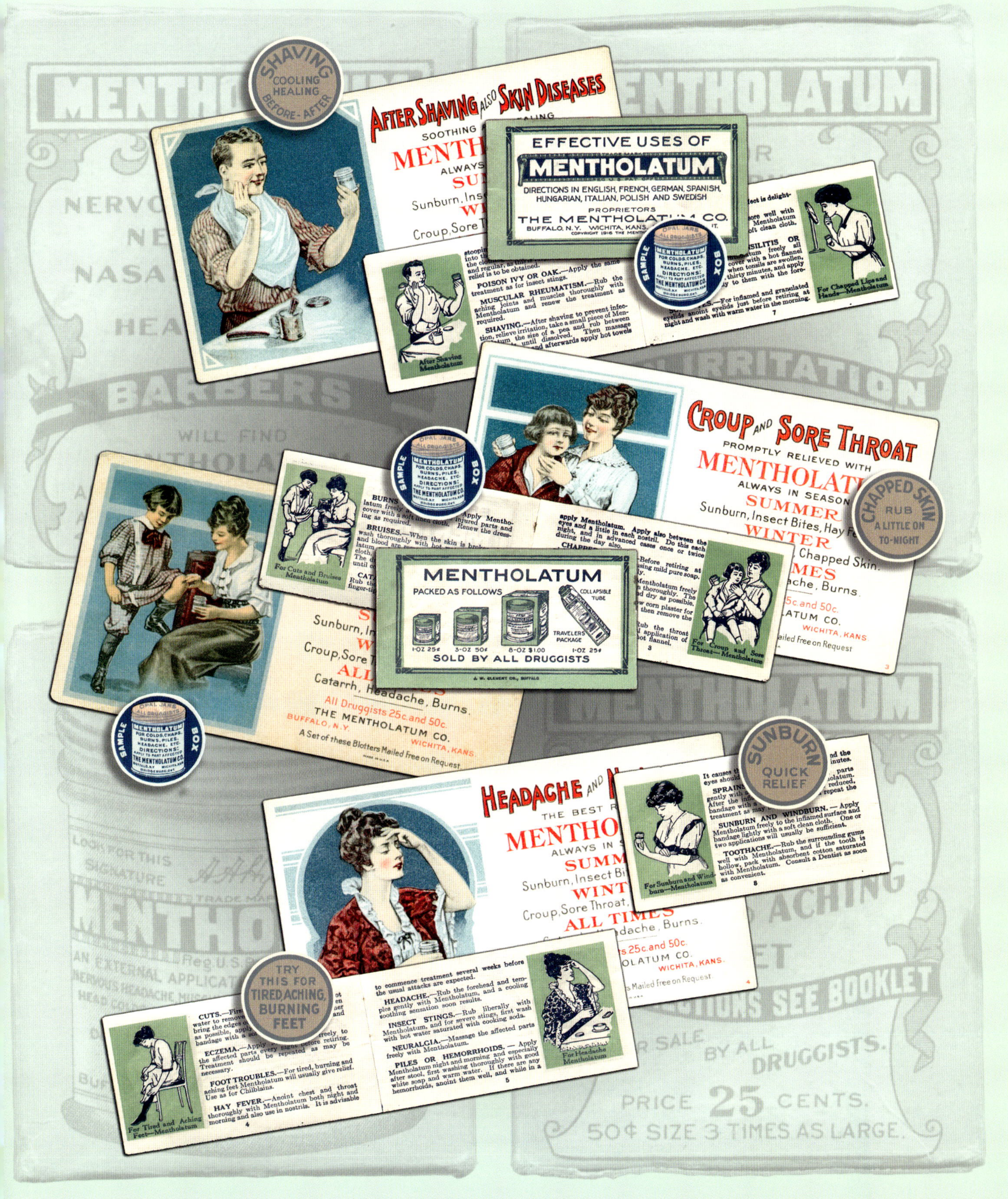

Little Nurse™—1917

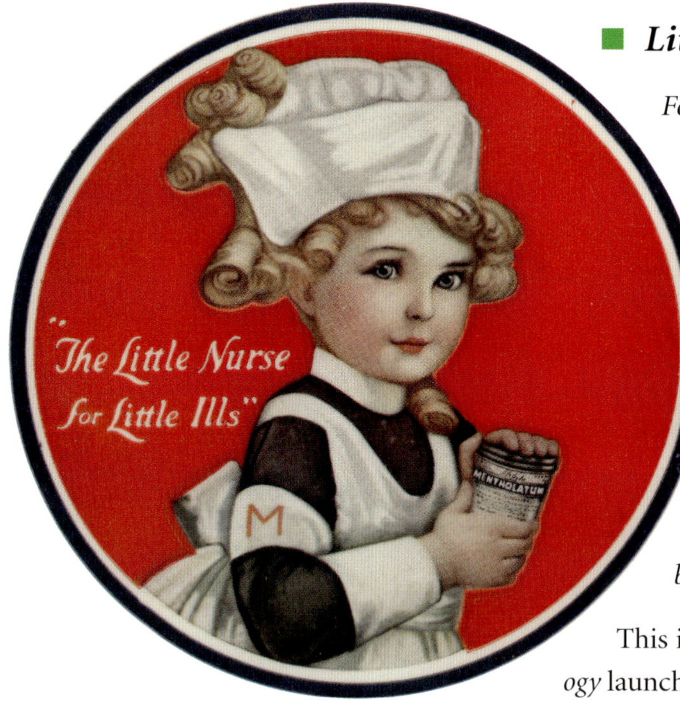

For several years we have been working on a campaign of magazine advertising for Mentholatum and have at last O.K.'d complete plans and copy. This started to run in the July issues of the Butterick trio and other women's magazines. The copy for this campaign has been most carefully prepared, and is exceptionally good, we think. In time the druggists should reap the benefit in largely increased sales.[27]

This inauspicious announcement in *Mentholology* launched the career of Little Nurse. The little girl with curly golden locks, short-short nurse outfit, and patent leather shoes captured the hearts of millions who saw her image on billboards, on posters, and in magazine ads. Her portrait graces one of the most sought after advertising tins in the collectors' market today. The "Blue Nurse" tin (as it is now called) was, and still is, a masterpiece of composition, charm, and color. It is a treasured cameo.

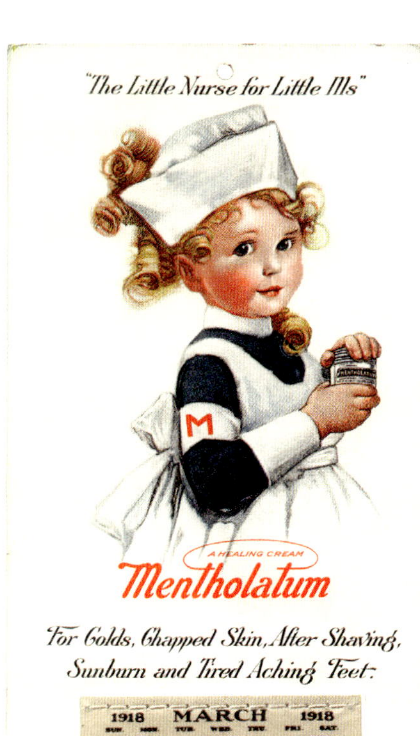

Limited-Edition Desk Calendar

This easel-back calendar is missing the first two months of the year because delays in printing kept distribution to druggists until March 1918. Pages for January and February 1919 were added at the end to make it a full year.

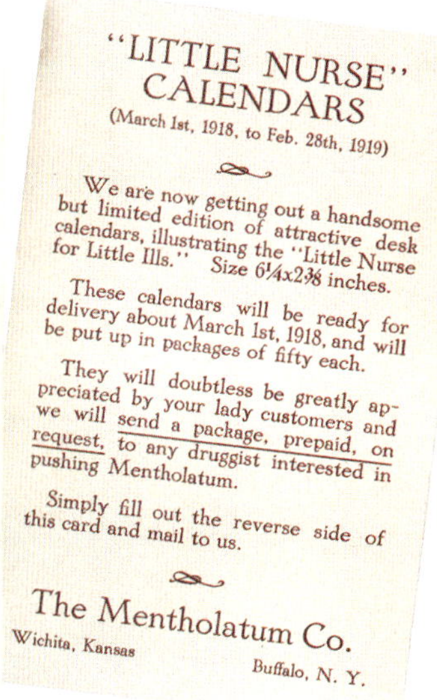

"LITTLE NURSE" CALENDARS

(March 1st, 1918, to Feb. 28th, 1919)

We are now getting out a handsome but limited edition of attractive desk calendars, illustrating the "Little Nurse for Little Ills." Size 6¼x2⅜ inches.

These calendars will be ready for delivery about March 1st, 1918, and will be put up in packages of fifty each.

They will doubtless be greatly appreciated by your lady customers and we will send a package, prepaid, on request, to any druggist interested in pushing Mentholatum.

Simply fill out the reverse side of this card and mail to us.

The Mentholatum Co.

Wichita, Kansas — Buffalo, N. Y.

The Little Nurse profile worked so well on the tin's circular format that her image remained in use on sample tins long after she had been retired from print.

Under a picture of the first Little Nurse window display, *Menthology* told the druggists, "This New Cut-Out on your counter or top shelf will tie up your store to the Magazine Advertising Campaign now running in women's magazines of National circulation amounting to Over Four Million Families." Then, almost as an afterthought, they introduced her at the bottom of the page: "'The Little Nurse for Little Ills' is featured in the campaign." Unfortunately, the magazine ad campaign "featured" Little Nurse for only seven years, from 1917 to 1923. After that, she had a few walk-on roles in handouts, remained in syndication through the 1930s on several sample tin variations, and experienced a comeback in Japan, where she is still employed and covered by trademark protection today. Throughout her magazine career she was called "The Little Nurse for Little Ills." Later on, by 1927, she became "The Little Nurse for Many Ills."[28]

People say that the young Shirley Temple looked a lot like Little Nurse. Although Shirley Temple was born in 1928, five years after Little Nurse's last magazine appearance, the woman who dressed Shirley for success, her mother, was an impressionable girl when Little Nurse was in the media spotlight. David Moore at the Mentholatum Company wrote in the spring 1997 employee newsletter, "it is rumored that Mr. Hyde's grand daughter was the model for the artist." Little Nurse looks to be about seven or eight years old, so the model should have been born around 1909. There are several Hyde girls who might fit the bill. A good candidate would be Betty Hyde, b. 1910, whose father Albert was A.A.'s oldest son. As far as influencing the artist is concerned, the Morton Salt Umbrella Girl, created in 1914, might be a consideration, but the 1912 easelback display "Don't Cry Mentholatum" (see page 68) clearly has the proper proximity pedigree.[29]

Portrait Tins

The Little Nurse image was so well suited to the circular format of sample tins that it continued to be used long after she was retired from print advertising. "Little Ills" was in use from 1917 to 1927 (top); "Many Ills" followed (center). The large tin was discontinued when the Wichita plant was closed in 1936. There was a smaller Little Nurse tin in use at the time as well as a thin green tin introduced in the late 1930s (right).

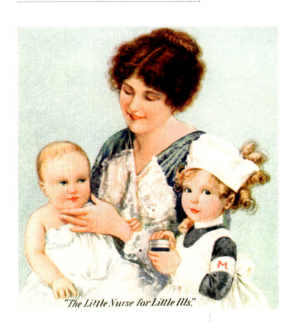

World events overwhelm the story at this point. The war in Europe was drawing the United States ever closer into its bloody grip. Then, on April 6, 1917, only a few months after German U-boats began hunting in the international shipping lanes, America declared war on Germany. The country shifted into high gear to train and supply troops to fill the trenches that lacerated France and Belgium. George Hyde, the youngest Hyde boy, joined up and saw the Hun in France where he was wounded by shrapnel. He returned home safely, to the relief of his family. While troops were fighting in Europe, the company had a minor skirmish on the home front. In 1918, Block & Co., a Brooklyn, New York, soap manufacturer, began marketing a product it called "Mentholanum," which provoked quick action to stop them. The Mentholatum Company took its complaint to the Federal Trade Commission, which was

"The Little Nurse for Little Ills."

The Artist's Contribution

Over the years several artists were responsible for interpreting Little Nurse. The unnamed artist of this remarkable painting, which was created for a blotter composition, captured a particularly sensitive portrayal of Mentholatum's sweetheart.

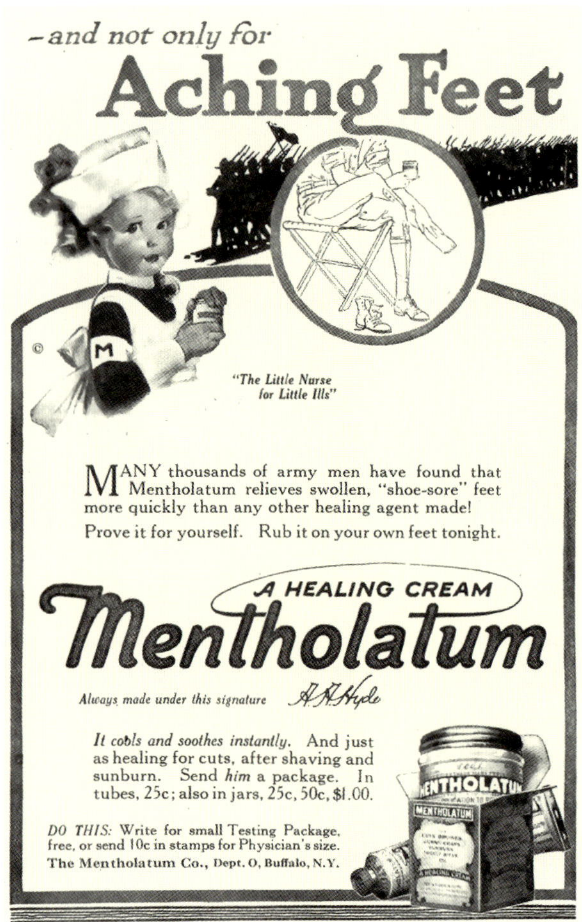

Little Nurse Aids the Troops

In 1918, World War I was on the mind of every American, and this ad suggests one more way to support the troops–send them Mentholatum!

founded by Woodrow Wilson in 1914 to safeguard against monopolies, unfair methods of competition, and false advertising. The case became the FTC's first drug-related action, and its decision ordered the Brooklyn-based pharmaceutical company to cease and desist from using the deceptive label.[30]

In April 1918, the factory had to be closed due to a wartime freight embargo. The spring edition of *Menthology* was shipped a month after its traditional April 1 due date. A jar of Mentholatum became a staple in the "comfort bags" sent by families to their boys in uniform. Private Tommy Cleves wrote to his sister from the Base Hospital in Deming, New Mexico, to request she send him a big jar of Mentholatum: "That is our first aid here, if it's a cut—'Mentholatum,' a cold or sore throat—'Mentholatum,' and the same with sore feet or after shaving a fellow uses lots of it where you have to take care of yourself to be up and coming." A letter sent in by Ralph Quackenbush, dated February 17, 1919, from Trier, Germany, related this story: "One of the boys of this squad—Goodwin of Terre Haute, Ind.—carried a jar of Mentholatum with him all thru the war. On the second day of November he gave first aid to a wounded Boche, applying Mentholatum to the wound. The Boche was so grateful that he reached under his coat for a cherished Iron Cross and presented it to Goodwin." Quackenbush went on to say, "The last copy [of *Menthology*] was received when we were holding the lines between Beney and Thiacourt after the St. Mihiel drive. We had been without printed matter of any kind for days so *Menthology* went the rounds, the boys waiting their turn to read it like men waiting in a barber shop for a shave Saturday night." Quackenbush was most likely a drugstore clerk before the war.[31]

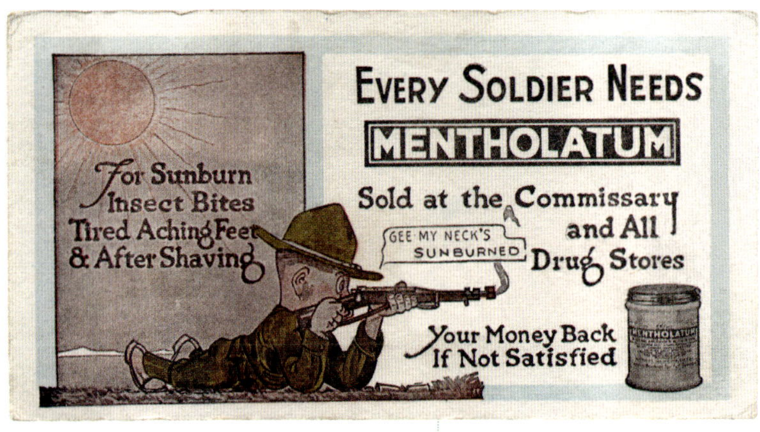

WWI Blotter

Considering this blotter's clean condition, it's safe to say it didn't see any "action" during the war.

A recipe for the best "Skeeter Beater" was printed in the summer 1918 issue of *Menthology*. It suggested adding "2 drams oil Pennyroyal with 2 drams oil Citronella" to Mentholatum. This might have been a hint that the company was thinking about, if not actively working on, a new

"Skeeter Beater"

Two brand names were in the running for the Mentholatum Company's repellant, and comps were printed in the type style to be used. Skeetolatum lost the vote and went into A. A. Hyde's scrapbook. Insectolatum won and went into production—when and for how long is not clear. Sample tin and envelope (left and below) promoted the one-ounce box and tin shown at right. Examples have been found only in Washington state.

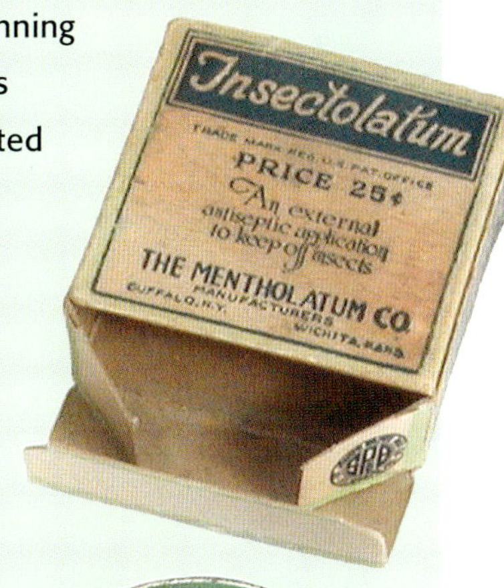

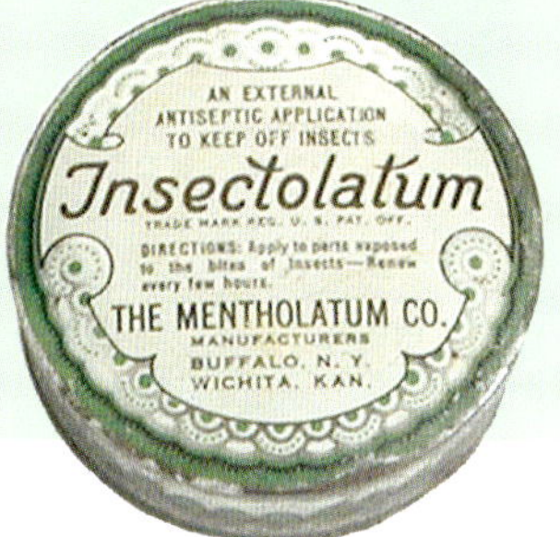

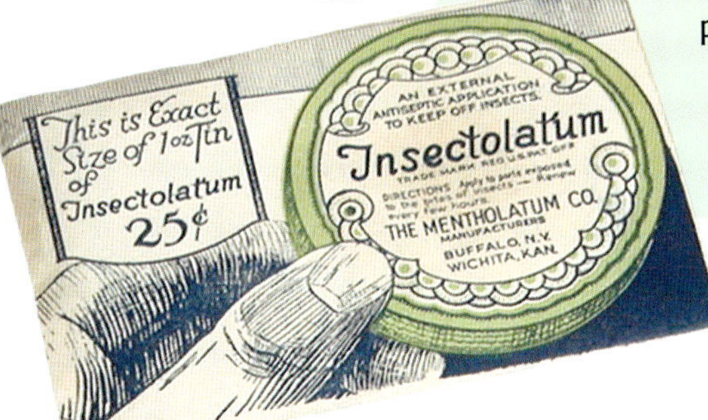

citronella-based product. One test label listed the contents: "6% Oil Pennyroyal, 4% Oil Citronella, as active repellents and 90% Mentholatum inert as a repellent."[32]

The Spanish influenza pandemic in 1918 struck millions of people worldwide. Twenty-five percent of all Americans fell ill, and 500,000 died. Although mentioned only briefly in *Menthology*, influenza was the subject of this letter sent to the company: "My wife, baby, and myself had influenza, but my daughter of four years was not afflicted. She has always had a great love for Mentholatum and while we were sick she kept her face covered with it. I really believe it saved her from taking the influenza. F. A. Evertsbusch, Ph.G., of Pateros, Washington." The editor noted that camphor had been highly recommended in the prevention of influenza. As letters from druggists and doctors came in on the subject, the editor printed the following recipe for the treatment of influenza and resulting pneumonia: "Melt contents of a 3 ounce jar (50¢ size) of Mentholatum, add 1 ounce turpentine. Apply thoroughly twice a day over the lungs, both front and back." Not much had changed since 1908, when the druggist in Willard, Ohio, doled out Vaseline, camphor oil, and turpentine for a cold.[33]

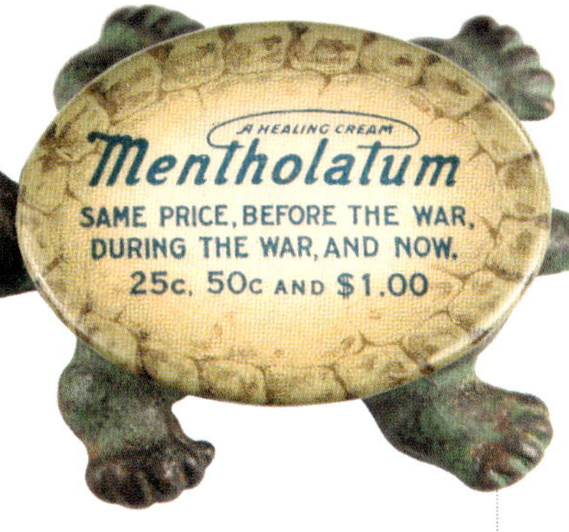

Paperweight Turtle

This cast-iron novelty with celluloid pinback shell announced the status quo.

Mighty Menthol

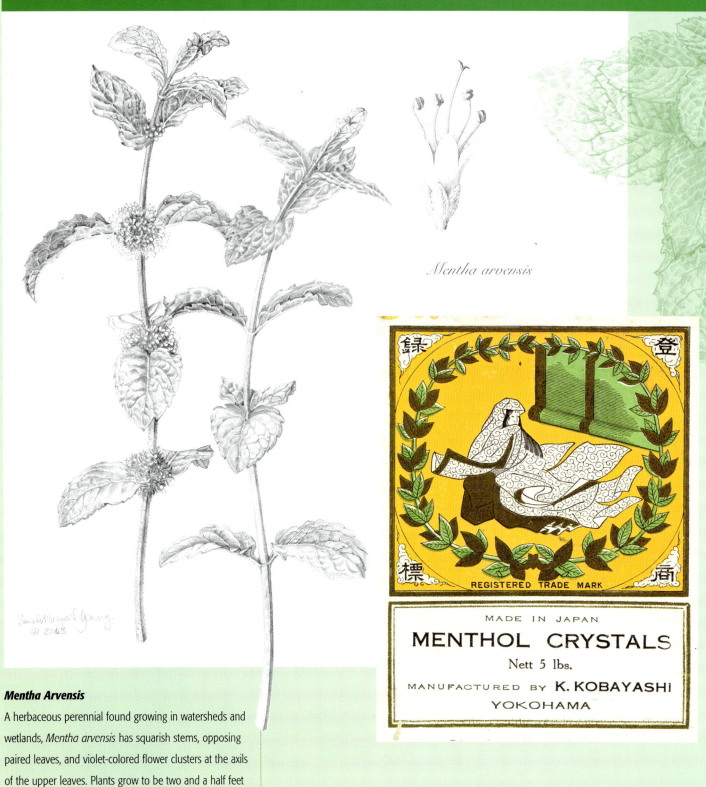

Mentha Arvensis

A herbaceous perennial found growing in watersheds and wetlands, *Mentha arvensis* has squarish stems, opposing paired leaves, and violet-colored flower clusters at the axils of the upper leaves. Plants grow to be two and a half feet tall from creeping rootstocks in low to midlevel elevations.

MENTHOLOGY

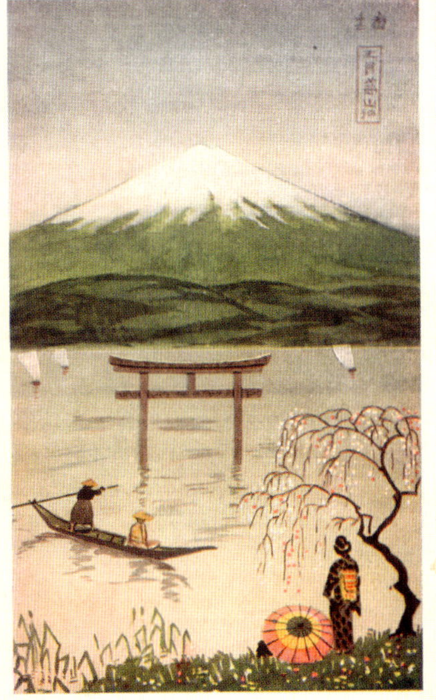

FUJI-YAMA---Almost in the shade of this sacred mountain, the fields of Japan produce the Peppermint Oil, from which comes the Menthol for Mentholatum. In the course of a year we import many tons of Menthol for the manufacture of Mentholatum.

Menthol

A crystalline organic compound of the isoprenoid family, menthol crystals liquefy when triturated (crushed) and mixed with camphor oil. Menthol's melting point is 42° to 44° Celsius. An original package label (opposite), c. 1900, is from A. A. Hyde's scrapbook. K. Kobayashi & Co., Ltd., an early supplier of menthol crystals to Mentholatum, was established in 1883 and is still in business today.

The two most obvious characteristics of peppermint are its strong, instantaneous smell and its cooling taste. This is why breath mints help us disguise the odor of bad breath and produce a pleasant, cooling effect on our taste buds. Both effects are produced by chemicals that are found in the oil extracted from a mint plant and are described as being "volatile" and "rubefacient." They are volatile, because their molecules quickly disperse into the air, creating the penetrating, sweet odor we detect with our nose. And they're rubefacient, or irritating, because when these active molecules touch the surface of our skin they stimulate the nerve endings that signal sensations of cold to our brain. Other rubefacient chemicals in oils from mustard and pepper act similarly by exciting the nerves that detect heat. Hot chili peppers don't really burn our mouth, and mint is not actually cold, but we are momentarily fooled by our senses to feel that they are. When cooled down to below zero, these hyperactive molecules crystallize and separate from their oily medium. The result is a mighty crystal called "menthol."

Menthol actually has more to offer than our senses tell us. *The Merck Index: An Encyclopedia of Chemicals, Drugs, and Biologicals*, states that menthol used topically is a mild local anesthetic and antiseptic. That means when rubbed on the skin it relieves pain and kills germs. *Herbal Drugs and Phytopharmaceuticals* adds that menthol acts as a spasmolytic (antispasm) agent on the smooth-muscle tissue found inside the nose, throat, sinuses, and nether regions. For example, menthol has been used by tobacco companies as an additive in their products ostensibly to make the harsh smoke feel "cool" and "mild," but more important to reduce coughing spasms. The fact that the tobacco kills off their customers is one thing, but heaven forbid, how would it look if they were walking around coughing all the time![1]

ANTI-INFLAMMATORY
ANTISEPTIC
ANESTHETIC
SPASMOLYTIC

The positive attributes of mint have been known for a very long time. According to Mentholatum's house organ, *Menthology*, ". . . the marvelous healing properties of Menthol, the chief ingredient of Mentholatum, have been known for centuries to the wise medicine men of Japan, where it first was extracted as oil from peppermint plants." The makers of Vicks VapoRub praised the virtues of peppermint in their 1930 circular titled *Directions for Using*: ". . . 3,000 years ago in Egypt, [oil of peppermint] perfumed the baths of the Pharaohs and eased the hurts of the slaves who built the pyramids. Its virtues are described in Icelandic medical books of the thirteenth century."[2]

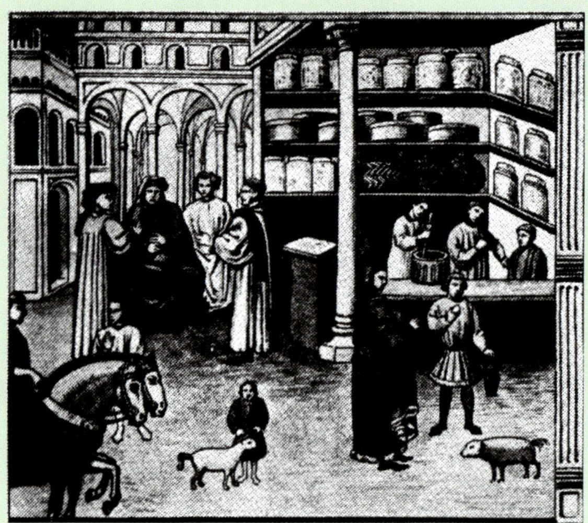

Ye Olde Corner Apothecary

Peppermint and other aromatic oils were prized among medieval apothecaries.

The seventeenth-century botanist John Parkinson listed the healthful applications of mint in his book *Theatrum Botanicum* (1640), in which he described some 3,800 plants. Parkinson, who was the apothecary to James I of England and later given the title Botanicus Regis Primarius by Charles I, observed that mint, "Applyed to the forehead or the temples of the head it easeth the paines thereof." He also recorded that mint applied to the heads of children "healeth the chaps of the fundament." Mint will "dissolve winde in the stomach, . . . help the chollick and those that are short-winded . . . the distilled water helpeth a stinking breath [and] helpe the scurfe or dandroffe of the head used with vinegar." Parkinson also recounted Aristotle's warning not to let soldiers use mint because it "abated their animosity or courage to fight." He also quoted Pliny when he told of mint being used "in the time of Great Pompey [*sic*]." The antibiotic effect of mint was also observed: "Divers have held for true, that cheeses will not corrupt, if they be either rubbed over with the juyce or the decoction of Mints, or laid among them."[3]

Menthology continued to explain that of the twelve varieties of mint, the "most important to be used medicinally is known as Mentha Arvensis or Japanese Menthol Mint." This mint is a perennial plant that was grown on "the bleak northern island [of] Hokkaido," and for half a century Japan held a monopoly on its production. Menthol mint fields were harvested by cutting the whole plant in June or July. A second and third cutting were also possible before the season ended. The harvested "herb" was shocked in the field to dry out and then placed in covered vats to be steamed. The steam extracted the volatile oil from the herb and carried the "strongly impregnated vapor" to a condenser, called the "worm," where cooling oil dripped from the end into a "can" (visualize a moonshine

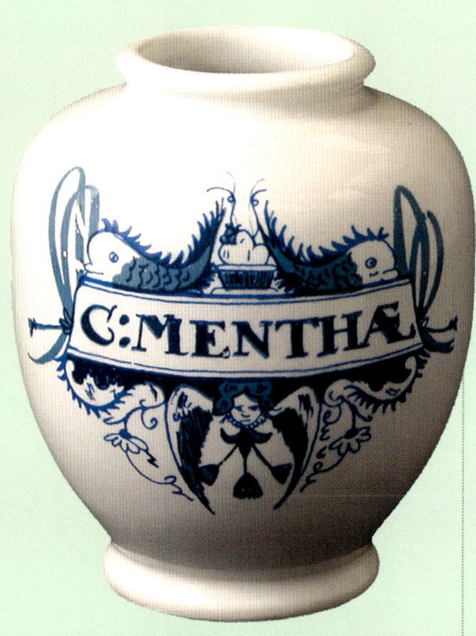

Reproduction Apothecary Vase

Gift of the Mentholatum Company, Ltd.

still). Finally, during the winter the oil was chilled with ice or snow and brine, "much the same as we freeze ice cream," and menthol crystals were formed. Crystallization extracted only the useful medicinal elements, leaving behind a depleted oil residue.[4]

Western chemists may have been aware of these crystals, which were known variously as peppermint stearescense, stearoptene of peppermint, and peppermint camphor, as early as the "later part" of the eighteenth century. Unfortunately, they didn't recognize the crystals' potential. Peppermint oil was what everybody wanted. A centuries-old commercial market for peppermint oil as a food flavoring already existed, and the oil was a familiar listing in the pharmacopoeias of the day. So, the crystalline form remained an obscure academic footnote throughout the first half of the nineteenth century. Progress was also delayed because Japan was "sakoku"—the closed country—prior to Commodore Perry's arrival there in 1853, and its production and use of the crystal was virtually unknown to the West.[5]

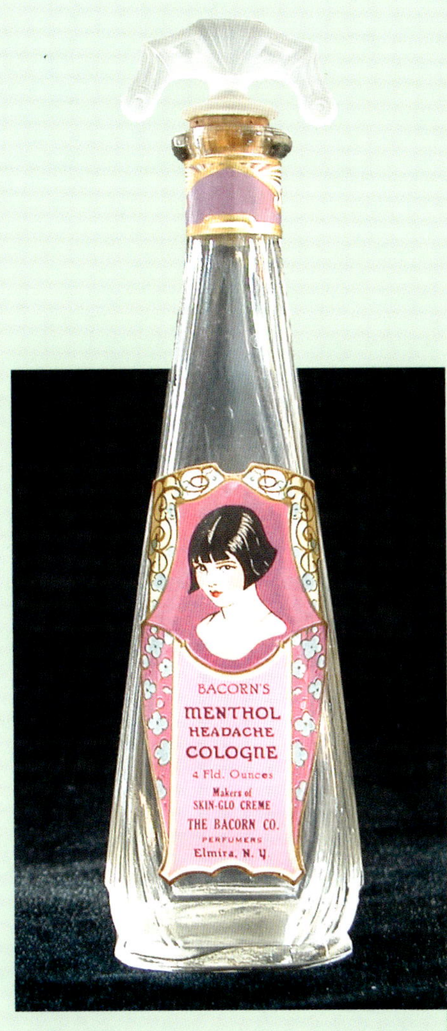

Menthol Perfume

It was an idea that lasted only as long as the factory did, when it burned to the ground in 1927.

As early as 1816 American farmers were cultivating native peppermint, *Mentha piperita*, and distilling it into oil in Wayne County, New York. The West's first encounter with the crystalline form in any quantity came when the Americans shipped their peppermint oil to Northern Europe to help fight a cholera epidemic and a large enough supply of the crystals could be produced and examined by the renowned French chemist Jean Baptiste Dumas, who in 1832 published the first chemical formulation of peppermint camphor.[6]

The Crystals Are Named

In the early 1860s the first shipments of Japanese peppermint camphor began arriving in America. This was a result of the historic trade treaty negotiated in 1858 by Townsend Harris, the first U.S. envoy to Japan, and it was the rudimentary first step in opening a worldwide commercial market for the crystals. The small white crystals were packed in "coarse earthenware jars protected simply by paper covers." The Japanese manufacturers, who only a few years before had been trading within the confines of a medieval empire whose borders were closed to the rest of the world, needed to learn more than just modern packaging standards. It was imperative that they seek out and develop relationships with chemical distributors in America and Europe who were willing to invent new products that would utilize

CH_3 OH H_3C CH_3

Menthol
$C_{10}H_{20}O$

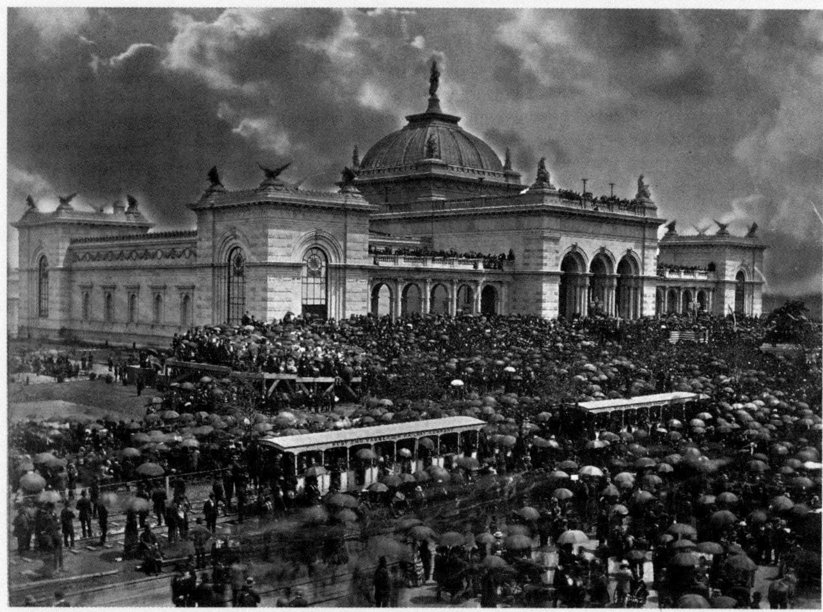

1876 Centennial Exhibition Opening Day

Fukui Makoto, Japanese Commissioner, in *Harper's Weekly*, July 15, 1876, commented, "The first day crowds come like sheep, run here, run there, run everywhere. One man start, one thousand follow. Nobody can see anything, nobody can do anything. All rush, push, tear, shout, make plenty noise, say damn great many times, get very tired, and go home." One of many proud American exhibitors was Hale & Parshall, Growers and Manufacturers. International Prize Medal, Oil of Peppermint. Lyons, Wayne County, New York (below).

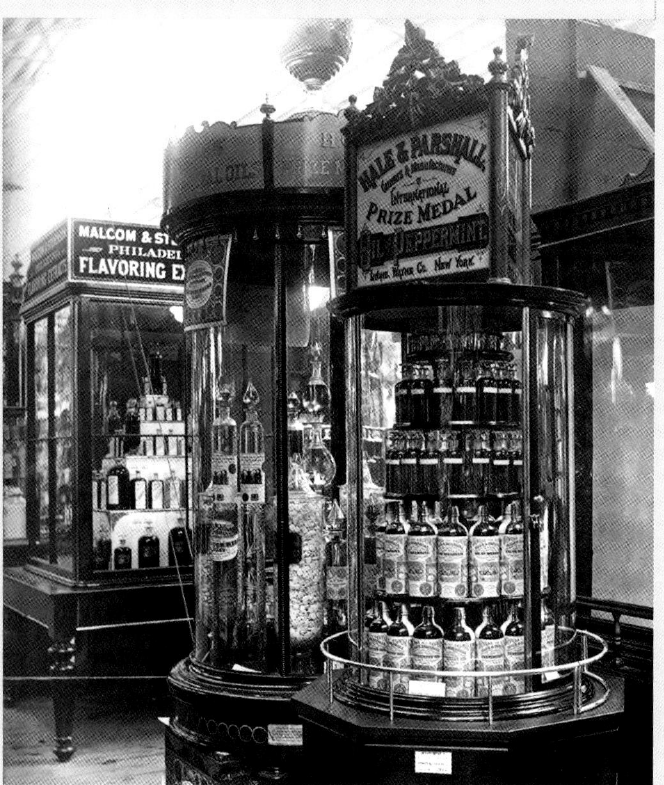

their crystals and generate awareness among Western consumers to create a new market from scratch. They also needed a better name for their healing crystals. That name was handed to them by A. Oppenheim. Upon receiving a supply of the Japanese *Mentha arvensis* crystals in 1862, Oppenheim conducted thorough tests, comparing them to Dumas's earlier work on the American *Mentha piperita*, and found them to be very nearly the same in composition. He then verified the formula to be a monatomic alcohol and proposed to the chemical and pharmaceutical community that the name "peppermint camphor" be dropped and replaced with "mentholic alcohol," or "menthol."[7]

Travelers returning from China and Japan occasionally brought home small vials of a viscous, semicrystalline, dark green or sometimes amber-colored oil called "Fook Chang Yong" that was used as a headache cure. In 1871, the long, flat glass vials of menthol remedy could be purchased at 744 Sacramento Street on the corner of DuPont in the heart of San Francisco's Chinese community. This, according to the Swiss professor of pharmacy Friedrich Fluckiger, from the University of Strasbourg, was similar to the "so-called *Menthol*" or "solid" Japanese peppermint oil, and was said to solidify in cold weather even in California. Awareness among druggists increased another notch. In 1876 menthol crystals were displayed at the Philadelphia Centennial Exhibition. Commercial interest rapidly increased as the exhibition attendees returned to their hometowns with a stack of exhibitor's cards in their pocket and began to think back over all the new products. By 1880, regular shipments of menthol were arriving in New York.[8]

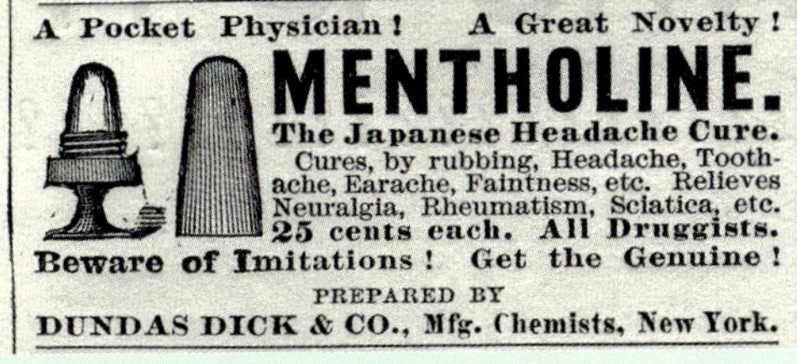

First Menthol Cone in America

The "Mentholine" brand name used by Dundas Dick & Co. in this September 1889 ad in *Frank Leslie's Popular Monthly* appears again after the turn of the century as a catarrh balm in the lineup of Rexall products. First sold as a novelty, menthol found a foothold in Western markets as an exotic Japanese headache cure packaged in attractive pocket- or purse-size containers. The Coffin & Wood Chemical Company (below) offered an attractive line of novelty products with oriental designs that were filled with menthol they manufactured themselves from American-grown mint. They, and every other American company that attempted to capture the menthol market from the Japanese, ultimately failed.

Menthol's First Commercial Success

In 1881, the New York–based Dundas Dick & Co., Manufacturing Druggists, introduced the menthol cone for relieving headaches. The novelty of this attractive beechwood treen with exotic Japanese menthol inside made it an overnight success. Within five years there were an estimated thirty different brands of menthol cones on the market. The July 1886 issue of *The Druggists Circular* published an article on menthol cones by C. L. Coffin of Coffin & Wood Chemical Co., Detroit, Michigan. Mr. Coffin made a survey of twenty-two brands, of which five were pure white menthol, one was pure brown, three were 95 percent pure, three were 90 percent, seven were 80 percent, two were 25 percent, and one contained no menthol at all. Coffin's investigation discovered that various cements were used to fasten the cones to the base, including common glue, gum arabic, gelatin, and paraffin. Some cones were found to be hollow, and others had a core made of different material. Wood cases were found to be superior to metal because wood did not conduct heat and provided insulation that helped reduce volatilization of the menthol. Be that as it may, Coffin's unbiased conclusion was that "As an anodye application for pain, as a local and mild anaesthetic, and in its many valuable and homely uses, menthol is *par excellence* a domestic remedy, and in these uses it is as yet in its infancy . . . we may predict for menthol a valuable and prominent position in the future of medicine."[9]

160 McKESSON & ROBBINS' PRICES CURRENT.

MENTHOL NOVELTIES.

MENTHOL CONES.

CARTRIDGE CONE
DRAUGHTSMAN STYLE
FRENCH
CREEDMORE
DEMI-JOHN
BEEHIVE
ORIENTAL

AMBER WOOD

Our Cones in Boxwood and Amberwood are Elegant NOVELTIES.

MENTHOL PUNGENT.

This very attractive novelty meets with unusual sales and is rapidly becoming popular, serving as it does all the offices of the Menthol Cone and being much more elegant in appearance.

HAK-KA VINAIGRETTE.

Our Hak Ka Vinaigrette is really the most beautiful novelty ever produced, and commands immediate sale. Its unique and elegant appearance makes it a taking article with the ladies.

Price Per Doz., $2.00.

PERFECT INHALER.

We have discontinued the manufacture of our small style Inhaler but continue to manufacture our larger size. The unprecedented success of our Menthol Inhaler in the treatment of Hay Fever, Asthma, Bronchitis, Coughs and Colds has has led to a lively demand for this valuable article. It finds steady sales, once having been seen and tried.

Larger Size retail at 50c. each; Per do

THE COFFIN & WOOD CHEMIC

DETRO

MENTHOL
An External Application
For Neuralgia,
Tooth-ache & Nervous Head-ache
DIRECTIONS.
To be rubbed over the forehead
and
the course of the nerves affe

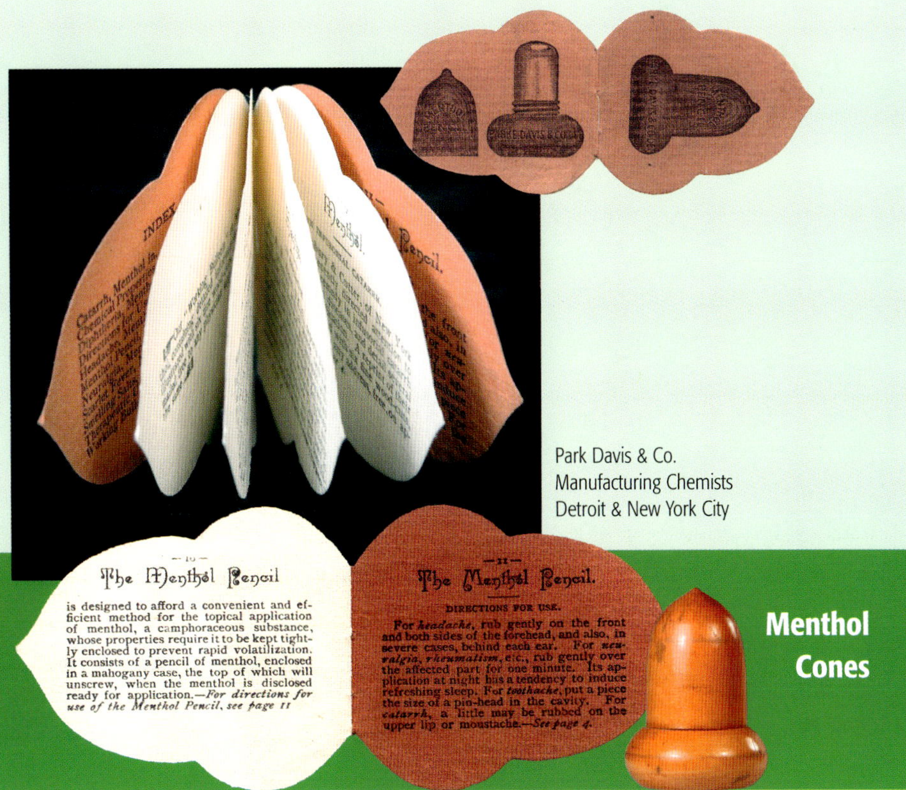

Park Davis & Co.
Manufacturing Chemists
Detroit & New York City

Menthol Cones

Eucalyptus

Eucalyptus oil comes from a deciduous tree that is indigenous to Australia and is now cultivated in the subtropical regions of southern Europe, Africa, Asia, and America. The colorless and highly volatile oil is extracted by distillation of the tree's leaves and branch tops. Eucalyptus oil's primary medical constituent is cineole, which has an antibacterial and fungicidal effect. It is also known as blue gum and fever tree.

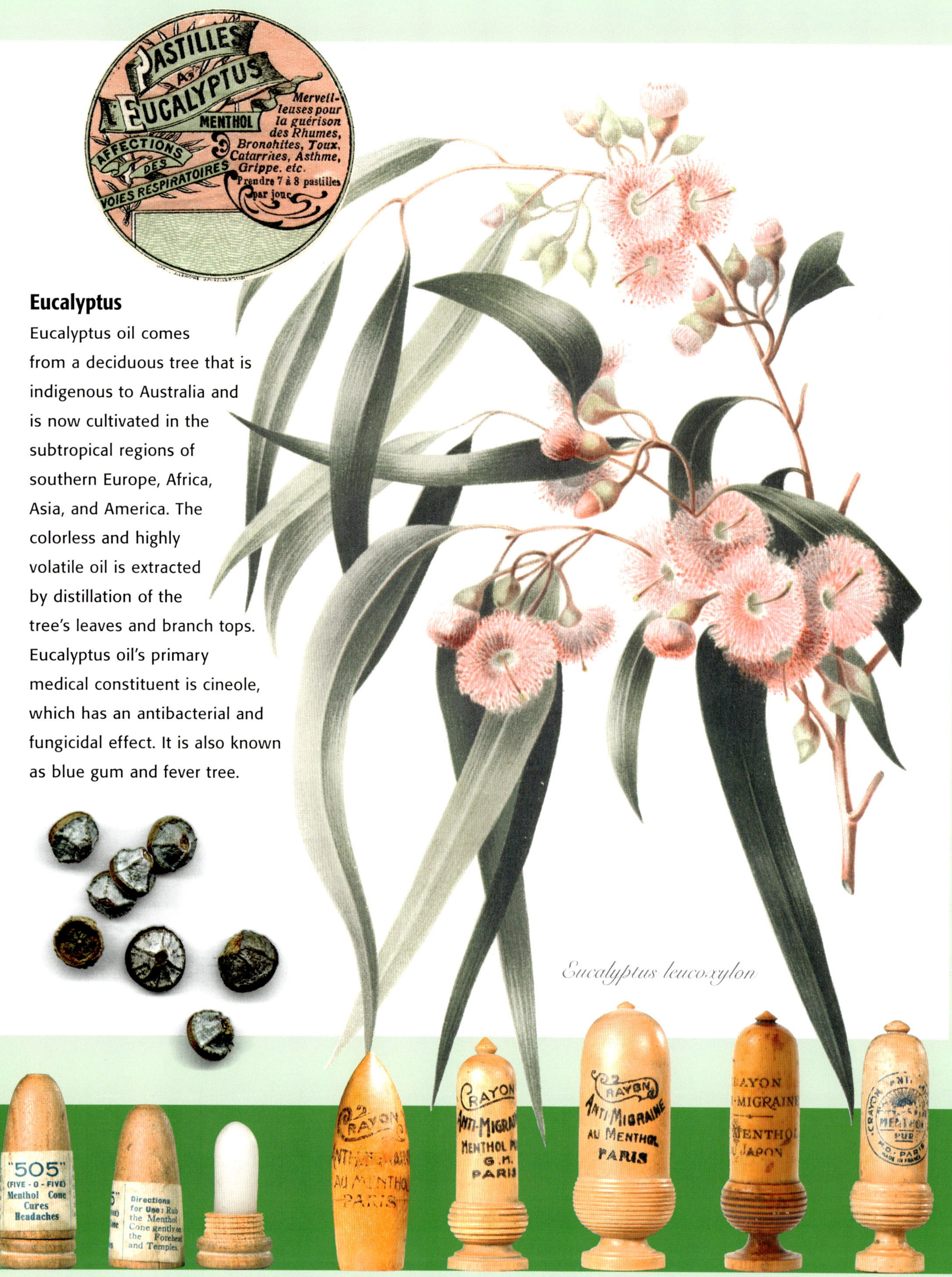

Eucalyptus leucoxylon

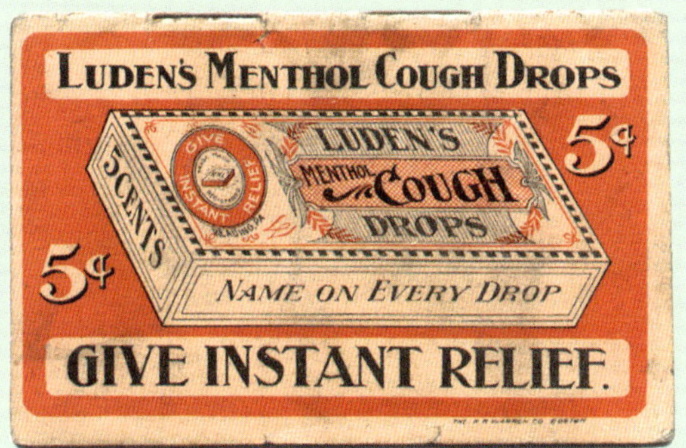

Novelty Spelled Success for Luden's

Luden's was the first hard-candy "drop" to be molded into a distinctive shape and the first to contain menthol, both novel ideas in 1881.

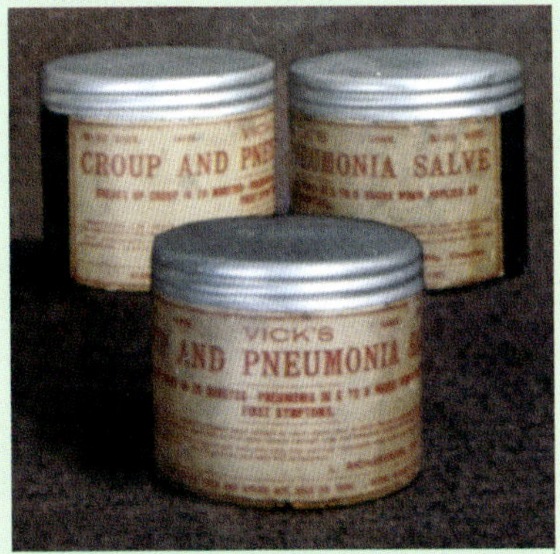

Where Is the Menthol?

Unlike other brands that extolled the use of menthol, Vicks Croup and Pneumonia Salve remained an anonymous brand among several dozen other Vicks medical products. Then Smith Richardson came to work for his father in 1907 and began a thirteen-year marketing campaign to make the salve a national brand without ever praising the virtues of menthol over camphor or any of the other volatile ingredients.

At the same time that Dundas Dick was introducing the menthol cone in New York, William H. Luden was adding menthol to his candy drops in Reading, Pennsylvania. By the end of the decade Luden's Menthol Cough Drops were sold nationwide. Another innovation, Menthol Plaster, "The Most Wonderful Plaster Made," came out in 1885. Plain menthol crystals were also tried out in glass inhalers previously used for other medications, and the next big menthol-delivery product was discovered. Cushman's Menthol Inhaler, which filed for a trademark patent in 1886, was the most heavily promoted of the new menthol inhalers.

The Druggists Circular reported in 1886 that there were two U.S. manufacturers of menthol crystals actively competing with the Japanese. It also reported that imports of Japanese menthol for the previous year had been five thousand pounds. According to the 1884 *American Journal of Pharmacy* (p. 405), Mr. A. M. Todd of Nottawa, Michigan, was the first person in America to produce menthol crystals from local mint. Albert M. Todd, was a grower, distiller, and refiner of essential oils who claimed in an advertisement in the 1887 McKesson & Robins' *Drugs, Chemical and Pharmaceutical Preparations* catalog (p. 192), that his company was "the most extensive producer of Oil of Peppermint in the World." Todd was not only extensive, he was thorough, for in 1886 he published his menthol findings in the *American Journal of Pharmacy* (p. 159). Todd's registered trademark was "Crystal White." A. A. Hyde blended his first menthol cough specific in 1890. He completed work on Mentholatum salve by 1893 and declared it to be ready for market in 1894. Lunsford Richardson, a North Carolina druggist, also made a menthol salve in 1894 that he called Vicks. In 1911 it would be renamed Vicks VapoRub.

Menthol steadily carved out a market in America, as well as in Great Britain and Northern European countries. Earlier attempts by American companies to produce their own menthol crystals

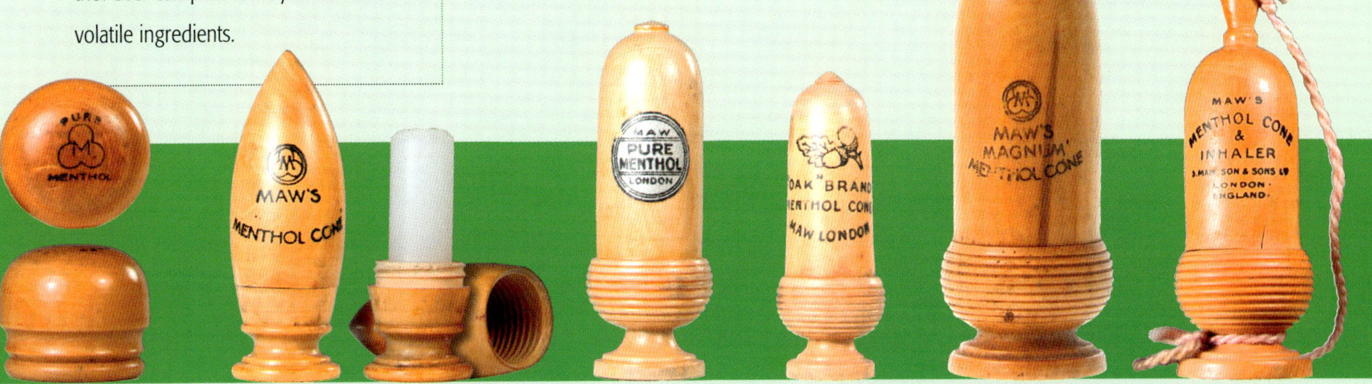

MENTHOLOGY

THE Camphor Trees of Formosa produce most of the world's supply of Camphor. Thousands and thousnads of pounds of Camphor are imported each year for the manufacture of Mentholatum.

Camphor

The camphor tree is an evergreen found in southern Japan, China, and Vietnam. Camphor trees grow to be hundreds of years old with trunks upward of fifteen feet in diameter. Natural camphor crystals are produced by cutting the entire tree trunk into small chips and then steam distilling them followed by a cold sublimation of the vapor. Camphor is quickly absorbed into the skin, and it causes a warm, painkilling sensation. This and its ability to ward off bugs made gum camphor a staple of the China trade since the fifteenth century.

In their 1893 booklet for the Chicago World's Fair, the Japan Camphor Company's New Jersey owners wrote, "The annual export of crude camphor from Japan averages about five million pounds weight, of which about one-fourth comes to the United States and the remainder to Europe." It took two hundred pounds of wood to make ten pounds of crude gum, and that was reduced even more when refined into crystals. The booklet stated that many districts in Japan were already denuded of camphor timber and that steps were being taken to renew the depleted forests by planting and carefully tending new trees. With the three-hundred-year-old trees already cut down, the company was projecting good results from twenty-year-old trees and felt that it was important to point out that there was a higher quantity of camphor in the roots of the trees. "Although enormous inroads have thus already been made upon the camphor forests of Japan, the remaining supply is still very large, and the trees belonging to the government are said to be alone capable of maintaining during the next twenty-five years the present average annual supply of camphor from Japan."

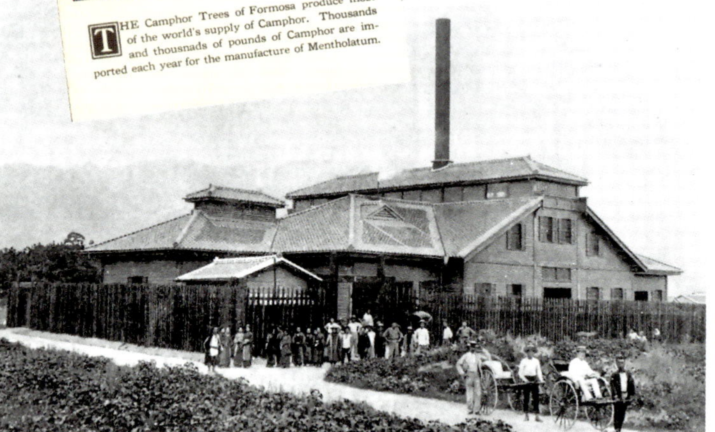

Top: Cover of 1926 *Menthology* (vol. 11, Fall 1926, no. 4). **Above:** The American-owned factory in Kobe, Japan, could produce fifty thousand pounds of refined camphor per month.

In 1920, *Menthology* (vol. 5, no. 1) revealed that "many tons" of camphor were used annually in making Mentholatum. Mentholatum acquired its camphor from the island of Formosa, now called Taiwan. Today, 75 percent of the camphor used in the United States is produced synthetically. Because camphor has been found to be poisonous if used in large quantities, it has been limited to no more than 11 percent as

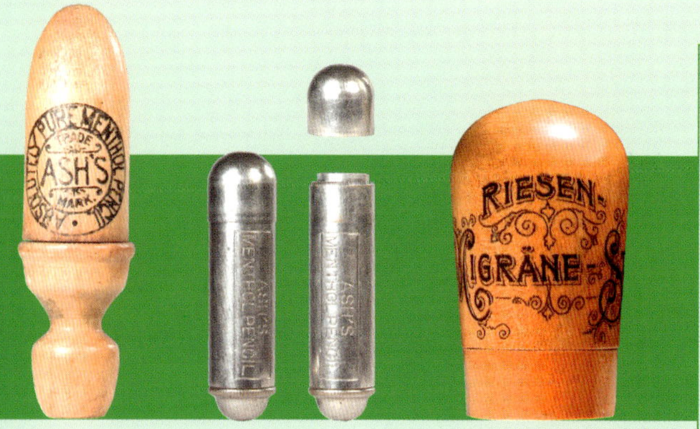

Victorian Treens

Victorian treen ware is the collector's category for these small boxwood containers, which are often mistaken for thimble and needle cases. **Page 93** (left to right): possibly the oldest menthol cone in this collection, a "Migran-Stift" (stick) made by "M. Badig" at the "Kem. Tekn. Fabrik" (Chem. Tech. Factory) in Malmo, Sweden; two examples of MENTHOL Trade Mark for "Neuralgia, Tooth-ache & Nervous Head ache," Bartlett Hooper & Co. Chemists, London (bullet shape collected from Montevideo, Uruguay, ton shape found in Capetown, South Africa); Park Davis & Co. acorn-shaped menthol pencil.

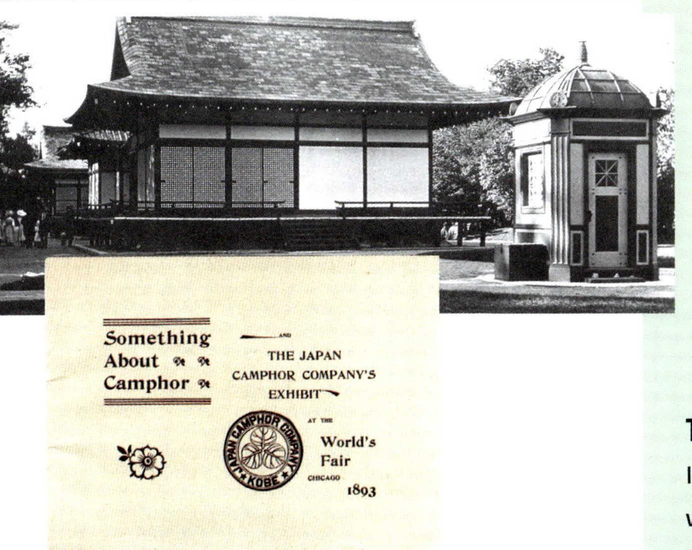

eventually were abandoned. It was simply not profitable when the Japanese consistently produced the highest-quality menthol, in abundant supply, at a reasonable price. The wholesale price in 1885 for one ounce of menthol in Chicago from a St. Louis importer was $1.04. By 1887, the New York price was 65¢. The Japanese would hold what might be called a benevolent monopoly on menthol production for many decades to come.

an active ingredient in manufactured topical lotions and astringents. In 1980, the Food and Drug Administration banned its use as camphorated oil, camphor oil, camphor liniment, and camphorated liniment. Oral ingestion may cause camphor poisoning within five to ninety minutes. Symptoms include mental confusion and jerky movements of the extremities, sometimes resulting in seizure.[10]

Top: The Japan Pavilion in Jackson Park at the 1893 Chicago World's Fair.
Above: The Japan Camphor Company's sixteen-page exhibit booklet.
Right: Vintage tin of one-ounce refined camphor tablets manufactured by the Camphor Refinery in Kobe, Japan, later named the Nippon Camphor Co., Ltd.

The Mint Ranch Saga

In 1920, Mentholatum's supply of menthol was threatened when Japan cut its production in half, causing the price to jump from $3 per pound to $15. It turned out that Hokkaido mint fields were being plowed under to make room for mulberry plants whose leaves were used as food for silkworms. This provided new incentive for American farmers to try to break Japan's monopoly. By 1923, experiments were being conducted to find the ideal climate and soil to grow menthol mint. California proved to be the best location, and farmers in Fresno and Kern Counties became the principal producers. Menthol mint was also grown in Michigan, northern Indiana, and western Oregon. By 1927, the Mentholatum Company announced that it was refining "many thousand pounds of Menthol" at its plant in Buffalo, from American-produced mint oil. In 1928, Albert T. Hyde, A.A.'s eldest son, purchased 514 acres to grow menthol mint on the west bank of the San Joaquin River in central California. The Dos Palos operation, which included a distillation plant, was appropriately named the "Mint Ranch."[11]

However, *Menthology* prematurely announced that American-grown mint had broken

Page 94 (left to right): "505" from Australia; five examples of French-made Crayon-brand antimigraine menthol "pur." **Page 95** (left to right): Pure Menthol from Maw & Son's of London, makers of the world's first baby bottle nipple (c. 1807); Maw's Menthol Cone; Maw's Pure Menthol; Oak Brand Menthol Cone; Maw's Magnum Menthol Cone; and Maw's (combination) Menthol Cone and Inhaler (found in Australia). **Page 96** (left to right): Ash's Absolutely Pure Menthol Pencil; Ash's metal twist-up Menthol Pencil; Riesen Migrane Stift. **Page 97** (left to right): Pierre de N. D. de Lourdes Docteur Acard de Paris Menthol Pur Calme Douleurs; Pierre Calme Douleurs de Saint-Vincent-de-Paul.

Japan's "age-old monopoly." Albert Hyde made a good start when he hired a Japanese foreman with expertise in cultivating menthol mint. The quality of the mint oil was measured by "proof" (80 proof, 90 proof, etc.), and the mint crop had to be free of wild grass and weeds, which might pollute the harvest. Water from the canal system had to be protected from contamination as it passed by other crops and from weeds that grew along its banks, so cement-lined canals were built. Only two hundred acres of the ranch were ever in mint, the rest being planted in other crops. In spite of "modern labor-saving machinery," American mint farms remained small and had trouble producing the high-proof oils that the industry demanded. Albert's operation produced quality oil but at great cost, and he was never able to compete with the Japanese monopoly.[12]

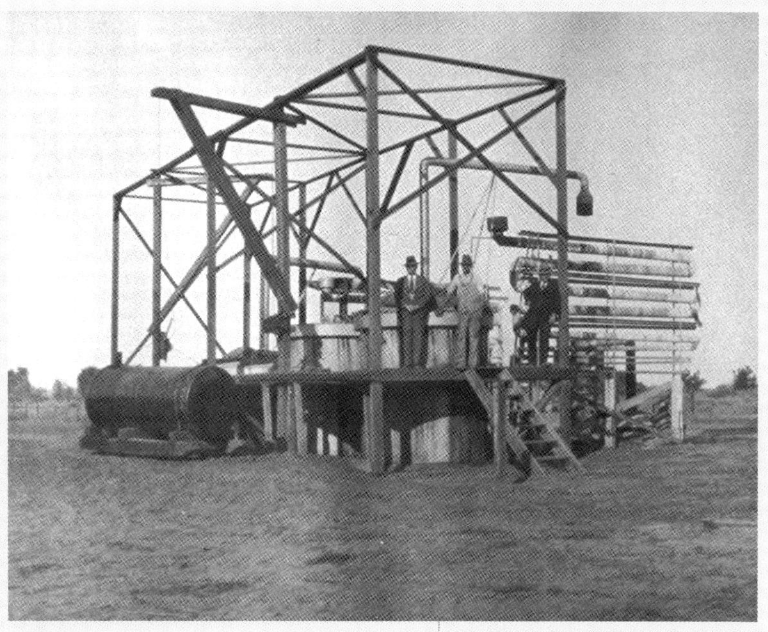

Distillation Plant

Bert Hyde (1915–2003), retired president and chairman of the board of the Mentholatum Company, remembered working summers for his father on the Mint Ranch when he was a student at Stanford University. He described the ranch's distillation plant having high-pressure steam tanks connected to a row of cooling pipes that dripped condensed oil into milk cans from the end. The picture shown above was taken before all six of the tanks were completed. After a lifetime's work dedicated to the company, Bert confessed that he never learned how menthol crystals were made from the mint oil. As far as he and the company were concerned it was an industrial secret (although he knew that it somehow involved a centrifuge). It is interesting to note that when his uncles were running the company they published each step of the process in a 1929 *Menthology*.

Albert's younger brothers in Buffalo eventually questioned the viability of the ranch. After all, it was producing only a small percentage of the menthol they consumed. Albert made the argument that the Japanese would eventually drag America into a war, at which time his operation would become valuable to them. Then matters took a turn for the worse when the foreman was threatened by a wealthy Japanese gentleman who arrived at the ranch one day in a black limousine, spoke harshly to the foreman, and sped away. When the loyal farmer refused to stop working, nighttime saboteurs torched the building where the rows of ten-gallon milk cans, filled with refined oil, were stored. They also flooded the mint crops and stole valuable equipment and tools. Finally, after all his hard work and dedication, the directors notified Albert that they would no longer buy his oil, and his spirit was broken. Albert Hyde died not long after of a stroke in 1935, and his family never again planted mint at the ranch.

Albert was right about the coming war with Japan, but he could not have predicted that the Japanese would continue selling menthol to the West through their business agents in Brazil. Today, the largest suppliers of natural menthol are located in China and India. *Mentha arvensis* L. is common in Asia, Europe, and North America, where it is known as corn mint, field mint, wild mint, Japanese mint, common mint, and menthol mint. It is typical to see peppermint (*Mentha piperita*) given credit as the source of menthol, but this is misleading. Both peppermint and corn mint contain L-menthol and D-menthol isomers, corn mint having the highest levels, but peppermint is used primarily for food flavoring and corn mint for pharmaceuticals and hygiene products. Of the two isomers, only L-menthol causes cooling. Known as optical isomers because they polarize light in crystal form or in solution, both menthols kill disease-causing organisms and promote healing. *Mentha arvensis* L. is the source of most of the natural menthol produced in the world today, and China is its fastest-growing producer's market. Menthol crystals have superceded vanillin as the aroma chemical with the highest annual world sales. Although synthetic menthol can also be made, natural menthol is still created in much the same way it always was. The herb is placed in high-pressure steam distillers to remove the oil, which is then refrigerated to crystallize the menthol. After cooling, the dementholyzed oil is drained off, and the crystals are placed in a centrifuge to spin off any residual oil.[13]

The First Menthol Cigarette

After WWI, cigarettes surpassed cigars as the preferred nicotine-delivery system in America. Veterans had acquired the "habit" during the war when a 15¢ civilian pack of Camels could be purchased for 7¢ at the YMCA canteen. Demand for cigarettes jumped dramatically after the right to vote amendment (XIX) passed in 1920. Young women were motivated to smoke first as a symbol of their new-found independence and later by simple teenage rebellion and Hollywood fashions. By 1923, Phillip Morris was marketing its Marlboro brand to the female demographic with the slogan "Mild as May."[14]

Inhaling cigarette smoke in the 1920s was no different from inhaling cigar smoke. It could be a harsh and often painful experience. Because they were smoking for show, most women puffed their cigarettes and thus avoided or delayed addiction to the nicotine. Puffing was not good enough for the manufacturers. They wanted users to inhale, so they searched for a milder tobacco. Independent of the big tobacco companies, Lloyd Hughes, the asthmatic son of a restaurant owner in Mingo Junction, Ohio, discovered what was, and still is considered to be the best solution to the problem. In spite of his asthma, Hughes enjoyed smoking an occasional cigarette, and he kept a pack in a tin box where he also stored his menthol inhaler. After prolonged storage in the airtight box, he noticed that menthol vapors had permeated the cigarettes. As a result they tasted better and smoked cooler. (Although not a part of the legend, it is very possible and easy to imagine that he and

Minty Clean Beats Listerine

Ricqlès brand "Alcool de Menthe" (c. 1895) was a "Produit Hygienique exquis," or an exquisite hygenic product for "Les Dents Labouche et La Toilette," the teeth, the mouth, and the toilet. This sounds like the nineteenth-century French equivalent of Listerine and at the time was certainly more accessible as Ricqlès was sold in "les Pharmacies, Parfumeries, Epiceries, fines et Herberisteries." Listerine was first formulated in 1879 as a surgical disinfectant having been named for the famous English physician Sir Joseph Lister. It wasn't until 1895 that Listerine was marketed as an oral antiseptic to dentists and 1914 before it became available as an over-the-counter product to the public. The shocker is that it took another seventy-eight years for Warner Lambert to introduce CoolMint Listerine.

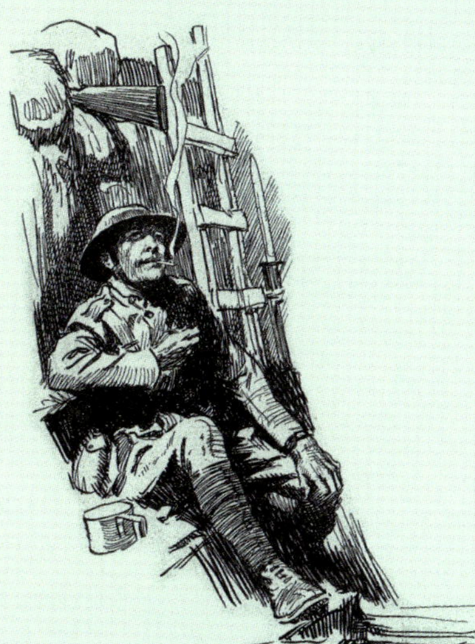

A Casualty of War . . .

If the Germans didn't kill him, the smoking addiction just might . . .

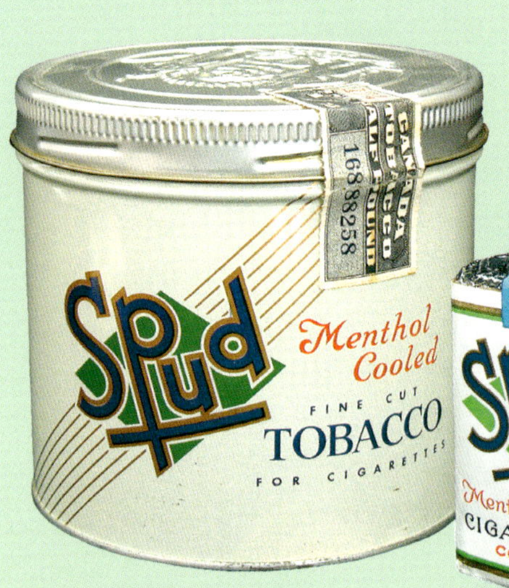

The Fifth-Largest Brand

Pictured above are a half-pound tin of cut tobacco for rolling your own and a pack of twenty factory-rolled cigarettes. Spud packaging remained unchanged throughout the 1930s.

Spud Advertising Was Eccentric (right)

Perhaps he needed something stronger than a menthol cigarette . . .

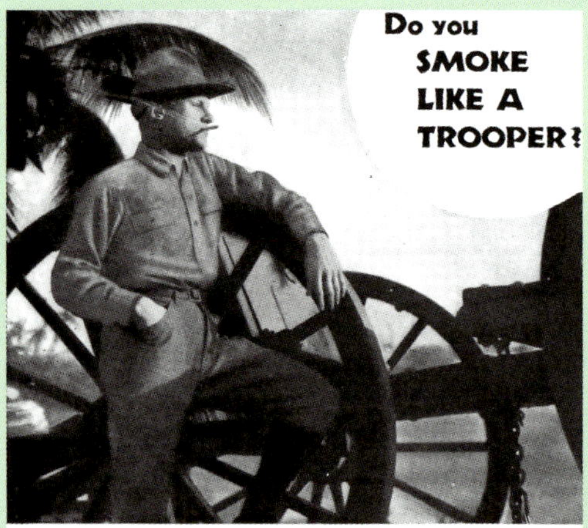

Big "show" tonight... better have Spuds!

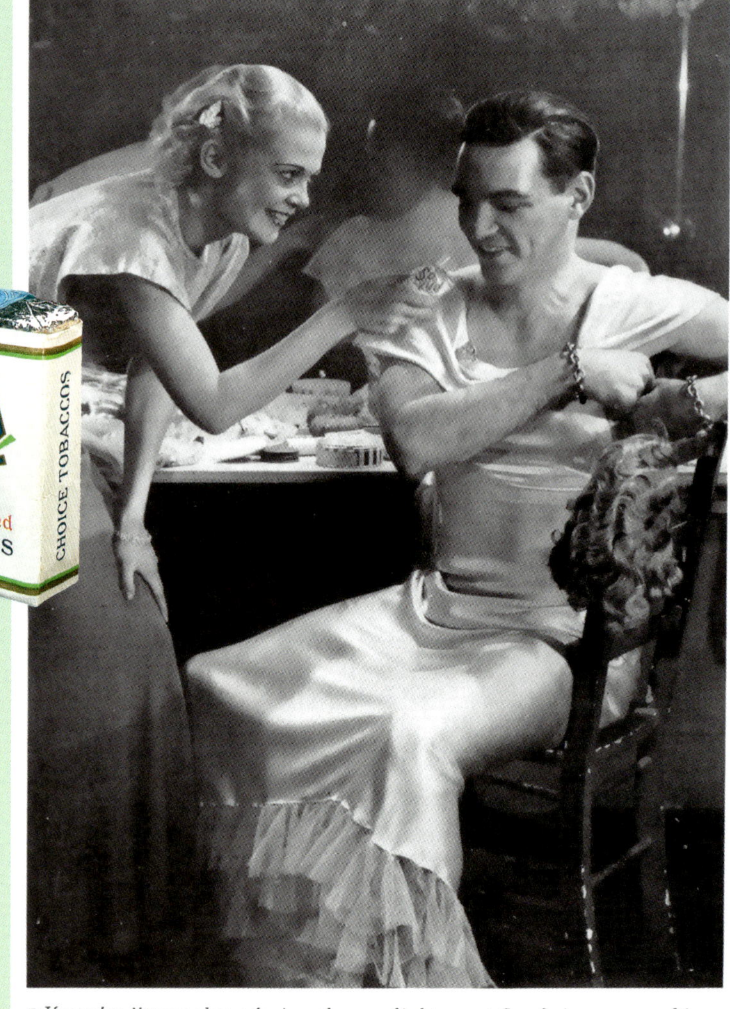

• If you're jittery about facing the spotlight—cast Spuds in your smoking-role. They keep heat out of smoke—so you keep a fresh, clean mouth. They taste better, too. With a natural tobacco fragrance unmarred by heat.

OPEN A PACK OF SPUDS and smell them. Notice that Spud's process doesn't change the fragrant odor of fine tobacco—though it takes the heat out of smoke.

Cork tips or plain. Cork tips are packed *down* so that even your own fingers don't touch them.

20 FOR 15c

(25 for 25c in Canada)

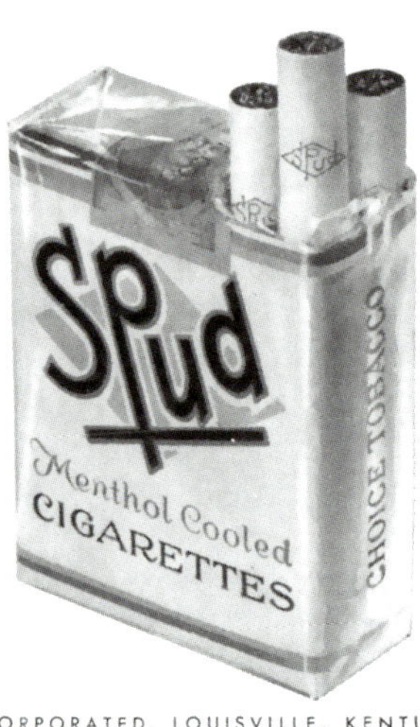

THE AXTON-FISHER TOBACCO CO., INCORPORATED, LOUISVILLE, KENTUCKY others could have placed a cigarette into the end of a glass tube inhaler and used it as a menthol filter.) On July 31, 1924, Hughes applied for a patent on a process he developed for spraying a solution of menthol, diluted in alcohol, over the cut tobacco before it was rolled into cigarettes. Hughes's patent (US 1,555,580) was issued on September 29, 1925. It claimed to produce "a cigarette tobacco which, while cooling and soothing to irritated membranes of the mouth and throat of the smoker, is absolutely non-injurious and is pleasant to the taste."[15]

Hughes named the new mentholated cigarettes "Spud" and contracted with Bloch Brothers Tobacco Company in Wheeling, West Virginia (makers of Mail Pouch chewing tobacco), to manufacture them. In May 1926, he sold his patent to the Axton-Fisher Tobacco Company, Inc., in Louisville, Kentucky, for $90,000 and promptly retired to spend it all. Axton-Fisher added a "cork tip" filter and hired a New York ad agency, which made Spud one of the top-five national brands by 1932. When smokers could no longer afford "store bought" cigarettes during the Depression, the company made a mentholated, fine-cut tobacco, which was packed in half-pound tins so that people could roll their own. Philip Morris acquired Axton-Fisher in 1944, and in 1966 the Spud brand was retired from commerce.[16]

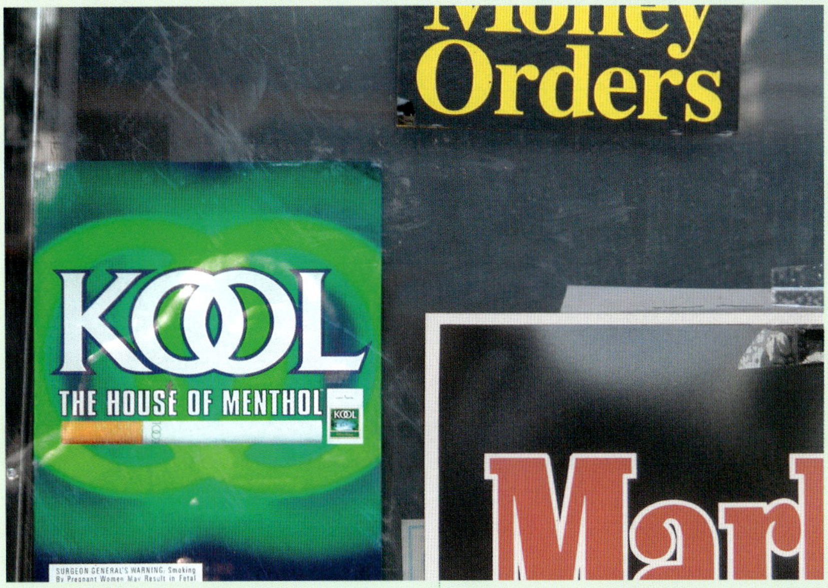

Menthol cools down the act of smoking and in turn heats up the sale of cigarettes. It helps a new smoker to inhale deeper and longer by damping the reflex to cough. More nicotine is then absorbed so that a dependence can be established before the smoker gives up in disgust. The sweet minty smell even helps to mask some of the nasty odors that foul the smoker's breath and clothing. If this weren't bad enough, menthol's abilities to reduce inflammation, kill off germs, and relieve pain are also masking the early symptoms of lung cancer in older smokers. Mentholated cigarettes are popular only in Asia (including China, India, Indonesia, Japan, and the Philippines) and North America (including Canada and Mexico). They account for 40 percent of the annual L-menthol consumption in the United States compared to only 10 percent worldwide.[17]

The House of Menthol™

This Brown & Williamson advertising campaign for KOOL cigarettes, a popular brand of menthol cigarettes since 1933, ran from 2000 to 2002. The story of menthol's role in the chemistry of cigarettes as revealed by ex–B&W research director Dr. Jeffrey Wigand was told in the 1999 movie *The Insider*.

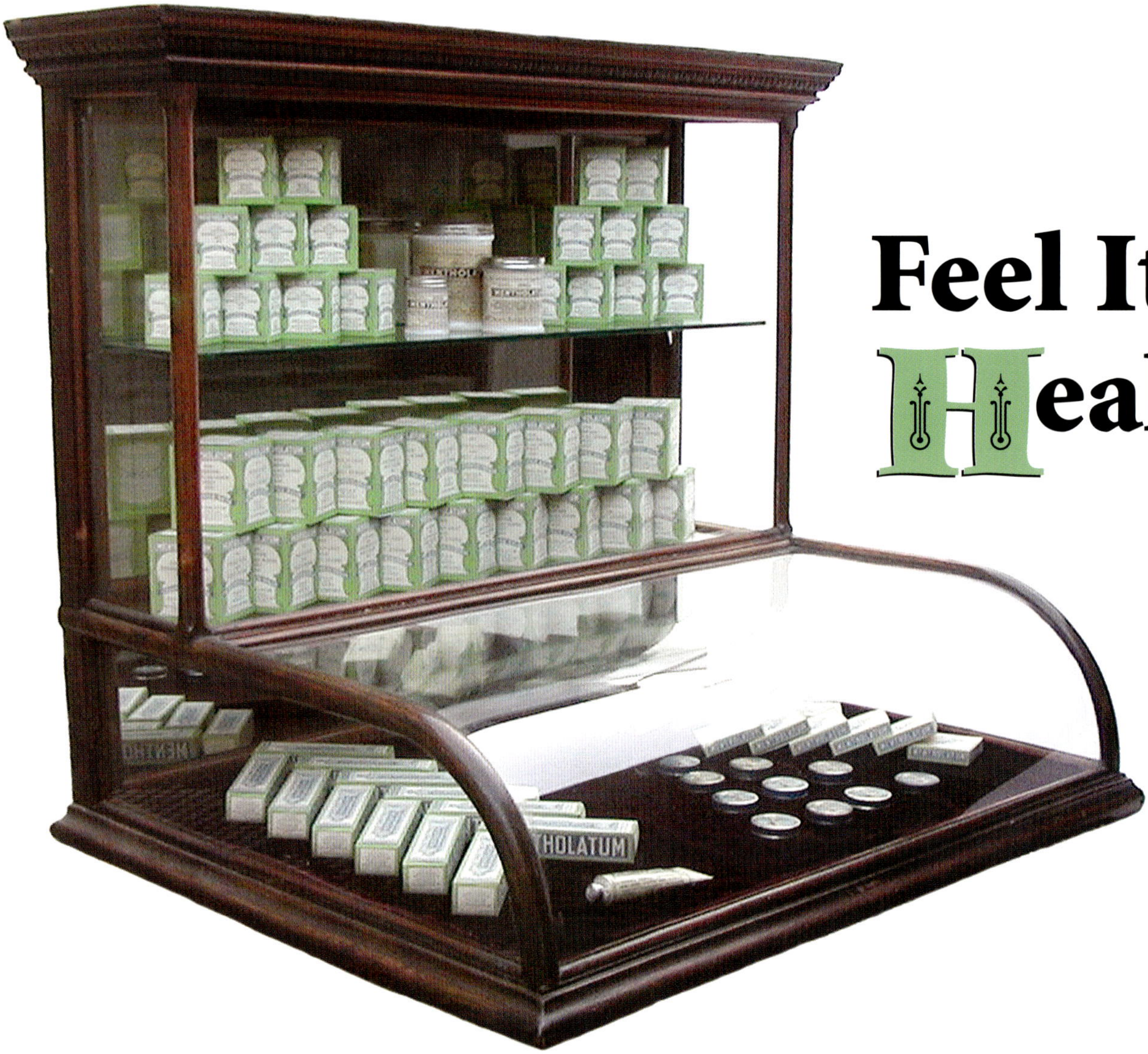

Feel It Heal

Ethel was twenty years old when she started work at the Mentholatum Company. She moved to Wichita in 1921 after her parents sold their farm near Andover, a few miles east of town. Her father, John Smith, and many of his rural neighbors came to take part in the city's booming economy and to enjoy the higher wages and shorter working hours offered there. The Smiths had moved to Kansas from Illinois in 1907 and participated in what is now considered the golden age of western farming, a period of prosperity that lasted from 1900 to 1920. Their departure from the arid land marked the beginning of a decline in small family farms, which were gradually replaced by highly mechanized, large-scale commercial operations.[1]

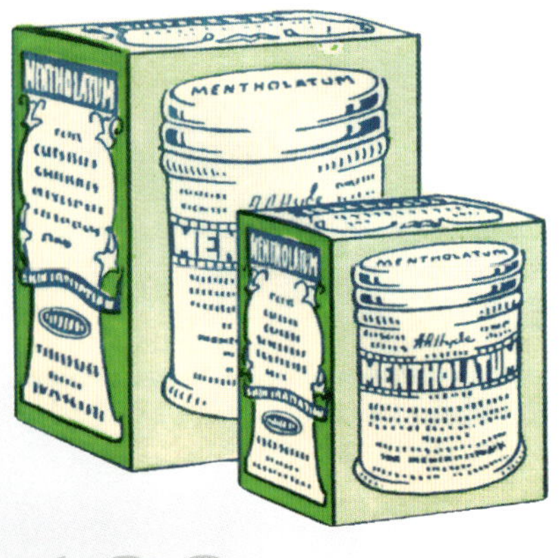

War-ravaged European markets were depressed and desperate for American food and products. But American workers were demanding more pay and fewer hours, which resulted in a decrease in productivity. The captains of industry saw a 25 percent decrease in production when hours were cut from sixty to forty-four a week. Men like A. A. Hyde, who had struggled against privation and had succeeded by hard work and long hours, were worried that a great opportunity for American industry would pass them by if labor did not step up to the challenge. The drain of farm labor into the city threatened an agricultural crisis, and yet Mentholatum and Wichita's other manufacturers needed more workers to meet the increased foreign demand for their products. For Mr. Hyde and his sons, who now managed the company, the problem boiled down to work ethics. They felt that "good, hard, honest service" was the only remedy. The Hydes also thought that labor unions had done a great deal of good for workers in industries not as benevolent as Mentholatum, but for them to exclude nonunion workers was wrong, and for them to threaten nonunion businesses was un-American. They endorsed the view of the *Parchment Prattler:*

> *There never was a time in the history of the world when it was more essential that we produce—that we produce to the maximum of our energy!—and there never was a time in the history of the world when, as individuals, we produce less than to-day. The wrist watch symbolizes [this] abnormal era.*

It was agreed that too many men back from the war were using their new wristwatches to check the time until the whistle blew instead of devoting themselves to their work. The solution: put the wristwatch away and place a "faithful alarm clock . . . on the bureau."[2]

In spite of the loss of farmers to the city, agriculture continued to be Sedgwick County's primary economy. The farming of wheat, corn, and oats supported a large milling and agricultural supply business that included one of the largest grain elevators in the country and three local tractor manufacturing plants. Another important crop at this time was broomcorn, which was used at the working end of brooms. Wichita dealers handled 65 percent of the nation's trade in this sturdy fiber. The local feed and meatpacking businesses continued to be strong at the Dold and Cudahy plants. Wichita's two other internationally ranked

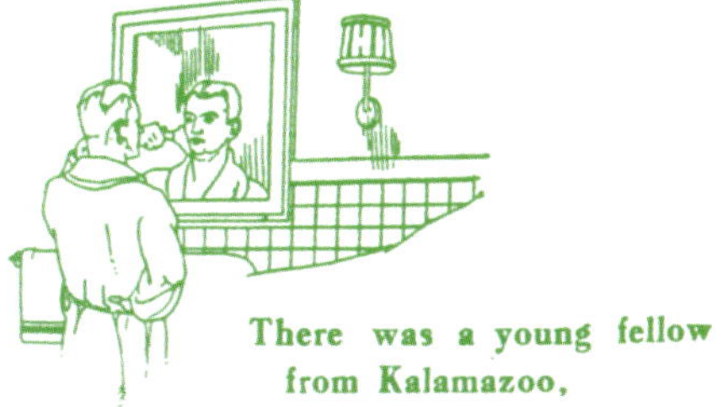
There was a young fellow
from Kalamazoo,

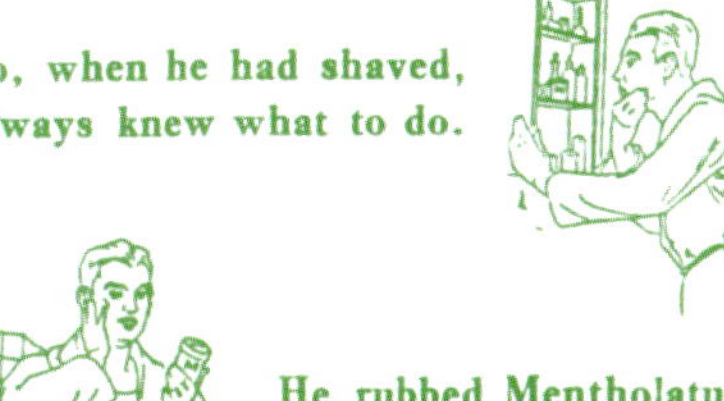
Who, when he had shaved,
always knew what to do.
He rubbed Mentholatum
all over his chin,

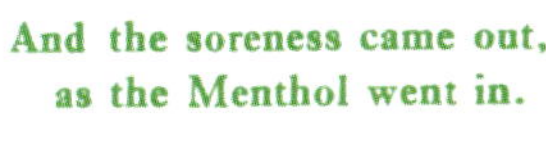
And the soreness came out,
as the Menthol went in.
Alfred I. Tooks.

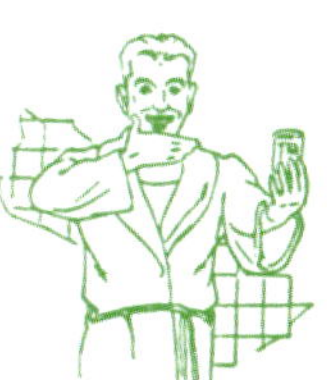

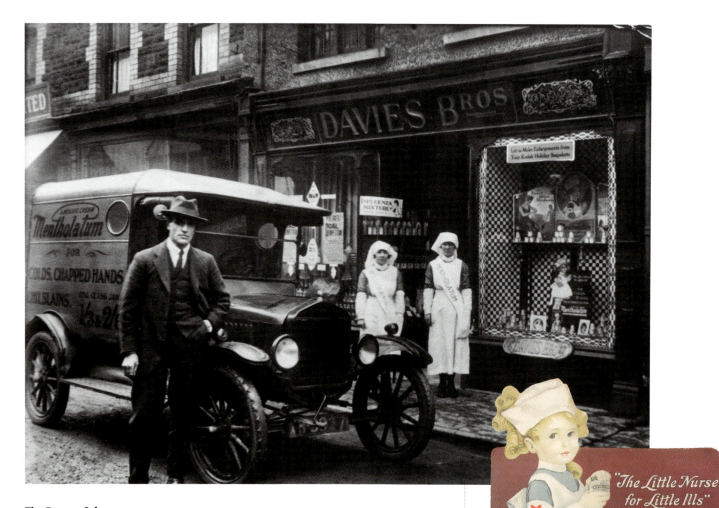

The Dapper Salesman . . .

and his Little Nurse assistants kick off a store promotion in front of a typical Victorian shop found in London or any other industrial town or city in Great Britain. The prices painted on the side of the truck were in old English currency. 1/3 was 1 shilling and thrupence–approximately the equivalent of today's 15p. 2/6 was half a crown (one crown was made up of five shillings)–approximately the equivalent of today's 30p.

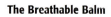

"The Little Nurse for Little Ills"

FOR COLDS, BURNS, SKIN IRRITATION

A HEALING CREAM

Mentholatum

TUBES 25¢ JARS 25¢ 50¢ $1.00

FOR CATARRH: APPLY INTO THE NOSTRILS. FOR CHEST COLDS: RUB ON CHEST AND BACK

TRADE MARK

MENTHOLATUM

REGISTERED

THE MEDICATED BREATHABLE BALM

FOR COLDS IN THE HEAD, NASAL CATARRH, HAY FEVER, CHEST COLDS, CHILBLAINS, CHAPPED SKIN AND SKIN IRRITATION, Etc.

DIRECTIONS: APPLY TO THE PARTS AFFECTED.

Made by THE MENTHOLATUM CO.,LTD.,AT SLOUGH BUCKS.

Contains: MENTHOL. 1.66 ACID. BORIC. 10.00 CAMPH. 10.00 OL. EUCALYP. 0.66 OL. PINI PUMIL. 0.66 METHYL. SALICYL. 0.66 PARAFF. MOLL. FLAV. AD. 100.00

The Breathable Balm

The U.K. label did not include A. A. Hyde's signature above the banner. There was an advertising slogan above a short list of remedies in the center; instructions for "Catarrh" and "Chest Colds" replaced "For Piles," and "Contents" replaced "Barbers" found on U.S. labels.

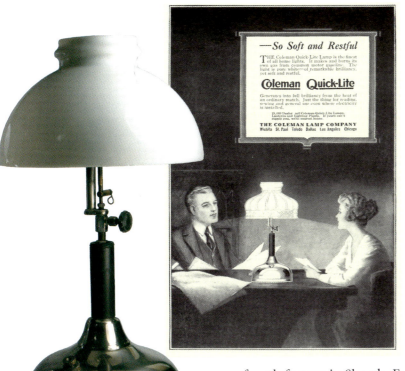

manufacturers were Coleman and Mentholatum. Coleman sold 600,000 lamps in 1920, and China was its largest foreign market.[3]

Labor issues aside, rising consumption and easy credit eventually combined to shift America's industry into high gear. In 1920, after a year under construction, Mentholatum's flagship factory was in full production in Buffalo. The eighty-thousand-square-foot, state-of-the-art plant could manufacture a boxcar load of product in a day. (See more about the Buffalo factory on pages 114–117.) In 1923, the company opened its fourth factory in Slough, England, an industrialized area outside of London. This was a tiny boost to Great Britain's depressed industry and high unemployment. The company's four factories were now distributing product to the four corners of the world. By 1926, they were selling twenty million units annually.[4]

(Text continues on page 107.)

Coleman Lamp

The Coleman CQ329 Quick-Lite lamp depicted in the February 1920 *Delineator* magazine ad was the most popular in the Quick-Lite series. Between 1917 and 1923, the Wichita factory manufactured more than two million of this style alone. Pictured above is a Quick-Lite CQ fount and handle with a No. 306 reading shade (ten-inch opal dome). The original coil generator has been replaced with a newer rotary generator.

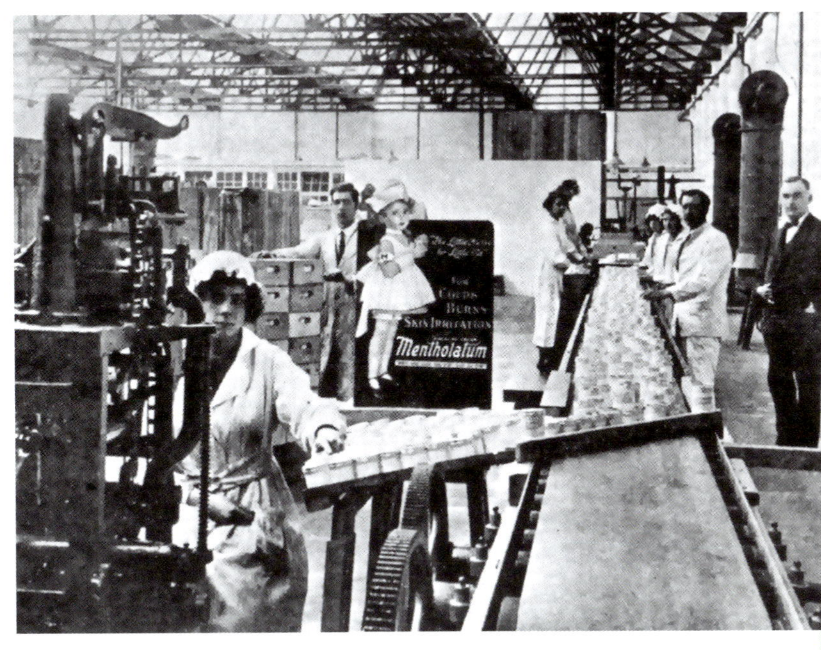

Slough, Bucks, England Plant

The Slough plant produced product for Europe, Africa, the Middle East, and Asia.

The Electrification of Room Vaporizers

Room vaporizers, as opposed to atomizers, provided an ambient dispersion of cool vapors within the vicinity of the bedridden patient. Vaporizers, like the ones pictured on page 36 and here, could quickly fill a room with the smell of menthol and other oils that would have been added to the water in their boilers. Although not designed to build up pressure like the atomizer, they often had spouts that could focus the steam toward the patient lying in bed. They worked best when placed on a nightstand and aimed out over the center of the bed so that the patient could breathe from the edge of the mist cloud. If the vapor was aimed at the patient's face, water would condense on the skin causing the patient to become wet and cold.

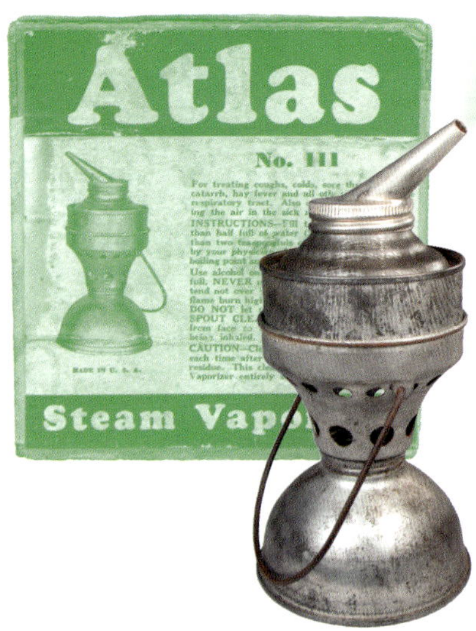

Oil-fired vaporizers, used well into the 1920s, are represented here by the utilitarian Atlas No. 111, a galvanized-tin unit built by DeVilbiss. The No. 111 was inexpensive to buy and was at home in sickrooms in city flats and farmhouses alike. Its handle allowed it to be moved when the patient changed locations, and the nozzle could be aimed so that the steam would have the best effect.

In addition to lamp oil, another portable fuel source was Sterno, a product used primarily in cooking and chafing dishes since 1893. The Sterno Company manufactured this graniteware vaporizer, which fit over a standard heating frame (not shown).

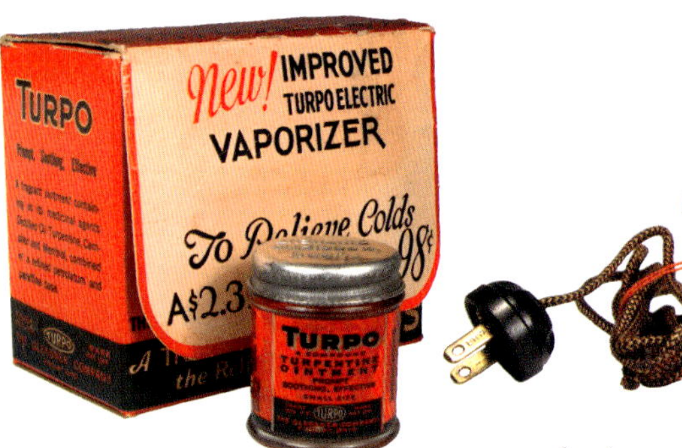

The "New Improved Turpo Electric Vaporizer" was only as portable as its four-and-a-half-foot cord would allow, but its electrodes were the future of vaporizer design. If there really was any "improvement," as the box claimed, it was overshadowed by a host of design flaws. The little device directed the hot steam only straight up and failed to provide a safe way to handle the glass jar when it became hot. There was no on/off switch, and the electrodes threatened dangerous meltdown when the water evaporated. Using it as a loss leader, the Glessner Company of Findlay, Ohio, claimed "a $2.35 value for only 98¢" and thus the sales of Turpo ointment and the conversion to electricity were its true benefits.

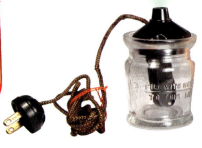

In 1927, two patents were issued that addressed the failures of the jar vaporizer. Max Katzman's KAZ brand and Nicholas Lawner's American Electric Vaporizer introduced the directional spout, safety handle, and, best of all, an automatic shutoff that engaged when the water level dropped below the electrodes. By now the sales pitch had been worked out: "no more open flame to worry about." The '20s was the decade of household appliance electrification, the room vaporizer not excepted.

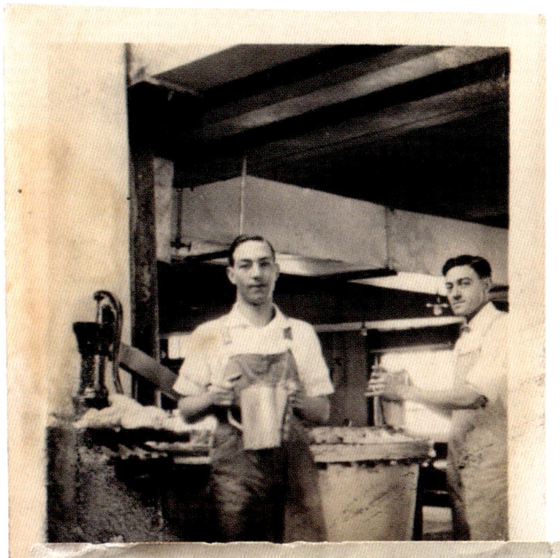

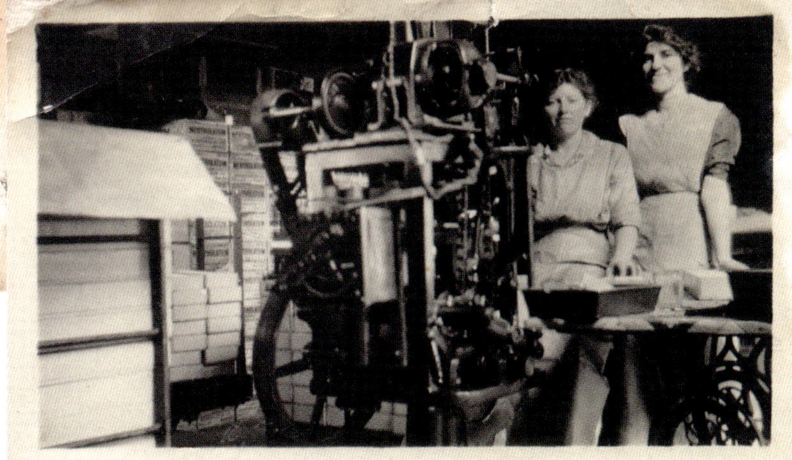

Ethel Smith had two country friends who preceded her to town and were now working at the Mentholatum Company. Clara Smith (no relation) and Ethel Chase were taking advantage of the new economic freedoms women had gained after the war (benefiting mostly educated, single, white women), and they heartily encouraged Ethel to fill out an application. Having done only farmwork, Ethel possessed no office training. Nevertheless, her friends knew she was smart and recommended she ask for office work anyway. Ethel was hired by the office manager, Margaret Saxe, a single woman who had worked for the company since 1905. The company's policy toward hiring women required them to leave once they married. Women were still expected to marry and raise a family, and men were to provide for them. Thus, the female employees who constituted the majority of workers there were either single "girls" or "spinster" women. New hires without business schooling were placed in the packing department to start with. If they could acquire the necessary typing skills, they might later be considered for a position upstairs, when and if one became available. Ethel's eight-year experience at the Mentholatum Company was typical: when someone above her married and left, she moved up until she too married and left. The other route was to remain a spinster and work there until retirement, which many did.

The Wichita Plant

The photographer forgot to indicate which one was George Simon, the "cooker," or record the identity of the other man (top). The kettle they were adding ingredients to was located at the back end of the factory floor, surrounded by plenty of natural light. Above, Carrie Stutsman (sitting) and coworker (standing) pose at a packing machine.

Ethel rode the streetcar to work each morning for a nickel fare. She and Clara and some of the other employees carried their sack lunches in their laps if they were lucky enough to find a seat. During the previous decade, Wichita's streetcar system had been allowed to deteriorate to such a poor state that standing up in the rattling "collection of junk," as it was referred to in the press, was a test of one's fortitude. Upon entering the factory building for the first time, Ethel was overwhelmed by the smell of menthol and camphor, but she soon became accustomed to it. Eighty years later, Ethel would fondly recall that the factory odor had an addictive quality, and afterward whenever she smelled a jar of Mentholatum, it reminded her of the best years of her life.[5]

(Text continues on page 109.)

The Physician's Knife

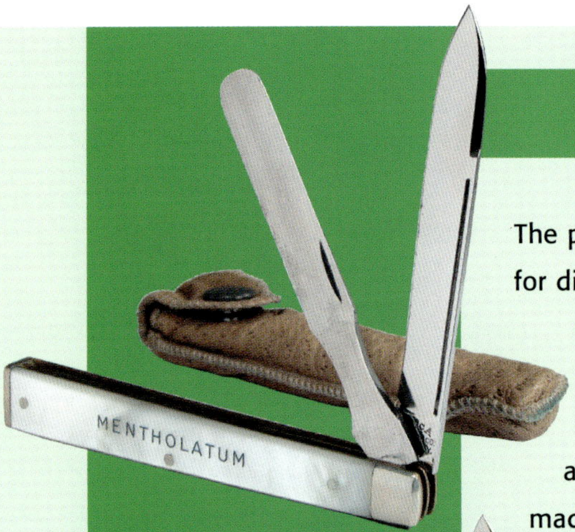

The physician's knife, so-called for its specific design as a tool for dispensing pills and powders, was given as a thank-you by the company for large orders from druggists. The knife has a distinctive spear-shaped master blade and a spatula blade in the secondary position. There is a heavy butt cap at the other end for crushing pills. The first knives were made by Utica Cutlery Company prior to 1921. The example top left has a pearl handle and came in a leather "purse."

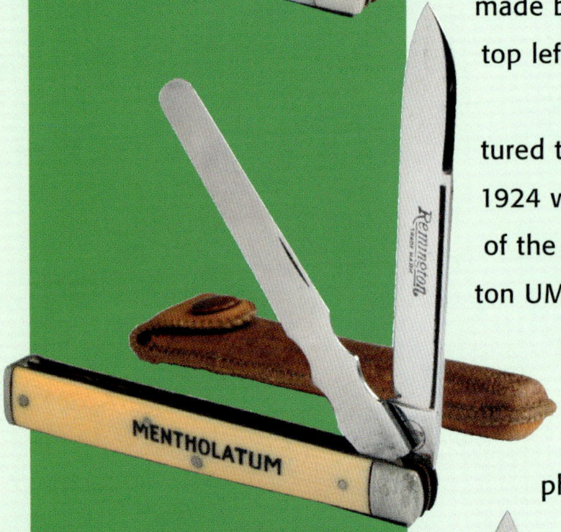

After 1921, the Remington Arms Company manufactured the physician's knife. Knives made between 1921 and 1924 were marked "REMINGTON UMC" inside a circle at the base of the master blade. The example at center left is a Remington UMC with a celluloid, faux ivory handle, and below it is the pearl version and purse with an embossed Remington snap. Knives with "MADE IN USA" outside of the circle were made from 1924 to 1933. The Mentholatum physician's knife is highly prized by knife collectors.

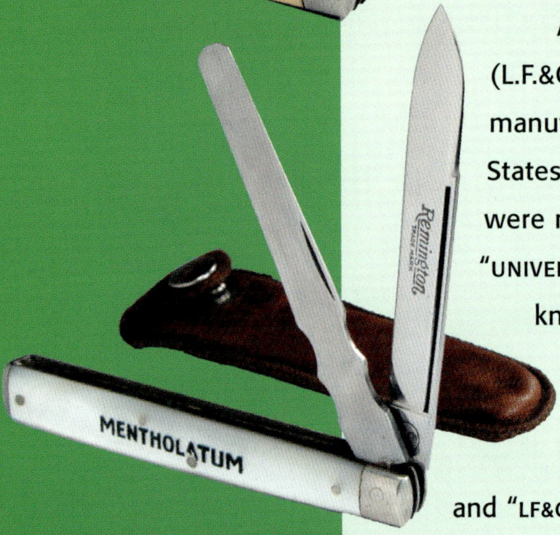

At the turn of the century, Landers, Frary & Clark (L.F.&C.) was the largest knife manufacturer in the United States. By the 1930s they were manufacturing the "UNIVERSAL" brand pocket knives. The example at right is an equal-end pocket knife with a bone handle, marked "UNIVERSAL STAINLESS" on the master blade and "LF&C USA" on the tang. The Mentholatum lettering style is from "A Healing Cream," which lasted from 1917 to 1926. This knife most likely was made in 1926.

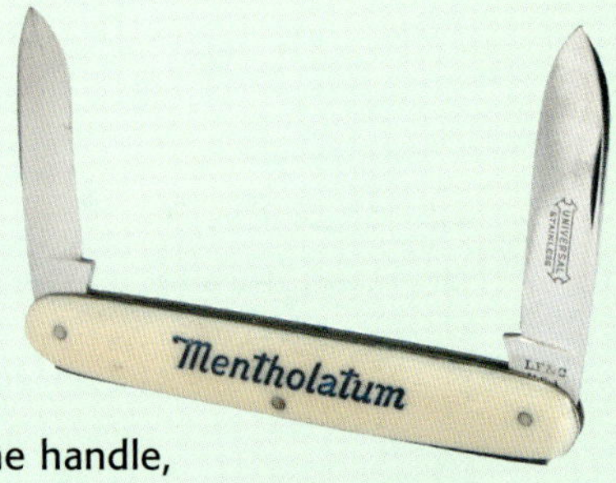

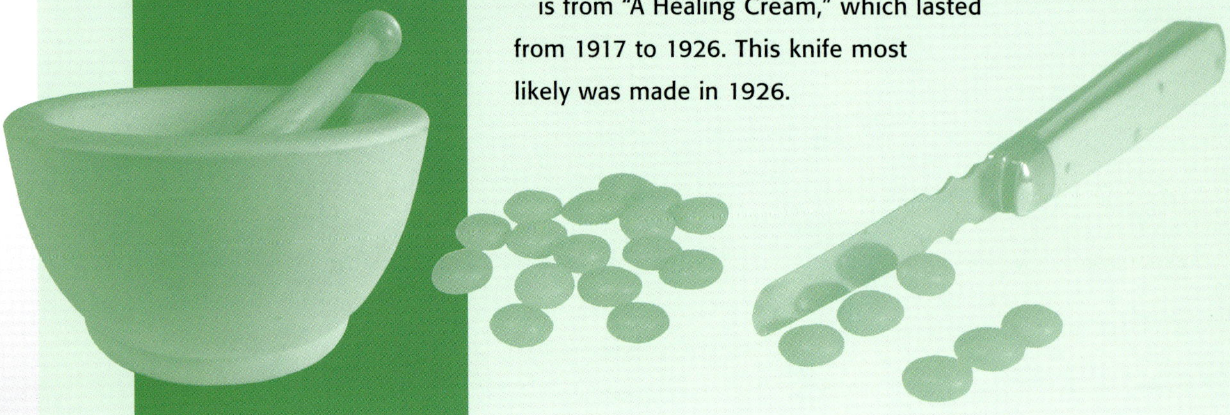

The business office was located at the front of the building. At the back was the copper kettle, the source of all the odor. Here, George Simon, the "cooker," prepared the salve, which was loaded into jars and tins by machines that poured an exact amount into each. The full jars were then placed into trays on a cart to cool down with the help of fans. When cool enough to handle, the jars were capped and run through a mechanized label machine that stood nearby. From her short stint on the factory floor, Ethel remembered that jars were placed into divided cartons, which were then packed into a wooden crate. (See page 116.) The crates were stacked inside the Douglas Avenue entrance by the shipping manager, Horace Brown, for transport to the train depot. Thousands of "trial-size" and the smaller "sample-size" tin "boxes" were also packed. Mary Plumlee, the manager of the packing department, once let Ethel run the labeling machine, and for a day or two she fed hundreds of the large eight-ounce-size jars through. (The large jars were produced only between 1916 and 1927.)

Ethel worked only a few months in the packing department before her friend Ethel Chase married and she moved up to the office to help with filing and mailing. Ms. Saxe offered to teach typing to the girls if they would come in an hour early each morning. Ethel learned quickly and was given advertising letters to type. When her friend Clara decided to marry a few years later

The Wichita Plant Floor Plan

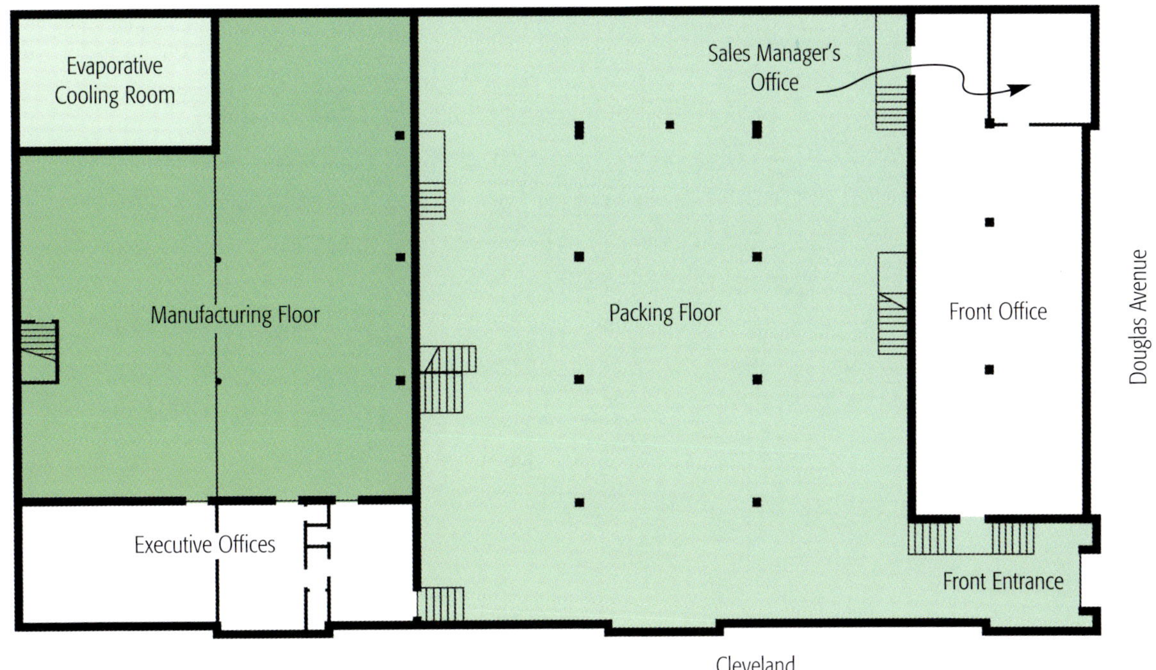

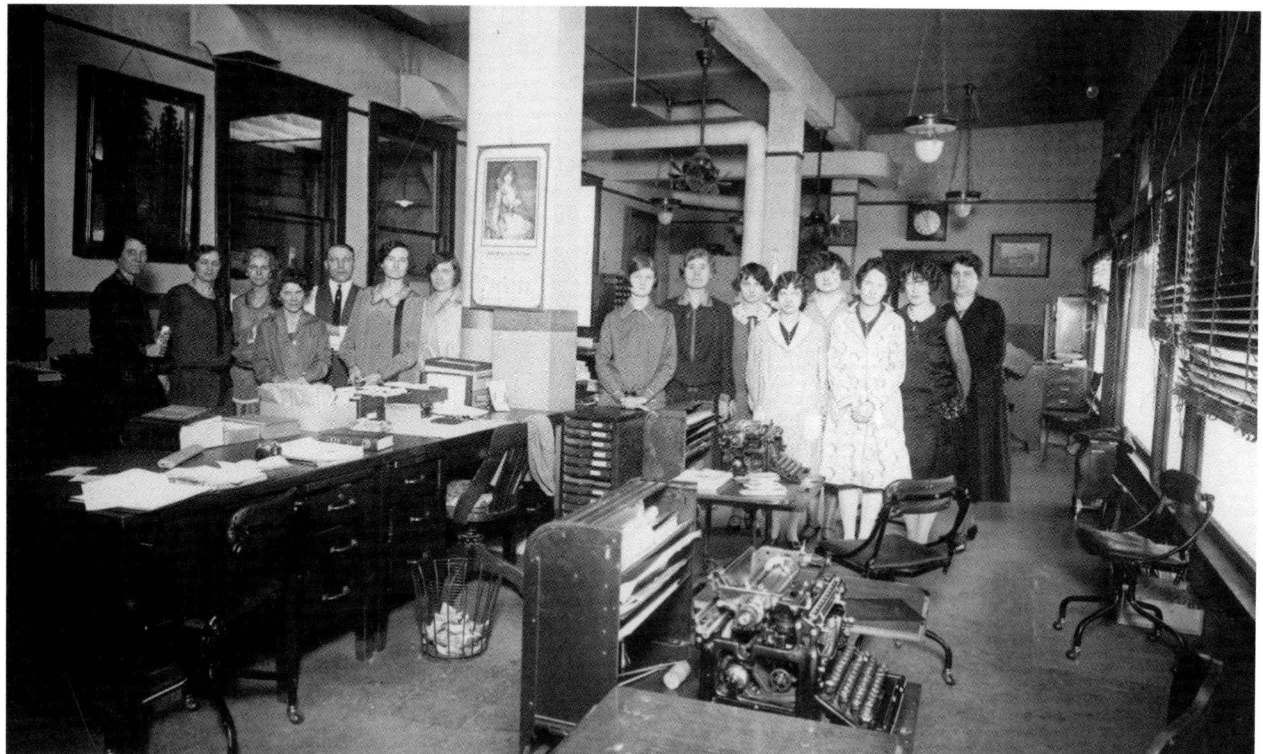

The Front-Office Staff in 1925

Ethel Smith is leaning on the left side of the column with the calendar. Turn to page 204 for a list of names.

(after the 1923 flood), Ethel was offered her position as the rebate clerk. This job required her to calculate the amount a druggist could claim for a rebate based on the size of his order and then issue him a check.

The Wichita office took care of sales west of the Mississippi, and the Buffalo office covered the eastern territory. The Wichita office had seven salesmen who traveled the western states and wrote up the druggists' orders. Their sales manager was Walter Taylor (1889–1936), and his office was located at Ethel's end of the floor. Walter was the son of A.A.'s partner in the Maple Grove Cemetery, and his first job out of school was as a salesman for the company sometime before 1910. He traveled eastern Kansas in his Ford Model-T until becoming sales manager a short time later. The other salesmen Ethel got to know were Mr. Kendrick, Mr. Galligher, Mr. McPhetridge, and Mr. Jones. Jones was notorious for his poor penmanship, and the girls who handled his orders let him know it. Each Christmas, Jones would give them a five-pound box of chocolate, which he thought might help amend his shortcoming.

Worker benefits at Mentholatum were progressive for that day. Ethel preserved the employee handbook she was given. It said that the rules and regulations were, for the most part, developed by the employees themselves. Hours for the manufacturing department were 7:55 A.M. to 5:00 P.M., with one hour for lunch,

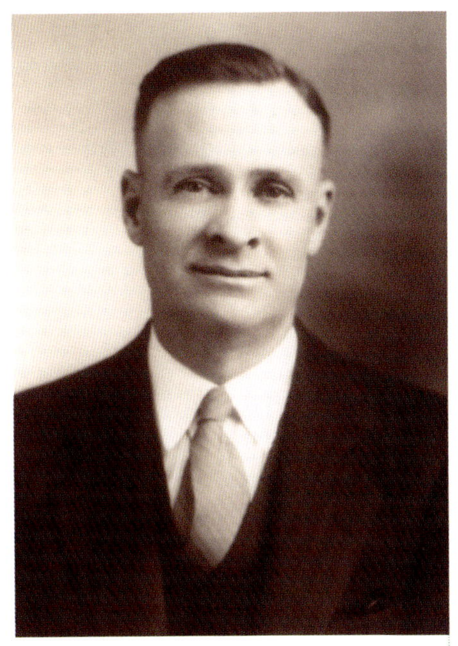

Lifetime Employee

In 1922 Walter Taylor (no relation to the author) moved his family to Buffalo to manage East Coast sales. Five years later he returned to Wichita when he was promoted to national sales director. He spent his entire career in the employ of Mentholatum.

and for the office, 8:25 A.M. to 5:00 P.M., except Saturdays, when both departments closed at noon. Half pay was allowed for "incapacitating sickness" up to four weeks. A.A. wanted to encourage a habit of saving for a rainy day, "which comes to each of us at one time or another," so he paid a quarterly bonus starting at 4 percent of the wages paid for the first year, 8 percent the second, and so forth, not to exceed a maximum of $250. In 1919 he built a building behind the factory that housed a new furnace for the factory and upstairs, a lounge, dining room, kitchenette, and shower bath for the employees. He also hired a "house mother" to prepare lunches for the staff. Ethel said he told the girls, "'Now you've got to learn how to cook so she'll help you make out the menu but you help her serve it,' so we'd have to go a little early before lunch and help Mrs. Hennington put the food out. Oh, she was a good cook, and a lovely lady. We also had what were called the club rooms up in the same building. So, Mrs. Hennington took care of the club rooms and kept them clean and we had hot lunches."

Vacation was two weeks with pay after the first year and could be taken at the beginning of "the vacation season—June 1." The employee handbook read:

> *The Chairman of the Board of Directors has a deep love of the mountains, and spends most of every summer in Estes Park,*

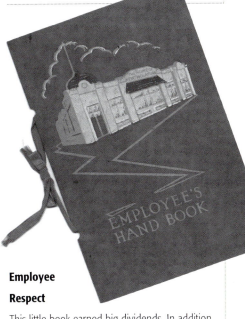

Employee Respect

This little book earned big dividends. In addition to listing work hours, regulations, vacation, and "workmen's" compensation insurance information, it described a quarterly bonus plan to assist employees in saving for a "rainy day."

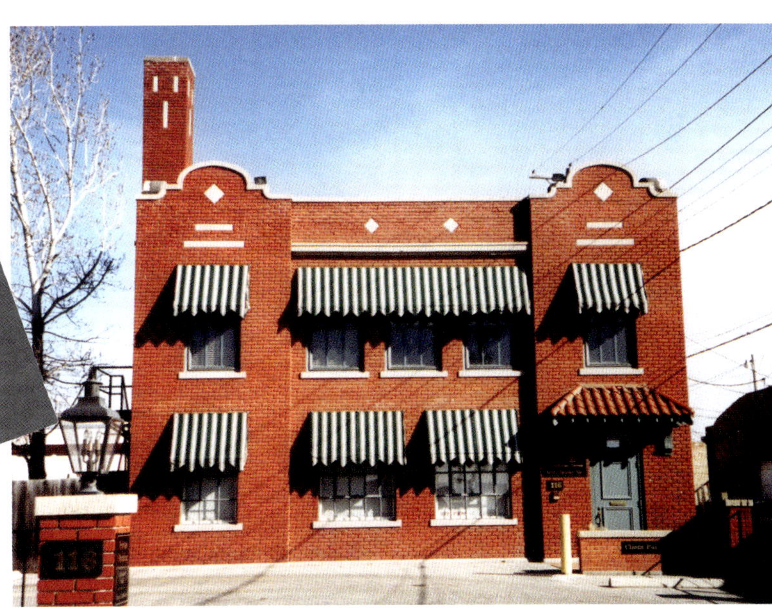

The Club House

Not a lot has changed over the years to this present-day view of the building where employees ate their lunches and held club meetings.

Colorado, and in order to share the inspiration received there, and recognizing the value of a change in environment and climate, in building up the tired bodies—making them fit for another year's work, he has made the following alternative possible: Employees having been with the Company one year or more may choose a trip to Estes Park in lieu of the two weeks' vacation with pay. The Company pays for a round trip ticket to Estes Park, Pullman ticket one way, board and lodging for ten days at the Western Conference [YMCA] grounds in Estes Park, and $25 for incidental traveling expenses.

Ethel took the trip as often as she could. She traveled with a typical group of six to Denver, where Billy Mitchell, Hyde's driver, would pick them up at the station in a seven-passenger "White" and drive them up to the mountain camp of the YMCA. The girls all wore the standard outdoorwear of the day: black "sateen" bloomers with elastic in the bottom and white "middy" blouses. Meals were provided at the Y-Camp dining hall, and box lunches were available if they went for a hike, horseback ride, or sightseeing trip in the car with Billy.

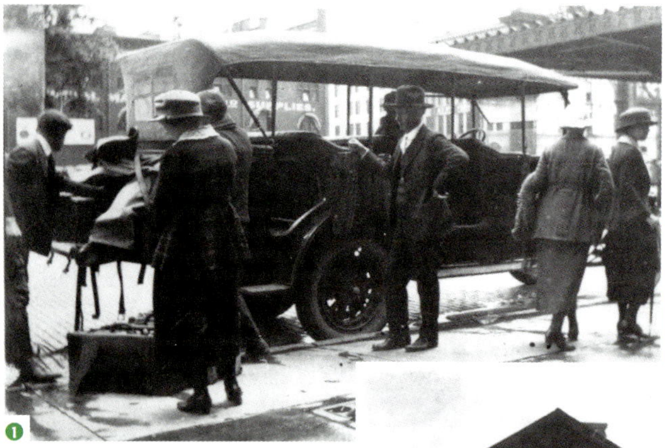

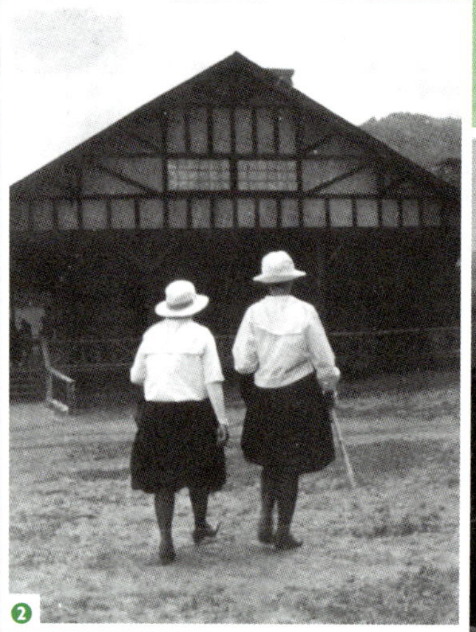

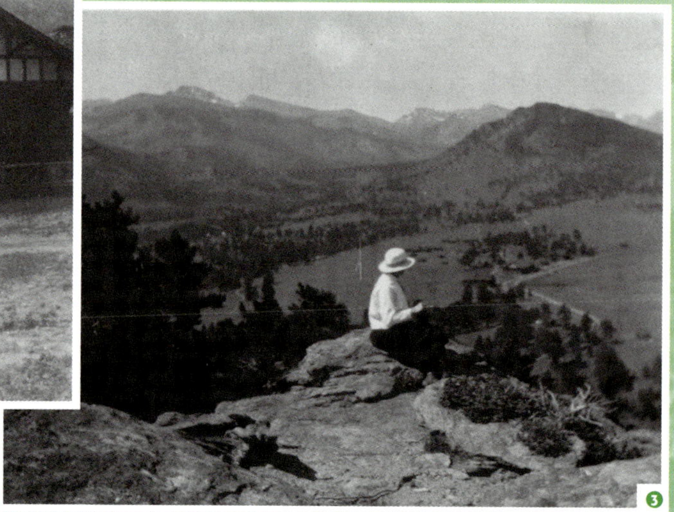

1

2

3

Y-Camp Vacation

Billy Mitchell loads up the seven-passenger White at the Denver train station in preparation for the drive up to Estes Park (1). Ethel and friend walk toward the Administration Building where events for the day were planned (2). Ethel overlooks the YMCA conference grounds in the valley below and the Front Range of the Rocky Mountains in the distance (3).

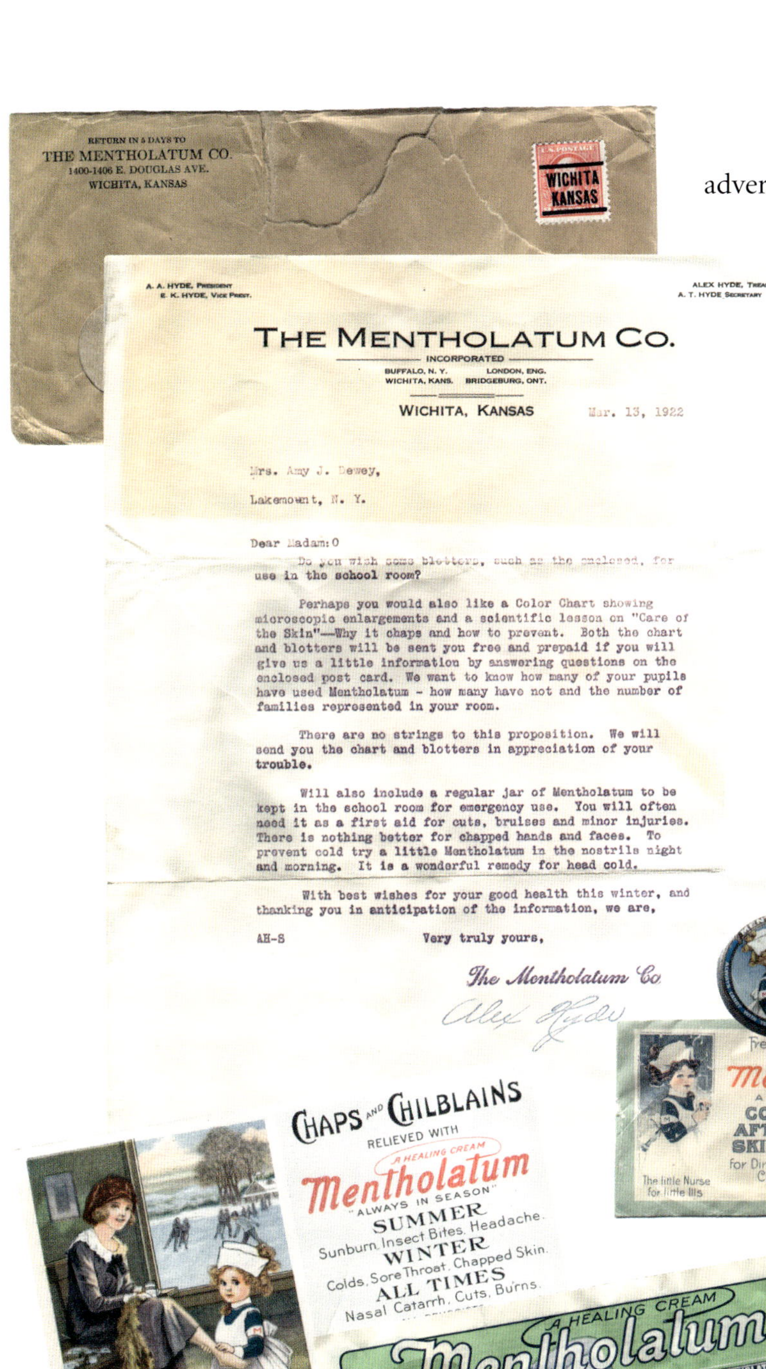

RETURN IN 5 DAYS TO
THE MENTHOLATUM CO.
1400-1406 E. DOUGLAS AVE.
WICHITA, KANSAS

A. A. HYDE, PRESIDENT
E. K. HYDE, VICE PREST.

ALEX HYDE, TREASURER
A. T. HYDE SECRETARY

THE MENTHOLATUM CO.
INCORPORATED
BUFFALO, N. Y. LONDON, ENG.
WICHITA, KANS. BRIDGEBURG, ONT.

WICHITA, KANSAS Mar. 13, 1922

Mrs. Amy J. Dewey,

Lakemownt, N. Y.

Dear Madam:O

Do you wish some blotters, such as the enclosed, for use in the school room?

Perhaps you would also like a Color Chart showing microscopic enlargements and a scientific lesson on "Care of the Skin"—Why it chaps and how to prevent. Both the chart and blotters will be sent you free and prepaid if you will give us a little information by answering questions on the enclosed post card. We want to know how many of your pupils have used Mentholatum - how many have not and the number of families represented in your room.

There are no strings to this proposition. We will send you the chart and blotters in appreciation of your trouble.

Will also include a regular jar of Mentholatum to be kept in the school room for emergency use. You will often need it as a first aid for cuts, bruises and minor injuries. There is nothing better for chapped hands and faces. To prevent cold try a little Mentholatum in the nostrils night and morning. It is a wonderful remedy for head cold.

With best wishes for your good health this winter, and thanking you in anticipation of the information, we are,

AH-S

Very truly yours,

The Mentholatum Co.

Alex Hyde

CARE of THE SKIN

FROM THE LONDON TIMES

"The importance of the care of the skin has always been underestimated. Every year, various breakages, scrapes and inflammations of the skin place vast numbers of people on the sick list. Most of this might have been prevented.

The enemy in the shape of germs of suppuration and blood poisoning is always at the gates. It has been calculated that even a moderately clean human skin carries millions of bacteria to the square inch. While the skin remains unbroken, these bacteria are harmless. They cannot pierce the strong, resistant texture, but even a small scrape or cut allows them to effect an entry.

The course of the case after entry of the germs depends upon two things—the power of resistance and the virulence of the germ.

Personal health is so important that its absence is sufficient to result in inflammations arising at places where the agent of injury may be no more severe than a frayed collar or a razor. The outer or horny layers of the skin are rubbed away and presently a boil or other trouble appears.

Careful washing with good soap is of first importance. This gets rid of some of the germs and cleanses small abrasions before they become infected. There can be no doubt that clean hands and hands often washed are much less liable to inflamed wounds than dirty hands. It is not necessary to use strong and irritating soap which, instead of protecting, injures the skin."

The Times might well have added that an application of Mentholatum after washing acts as an antiseptic and lubricant to the outer layer of the skin. Mentholatum keeps the skin soft and pliable, avoiding cracking and chapping, even in severe weather.

Post Card

THE MENTHOLATUM CO.

1400-1406 E. DOUGLAS AVE.

WICHITA, KAN.

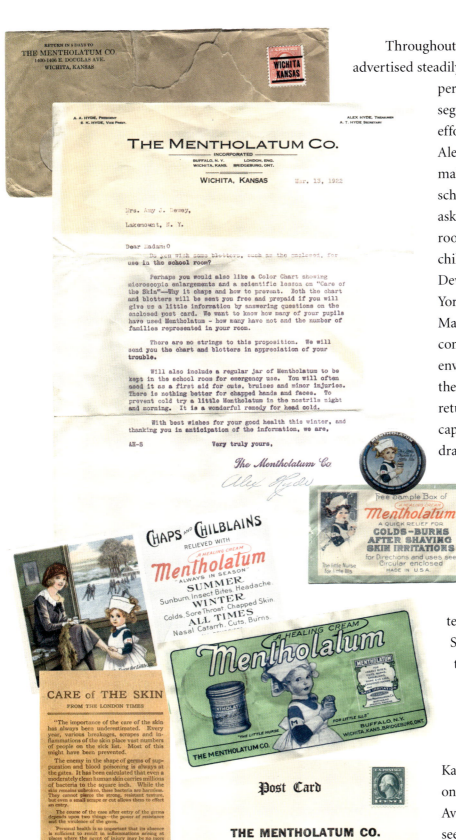

The 1922 Dewey Packet

Throughout the decade, Mentholatum advertised steadily through magazines, newspapers and mailings. One market segment they spent a great deal of effort on was schoolchildren. Alex Hyde's office regularly mailed personalized letters to schoolteachers across the country, asking for a count of their classrooms so he might send each child a blotter. Mrs. Amy J. Dewey from Lakemont, New York, received such a letter dated March 13, 1922. The envelope contained a cover letter, sample envelope and tin, blotter, "Care of the Skin" handout, and stamped return postcard. This time capsule was found in a dresser drawer at an estate sale by an alert antique dealer who recognized its historic value and did not salvage it for the tin and blotter. The Dewey letter dated the tin and blotter.

When shown the contents of the Dewey letter, Ethel Smith Willard recognized the tin but could not recall ever seeing blotters during her time at the company. The outer envelope was postmarked Wichita, Kansas, and the return address on the postcard was Douglas Avenue. Because Ethel did not see these items in the front office, it might indicate that they were handled in Alex's office at the back of the plant, where she seldom ventured.

(Text continues on page 118.)

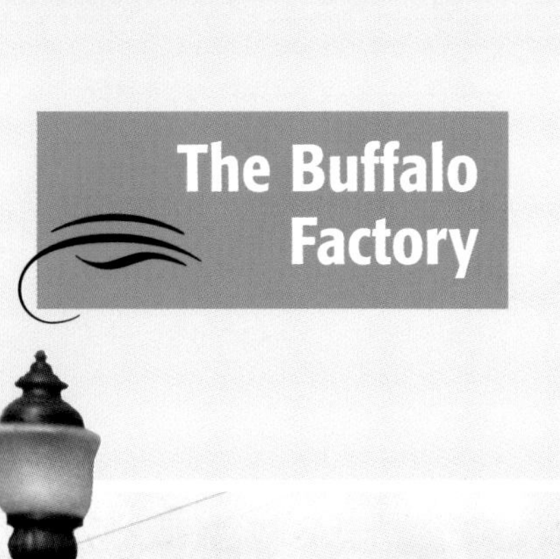

The Buffalo Factory

Located at 1360 Niagara Street overlooking the Niagara River (A and B, below) the eighty-thousand-square-foot, four-story Mentholatum factory was a state-of-the-art facility when it was completed in 1919. The rectangular concrete and brick block had windows inside each frame of the grid-patterned facade that opened to bathe the production floors with light and cross ventilation. An artesian well provided enough water for manufacturing needs, a ceiling fire sprinkler system that was ahead of its time, and air-conditioning for the entire building.

The following selection of photographs, some with known dates and others that are unknown, illustrate how the factory manufactured Mentholatum during the plant's first decade.

The front-office photograph (C, below) was taken in February 1926, based on the Denver & Rio Grand Western calendar hanging on the window frame in the back, left-hand corner of the room. This photograph also helped to date a stack of

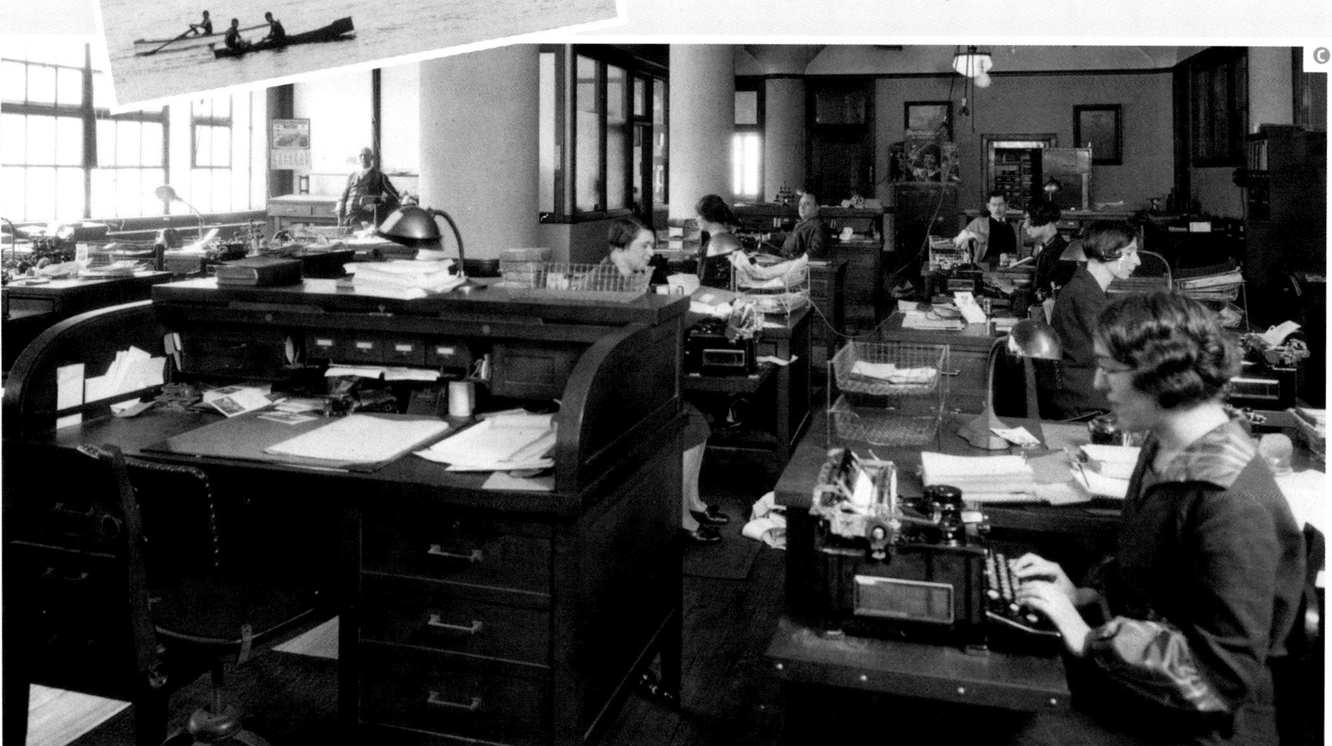

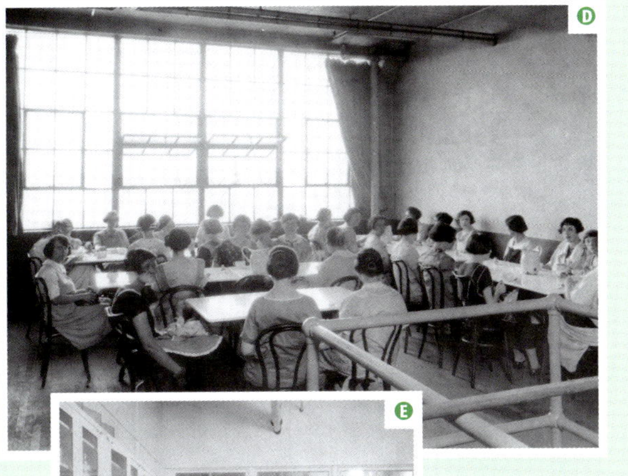

blotters that can be seen on the unoccupied desk in the foreground. With their hair styled in the fashion of the day, these working "girls" (D, left) were probably asked to go sit in the lunchroom and pose for the photographer.

Hundreds of thousands of pounds of petrolatum a year started the process on the top floor in the "Hot Room," where it was heated by steam pipes and held in a large tank until the cooker needed it. In the "Kettle Room" on a floor below, the ingredients were mixed with the petrolatum in a row of kettles (shown at left in two photos from the 1940s, E and F) and the hot Mentholatum was then pumped through insulated pipes from one kettle designated the "holding kettle" to where it was needed. From the warehouse on the top floor the jars were cleaned and placed in open wood boxes to be pushed down the spiral slides to the floors below.

This early photograph (G, below) shows two filling lines in action. At the base of each spiral slide was a filling machine that was hooked up to an insulated pipe from the holding kettle. As the boxes arrived, the jars were emptied out on a sorting platform by a worker, lined up, and fed into the machine where each one was filled with a pre-measured amount of hot Mentholatum and then ejected onto the conveyer. The conveyer belt ran the full length of the floor to allow the jars to cool. Fans were located at intervals along the line to help speed up the cooling if necessary.

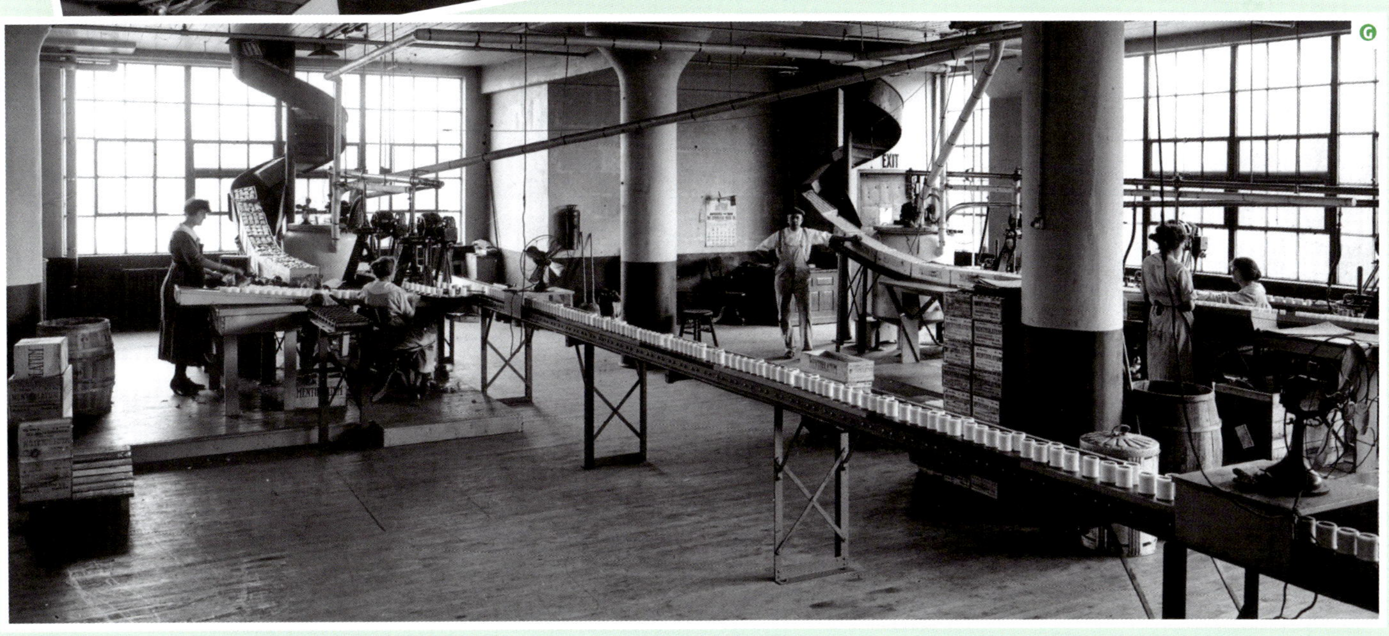

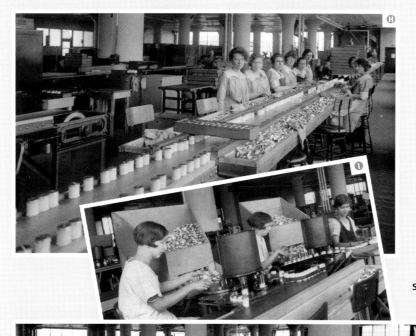

Caps were placed on each jar by hand (H, left) until the very first "Capem" capping machine (I) was developed for the company by Consolidated Packaging Machinery Corp. sometime before this picture was taken in 1926.

The capped jars passed through a labeling machine and were then placed by hand into boxes with an insert. This photograph (J) shows that the Little Nurse inserts were stacked on the table over the conveyor belt and the prefolded boxes were inside the cages beside each employee. The filled boxes were then placed inside a carton (seen stacked behind the cages), six three-ounce jars per carton and twelve one-ounce jars per carton. The next photo (K) shows a box-packing machine that replaced the hand method.

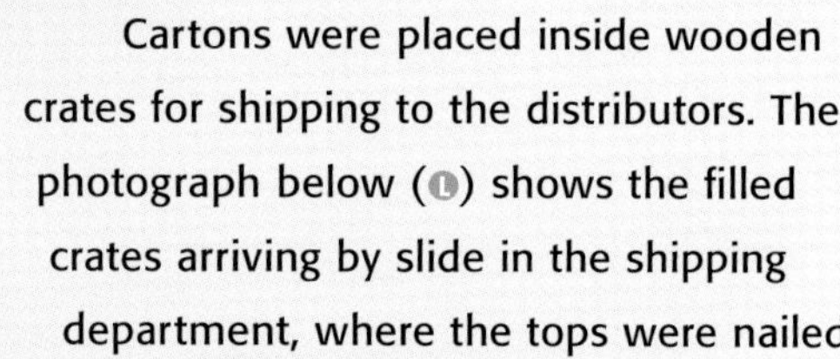

Cartons were placed inside wooden crates for shipping to the distributors. The photograph below (L) shows the filled crates arriving by slide in the shipping department, where the tops were nailed

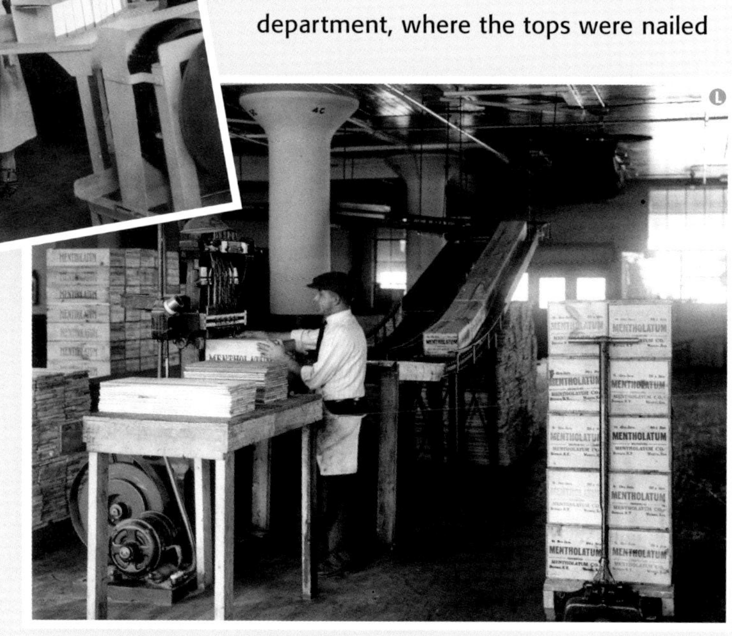

closed before they were stacked for storage and shipping. The ground floor (M) conveniently opened in the back to a rail line that ran along the river's edge. Truck loading could be accommodated from a side entrance.

Tube manufacture evolved from filling the tubes at one station and closing them at another (N) to one continuous revolving system (O).

The sample tin filling system (P) started with the woman sitting at the top left side of the rig where the cup or bottom half of the tin box was filled with a measured amount of Mentholatum. The cup then slid down the ramp and was deposited onto the outer edge of the conical cooling wheel. After one full rotation of the wheel, it was diverted onto the sorting table, where a lid was placed onto it and it was thrown into a box with hundreds of others ready to be slipped into an envelope or sample box.[6]

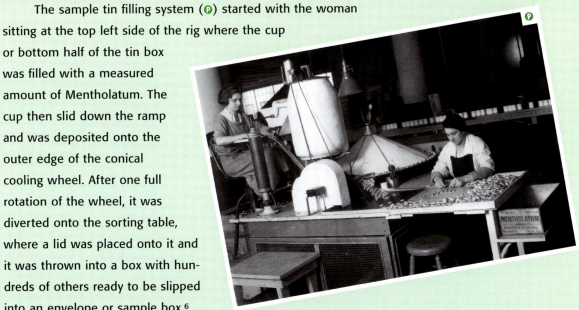

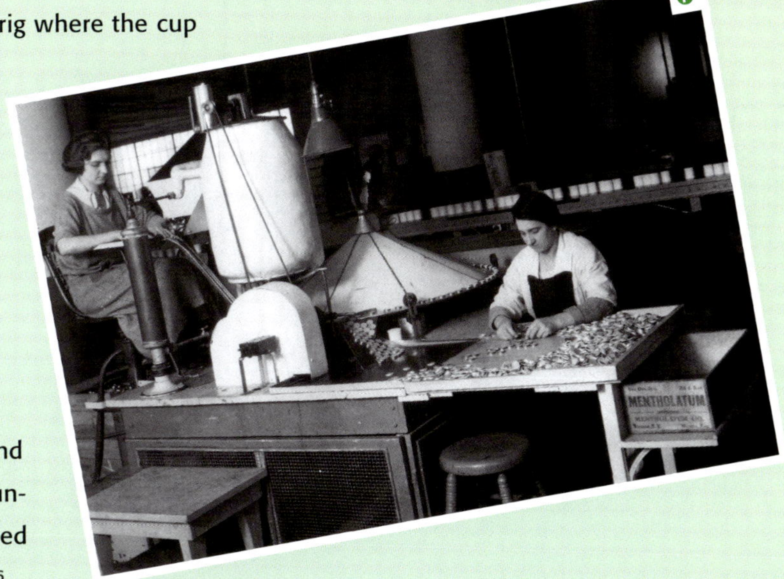

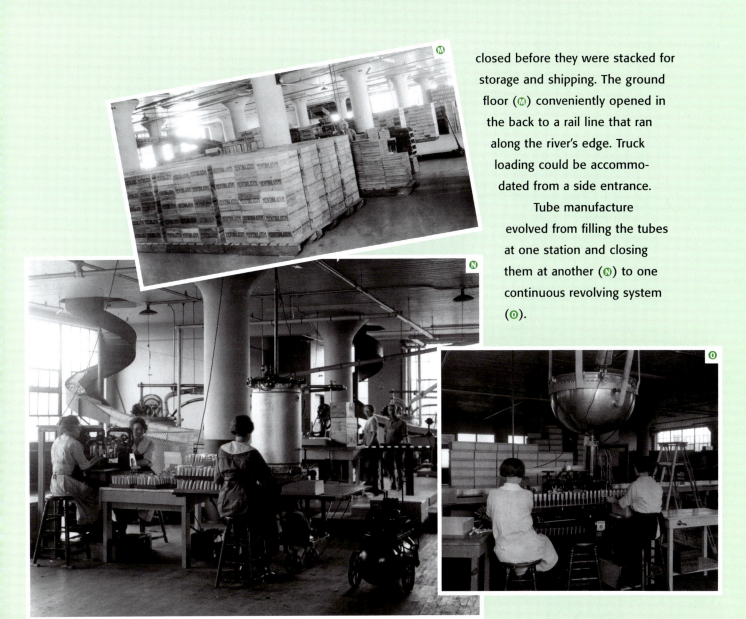

Mimics

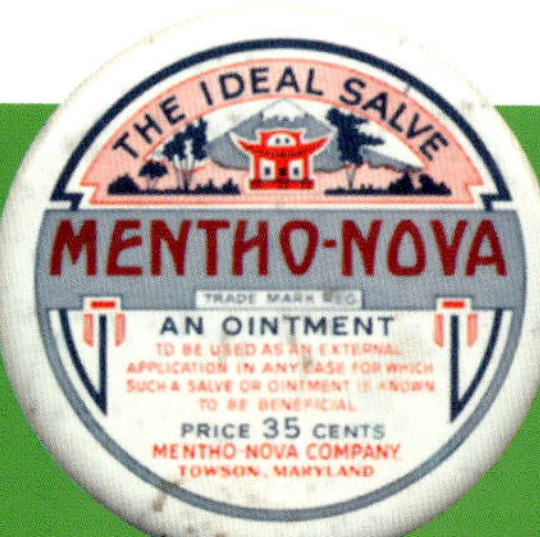

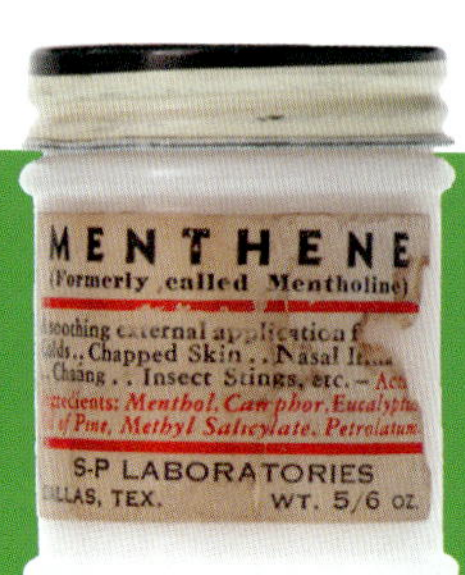

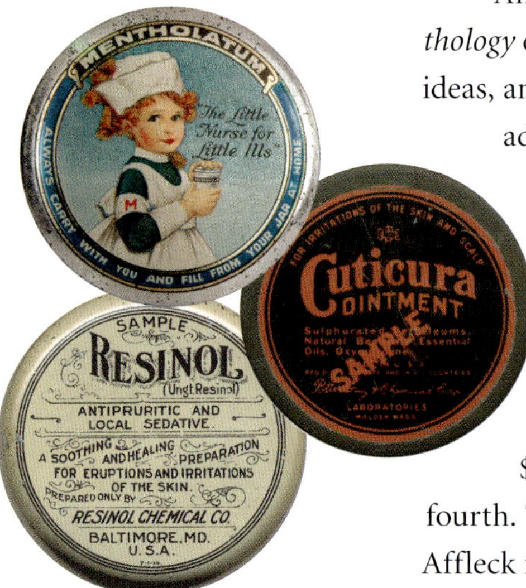

▲ Top Sellers

Another item that Ethel was unaware of was Alex's *Menthology* quarterly. During the early 1920s, Alex asked for sales ideas, and a steady flow of them were sent in. One druggist advised his customers who owned chickens to use Mentholatum for roup. Another suggested that on Fridays barbers use it when shaving their customers—who will miss it over the weekend and surely ask the druggist for some of their own to use at home. Alex decided to turn it into a competition in 1921 by offering $50 for the best advertising suggestion of the year, $25 for the second best, $15 for the third, and $10 for the fourth. The winner, announced in January 1922, was W. R. Affleck from Orofino, Idaho. Affleck, the president of the Idaho Board of Pharmacy, suggested placing a $1 bill into one jar in a stack of many jars as a "try-your-luck" scheme to boost sales of the jars. The second-prize winner, Seitz Drug Store in Ellsworth, Kansas, had the customers guess the number of jars stacked in the window display for a reward of an eight-ounce jar.[7]

▼ Top Advertisers

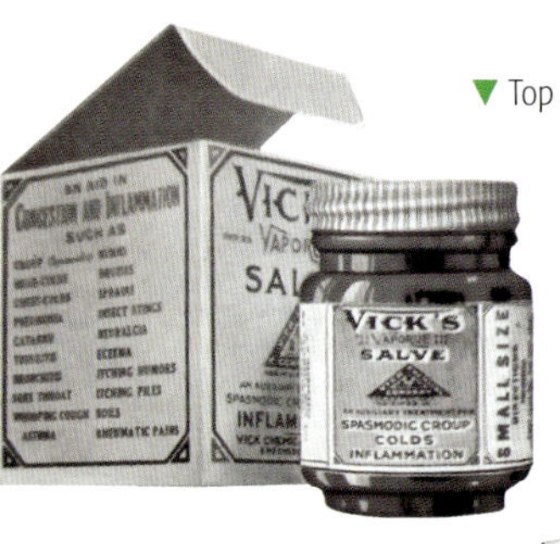

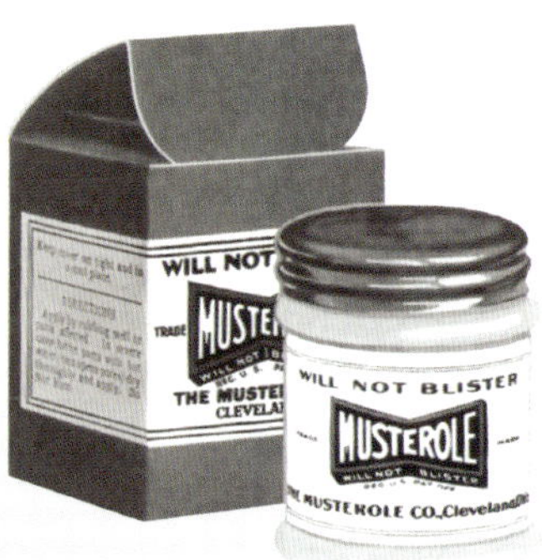

A nationwide survey published in the January 1922 issue of *The Druggists Circular* asked leading druggists throughout the United States to list the top-selling proprietary toilet articles in their stores. They concluded that "Mentholatum, Cuticura and Resinol ointments are, in the order named, the best selling ointments in all parts of the Country." The most conspicuous advertisements for cold remedies in national magazines at the time were Mentholatum—"The Little Nurse for Little Ills," Musterole—"Better Than a Mustard Plaster," and Vicks VapoRub.[8]

Menthology recommended that the men who worked the soda fountains, filled the prescriptions, and developed the film might find relief for their sore hands in a jar of Mentholatum. It also advised the druggists to sell to policemen, postmen, campers, and clerks for their "Tired, Aching Dawgs."[9]

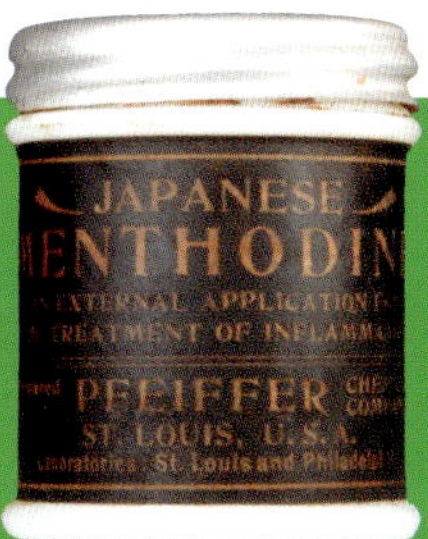

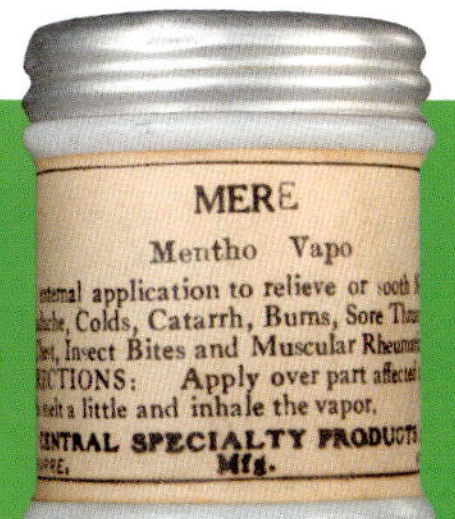

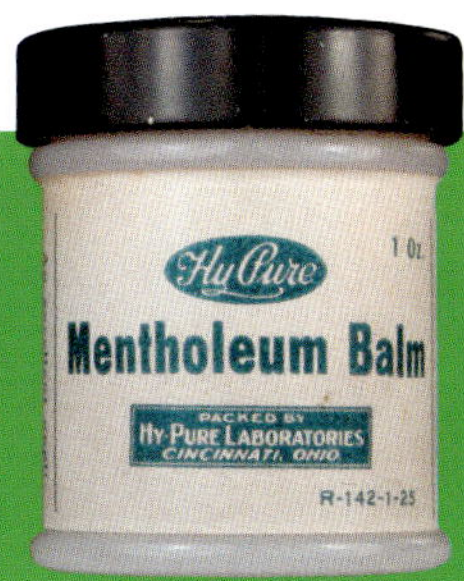

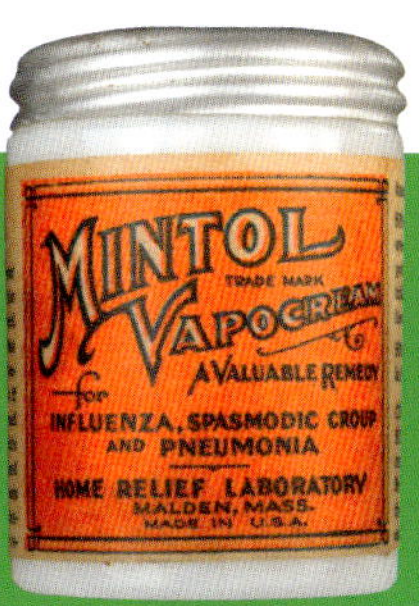

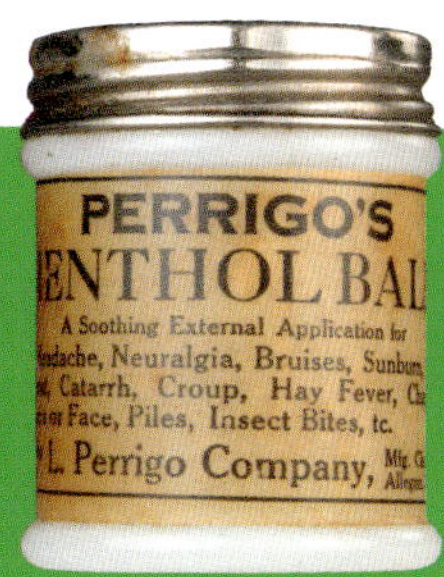

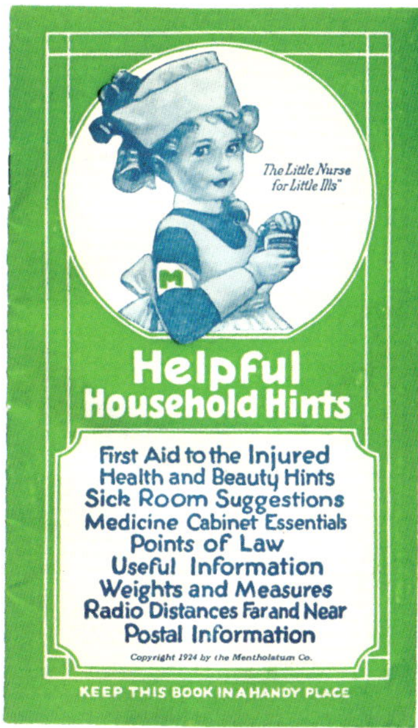

Helpful Household Hints

This is a 1924 promotional handout.

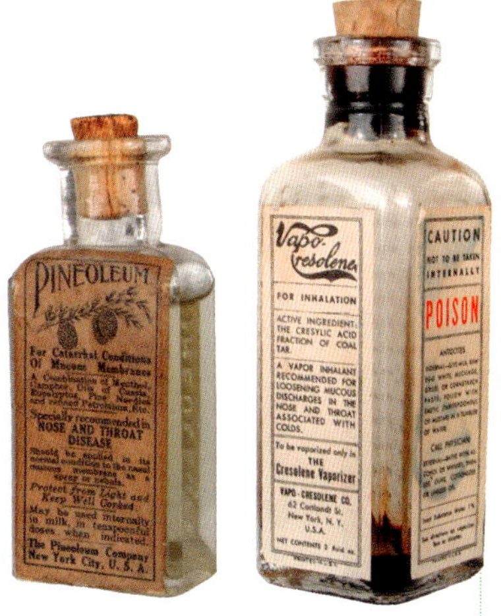

Name Your Poison

Pineoleum and Vapo-Cresolene were popular for use in vaporizers.

Ever on the lookout for creative new ways to use Mentholatum, the company continued to publish ideas in *Menthology*. In the mid-1920s, it recommended using Mentholatum as a cleansing night cream. Another suggestion was to use it as a scalp treatment for dandruff. The most exotic new use of the decade came from a missionary who recounted how he had used Mentholatum to tame ruthless Chinese river pirates. After he and his crew had been robbed, Rev. Ray treated the bandit chief's wounded leg with Mentholatum and was spared his life in gratitude. One of the company's oldest claims, the use of Mentholatum to relieve mosquito bites, came into question in 1926 when *Menthology* reported that there was some difference of opinion as to whether or not it would also keep mosquitoes away.[10]

After the introduction of automated filling machines into the factory at the end of the war, sales of jars began to drop, while the sales of tubes increased. Previously, glass jars (called pots) had been filled by hand to their tops. When machines that could fill measured amounts of salve were installed, problems arose due to variations in the size of the jars. Glass manufacturers were unable to make one unified size, causing a slightly undersized jar to overflow and a slightly oversized jar to look partly full. Customers had no way of knowing this, and because they were unable to account for the various levels, they decided it was safer to purchase a tube. When the company realized this, *Menthology* asked the druggists to explain it to their customers personally, and jar sales picked back up. Then, in 1927, a reverse perception began to circulate that the one-ounce jars held more salve than the one-ounce tubes, and once again *Menthology* asked for the druggists' help to set things straight. *Menthology* also suggested a way to boost Mentholatum's strength by just adding one ounce of turpentine to three ounces of Mentholatum. This is considered dangerous to us today, but products like Pineoleum, which was mostly turpentine, and Vapo-Cresolene, made of a caustic and poisonous isomeric phenol called cresol (a variant of creosol), were popular brands that were challenging Mentholatum.[11]

On June 10, 1923, a dam on the Arkansas River near Pueblo, Colorado, broke, and the resulting surge of water flooded the center of Wichita. The factory's front basement—where the print shop was located along with the company's old files—and the back basement were submerged. The *Menthology* mailing list was lost, as were most of the company's early historic documents. (Early copies of *Menthology* in the Hyde Collection have slight water damage and mud residue from this flood.) Shortly after the flood, Ethel and Clara left for their vacation in Estes Park, and as they passed through Pueblo, they tried to locate the broken dam from their Pullman window, but it was too dark to see anything.[12]

When a Kentucky druggist in 1925 requested extra copies of *Menthology* with his own advertisement printed on the back mailing cover, Alex Hyde gave him and the readers an idea of what that might cost. Alex revealed that sixty thousand copies of *Menthology* were sent out each quarter and the cost to the company was $2.75 per hundred for a two-color cover ($1,650) and $3.45 per hundred for a four-color cover ($2,070). *Menthology* periodically

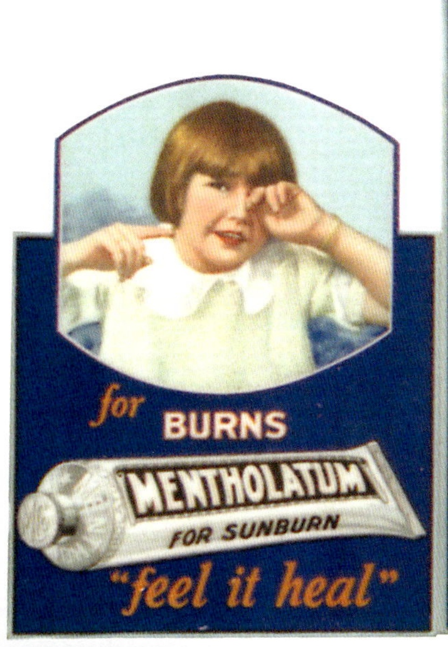

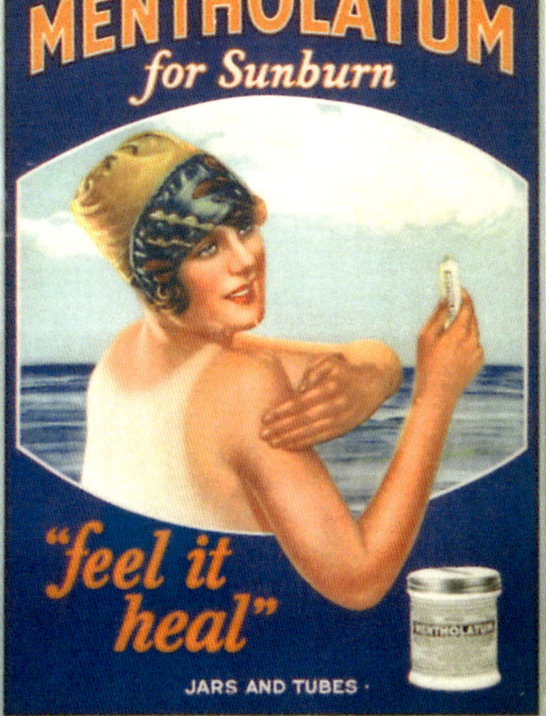

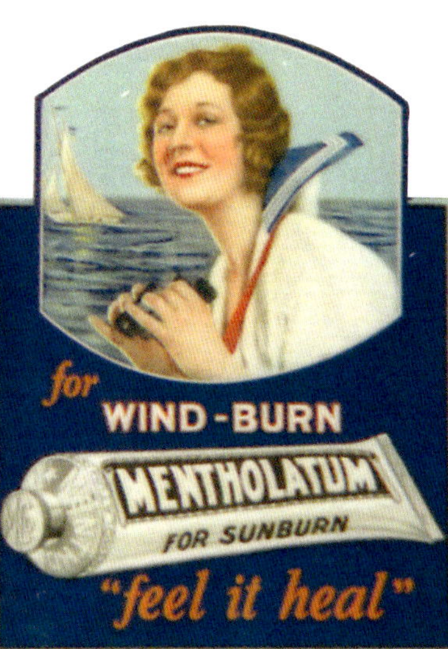

The Sunburn Triptych

Three easel-back panels for window or indoor display were sent free upon request to druggists during the 1928 summer season. (See Catalog page C124.)

reminded druggists about the benefits of selling Mentholatum. As an example, the company warranted each sale with a money-back guarantee as well as provided free replacement insurance for a portion of Mentholatum stock damaged or destroyed in drugstore fires. *Menthology* also introduced the upcoming season's window displays, which could be obtained by mailing in a return postcard. To help druggists improve their presentations, they offered in 1927 a free booklet titled, "Art in Window Decorating."[13]

A Rare Roll

Beyond the existence of this one roll in a collection in South Dakota, nothing else is known about the fate of the product after it was launched in 1925.

Cough drops were introduced in the fall of 1925. The next year twenty-six million packages were sold. In 1927, a hemorrhoid applicator for the tube was introduced, and the trouble-some eight-ounce jar was discontinued. The company said this was to fall in line with the movement toward the standardization of packages as sponsored by the National Wholesale Druggists' Association. But the large jar had always been a slow seller; after all, a little Mentholatum went a long way.[14]

(Text continues on page 124.)

Highway Signs

"For years we used Highway Signs and felt they were effective advertising. In 1925 this subject came up for discussion and the directors of the Company agreed that this form of advertising was unfair to the Public. All of our supply of signs was destroyed and from that time we have never put up any outdoor advertising."

Mentholatum's decision to remove its highway signs came at a time when the number of automobiles traveling on America's roads had more than doubled in the past five years and would eventually triple by the end of the decade. Road construction was booming. How many other businesses had the moral strength and aesthetic integrity to argue that billboards ruined the natural vista and were a blight upon the landscape? Advertising agencies, and no doubt the rival brands, must surely have thought Mentholatum was nuts to condemn billboards, labeling them a clear invasion of common rights and an expression of private gain and public loss.[15]

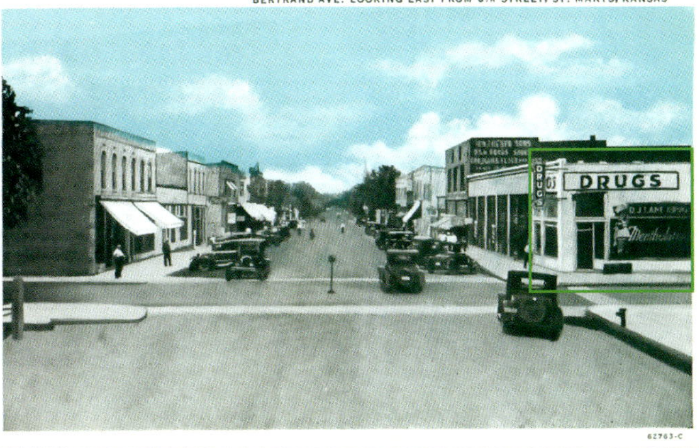
BERTRAND AVE. LOOKING EAST FROM 6TH STREET, ST. MARYS, KANSAS
DRUGS

Postcard Commercialized

Did Mentholatum's wall sign invade the integrity of this promotional postcard for St. Marys, Kansas?

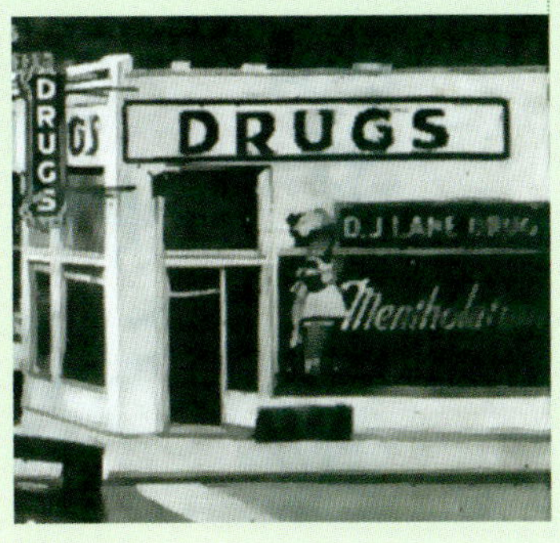
DRUGS

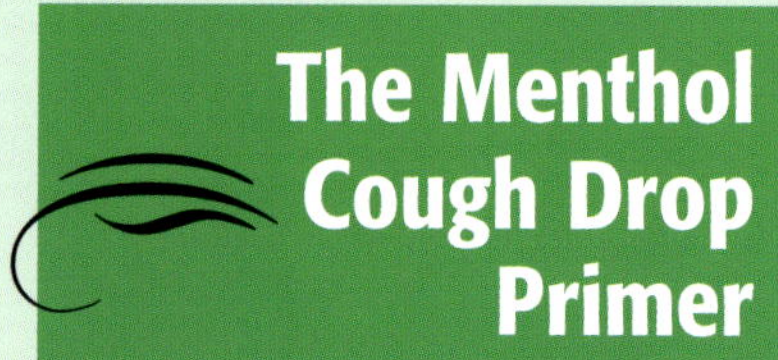

The Menthol Cough Drop Primer

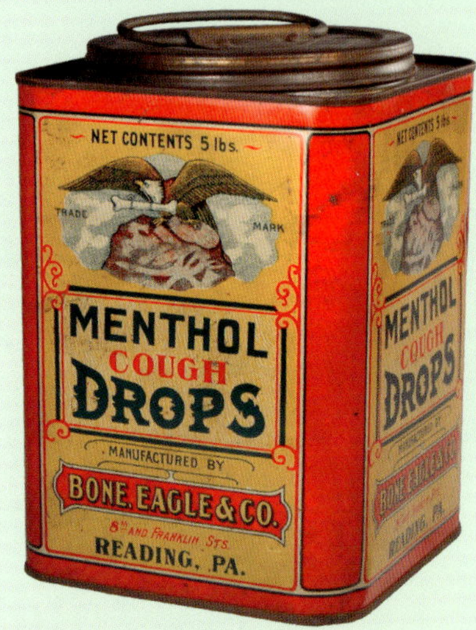

Before 1881, a traditional cough drop was either red, cherry-flavored hard candy or black licorice candy. "Drops" were made by pressing warm candy syrup into gang molds and then "dropping" the cooled and hardened casting onto a table to break apart and separate the candies. As to the candy drop's effect on coughs, that was another matter.

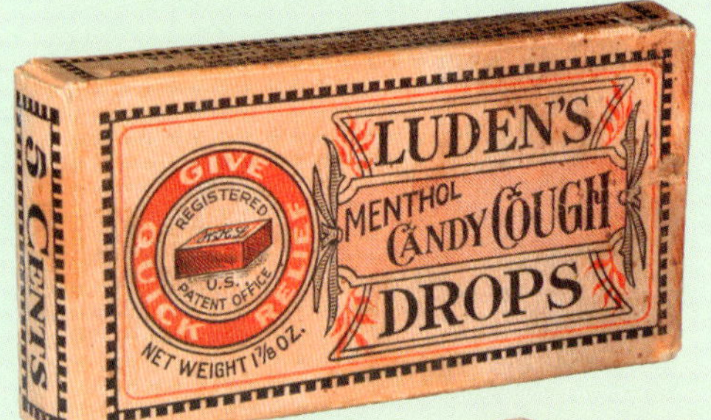

Luden's Cough Drops were one of the first American products to contain menthol. In 1881, William H. Luden combined the traditional candy cough drop with the art of molding toy candy, added the exciting new menthol crystals from Japan, and synthesized a yellow menthol-flavored hard candy pastille with his name molded on top. The components of W. H. Luden's first-ever menthol cough drop, in spite of changing mold designs, flavor recipes, and coloring by other companies, have remained the same since that day more than a century ago. The meaning of the word *drop* has also continued to mean molded pastille or lozenge even though the technology has become automated.

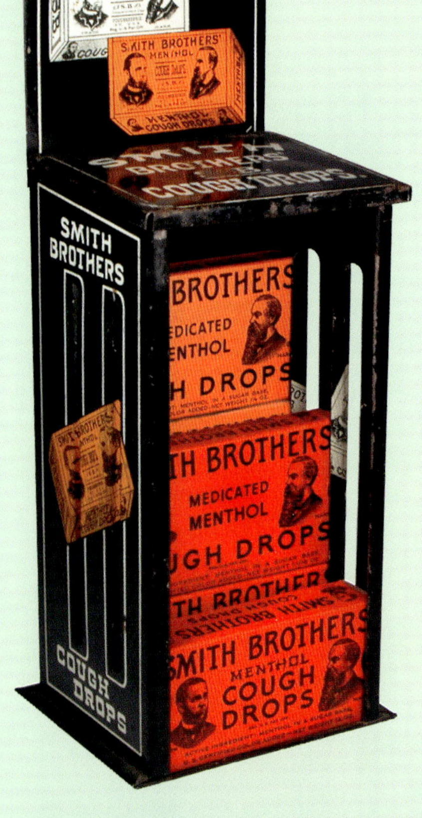

Traditionally, cough drops were sold in drugstores from a glass bowl on the countertop where the druggists would count out the number of drops in a customer's purchase and place them in a bag. This five-pound can (upper right) manufactured by Bone, Eagle & Co. in Reading, Pennsylvania, is an example of how bulk cough drops were shipped to the drugstores and general stores.

By the turn of the century, the Luden's Company was packaging their drops in the familiar two-by-three-and-one-half-inch box, which they lined with waxed paper to keep the drops fresh and clean and to prevent them from sticking to the cardboard. The Luden's box pictured in the upper left was in circulation after 1906. Molded hard-candy drops packaged in boxes soon became the standard for all national competing brands.

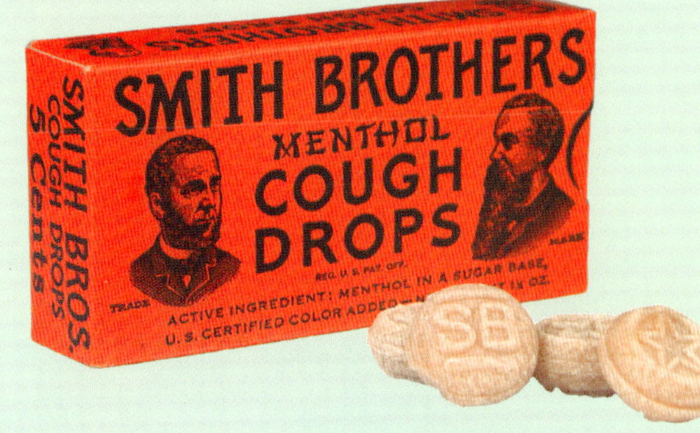

■ **Smith Brothers** Founded in 1847, Smith Brothers began marketing a black licorice cough drop in 1852. At first it was sold like bulk candy, and then in 1872 it came in a "factory filled package" so that the customer could be sure that there were no substitutes made behind the counter. After the demonstrated success of Luden's, Smith Brothers began molding their drops into a distinctive shape. It wasn't until 1922 that they developed and introduced a menthol cough drop (Wild Cherry was introduced in 1948). The metal countertop display (above) could be used to dispense both black and menthol products.

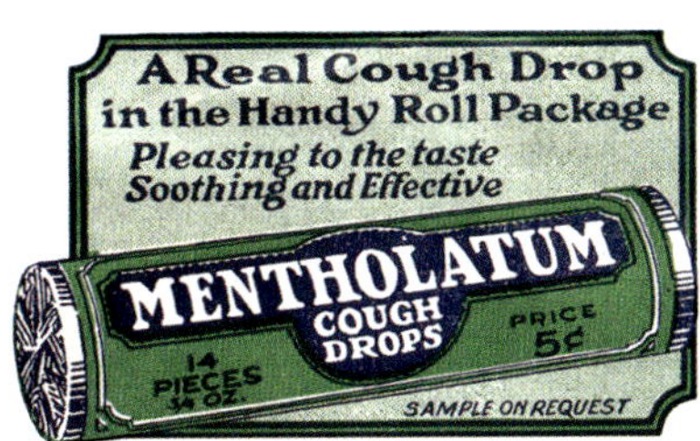

■ **Mentholatum Cough Drops** Rolls of candy lozenges were introduced in *Menthology* in 1925. It is safe to assume that the company outsourced the manufacture of the product to a candy manufacturer. The rolls were 2⅝ inches long and ¾ inch in diameter.

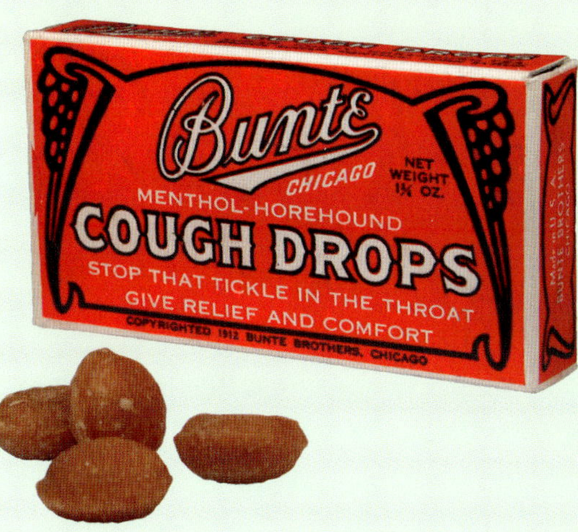

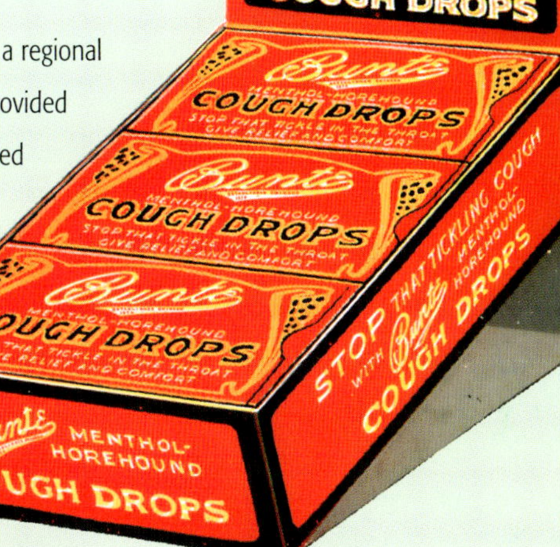

■ **Bunte** In the mid-1930s Bunte, a regional Chicago brand founded in 1876, provided this cardboard box display (illustrated right) to druggists for their menthol cough drops.

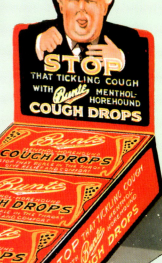

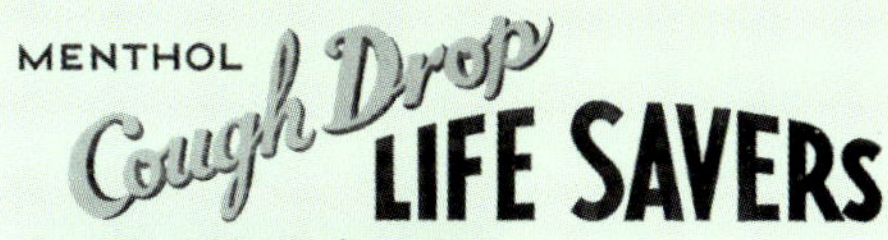

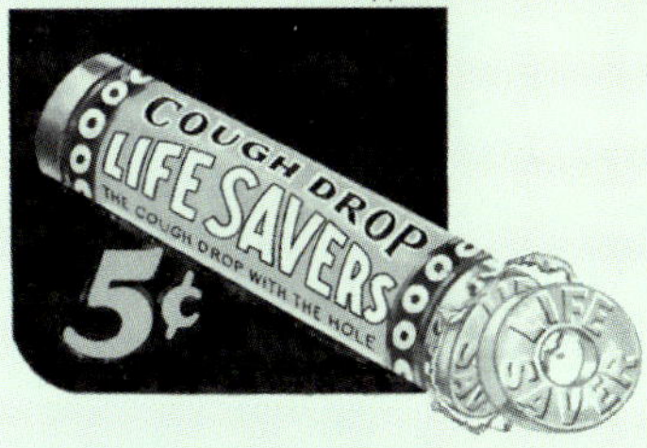

■ **Life Savers** Founded in Cleveland, Ohio, in 1912, Life Savers was the first roll candy and the first to use tin-foil wrappers. Menthol cough drops were advertised in *The American Magazine,* December 1931.

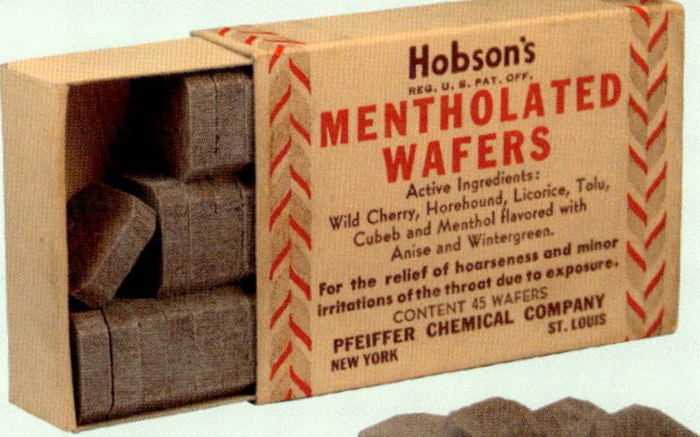

■ **Hobson's** The wafer was a less popular form of cough candy represented here by Hobson's.

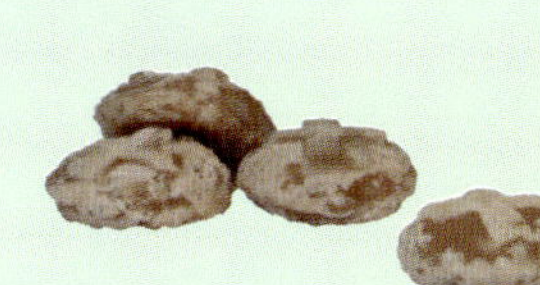

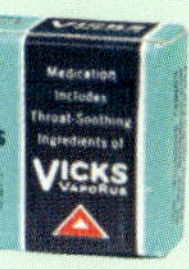

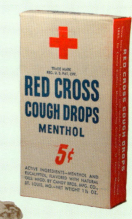

■ **Red Cross** This c. 1898 brand of cough drops was popular during World War II.

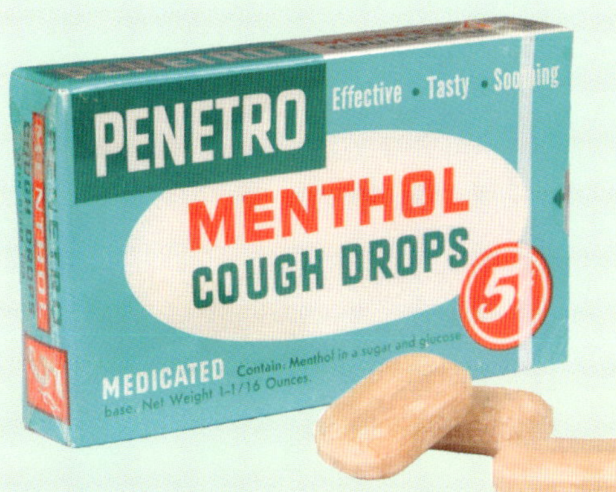

■ **Penetro Menthol Cough Drops** These were a product of the 1950s.

■ **Vicks Sample Box Held Just Two Cough Drops** In 1931, Vicks announced the launch of their new Vicks Nose & Throat Drops (Va-tro-nol) (this product failed) and Vicks Medicated Cough Drops in 1,300 daily newspapers and distributed ten million free samples along with inserts in twenty-six million VapoRub packages.[16]

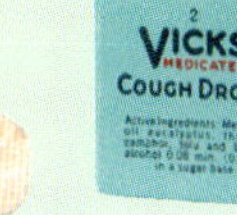

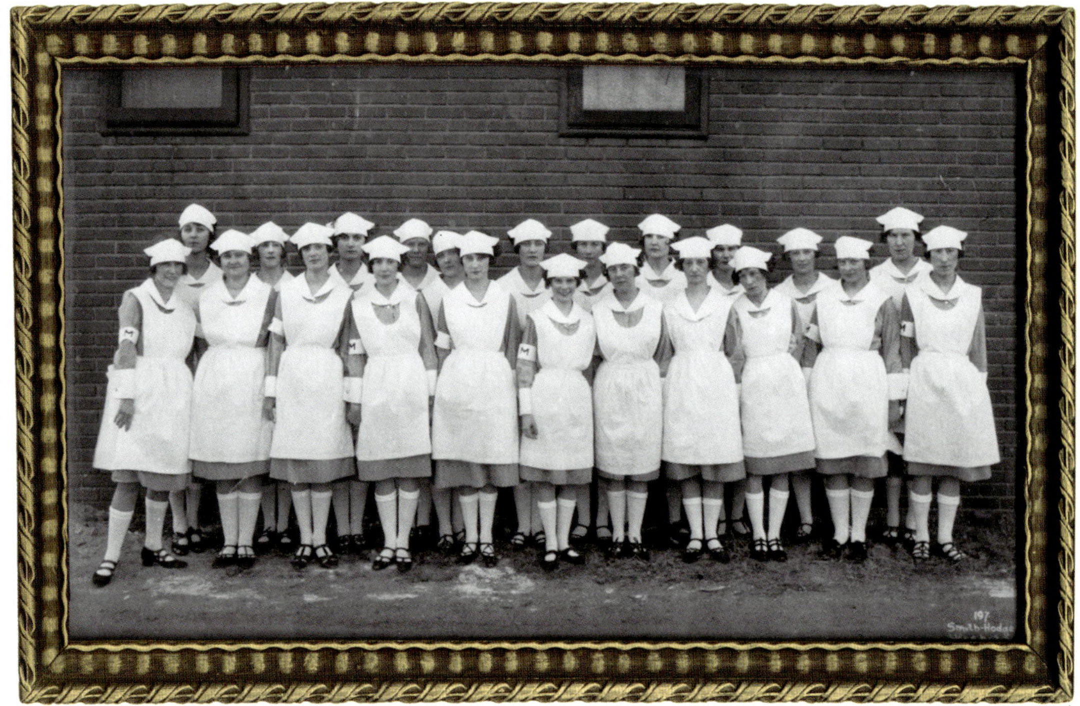

The Not-So-Little Nurses

In spite of their shockingly short hemlines, the women were still disappointed not to be able to keep the custom-fitted costumes.

On March 2, 1925, the city of Wichita threw a huge party at the Forum for A.A.'s seventy-seventh birthday. More than twelve hundred dinner guests were seated, and two thousand looked on from the balcony to honor Wichita's most famous philanthropist. Twenty-two girls from the factory served as usherettes dressed up in custom-fitted "Little Nurse" costumes. Earlier in January, when Mr. and Mrs. Hyde celebrated their golden wedding anniversary, the employees and salesmen of the three factories chipped in and gave them a bouquet of American Beauty roses at a private ceremony held in the Wichita office. After the presentation by George Simon and comments of appreciation from other employees, Mr. Hyde asked to speak. His speech was recorded by a stenographer, and copies were sent out to the other factories.

Mrs. Hyde, Mentholatum employees, friends: Possibly a couple of tear drops would better express our appreciation than words. We have known poverty, probably as bitter as any of you have ever known, and we hope to never forget the relationship that exists between capital and labor. The Mentholatum business was started in a very small way and developed little by little and we have always felt interested in each one of

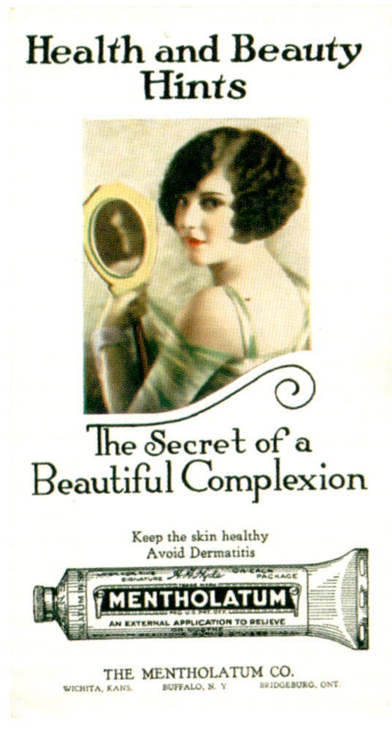

Better than French Creams

This testimonial promoted Mentholatum as a treatment for delicate complexions, dandruff, and dermatitis. "Mentholatum is wonderfully refreshing and exhilirating and used every day, is the real secret of beauty."

you. Some we know well enough to call you by your first name and others not quite so intimately.

I think you all know that I enjoy being with you at your Club meetings and dinners and Mama feels the same way—that it is more like being with our own "blood-relatives."

I want you all to feel perfectly free to come to me at any time with your personal problems or to discuss with me anything which you think might be to the interest of the business of the Company.

It is my earnest desire that a most hearty co-operation shall continue to exist between the employers and employees of the Company.

And now from the bottom of our hearts, we offer our thanks and appreciation.

Ethel was an active member of the Mentholatum Club. She sang with the Girls Glee Club and wrote songs for their performances at church and social occasions. Her skill and devotion to her work and her creative contributions to the club didn't go unnoticed by the Hydes. Ethel had become good friends with Ida Doffelmeyer, who was A. A. Hyde's secretary. Through Ida, Ethel became aware of the interesting and worthwhile philanthropies Mr. Hyde was working on. "Ida told me at different times how

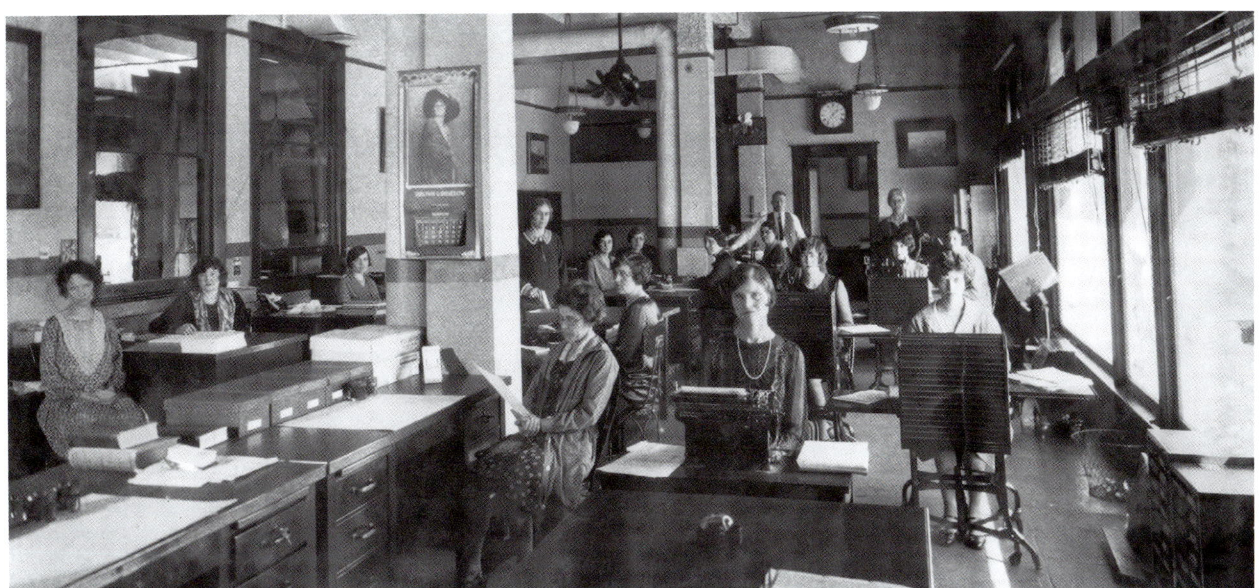

The Front-Office Staff in March 1928

Ethel Smith Willard is seated third from the left, and office manager Margaret Saxe is front center looking at a paper. Turn to page 204 for a listing of names.

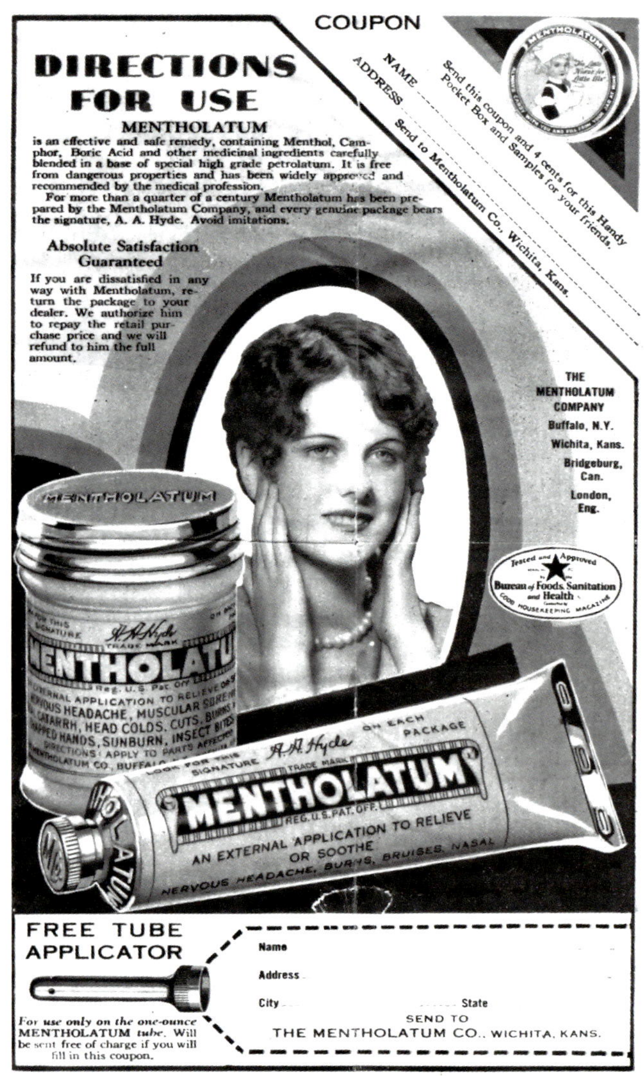

1929 Products Roster

As the decade came to a close, the packaging looked the same as it had in 1916.

particular A.A. was of where he sent donations. He spent a lot of time learning about the group or individual he sent money or help to. He'd get all the details down before he gave them a nickel."

When A. A. Hyde learned from Ida that Ethel was getting married, Ethel remembered, "I was going back from the lunchroom one day to the office, and Mr. Hyde had his door open and saw me go by and he hollered 'Ethel come in here,' so I went in and he said, 'sit down over there,' and I sat down right in front of him. He said, 'I want you to tell me all about this young man you're going to marry,' so, I told him all the things I appreciated about him, and then Mr. Hyde gave me his blessing and I left. That was Mr. Hyde." With a heavy heart, she left her job in June of 1929. Seventy-one years later, Mrs. Ethel Smith Willard told the author at her home in Newton, Kansas, "I live the Mentholatum Company over about every day, Alex."

The 1920s had started out with labor unrest and low industrial productivity. As the decade progressed, productivity improved, social standards for women and workers improved, and the economy roared. Mentholatum's retail price standard came under pressure from inflated costs in materials and advertising. The Hyde boys had hoped that overhead would level off or possibly return to prewar levels, but now they could no longer afford to wait, and on July 1, 1929, they announced the first price increase in more than thirty-four years. In spite of A.A.'s opposition to the plan, his sons voted to increase the retail price of one-ounce jars and tubes to 30¢ and three-ounce jars to 60¢. Hyde recalled several years later that this was the greatest mistake the company ever made.

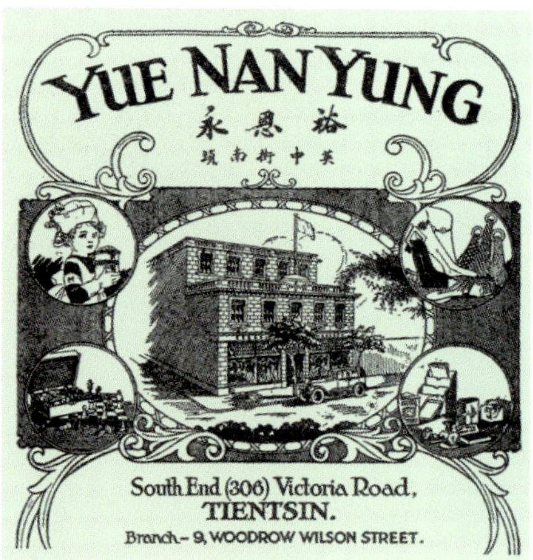

China Rep

The company was represented in Tientsin, China, by Mr. Yue Nan Yung, importer of fine silks, perfume, stationery, and games.

What goes up must come down. The prosperity was not destined to last for long, and throughout the summer of '29, the boom that had characterized the decade began to falter. Economic indexes took a downturn, and stock prices began to slide. By October, Wall Street was in a full panic as the stock market crashed.

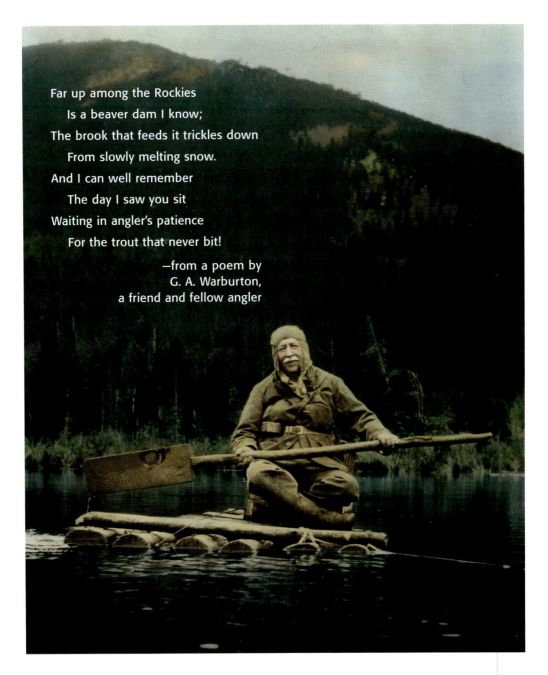

Far up among the Rockies
Is a beaver dam I know;
The brook that feeds it trickles down
From slowly melting snow.
And I can well remember
The day I saw you sit
Waiting in angler's patience
For the trout that never bit!
—from a poem by
G. A. Warburton,
a friend and fellow angler

A. A. Hyde's Favorite Photo

This cherished image of Hyde was taken in August 1929 by Margaret Plagge. The happy eighty-one-year-old is on a raft in the middle of the "Old Beaver Dam in Hidden Valley," Rocky Mountain National Park, Colorado.

"Make the Passer-Buy"

It took several years before most Americans comprehended the severity and magnitude of what is now called the Great Depression. Conservative business leaders thought it was simply a downturn in the business cycle and told everyone the economy would correct itself. But by 1932 they could no longer be certain it would, as they watched wages drop 33 percent in 1931 and 60 percent in 1932 and saw unemployment reach 24 percent and continue rising. The gross national product fell almost 50 percent during Herbert Hoover's laissez-faire administration. The president's inaction, combined with the Republican-led Congress unwisely passing the Hawley-Smoot Tariff Act (1930), which sparked an international tariff war, spread the Depression worldwide. A. A. Hyde must have also thought the "downturn" would run its course in a few years based on his experience in 1890. He attempted to calm the druggists' fear and encourage confidence with a signed statement printed in *Menthology*:

> *The Mentholatum Company, during the first three quarters of 1931, has had a very normal business. Some months have been ahead of last year and some months have been behind. Frankly, we are greatly pleased and feel fully justified in having launched the largest advertising campaign in our history. This is just to try to express to you our sincere appreciation of your continued cooperation and good will.*[1]

In the spring of 1932, when by all reasonable forecasts the Depression should have been over, *Menthology* published a homily entitled "Depressions End." A "Source Unknown" wrote: "Have I told you what caused this and all other depressions? . . . All values, in the final analysis, are measured in terms of human

Tired aching feet ? MENTHOLATUM soothes,cools and relieves.

Swirl Logo

The swirl logo first appeared in 1931 magazine ads and was in use until the J. Walter Thompson advertising agency was hired in 1942. This engraved block was used in a letterpress.

The title for this chapter is taken from an ad in *Menthology,* vol. 16, 1931, no. 1, p. 6, promoting the 1931 window display.

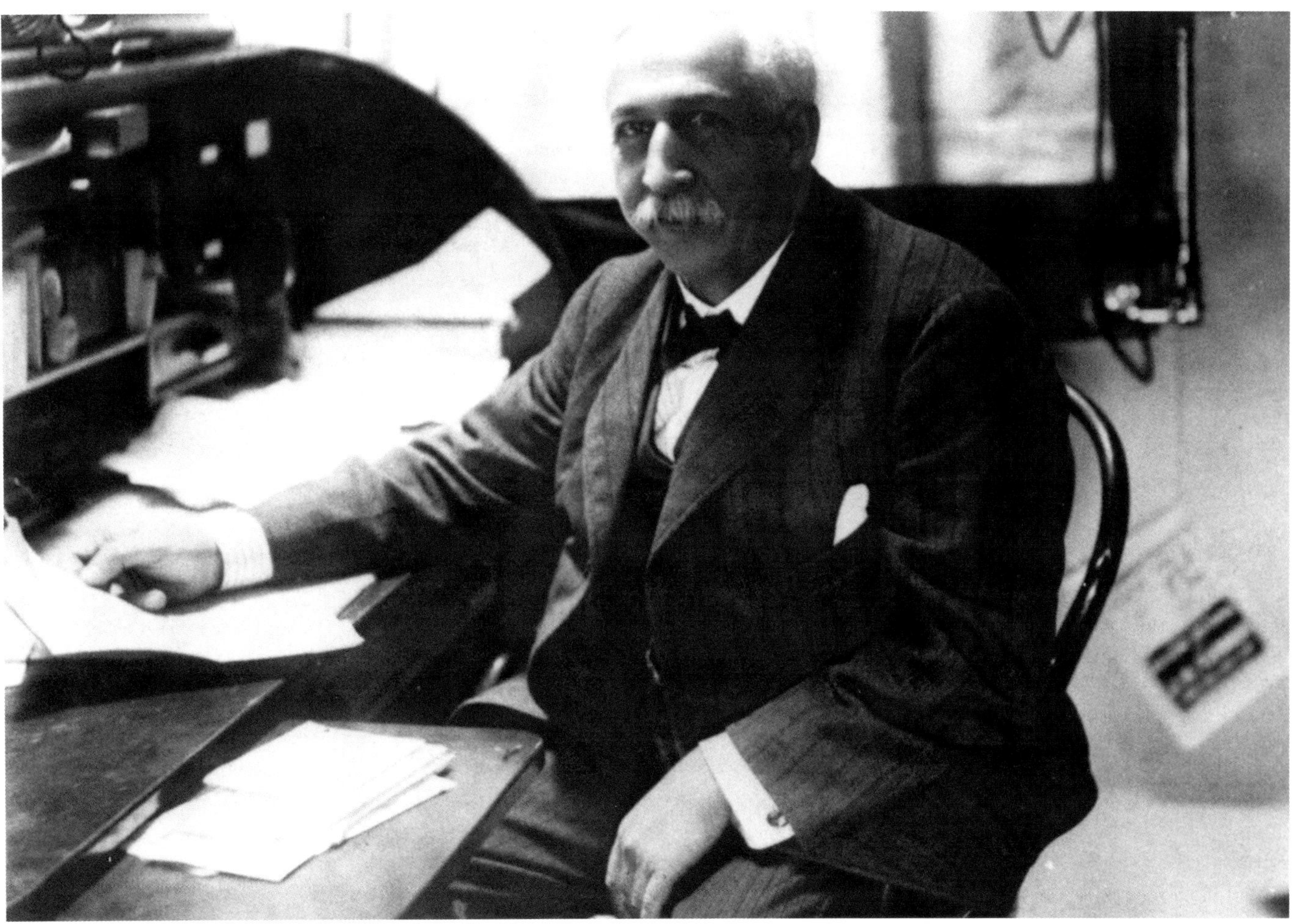

A. A. Hyde at His Desk

"I could not name one of the fifty-eight nations of the world which I travelled over in the past twenty years where I have not seen the great influences which have come forth from the life of A. A. Hyde. It is inspiring to think that a man can sit in a Wichita office, and cause streams of service to flow forth to every continent on earth. His gifts to the world, I say, have been omnipotent—and eternal."

John R. Mott, Secretary of the International Committee of the YMCA[2]

happiness. And our total trouble is that we have, in America, given money a bloated value as a bringer of happiness. . . . Happily I learned that the things that bring us most happiness require no money. I have discovered there is greater joy in walking by a brook than listening to 'Amos and Andy.'" (Was this A. A. Hyde's voice recalling his experience in 1887–1889?) By the fall issue, though, the editor's tone was more resigned: "A friend was philosophizing on the blessings of these times and the changes in his family resulting from our much maligned depression." His friend said his family had "changed from a 'want more' family to a 'want less' family and from selfishness to an interest in each other and others outside less fortunate." The editor concluded that this was also true for a cross section of the country and said, "The good Lord often gives us a boost which at the time, feels a lot like a common kick." In the same issue he provided an alternative definition of *depression*: "A period when people do without things their parents never had."[3]

The hardships faced during the first half of the decade were not just economic, they were also ecological, particularly for the people living in the West. Drought hit the Great Plains in 1930 and moved around the western states for most of the decade to come. In 1931, the Midwest suffered a devastating plague of grasshoppers that destroyed the crops on countless acres of rich farmland. The southern plains were hit the hardest, when on April 14, 1935, a dust storm blocked out the sun in much of eastern Colorado, western Kansas, and the panhandle region of Oklahoma, Texas, and New Mexico. During "Black Sunday," an estimated three hundred million tons of topsoil blew away and was scattered by the jet stream across the northeastern states all the way to the Atlantic. Dust storms continued to blow until 1940, giving the era its name, "the Dust Bowl." By mid-decade, 750,000 farms had been foreclosed since the start of the Depression. The second half of the decade saw flooding in the Northeast and Ohio River Valley and killer tornadoes in the South. So the primary challenge for Mentholatum during the 1930s was to help keep the beleaguered drugstores open.[4]

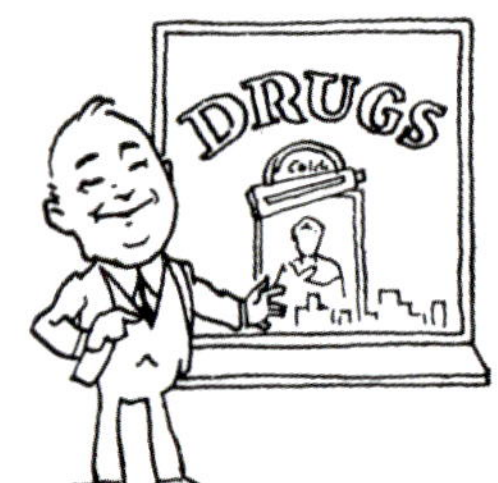
DRUGS
You have a
Sales Idea that
is Profitable

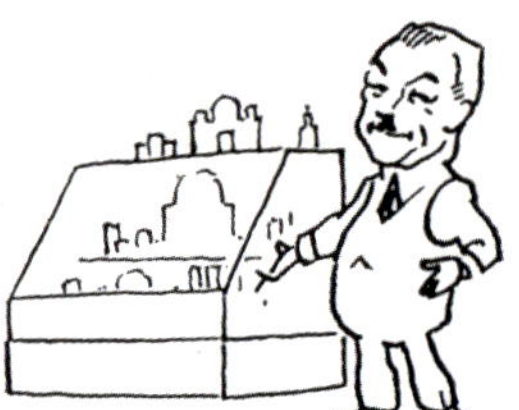
I have one
that makes
me a Profit

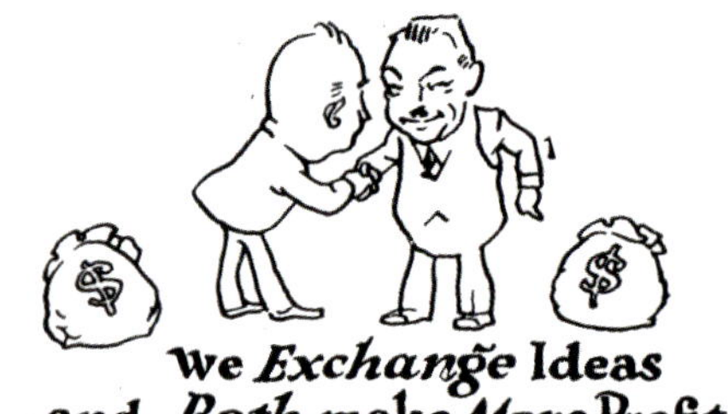
We Exchange Ideas
. . and Both make More Profit

Common Cents

Fortune magazine (vol. 6, no. 4, Oct. 1932, p. 88) reported that Mentholatum's 1931 advertising budget was $96,000. This illustration is from *Menthology*, vol. 16, 1931, no. 2, p. 4.

"Sales Suggestions" and "Drug Store Hints" were collected from all over the country and printed in *Menthology*. The concept was, "if two men each have one dollar that they exchange with one another, they both end up with only one dollar each. But, if two men each have an idea that they exchange with one-another, then they both end up with two ideas each." Some of the best suggestions shared by druggists from around the country included these:

■ "A good many of us can use leisure time to paint and brighten our stores, make little conveniences for waiting customers, changes in goods, displays, etc. Such employment costs little and is a thousand times better for depressed spirits and to encourage business than being idle and in the dumps. 'Where you can not branch out, deepen.'"

Laurence C. Jones, Piney Woods School, Mississippi

■ "Do you ever get sleepy when driving? Most people do. Try rubbing a little Mentholatum on your eyelids the next time you get drowsy while driving. Numbers of friends have told us that it is almost a sure cure. We assume that you always carry Mentholatum with you."

■ "A simple yet effective way to boost Mentholatum sales is to display on your show case, nearest your wrapping counter, a number of the tubes, and different sized jars. Have it handy so your customers can pick it up, handle it, and read the directions while waiting for their packages to be wrapped."

Dubuque, Iowa

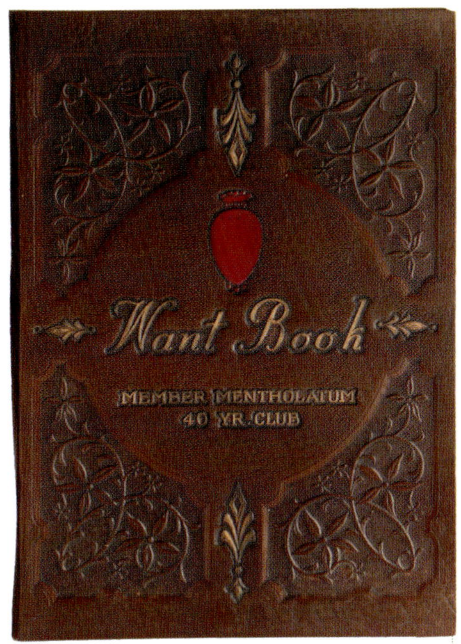

40 Year Club

In 1931, *Menthology* announced that there were 976 members in the 40 Year Club. Pharmacists with forty years' experience in the trade were invited to become members and given a commemorative gift by the company. In return, members were occasionally asked to answer product survey questions, thus becoming a brain trust for Mentholatum's marketing department. See Catalog pages C190–C193 for more club gifts.

■ A Louisiana druggist set up a Mentholatum window display, then covered the glass with Bon Ami, leaving a peek hole in the middle. He painted a sign on the outside of the window that said, "Keep Your Eye on This Window." "It is surprising, how many people even get out of their automobiles to peek in."

Ferriday, Louisiana

■ "Tip to drug stores near schools. Place a pencil sharpener near the door. Many sales will result from adults as well as children, who drop in to sharpen their pencils."

■ A Kentucky druggist displays Mentholatum on the fourth of July, when there are lots of firecracker burns. "We have learned that if Mentholatum is applied to a minor burn and rubbed in well, as soon as it is done, that in most cases there will be no blister, and should there be one, it won't be nearly so painful. This knowledge is especially useful around holidays."

Hopewell's Pharmacy, Paducah, Kentucky

■ "Display in a prominent place a medicine cabinet such as is in modern bathrooms, equipped with the necessary articles of a medicine cabinet. This will attract the customers' attention and remind them of articles needed in their own medicine cabinet. Put a sign over it reading: 'What Your Cabinet Should Contain.'"

Coleman's Drug, Asheville, North Carolina

Probably the best sales suggestion during these troubled times came from Albert E. Branch in 1935:

■ "I had a number of 'dead loss' accounts from former loyal customers. Unable to pay me, they felt uncomfortable in my store and took their cash business elsewhere. Removing their accounts from my loose-leaf ledger, I marked them paid and mailed them to my former customers with a note explaining that I was giving them the old account and asking them frankly to come back and trade with me. This has brought my old customers back to spend cash with me, in many cases to pay their bills, and given me valuable good advertising."

Albert E. Branch, Ettrick, Virginia[5]

Another way that *Menthology* helped the druggists was by providing instruction on basic display techniques. Druggists were urged to question if their window trim "invite[s] the eye? Is it easily read? Is it easily understood? Does it carry the message?" *Menthology* provided a section explaining primary colors and another on the meaning of colors, for example: "blue = truth, green = envy," etc.[6]

Menthology made several important announcements in the early part of the decade:

The Hydes

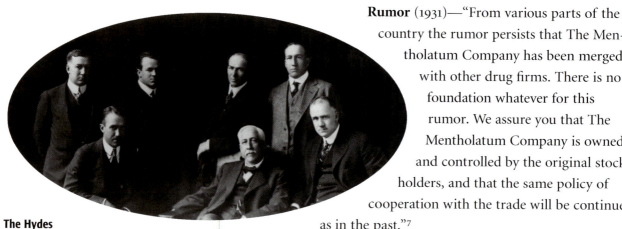

A. A. Hyde and his adult sons.

Rumor (1931)—"From various parts of the country the rumor persists that The Mentholatum Company has been merged with other drug firms. There is no foundation whatever for this rumor. We assure you that The Mentholatum Company is owned and controlled by the original stockholders, and that the same policy of cooperation with the trade will be continued as in the past."[7]

Our Policy (1932)—"We have undertaken to maintain a strictly impartial, but at the same time friendly, relationship with each one of the 60,000 druggists throughout the country. You can readily understand how impossible it would be for us to do co-operative advertising with individual firms, no matter how special the request or worthy the opportunity. We believe that such advertising tends toward individual rather than collective relationship with the drug trade, and this we wish to avoid. Therefore, please do not feel that we are discriminating against your firm if we refer you to this statement from time to time, as the above has long been our established policy from which we do not make exceptions."[8]

Our Advertising Policy (Winter, 1932–1933)—"Mentholatum's advertising has always been conservative. We never make a claim that is not substantiated by the leading textbooks on medicine and pharmacology. As a result, when a customer purchases Mentholatum from you after reading our advertising he obtains the therapeutic results for which he bought it, and is, therefore, most apt to become a satisfied user and regular customer. Such a conservative advertising policy may at times appear to be less productive of consumer sales than more extravagant advertising, but it is steadfastly building respect and prestige for Mentholatum and increasing its host of satisfied users."[9]

National Recovery Administration (August 25, 1933)—"The Mentholatum Company has very willingly signed up under the blanket code of the N.R.A. This change has not been difficult, for we adopted a five day week several years ago, and all of our regular employees are paid above the minimum required under the code. Another feature of which we are quite proud is the fact that not one of our employees has been dropped on account of the so-called depression."[10]

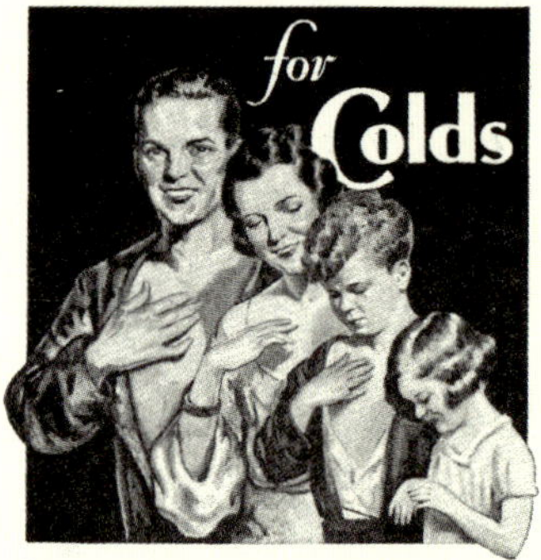

▲ February 1933, *The American Magazine*, 6⅜"H × 2¼"W

Ephedrine—the New Menthol

Ephedrine was the hot new wonder drug in the early 1930s. First synthesized by a German chemist in 1887 and later rediscovered by an American chemist named K. K. Chen working for Eli Lilly, ephedrine was a derivative of the Chinese herb ma huang (*Ephedra equisetina*). It was found to be an effective bronchodilator, a fact that Chinese healers had known for thousands of years.[11]

▲ Free sample box

Ephedrine and menthol were the power ingredients in the 1931 introduction of Vicks Medicated Cough Drops and Vicks Nose & Throat Drops (shown at right), which was later named Va-tro-nol. Ephedrine made the cough drops "Medicated" and the nose drops "A Scientific Preparation to Fill a Modern Need." Retailers handed out ten million small sample boxes of Cough Drops (see page 123), and twenty-six million more were placed inside packages of VapoRub.

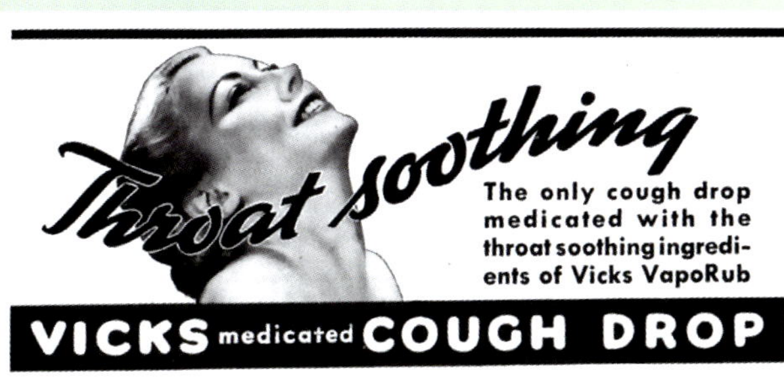

Several million two-inch-tall sample bottles of Throat Drops were also handed out by the retailers.

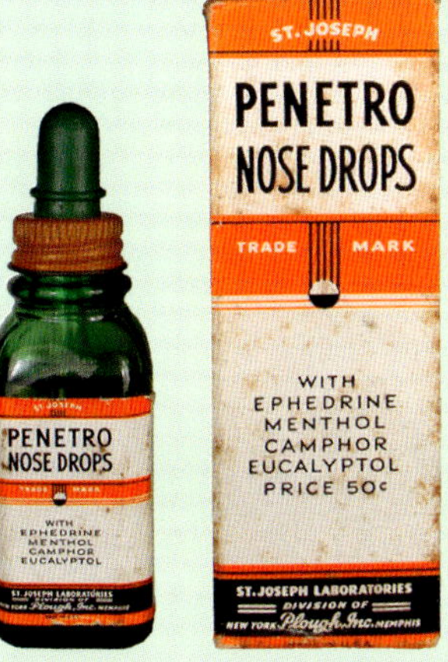

New trademarked products with ephedrine in their name hit the market, including Metaphedrin Inhalant from Abbott Laboratories (1932), Adrephine Inhalant from Parke-Davis & Company (1932), and Efedron Nasal Jelly and Efemist Inhalant from Hart Drug Corporation (1932). Eventually the excitement over ephedrine faded. Ephedrine followed menthol's path, becoming a common ingredient or generic exemplified by Penetro Nose Drops (1935) and Rexall Nasal Jelly with Ephedrine (shown above left and at right).[12]

Ma huang was hard to obtain in commercial quantities so chemists worked to develop a synthetic ephedrine. Sometime during the search one of them discovered amphetamine. It wasn't until more recent times that ephedrine began to be used in large doses to promote weight loss and enhance athletic performance. Today the government regulates synthetic ephedrine because of its use in synthesizing crystal meth.

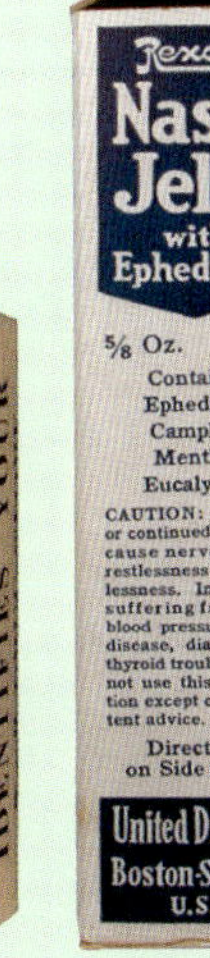

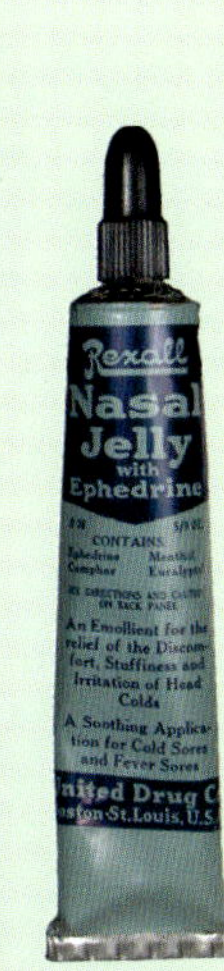

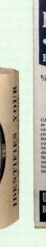

More Federal Regulation

Then, *Menthology* reprinted an editorial from the November 1933 edition of the trade magazine *Printers' Ink.* "The enclosed clipping . . . points out clearly the evils of the Tugwell Bill." The editorial warned the druggists about the bill before Congress that:

> *places the manufacture, distribution and advertising of all food, cosmetics and drugs under the supervision of a political branch of the Government. It puts a scientific matter into the hands of a political agency. It grants sweeping power to a political officer to set up scientific standards and professional ethics, and to interpret as he sees fit every activity involved in manufacturing, processing and marketing foods, cosmetics and drugs. It gives these industries no recourse to the courts in questioning the decision of this political officer. His word becomes the law of the land. One ignorant or stupid administrator could practically destroy an entire industry.*[13]

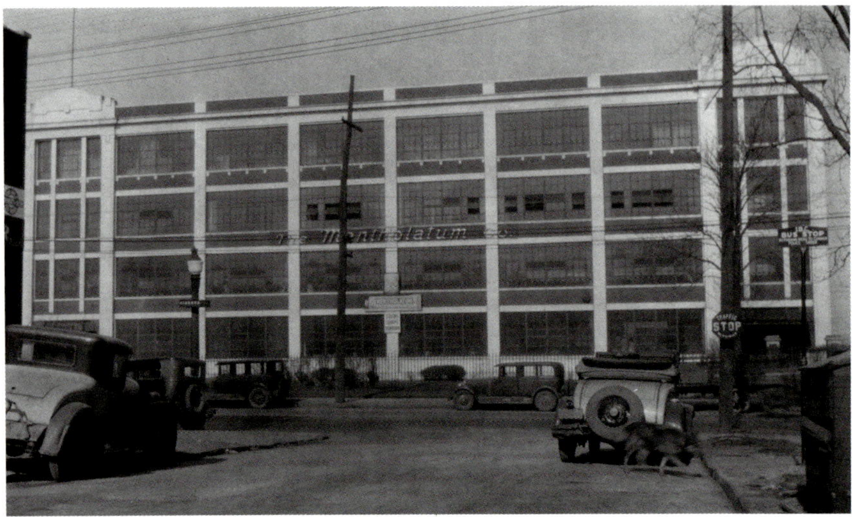

Buffalo Plant

This early-1930s-period view shows the Buffalo plant from the corner of Penfield and Niagara.

A matter of days after his inauguration in 1933, Franklin D. Roosevelt initiated a revision of the 1906 Pure Food and Drugs Act. The last time Congress had visited drug safety was back in 1912, when it passed the Sherley Amendment. Walter Campbell, Chief of the Food and Drug Administration, and Rexford Tugwell, Assistant Secretary of Agriculture, began the onerous task of drafting reform policies to regulate the manufacture and sale of food and drugs, including, for the first time, the cosmetics industry. Their fight in Congress took five years and was in many ways like the fight to pass the 1906 Act. Both efforts required many years of debate and compromise, only to result in weakened legislation.[14]

Tugwell was an economics professor at Columbia University before becoming a member of FDR's New Deal "Brain Trust." His and Campbell's initial goal was to expand existing controls to include brand advertising, an obvious extension of labeling. In addition to regulating advertisers, they wanted to initiate FDA factory inspections, require interstate permits, and enforce stronger penalties for violations. When the nostrum makers got

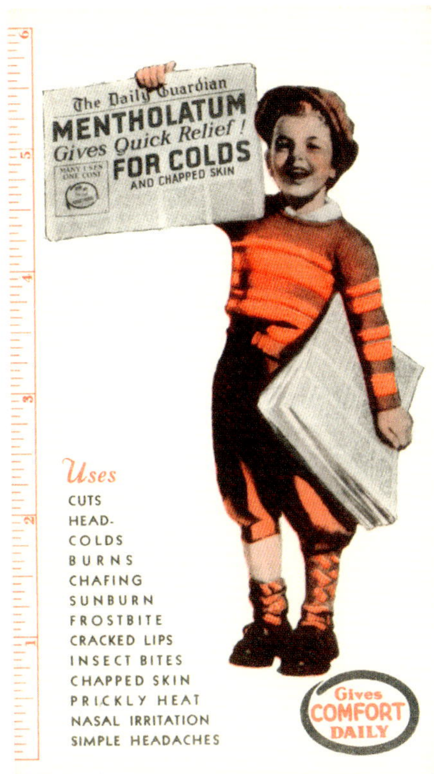

Newsboy Ink Blotter

It was given out during the winter 1933–34 cold season. The illustrator was Andrew Loomis (1892–1959), a premier figure and portrait painter in the 1930s and 1940s. In addition to his commercial work, Loomis was also a teacher and author of instructional books for artists. (See Catalog page C71.)

wind of this, they cried foul, said this was "un-American," and branded Tugwell an evil villain.[15]

The politics were as fierce in 1933 as they had been in 1906. But this time around, the complexities of regulating the industry were far greater, providing more opportunities for opponents to stall drafts in committee and force revisions. The Proprietary Association and the United Medicine Manufacturers represented the sentiment of a majority of proprietors who wanted the bill killed. Opposition also came from advertising, publishing, fruit growers, food processors and canneries, and cosmetics and pharmaceutical manufacturers, who formed "one of the noisiest and most determined lobbies of modern times." Opponents called the bill "grotesque in its terms, evil in its purpose, and vicious in its possible consequences." The drug companies protested that if they were required to say "does not cure" on their label, then doctors should also be required to hang a sign over their door saying, "I do not cure." One supporter of the bill characterized the patent medicine advertiser and manufacturer as "the vilest man on the face of the earth." The first bill that Tugwell and Campbell drafted became so compromised in committee that *Consumer's Research* said it was "a more adulterated and misbranded product than anything marketed." Those that testified against the bill included the owners of Lydia Pinkhams and Vicks VapoRub. Tugwell called the final draft "a subverted thing," the result of "a cause . . . betrayed." President Roosevelt finally signed the Food, Drug, and Cosmetic Act on June 25, 1938, as one of his last enactments of the New Deal.[16]

The new law might not have done all that the scientists wanted it to do, but it still had some teeth in it. They had managed to strengthen misbranding provisions by outlawing

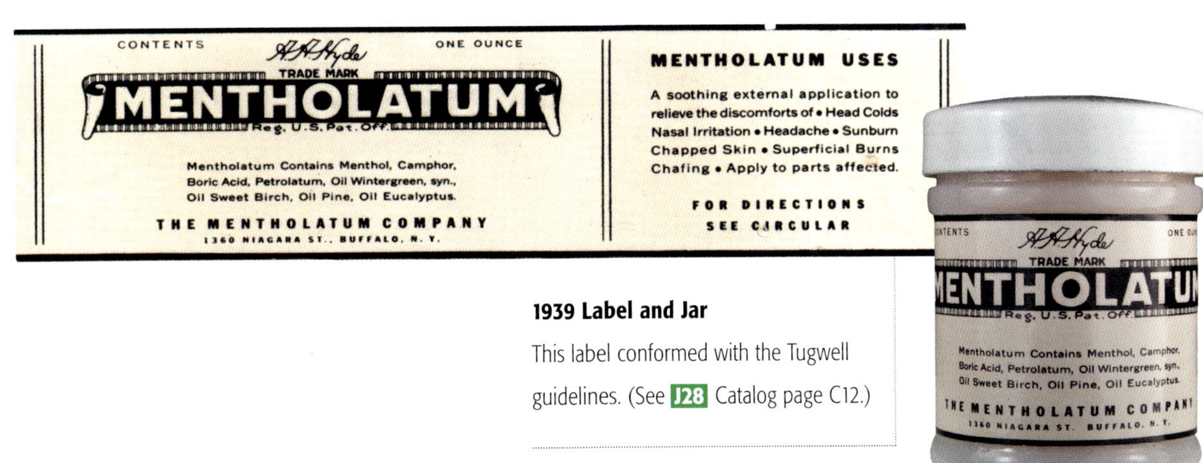

1939 Label and Jar

This label conformed with the Tugwell guidelines. (See J28 Catalog page C12.)

"Mr. William Mahon, our California representative, once falsely accused of having talked both arms off the statue of Venus de Milo, found facts of more avail than eloquence with a Department of Justice Agent (G-man to you). Summoned to the door of his room in a California hotel, Our William was face to face with a stern individual who kept his right hand in his coat pocket and requested his victim for full particulars as to his identity, occupation, collar size, and golf handicap. He was looking for William Mahan, infamous for the Weyerhaeuser kidnapping. With his credentials, and all the oratory his Kentucky ancestry and a cold sweat could inspire, Bill managed to convince the federal agent that it was a case of mistaken identity, that he had worked for The Mentholatum Company thirty-one years, that he had a heart of eighteen carat gold and loved dogs and little children. The bloodhound of the law departed with several samples of Mentholatum to apply to his feet and oil up his Tommy-gun."

–*Menthology*, vol. 20, 1935, no. 4, p. 10

false and misleading statements, erroneous positive statements, omission of warnings when a medication might be hazardous, and drugs dangerous to health when used according to directions. Common names of active ingredients were required on the label as was a list of any habit-forming drugs and narcotics. Penalties were stiffened, and the FDA was given the power of injunction to add to its seizures and criminal actions. Mentholatum made the appropriate changes to its label by 1939, moving the ingredients from a side panel to the center under the trademark banner. The controversial advertising component of the bill had earlier been cut out and put under the jurisdiction of the Federal Trade Commission in the Wheeler-Lea Act. The 1938 fall edition of *Menthology* contained a hint of sour grapes when the editor defended advertising:

> *Of the hundreds of thousands of ads examined by the Federal Trade Commission, a percentage of .0059 warranted corrective action. Not bad for an industry purportedly seething with villains armed to the teeth with split infinitives ready to pop out and jab the unsuspecting public in the pocketbook.*

Compare this statement with the one A. A. Hyde sent to the druggists c. 1903 (see page 20). No doubt, the Hydes were truly unaware of the number of lethal and injurious products their "industry" continued to sell through misleading advertising. The Tugwell Act helped the FDA stop the use of deadly dinitrophenol in weight-reducing drugs and force analgesic manufacturers to reduce the levels of cinchophen, aminopyrine, and mixtures of bromides and acetanilid in their formulations.[17]

Looking back, it was inevitable that the government was going to clamp down, as it did little by little, on every aspect of the proprietary medicine and pharmaceutical industries. Despite this outcome, the writer James Harvey Young claims that quackery has become more prevalent today than ever before. For Mentholatum it was not a matter of dangerous ingredients that had to be removed, but a matter of editing down its general-use identity. Mentholatum's good reputation kept it out of the quack and nostrum catagories, but that would not stop the federal magnifying glass from eventually scrutinizing the friendly salve. In 1955, the FTC created a special task force to monitor radio and TV advertising. Instead of simply reading the scripts of remedy ads as they had done before, they were now charged with listening and watching for "tone of voice" and "facial expression." As a result of their survey, complaints were

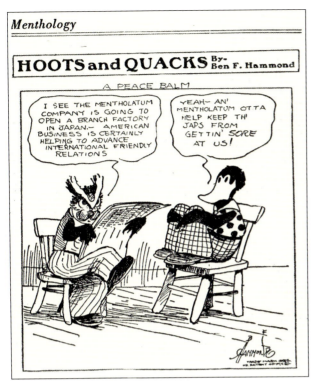

▲ *Menthology*, vol. 15, 1930, no. 4, p. 8

issued, among others, against Mentholatum, Infra Rub, and Heat for running misleading arthritis and rheumatism ads. Today's label claims only an aromatic relief for colds and chapped skin, and in the case of Deep Heating, relief of sore muscles.[18]

The World Market

At the start of the decade, Mentholatum was marketed in more than one hundred countries. The *Wichita Eagle* reported in June 1930 that, "Today the largest foreign proprietary imported into Japan is the Wichita Mentholatum. Here is the latest chapter in the story of Mentholatum—the conquest of Japan. It renews an old lesson—that wide as the world is, distance does not exist between demand and supply when the article of exchange is right."

Several million jars were sold in Japan in 1931, the year imperial troops occupied Manchuria, claiming to bring stability to the region. In 1932, Japan attacked Shanghai, and the League of Nations branded Japan the aggressor. When Japan (and Germany) withdrew from the League of Nations in 1933, the Omi-Hachiman factory was completed at a cost to the U.S. company of more than 100,000 yen. (For more, see "Omi Mission Factory" on pages 155–160.) In spite of strained international relations with Japan, the Mentholatum Company continued its close ties with the Omi-Hachiman plant through the mission's founder, William Merrell Vories. The mission newsletter, *Mustard Seed*, reported in 1935 that Mentholatum was being used by the members of the famous all-female Takarazuka Opera beneath their makeup to protect their skin from the greasepaint. A Japanese soldier, Jo Takeda, returning from his conscription service in 1936, told the *Mustard Seed* that he had run across empty Mentholatum jars along the far borders of Manchuria. He said that seeing the jars made him feel homesick. On the other side of the Japanese/Chinese front, the American Presbyterian Mission in Shunteh, North China, was receiving annual shipments of Mentholatum ointment and Brushless Shave.[19]

Despite the hysterics of organizations like the "Buy American League," that represented merchants who felt threatened by competition from Japanese imports, Japan was America's third-largest trading partner in 1937. The United States was Japan's largest customer, receiving 25 to 30 percent of exports. Raw silk

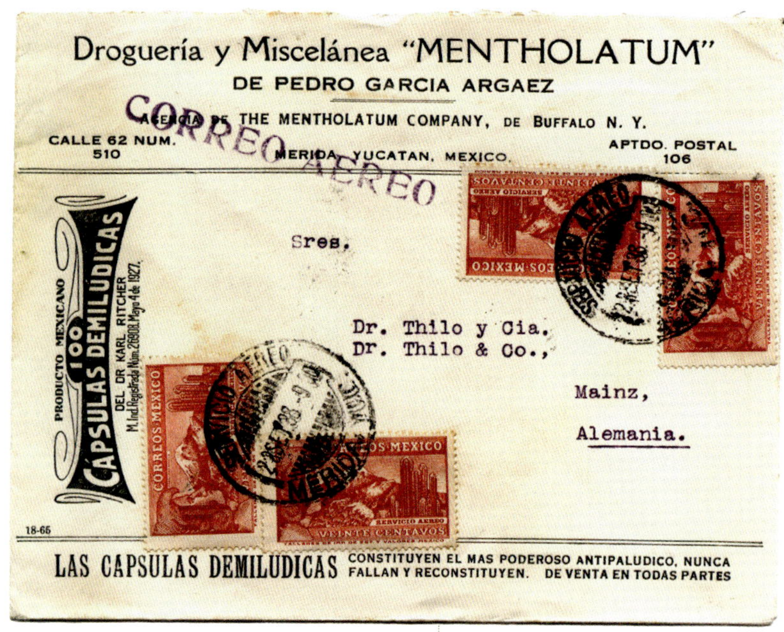

Pedro Garcia Argaez

He was Mentholatum's agent in Merida Yucatan, Mexico, in 1938.

and cotton made up 60 to 80 percent of the Japan-America trade. Menthol production for the year was 10,320,000 kilograms, and 90 percent was exported with the United States receiving half. According to the Japan Foreign Trade Federation, menthol was an important ingredient in the "preparation of tooth-powder, mentholatum, chewing gum, candies, etc." The United States also received half the export of Japanese camphor, which was used in the manufacture of celluloid, medicine, perfumes, insecticides, and incense. The Trade Federation was quick to point out that Japanese camphor-based celluloid film made the American motion picture industry possible.[20]

In Bogota, Colombia, the daily newspaper, *El Tiempo*, reported on December 13, 1932, that Lieutenant Colonel Carlos J. Villar included Mentholatum on a list of items he wanted families to send in their Christmas packages to the troops on the Peruvian front. The Nicaraguan Ministry of Public Health and Welfare announced in Managua on November 15, 1934, "It is known in this Office that various pharmacies and drug stores of the Republic have been making products analogous to Mentholatum. . . . In no case can these be sold under the same name as legitimate preparations, under penalty of the law, which this Ministry will invoke against those who do not heed this warning." The Mentholatum agent in Bolivia wrote to the company on March 7, 1935, to say, "Referring to the Government decree regarding exchange at official rate for articles of first necessity; Mentholatum has always come

Home Faith

"Don't believe any family in the world uses as much Mentholatum as the family of the makers. Our parents started the making of it and I have had it put down my throat, up my nose, in my eyes, on my chest, on patches all over my anatomy for burns, cuts, sores—and during scarlet fever I had full body smears for several weeks. Our folks believed in it, and we believe in it—so do our children.

The Editor"

–*Menthology*, vol. 21, 1936, no. 2, p. 7

Note: camphor poisoning is a real danger. A recent poisoning occurred in 2000, after a mother applied Vicks to her two-month-old child's chest and neck three times a day for five days (Rx Remedy, Inc., 2000, www.ahealthyme.com). The *PDR* warns: "Camphor salves should not be administered to infants. . . . A lethal dose for children is approximately 1 g, for adults approximately 20 g (toxic dosage of camphor is 2 g)." [*PDR for Herbal Medicines*, first edition (New Jersey: Medical Economics Company, 1998), p. 751.] Mentholatum labels include a warning to keep out of the reach of children and use for adults and children two years of age and older.

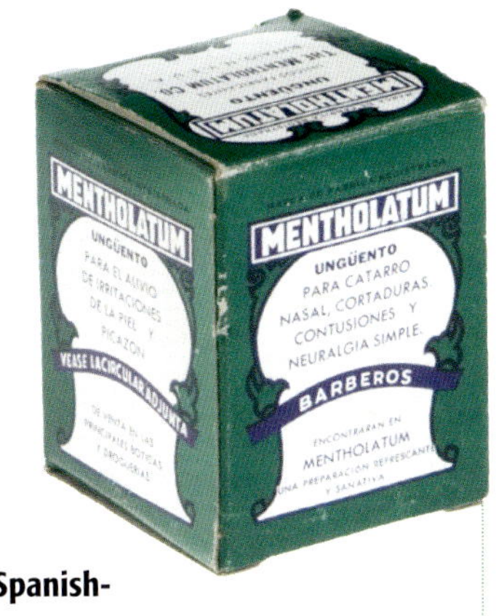

Spanish-Language Box

Mentholatum was registered in seventeen South American countries.

under this category. . . . Almost every soldier carries his small supply of Mentholatum in an all round first aid dressing, and [it is] a wonderful comfort in the treatment of insect stings. It is absolutely necessary. . . ." *Menthology* printed photographs of West African street markets in Sekondi, Gold Coast, and Lagos, Nigeria. The captions pointed out that the "Friends Post Card," which the Slough, England, factory included in each box of Mentholatum, had also become a marketable commodity. The coveted postcard was good for a free sample and was traded for the equivalent of one cent.[21]

Price cutting was a popular way for large buyers to beat their competition by selling items for less than the price marked on the label. "Cutting" threatened small concerns who could not qualify for the discounts awarded by manufacturers for large orders. Cutting gave power to a small group at the expense of the larger economic order and was deemed unfair. Although Mentholatum also provided discounts for large orders, it had always advocated price maintenance. California was the first state to pass a fair trade law (1931), and Mentholatum was one of the pioneer companies to qualify. They later obtained "contracts" with other states like Oregon, Louisiana, Ohio, Illinois, and Iowa, as each one passed similar laws. The company instructed its salesmen in a letter dated September 18, 1935, to encourage every druggist they called upon to join the National Association of Retail Druggists and add their influence to the passage of a federal fair trade law. The Proprietary Association also supported the proposed law. *Menthology* said: "We are wholeheartedly in favor of and are supporting the movement for Federal Fair Trade Legislation legalizing the maintenance of fair resale prices because with it we believe will come a New Era for the Retail Druggists, the Manufacturers, and the Public." Eventually, forty-two states convinced Congress to pass the Miller-Tydings Fair Trade Enabling Act (an amendment to the Sherman Antitrust Act) in 1937, allowing resale prices to be fixed by brand-name manufacturers.[22]

On January 4, 1935, an ailing A. A. Hyde made his way to the podium where he spoke for a few minutes to the Mentholatum salesmen who had assembled in Wichita for their convention. This was to be his last public appearance, for on January 10 the humble philan-

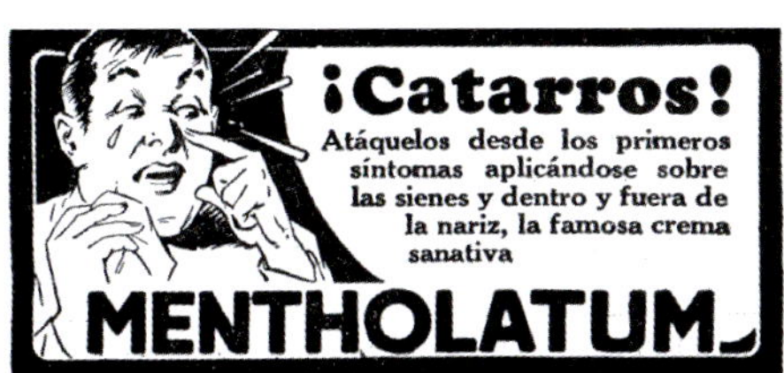

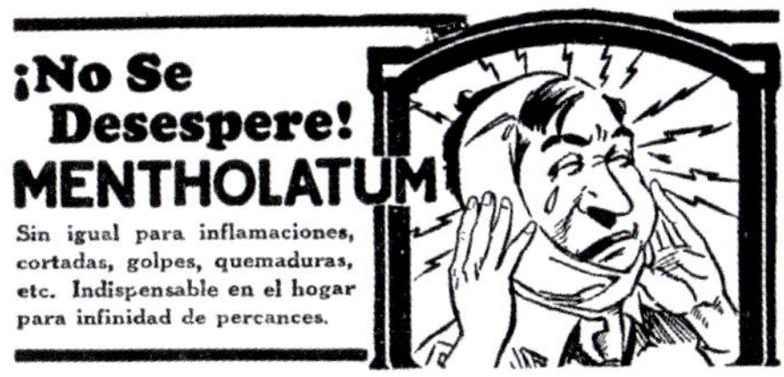

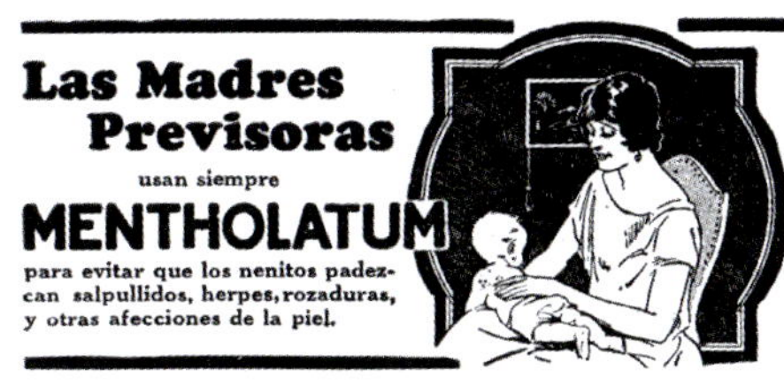

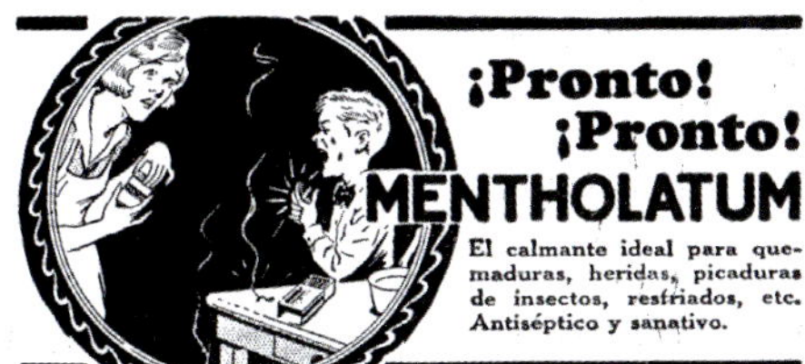

South American View

These energetic ads could be seen in the 1932 *Holger-Glaesel Pharmacy Almanac* in Guayaquil, Ecuador, and earlier in the 1929 *Leonard Pharmacy Almanac* in Lima, Peru.

thropist and father of the friendly salve died. In an obituary published the next day, the *Wichita Beacon* wrote that the Sermon on the Mount "actuated Albert Alexander Hyde in his every act and kindly deed. . . . He gave of himself and his, and as he did so he was given stewardship of possessions which he held in solemn trust." In a reference to nature, "His vision was as broad as the vast plains that he loved." And of the citizens of Wichita, "He walked with the lowly as he stood among those of high estate. To A. A. Hyde the humblest was not less than such as commanded stores that a Midas might not buy. Harsh terms were never in his lexicon. His employees were his associates and his friends. His family was dear to him beyond all other mortal things. Children gathered at his knee. He was charitable as have been few men. *Well done, thou good and faithful servant . . .*"[23]

(Text continues on page 142.)

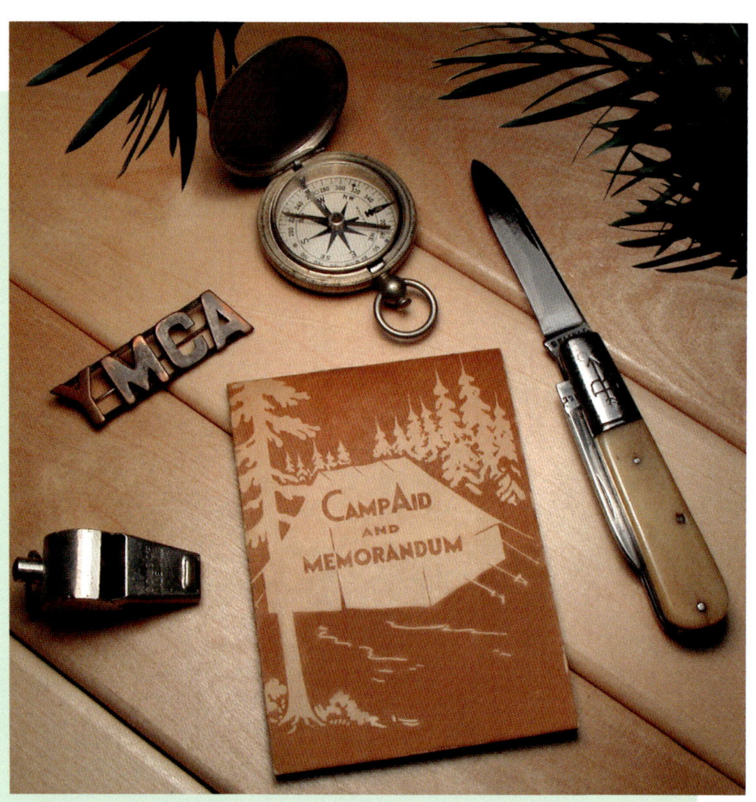

Camp Aid and Log Books

"For the eleventh year [started in 1930] hundreds of thousands of Camp Booklets and samples of Mentholatum [3,500,000 in 1941] will be shipped to our carefully checked lists of cooperating summer camps—one booklet for every camper and each containing a sample of Mentholatum in a pocket in the back cover. Designed to be carried easily in a shirt pocket, these little booklets have 24 pages of carefully edited, cleverly illustrated items on camp lore and first aid, with space for autographs, camp records, diary, etc.—even a blotter for pressing flower specimens. So popular has the Camp Aid and Log Booklet become that many camp directors tell us that they have incorporated their use directly into their camp programs. We believe that we are lending a hand in furthering the enjoyment of the opportunities of that Great American Institution, the Summer Camp, and that this aid in the name of the Mentholatum Company is of benefit to druggists everywhere." John Hyde said the Camp Aid and Log Book is "the most frequently mentioned source of knowledge about the product from people in my generation."[24]

Mr. A. A. Hyde's Last Message to His Salesmen

in Convention Friday, January 4, 1935

Looking back over the years of the Mentholatum Company and the Hyde family, I can't help but feel that the Lord has guided us in many ways. I think we have always had the loyal cooperation of the traveling men as indicated here in this meeting. I believe it has been quite a family cooperative organization from the time it started. I think you all know that we started without a cent; I was bankrupt, and the two men with me were both bankrupt—at least not worth anything. But somehow, we have gone ahead. The means we used in the beginning was the personal work of everybody we could get to help us. We succeeded remarkably well. We used our brains, our muscles, and all the help we could get, to put Mentholatum over. We thought we had a fine preparation; it did what we said it would do, and in many respects we had the best preparation on the market. It built up trade for itself in a wonderful way. Of course, there wasn't the competition then that there is now.

Here I am, approaching eighty-seven—wabbling around on my feet, and at the head of an organization that has made a real success in the world in a material way, and which supports a good many families. I, feeling the obligation I do to my profession of Jesus Christ and the spreading of the gospel, have used a good deal of time and money in spreading this gospel to the ends of the earth. I believe that with all the unfavorable conditions existing in the world today, the teachings of Jesus Christ should be spread as never before. If the teachings of Christ (for instance, His Sermon on the Mount) were adopted in the lives of men in any great proportion today, all the troubles that the world is facing would be done away with. The principles of Jesus Christ, as He gave them, would solve every one of these problems. I believe it and try to act on it.

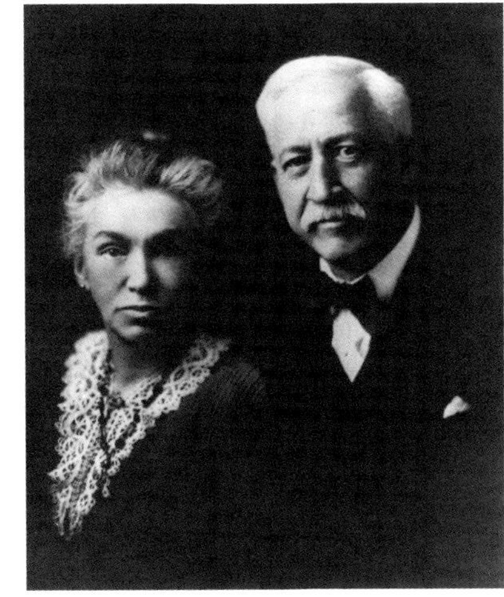

I have been put on a pedestal and complimented for simply doing what I think the normal man ought to do and what Christ taught that he ought to do—that we are not here to lay up worldly treasures but to be of service. I know a few men who have followed that principle and have lived up to it. They have had the joy beyond compare of the ordinary man. Most of us have been taught in our youth that success in life was obtaining power, wealth, ability, etc. This is a fool idea. Here I am, almost on the verge of the grave—you men may never see me again; I have no great ability; I sit here and cannot comprehend a great deal you men are saying; but I want to say to you that I look backward and find a great joy in having overcome a lot of temptations in the world and having done something toward making this world what it ought to be and having helped in the service of teaching the gospel of Jesus Christ here, at home, and abroad; and it is a real satisfaction to me.

I didn't expect to say a word of this character. However, I am glad of this opportunity of fellowship with you and of expressing what I believe to be the truth in regard to the Kingdom of God on earth and our loyalty to it, if we want to have joy and peace at the end of life. I hope you wont take this at all personally, for I feel my shortcomings one hundred times more than any of you men can see them. However, I have had a great joy and satisfaction in my work and profession, and I will enjoy it to the end. God go with you and bless you all.

Two new products were introduced in the winter of 1936: "Mentholatum Liquid" and "Mentholatum Brushless Shave." The liquid was produced for people who "prefer nose drops or spray." It came in a one-and-three-quarter-ounce green glass bottle with an eyedropper and wad of Kleenex® brand tissues. This was possibly the only time Mentholatum made a joint promotion with another brand product. Kleenex was first introduced in 1924 as "the disposable cold cream towel," then after 1930 it became "the disposable handkerchief." On the top layer of Kleenex folded inside the box was printed "MENTHOLATUM LIQUID Does Not Stain. These KLEENEX ABSORBENT TISSUES Are Included For Your Convenience." Brushless Shave, according to the company, was tested for several years and "has proved a repeater wherever it has been introduced." In 1938, a defensive-sounding *Menthology* said, "Now we know darned well that our new Mentholatum Brushless Shave won't satisfy every member of the shaving public." There is no evidence yet how long Mentholatum Liquid actually lasted on the market, but Brushless Shave was listed for sale at 35¢ a tube in the fall 1941 issue of *Menthology*, and the author has a carton of six tubes dated 1952.[25]

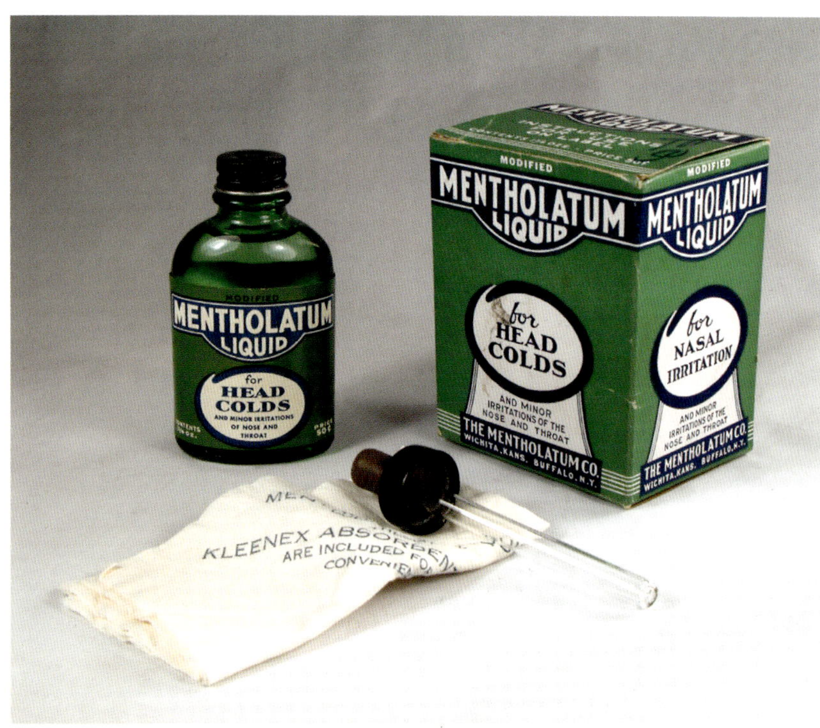

Mentholatum Liquid

Liquid was used in vaporizers and atomizers as an inhalant. There were approximately two dozen inhalant brands on the market at this time.

Starting in the fall of 1934, the Buffalo plant began hiring blind "girls" to work in the packaging department. Paul Hyde (1888–1956) made a plug in the winter 1935 edition of *Menthology* for other employers to consider doing the same. The company cooperated with the local Buffalo Blind Association and the New York State Commission for the Blind to "experiment" and see if sightless workers could succeed at factory work. Mentholatum was the first manufacturer in Buffalo to hire the blind, and by 1936 it had four full-time blind employees. Plant superintendent W. H. Peeples testified, "These girls are making good far beyond our expectation, and are doing better work than the average, sighted girls. In fact, one of the girls is rapidly becoming expert."[26]

(Text continues on page 146.)

Cold Tech

During the 1928–29 winter cold season, Mentholatum first advertised a twenty-one-page pamphlet titled *How to Get Rid of Colds: Written by a Physician*. This "sales help" gives us a view of the state of the art in cold prevention and treatment of the day. It defined a cold as an infection, with mucus discharge, of the membrane lining the nose and throat. It explained that the infection generally starts in the nose and progresses down to the throat and spreads into the respiratory tract. It is an infectious or contagious disease and "many people have several colds a year, some in the winter season, and some in the hot weather."

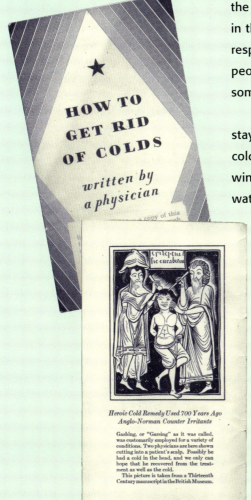

Heroic Cold Remedy Used 700 Years Ago
Anglo-Norman Counter Irritants
Gashing, or "Garsing" as it was called, was customarily employed for a variety of conditions. Two physicians are here shown cutting into a patient's scalp. Possibly he had a cold in the head, and we only can hope that he recovered from the treatment as well as the cold.
This picture is taken from a Thirteenth Century manuscript in the British Museum.

To prevent a cold it recommended avoiding poor ventilation, staying in good health, avoiding contact with people who have a cold and the things they touch, and after "a windy day in the city, in winter, . . . a mechanical cleansing of the nose and throat with a salt water snuffle and gargle (as) a good preventive measure. . . ."

Once you have a cold you go through three stages, and Mentholatum provides relief to all three, it said. Stage one is characterized by dryness to the nose and throat and often the eyes. This is a good time to rest, drink lots of water, and apply Mentholatum to the nostrils. Inhalation of Mentholatum vapor is also suggested and described by floating half a teaspoonful of Mentholatum in a teacup of boiling hot water and cupping your hands to create a funnel to breathe in the vapor.

Stage two is marked by abundant mucus discharge from the nose and sneezing. The throat becomes swollen. Continue the vapor treatment and rub Mentholatum on your throat and chest and wrap up with hot flannel before bedtime. Apply Mentholatum to sore nostrils to relieve chafing from nose blowing.

Stage three is when the body begins to "dry up" the infection. "The secretion becomes less profuse, but it is now definite pus." Use Mentholatum on sore nose and lips. In summary, if Mentholatum is used as directed at stage one, stage two and three can often be avoided. All it takes to treat a cold is "common sense, water, and Mentholatum."

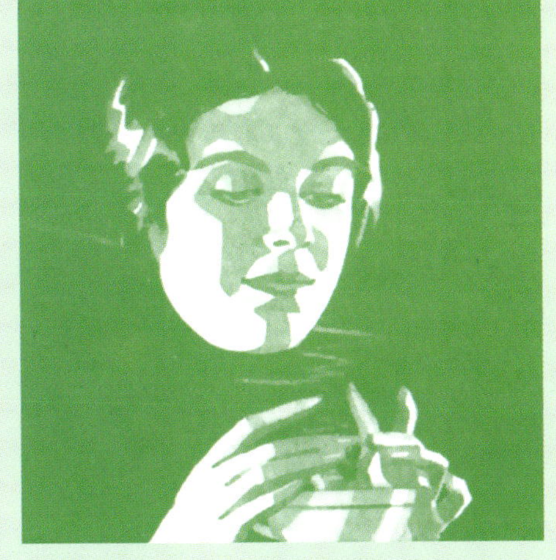

The last chapter is an interesting review of the old ways of treating colds. It warns against the practice of taking violent cathartics. Self-medication with drugs that treat the symptoms is discouraged. "Feed a cold" is now considered to be the wrong thing to do. Finally, "in the old days" when colds were thought to be caused by cold air, people stayed indoors with the windows closed. "Nowadays we know that fresh air helps a cold and that to be outdoors, if not subjected to long exposure and fatigue, is a good thing."

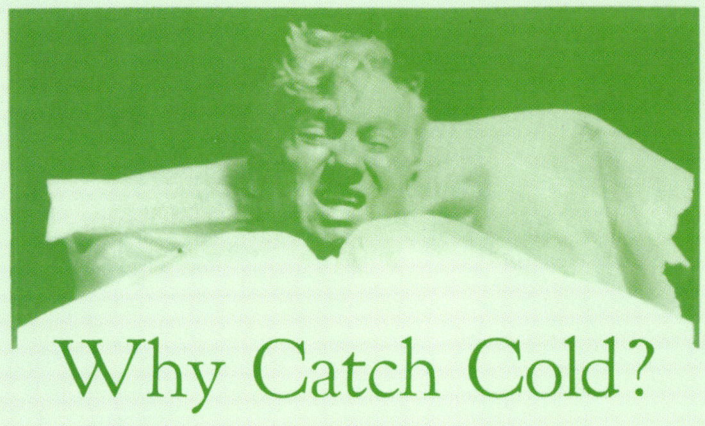

Why Catch Cold?

Feed a Cold

An article in the November 1932 *American Magazine* titled "Why Catch Cold?" by Walter A. Wells, M.D., covered the prevention and treatment of colds for the readership of the day. He claimed that most people had three colds a year, the first in November and the last in February. Colds cost industry $450,000,000 or ninety million lost work days—an imposing statistic at a time when there were forty-two million people "engaged in gainful industry." He speculated that if people would just learn to stay home at the first sign of a cold instead of going to work and spreading it among the other employees, "it wouldn't be long before the October and February epidemics were little more than an unpleasant memory."

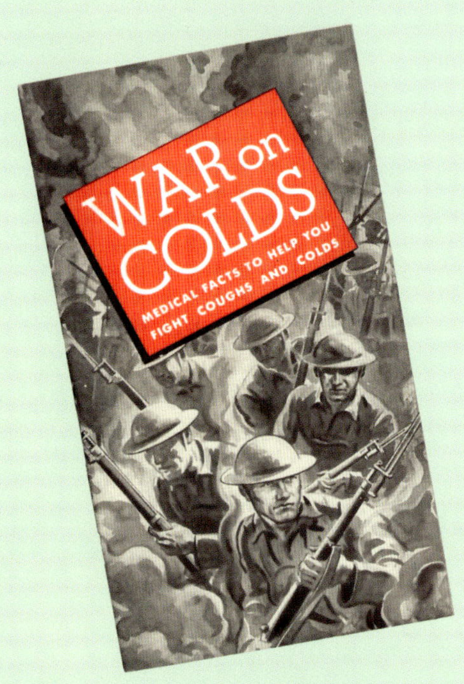

Wells wrote that the search for the cause of the common cold began in Germany in 1914 (see discussion of W. Kruse on page 33) and was now being carried out at the Rockefeller Institute Hospital in New York and at Johns Hopkins Hospital in Baltimore. Scientists there had found an organism smaller than any bacteria "heretofore known," invisible to the most powerful microscopes and capable of penetrating a porcelain filter. If this is the "long-sought cause of colds," he concluded, "the cure is not far off."

Dr. Wells recounted the recent discovery of vitamin A and recommended that a cold sufferer eat a diet rich in the liquid sources of vitamin A such as milk, orange juice, and cod-liver oil, with small portions of fruits, vegetables, and meat, and avoid fried foods, cheese, beans, pastry, and freshly baked breads. He suggested a half glass of water with a half teaspoon of bicarbonate of soda three or four times a day and a mild saline laxative: "No doctor ever said a wiser thing than the famous Dutchman, Boerhaave, when he wrote, 'Keep the head cool, the feet warm, and the bowels open.'"

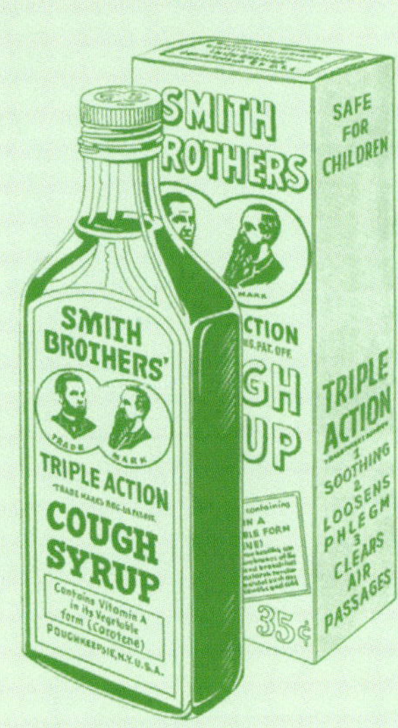

Treatment of a head cold starts with a spray douche of saline water to clear the nasal passages of mucus. For a sore throat, a simple gargle with a alkaline antiseptic solution will do. When the infection has reached the bronchial tubes, breathe steam with menthol using "Grandmother's method of placing a newspaper cone over a kettle of steaming water."

The author of the book *The Common Head Cold and Its Complications*, and a Fellow of the American College of Surgeons, Dr. Wells was critical of people for overdressing, overheating, and overeating. He thought that everyone should get plenty of outdoor exercise, take cold-water showers, and eat a diet rich in vitamin A.[27]

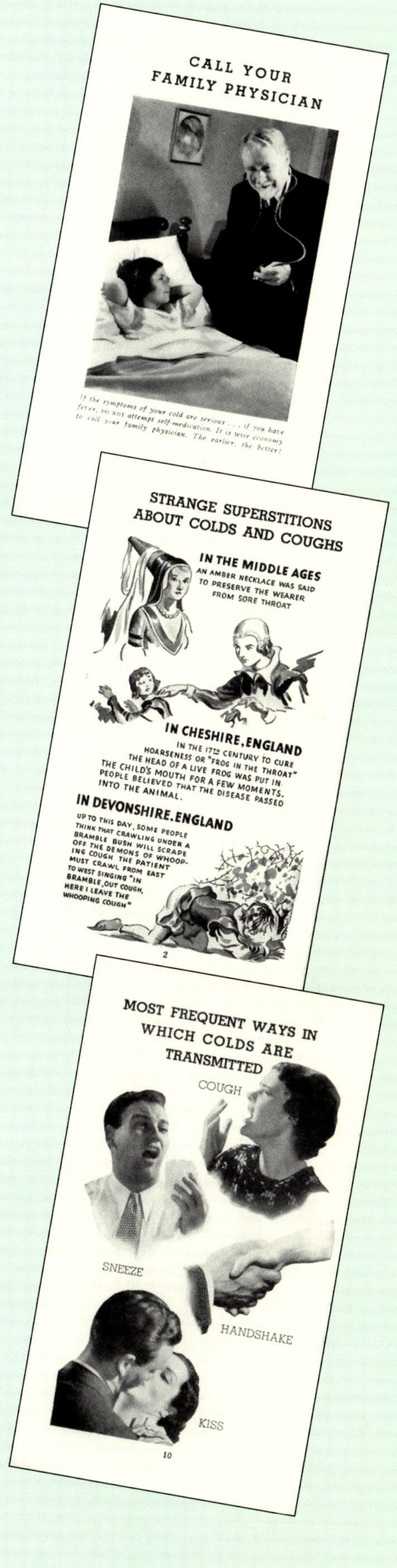
CALL YOUR FAMILY PHYSICIAN
If the symptoms of your cold are serious . . . if you have fever, do not attempt self-medication. It is wise economy to call your family physician. The earlier, the better!
STRANGE SUPERSTITIONS ABOUT COLDS AND COUGHS
IN THE MIDDLE AGES
AN AMBER NECKLACE WAS SAID TO PRESERVE THE WEARER FROM SORE THROAT
IN CHESHIRE, ENGLAND
IN THE 17TH CENTURY TO CURE HOARSENESS OR "FROG IN THE THROAT" THE HEAD OF A LIVE FROG WAS PUT IN THE CHILD'S MOUTH FOR A FEW MOMENTS. PEOPLE BELIEVED THAT THE DISEASE PASSED INTO THE ANIMAL.
IN DEVONSHIRE. ENGLAND
UP TO THIS DAY, SOME PEOPLE THINK THAT CRAWLING UNDER A BRAMBLE BUSH WILL SCRAPE OFF THE DEMONS OF WHOOPING COUGH THE PATIENT MUST CRAWL FROM EAST TO WEST SINGING "IN BRAMBLE, OUT COUGH, HERE I LEAVE THE WHOOPING COUGH"
2
MOST FREQUENT WAYS IN WHICH COLDS ARE TRANSMITTED
COUGH
SNEEZE
HANDSHAKE
KISS
10

In 1934, Smith Brothers produced a pamphlet titled *War on Colds: Medical Facts to Help You Fight Coughs and Colds*. As the title suggested, war was the metaphor used throughout this twenty-eight-page advertisement for Smith Brothers Cough Drops. It told us that colds cause a "money loss of over two billion dollars each year." It explained that "during the present century a great army of scientists has spent many years and large sums of money in an endeavor to find the actual cause of colds. Unfortunately, they have not been able as yet to put their fingers on the specific cause."

Some scientists believed that viruses, which are "ultra-microscopic bodies . . . too small to be detected by our most powerful microscopes," were the cause. Some thought that bacteria were the culprits. And, the latest theory was that the cause was a common bacteria that lives in the nose and enters a stage of life where it degenerates to become so small that it "can readily pass through a stone filter." The pamphlet provides a cross section of the nose and throat and describes how colds *attack* the mucous membrane and the body supplies it with extra blood and white blood cells causing the membrane to become inflamed.

Prevent colds, it warned, and "fight off the enemy" with a well-balanced diet and fresh air, and avoid contact with those who have colds. If you have a cold go to bed, drink plenty of water, don't overeat, keep your bowels open ("if you need it take a mild laxative"), call a physician, and "don't irritate your throat by coughing. Use a good cough drop or cough syrup—at the first sign of a cough."

The second half of the pamphlet was devoted to the case for vitamin A. Scientists discovered that vitamin A was the "vital substance necessary for the maintenance of a healthy, resistant mucous membrane," and this discovery "has been hailed as one of the most valuable achievements of modern medicine." Primary vitamin A (carotene) "until recently" was "one of the world's most precious substances. It cost $11,000 a pound . . . then a group of American scientists discovered how to produce (it) in commercial quantities." Smith Brothers Cough Drops and Smith Brothers Cough Syrup both have vitamin A, and Smith Brothers is the only brand to have it. The pamphlet ended with a history of the company.

The Pigmies *Books*

Throughout the 1920s and mid-1930s, the Mentholatum Company produced a series of small, pocket-sized booklets that were distributed to students in schools and promoted the use of its products. The booklets were entitled *Pigmies* and were exclusive of the company's other advertising. Sample tins were sometimes pasted onto a page in the booklet, or the two were placed together in a cellophane bag. The series consisted of four variations, starting with a simple twofold pamphlet, followed by three paperbound "books," as the company called them.

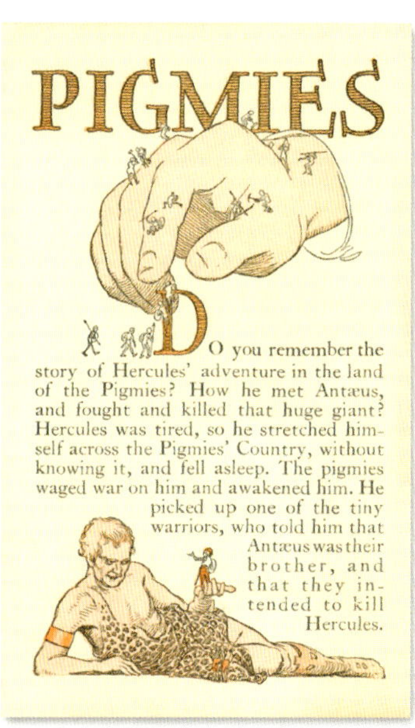
PIGMIES
DO you remember the story of Hercules' adventure in the land of the Pigmies? How he met Antæus, and fought and killed that huge giant? Hercules was tired, so he stretched himself across the Pigmies' Country, without knowing it, and fell asleep. The pigmies waged war on him and awakened him. He picked up one of the tiny warriors, who told him that Antæus was their brother, and that they intended to kill Hercules.

WASH the face and hands with warm water and good soap, rinse with cold water and dry thoroughly. This is of first importance, as it removes many of the germs and cleanses small scratches before they become infected. Clean hands, and hands often washed, are much less liable to inflamed wounds than dirty hands. An application of Mentholatum after washing keeps the skin soft and pliable and prevents chapping.
Cold Prevention
A little Mentholatum in the nostrils night and morning keeps the head clear, often preventing colds and is an excellent relief for stuffy head colds and catarrh. Try it.
MENTHOLATUM
THE MENTHOLATUM CO.
WICHITA, KANS. BUFFALO, N. Y. BRIDGEBURG, ONT.

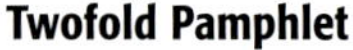

Twofold Pamphlet

Front and back pages, 3½″ × 6″, two-color litho., pre-1932.

The pocket-book format the company chose to use was patterned after the almanacs and recipe books that rival brands had placed on drugstore counters for the past fifty years or more. Inexpensive, paperbound books date back to the earliest days of the printing press. Full-sized, bound octavos were heavy and expensive to make and traditionally sold from bookshops in the larger towns. Alternatively, lightweight "chapbooks" containing poems, ballads, and stories were made to fit easily into backpacks and handcarts and carried throughout the English countryside by peddlers known as "chapmen." During the seventeenth and eighteenth centuries in America, itinerant frontier preachers carried small printed "tracts" containing bible verses and catechisms in their saddlebags to disperse among their far-flung congregations. The folded pages of early chapbooks and tracts were printed with black ink and hand bound with a piece of thread. Illustrations were limited to simple line engravings, with the option of adding hand-painted colors afterward. While the format of these small books had remained substantially unchanged from the archaic chapbook, the production values had improved remarkably by the 1930s.

New printing technologies introduced toward the end of the nineteenth century, such as one-color offset lithography, the linotype machine, and cheap sulfite papers, helped to reduce the costs of printing newspapers and magazines but did little to change the look of mass printing. Pages that required several colors were hard to keep accurately registered as they were

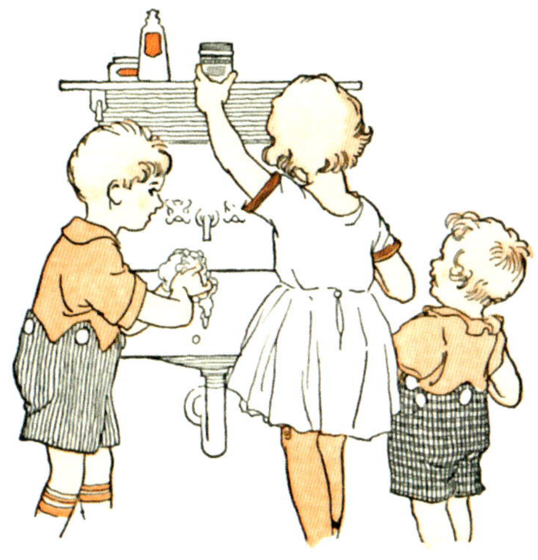

repeatedly passed through the press to add each new color. Early Mentholatum blotters are notorious for their sloppy color registration. Fine-art lithographs often required a dozen or more custom-mixed ink colors, each one carefully registered to pass through the printing press. Posters and die-cut display boards used fewer colors. Later, with the advent of photographic transfer and halftone screens, graphic artists could improve a simple one-color job by adding gray tones to their line art. They could also reproduce full-color illustrations with the use of only four ink colors (magenta, yellow, cyan, and black). Color printing was necessarily expensive and therefore was generally limited to cover art. By 1930, when the first two-color presses went into operation, four colors could be printed with only two passes instead of four, making it easier for advertisers to justify the cost of four-color handouts.

Mentholatum's 1932 *Pigmies* booklet is a colorful early example of this modern, automated printing and binding technology. Half of the book's pages were illustrated in color, and it was bound together with wire staples instead of thread. When the little books were first handed out, the country was in the midst of the Great Depression, and people considered them a rare and treasured keepsake. It isn't surprising, then, that so many perfectly preserved *Pigmies* books have survived to be traded on the market today.

The first in the series is an attractive little two-color handout in the William Morris style with freehand line illustrations done by a competent artist. It tells the story of Hercules's adventure in the land of the Pigmies. It instructs the children that just like the "wee pigmies" attacked the sleeping Hercules, "pigmy germs" are not afraid to attack us. "So, children, keep your skin in good condition by using Mentholatum every night before you go to bed."

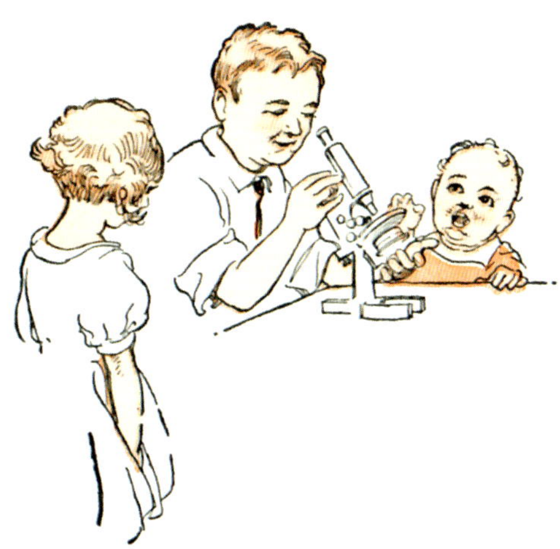

Following this is a lesson entitled "Care of the Skin, Why It Chaps and How to Prevent," accompanied by a cross-sectional illustration of the hair and sweat pore. The children were told that Mentholatum "supplies the oil and healing properties to keep the outer layer [of skin] in a healthy condition." *Menthology* first published an article from the *London Times* titled "Care of the Skin" in 1922. Based on the discovery of the 1922 Dewey letter and its contents (see page 113), we know that "Care of the Skin" was also being sent out to the schools in the form of a "color poster" (see Catalog page C144), and included a handbill, printed on both sides, that quoted the *London Times* article.[28]

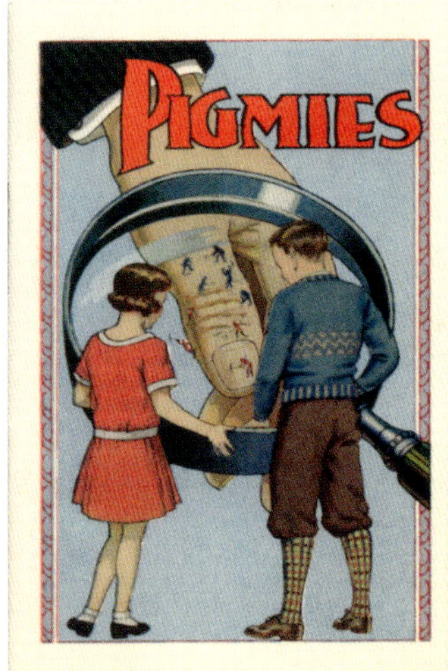
PIGMIES

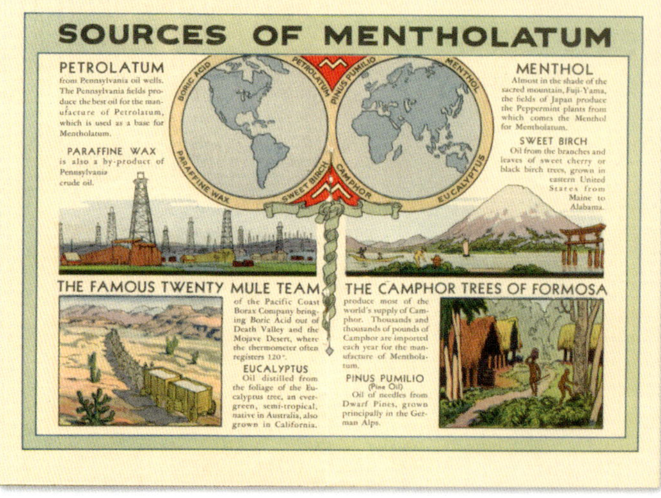
SOURCES OF MENTHOLATUM
PETROLATUM
from Pennsylvania oil wells. The Pennsylvania fields produce the best oil for the manufacture of Petrolatum, which is used as a base for Mentholatum.
PARAFFINE WAX
is also a by-product of Pennsylvania crude oil.
BORIC ACID
PETROLATUM
PINUS PUMILIO
MENTHOL
PARAFFINE WAX
SWEET BIRCH
CAMPHOR
EUCALYPTUS
MENTHOL
Almost in the shade of the sacred mountain, Fuji-Yama, the fields of Japan produce the Peppermint plants from which comes the Menthol for Mentholatum.
SWEET BIRCH
Oil from the branches and leaves of sweet cherry or black birch trees, grown in eastern United States from Maine to Alabama.
THE FAMOUS TWENTY MULE TEAM
of the Pacific Coast Borax Company bringing Boric Acid out of Death Valley and the Mojave Desert, where the thermometer often registers 120°.
EUCALYPTUS
Oil distilled from the foliage of the Eucalyptus tree, an evergreen, semi-tropical, native in Australia, also grown in California.
THE CAMPHOR TREES OF FORMOSA
produce most of the world's supply of Camphor. Thousands and thousands of pounds of Camphor are imported each year for the manufacture of Mentholatum.
PINUS PUMILIO
(Pine Oil)
Oil of needles from Dwarf Pines, grown principally in the German Alps.

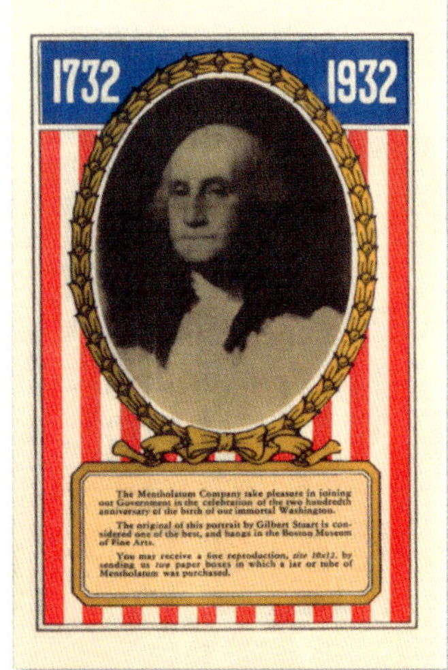
1732
1932
The Mentholatum Company take pleasure in joining our Government in the celebration of the two hundredth anniversary of the birth of our immortal Washington.
The original of this portrait by Gilbert Stuart is considered one of the best, and hangs in the Boston Museum of Fine Arts.
You may receive a fine reproduction, size 10x12, by sending us two paper boxes in which a jar or tube of Mentholatum was purchased.

The First Twelve-Page Booklet

Front cover, center spread, and back cover, 3⅜″ × 5¼″, four-color litho., stapled, 1932.

This pamphlet concluded with instructions to wash a scratch with soap and water to prevent germs from infecting it, then apply Mentholatum to keep the skin "soft and pliable and prevent chapping." The child was reminded on the back page to use Mentholatum "in the nostrils night and morning" to prevent colds and catarrh.

An examination of the product illustration on the back page shows the jar and tube that were used prior to 1930. Considering the pamphlet was not in use when the Dewey letter was sent in 1922, this narrows the publication of the twofold to sometime after 1922 and before 1930.

Next in the Pigmies series is a four-color booklet that also tells the story of Hercules in the land of the Pigmies. Similar line drawings appear, carried over from the first, with slight modifications made to them. The text is almost word for word the same as the twofold, with the exception of a few minor edits.

The color illustration on the cover depicts a girl and boy standing before a giant magnifying glass. Behind the glass is a giant's hand (in a business suit) with his thumb under the lens. The thumb, which is the size of the boy's torso, is the subject of the children's gaze. All over the thumb, they can see little people attacking the skin with pickaxes. The boy is wearing plaid knee socks, wool knickers, and a knit sweater. The girl is wearing a simple red, flapper-style dress, and her right arm is resting on the rim of the magnifying glass. Compared to the romantic cover art of the earlier edition, this contrived, scientific exaggeration leaves little to the imagination.

The illustration is symbolic of a transition time for the Mentholatum Company. A. A. Hyde's era of the home remedy was coming to an end. His sons, who now ran the company, saw

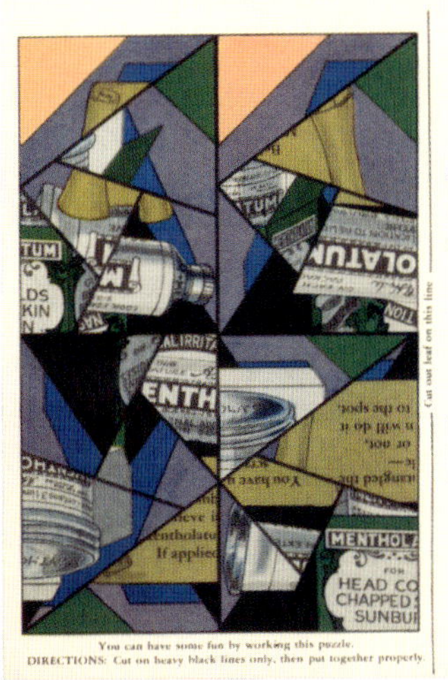

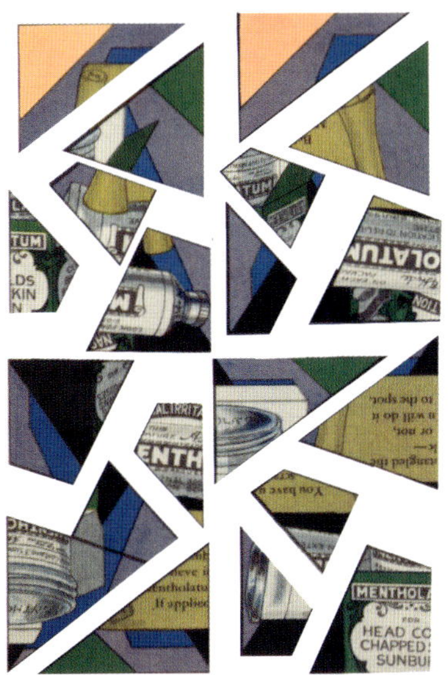

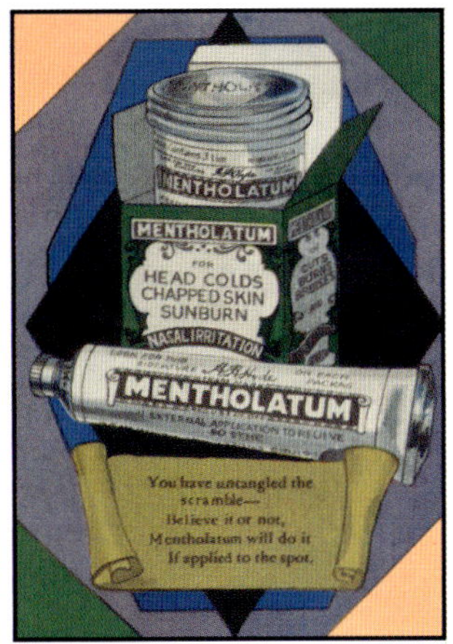

The Puzzle Page

The page as it appeared in the booklet (top), cut apart (center), and put back together (above)

that their future success was going to depend on science and how closely they could steer the public's perception of Mentholatum into a position similar to that of the truly scientific medicinal products coming onto the market. In the spring 1932 issue of *Menthology*, under the title "Enduring Strength," they wrote:

> *In arriving at the proper strength for Mentholatum, we have conducted numberless laboratory tests and consulted hundreds of pharmacists, doctors and chemists over a forty year period. During that whole time the blend and strength have remained the same, for this blend releases the proper strength slowly and with long continued effectiveness. The simple and convincing test is to rub a bit of Mentholatum on one temple and some of a similar product on the other. After an hour's time, compare them. We recommend this test to anyone questioning the strength of Mentholatum.*[29]

The booklet continued with "Care of the Skin," repeated from the earlier pamphlet, which was followed by one page devoted to "Cold Treatment." Here, children were instructed to drink "large quantities of water" to flush out the kidneys, and to insert Mentholatum into each nostril, "drawing long breaths after." A Mentholatum chest rub was recommended before going to bed.

Anyone who ever had this treatment applied was likely to never forget the experience. Before being sent to bed at night, the chest and throat were massaged with Mentholatum ("use about half a tube") and then wrapped up with flannel. Left in the darkened bedroom, his or her chest began cooking like a reactor core meltdown, and then the head began spinning from the fumes. All night, the cold continued on its merry way with absolutely no interruption. The only benefit from this draconian treatment was that the victim became so totally overwhelmed by the Mentholatum-induced symptoms that she or he forgot all about the cold symptoms. And herein lies one truth about A. A. Hyde's balm: although it had a nominal physiological effect, it powerfully distracted the senses!

"Sources of Mentholatum" was a four-color center spread featuring a map of the world framed by four painterly illustrations: oil wells in Pennsylvania, the "Famous Twenty Mule Team" in Death Valley, the camphor trees of Formosa, and Mount Fuji in Japan. The composition is symmetrical and masculine, and the colors are subdued. The next three pages were devoted to the treatment of chapped skin, windburn, nasal catarrh, nervous

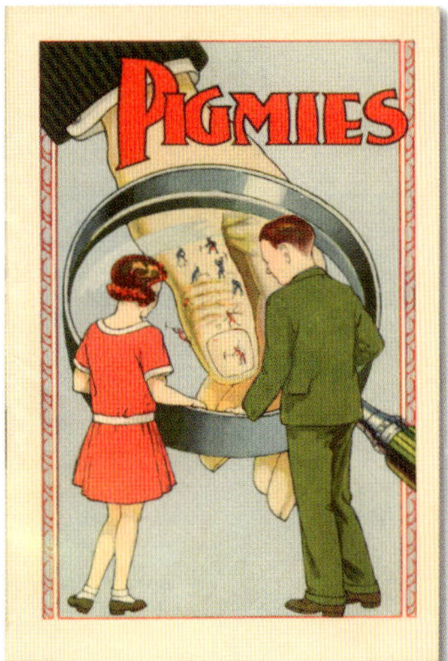

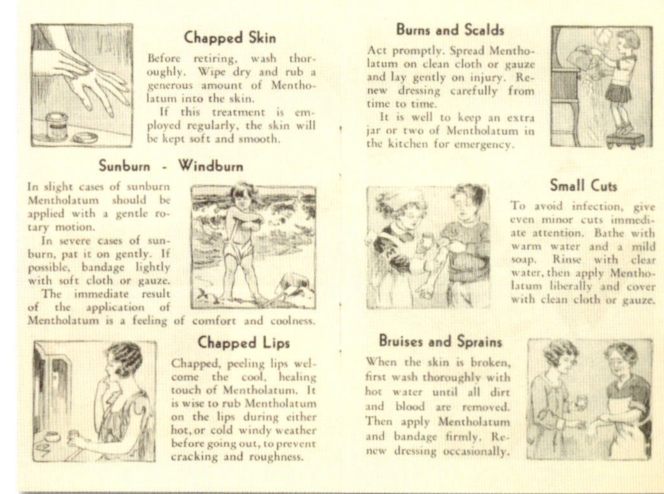

Chapped Skin

Before retiring, wash thoroughly. Wipe dry and rub a generous amount of Mentholatum into the skin.

If this treatment is employed regularly, the skin will be kept soft and smooth.

Sunburn - Windburn

In slight cases of sunburn Mentholatum should be applied with a gentle rotary motion.

In severe cases of sunburn, pat it on gently. If possible, bandage lightly with soft cloth or gauze.

The immediate result of the application of Mentholatum is a feeling of comfort and coolness.

Chapped Lips

Chapped, peeling lips welcome the cool, healing touch of Mentholatum. It is wise to rub Mentholatum on the lips during either hot, or cold windy weather before going out, to prevent cracking and roughness.

Burns and Scalds

Act promptly. Spread Mentholatum on clean cloth or gauze and lay gently on injury. Renew dressing carefully from time to time.

It is well to keep an extra jar or two of Mentholatum in the kitchen for emergency.

Small Cuts

To avoid infection, give even minor cuts immediate attention. Bathe with warm water and a mild soap. Rinse with clear water, then apply Mentholatum liberally and cover with clean cloth or gauze.

Bruises and Sprains

When the skin is broken, first wash thoroughly with hot water until all dirt and blood are removed. Then apply Mentholatum and bandage firmly. Renew dressing occasionally.

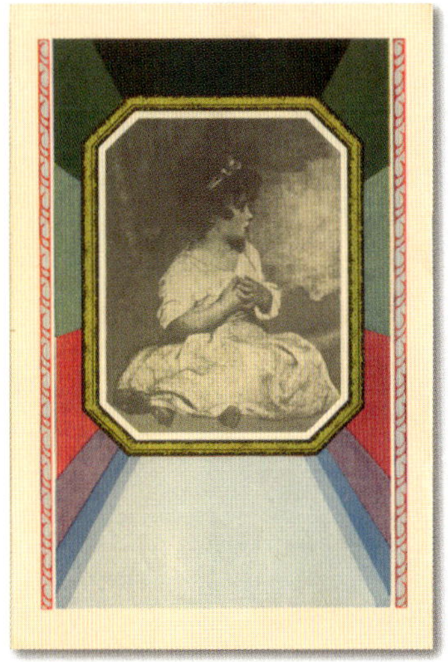

The Second Twelve-Page Booklet

Front cover, sample pages (with Little Nurse), and back cover, 3⅜″ × 5¼″, four-color litho., stapled, 1934.

headache, chilblains, and so on. Each treatment was accompanied by a one-inch-square black-and-white or color illustration. The Little Nurse also made a guest appearance in the "Small Cuts" department.

The tenth, unnumbered, page was the "Puzzle" page. Although this seventy-four-year-old document is too valuable to physically cut with scissors, it could nevertheless be re-created and cut out with a computer. See it on page 149. The jar and tube depicted in the completed artwork indicate an embossed tin lid on the jar and a metal cap and folded closure on the tube.

"Masterpieces of Art," located in the back, was a selection of ten color prints. "To secure one of these pictures make your selection by number, and with your request enclose the paper box that held either a jar or tube of MENTHOLATUM when purchased." The back cover celebrated, in patriotic red, white, and blue, the two hundredth anniversary of the birth of "our immortal Washington, 1732–1932." George's portrait, by Gilbert Stuart, is now a "fine reproduction" print and can be secured for "two paper boxes."

The third issue was a revision of the 1932 booklet. The front and back cover illustrations have been amended, the illustrations on the "Cold Treatment" page have been replaced, and there is minor editing throughout the text. The changes to the cover art are the most interesting. First, the boy has changed into a green suit coat and pants, obviously to create a more contemporary look. But his posture has become submissive, compared with the original boy's confident, legs firmly planted, stance. The girl has undergone a less dramatic makeover. Her right arm has been moved aside, probably so that it will not detract attention from the thumb, and her brown hair has been tinted red. The back

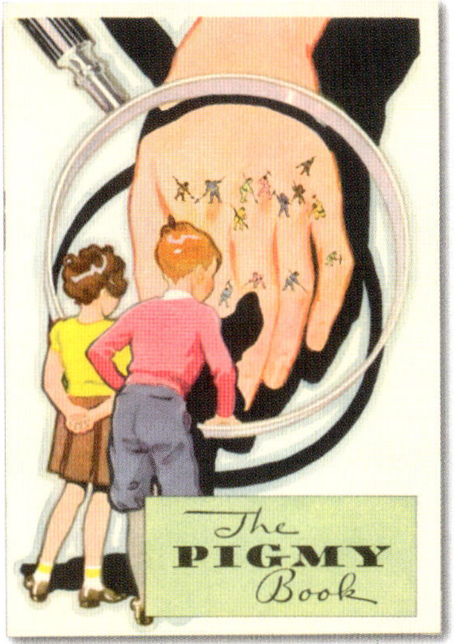

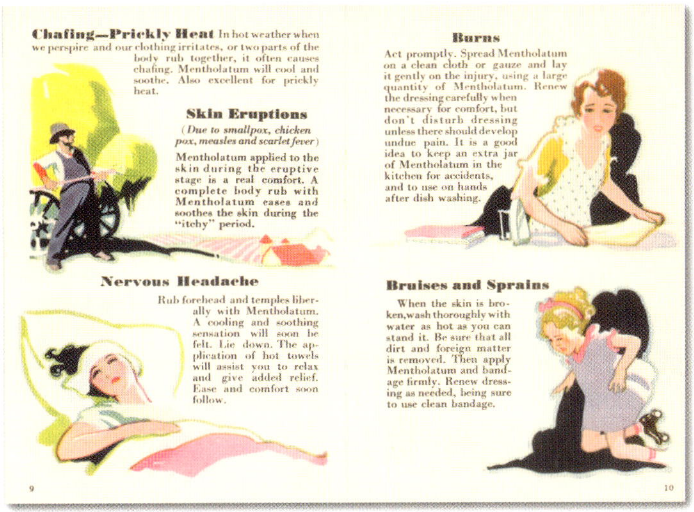

Chafing—Prickly Heat In hot weather when we perspire and our clothing irritates, or two parts of the body rub together, it often causes chafing. Mentholatum will cool and soothe. Also excellent for prickly heat.

Skin Eruptions

(Due to smallpox, chicken pox, measles and scarlet fever)

Mentholatum applied to the skin during the eruptive stage is a real comfort. A complete body rub with Mentholatum eases and soothes the skin during the "itchy" period.

Nervous Headache

Rub forehead and temples liberally with Mentholatum. A cooling and soothing sensation will soon be felt. Lie down. The application of hot towels will assist you to relax and give added relief. Ease and comfort soon follow.

9

Burns

Act promptly. Spread Mentholatum on a clean cloth or gauze and lay it gently on the injury, using a large quantity of Mentholatum. Renew the dressing carefully when necessary for comfort, but don't disturb dressing unless there should develop undue pain. It is a good idea to keep an extra jar of Mentholatum in the kitchen for accidents, and to use on hands after dish washing.

Bruises and Sprains

When the skin is broken, wash thoroughly with water as hot as you can stand it. Be sure that all dirt and foreign matter is removed. Then apply Mentholatum and bandage firmly. Renew dressing as needed, being sure to use clean bandage.

10

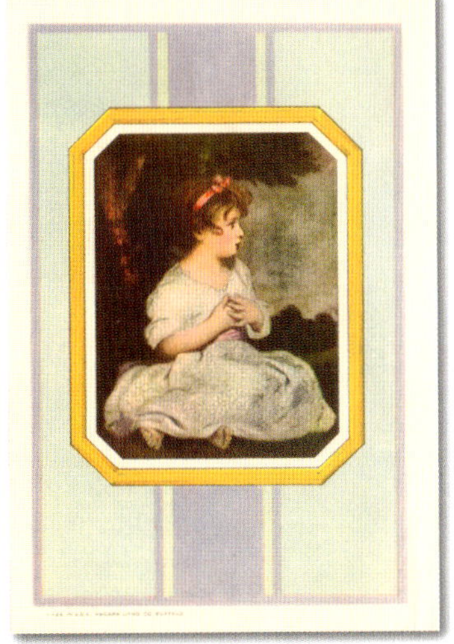

The Third Twelve-Page Booklet

Front cover, sample pages, back cover, and center spread (below), 3⅜″ × 5″, four-color litho., stapled, 1936.

cover depicts one of the masterpiece-for-box prints, graphically framed by some of the same geometry and muted colors that were used in the puzzle art.

A modernized version of the previous two booklets, the fourth in the series was completely rebuilt from the ground up. For the first time, the back cover is marked, "Made in USA Niagara Litho Co. Buffalo." The color illustrations are new, a modern type style is used, and the text is rewritten. The cover art depicts a much younger girl and boy looking through the same huge magnifying glass. This time, the Pigmy people are attacking a giant woman's hand. The girl's skirt is pleated, and the boy is back in knickers. The color in this watercolor illustration, as well as the others, is saturated and bright. The artwork is stylized by dramatic black shadows. What today looks like a gimmicky blue outline offsetting the figures might have been a totally new look back then.

A glaring yellow and blue world map covers the two center pages. Below the map is a listing of the ingredients, and this time it includes the locations of Mentholatum's five factories. Children were informed that a thirteen-by-twenty-three-inch copy of the map could be obtained in exchange for their address written on an empty jar box or tube box.

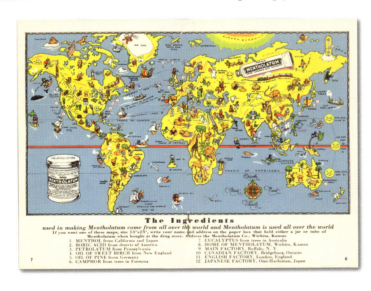

The Ingredients

used in making Mentholatum come from all over the world and Mentholatum is used all over the world

If you want one of these maps, size 13″x23″, write your name and address on the paper box that held either a jar or tube of Mentholatum when bought at the drug store. Address the Mentholatum Co., Wichita, Kansas

1. MENTHOL from California and Japan
2. BORIC ACID from deserts of America
3. PETROLATUM from Pennsylvania
4. OIL OF SWEET BIRCH from New England
5. OIL OF PINE from Germany
6. CAMPHOR from trees in Formosa
7. EUCALYPTUS from trees in Australia
8. HOME OF MENTHOLATUM, Wichita, Kansas
9. MAIN FACTORY, Buffalo, N. Y.
10. CANADIAN FACTORY, Bridgeburg, Ontario
11. ENGLISH FACTORY, London, England
12. JAPANESE FACTORY, Omi-Hachiman, Japan

7 8

This map was created by Robert Aitchison (1887–1964), a graphic artist and corporate

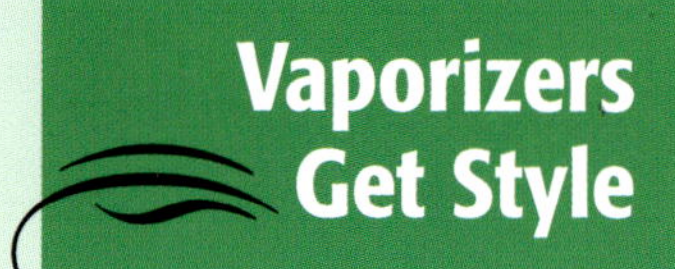

Vaporizers Get Style

Vaporizer design continued into the 1930s with improvements to function and style. The Vapo Cresolene Vaporizer that was once fired by kerosene was now replaced by a new electrified Bakelite model. The metal saucer, as suggested on the box, was also ideal for vaporizing perfumes, and extra saucers cost ten cents.

Max Katzman's 1931 patent application was an improvement over his 1927 electric vaporizer patent. When the new patent was issued in 1933, it supported an already successful line of KAZ Electric Vaporizers, represented here by a Model No. 70. This later-model KAZ located a separate "medicine chamber" above the electrodes, which produced a uniform mixture of steam and medication. It had a sixteen-ounce capacity and automatic shutoff. It came with a free one-ounce bottle of KAZ Inhalant fluid, a mixture of eucalyptus, peppermint, lavender, menthol, camphor, etc.

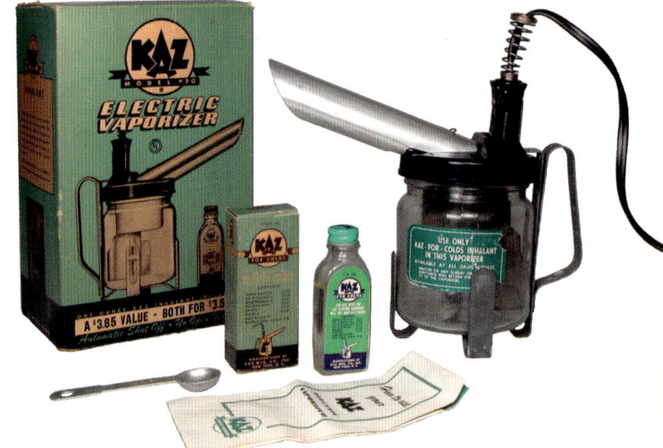

Aug. 15, 1933.
M. KATZMAN
ELECTRIC VAPORIZER
Filed Sept. 28, 1931

American Druggist

DeVilbiss Steam Vaporizer

63 *An effective improvement on the old croup-kettle has been announced by the DeVilbiss Company. An automatic device which cuts off the current when the water is evaporated is a special feature, permitting the machine to be used with safety while the patient is asleep. The machine is of simple, sturdy construction and is rustproof and sanitary. Detailed information will be sent on request*

April 1932

In the April 1932 issue of the *American Druggist* magazine, DeVilbiss introduced its new steam vaporizer in the new-products section. Later in December it filed for a patent, which it received on March 6, 1934. DeVilbiss, which had been making vaporizers since 1888, was now making one that looked just like the standard functional-looking KAZ vaporizer. Sometime after 1935 aluminum became popular and vaporizers like the streamlined DeVilbiss 46 were produced. The 46 had a few problems the earlier vaporizers didn't have. First, it would not shut off completely when the water ran out; second, it required a ball of cotton to be placed inside the head to filter the medication; and third, its heating element could not be submerged in water while cleaning the unit after use. This was clearly a case of function sacrificed for style.

The stylish and modern-looking Prak-T-Kal Electric Vaporizer operated on the same principals as the DeVilbiss 46 and it suffered the same failures. The "medication chamber" was much larger and

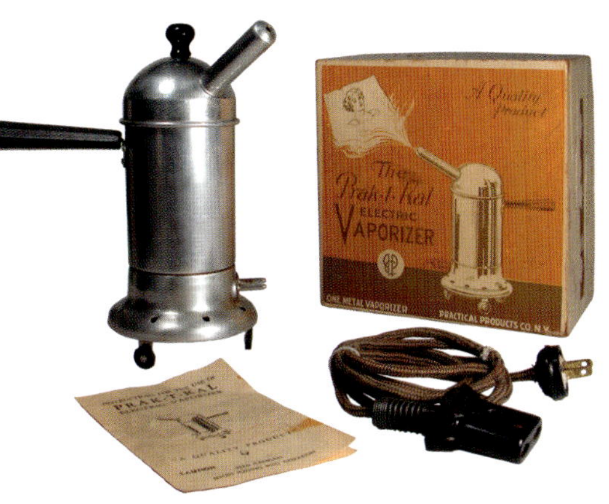

required more cotton, and its water capacity was much smaller. Practical Products Company of New York did not make such a practical vaporizer.

Eventually style and function came together. The DeVilbiss 148 was the ultimate in streamline simplicity when it was patented in 1944. Its carton opened to display the black plastic cone and explain its features. Although the sleek vaporizer safely shut off when the water ran out and could be submerged when cleaning, it still required a new ball of cotton every time it was used. This was a small inconvenience for an object of eye-pleasing style and practical function.

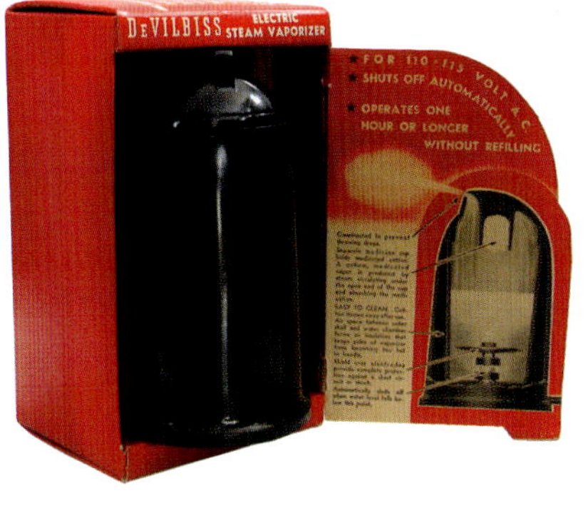

officer for the McCormick-Armstrong Printing Company in Wichita, Kansas. Aitchison's passion for maps and cartography led to his creation of a world map for the winter 1932–1933 cover of *Menthology* and, later, a wall-size world map by 1935. Aitchinson may have been inspired by the pictorial maps of Jo Mora (1876–1947), who had completed his Yosemite map in 1931. Between 1936 and 1943 Aitchinson created twenty-six state maps, which were less whimsical than the world map and were given out gratis to schoolteachers to hang in their classrooms. These fantastic maps are hard to find today without pinholes, tears, and chipped corners, and outside of the Hyde Family Collection, complete sets are rare. It is very possible that Aitchison also created the 1932 "Sources of Mentholatum" center page art, as well as many other illustrations for *Menthology*. There is a strong similarity in the drawing style of his 1940 Oregon Historical Map (see Catalog page C167) and the 1932 booklet illustrations.

It is paradoxical that the world map was covered with little black Sambo figures. In addition, there were Sambo jokes printed in almost every issue of *Menthology*. This lies in stark contrast to A. A. Hyde's legendary concern for civil rights, his philanthropic support for Piney Woods School in Mississippi, and his support for the national tours of the Piney Woods Gospel Singers. Perhaps it can be explained through the metaphorical layers of an onion. Hyde, compared to his generation, had peeled away many more layers of racism than most others, but he hadn't eliminated all. The remaining layers could be peeled away only by his children, grandchildren, and great-grandchildren to come. It might be added that he found humor at the expense of other groups as well. (The "Scotch" jokes, in particular, get the author's goat!) His all-time favorite jokes were the ones that were made at his own expense.

The little booklet ended with the "Masterpieces of Art" offer, but this time the examples were printed in color. This was the last advertising promotion to use the Pigmy theme. A copy of this booklet was found in an envelope sent to Miss Mary Elizabeth Wood of Chesterville, Ohio, containing a request to schoolteachers. It was postmarked January 28, 1935.

Streamline Effect

By 1932, the automobile had captured 40 percent of the passenger train business in America. New trains called "Streamliners" were introduced by the railroads to cut costs and lure riders back. The sculpted steel "Zephyr" was not as heavy as its cast-iron predecessors, so it could carry more material. Its diesel engines ran faster than the older steam-powered locomotives. The design of the Zephyr helped the railroad business and also ushered in the era of streamline aesthetics. Showcased at the 1934 Chicago World's Fair, streamlining symbolized a bright and modern future for a country in dire need of a vision of better times to come. Designers throughout the industrial and commercial sectors embraced the optimistic style of streamlining. Mentholatum introduced a new streamlined cap midyear 1939 that hid the twists from view. Streamline art also graced the cover of the spring 1939 issue of *Menthology*.

The company won the top award for display art at the 1938 All American Packaging and Display Competition sponsored by the trade journal *Modern Packaging*. The "window card" that won was titled "Winter 'Sports.'" In 1939, the Hydes marked Mentholatum's fifty-year anniversary with a special issue of *Menthology*. In it, they told the story of Ella B. Veazie, their first traveling agent, who was now almost eighty-eight years old. There was a brief history of the company. They assured the druggists that although A. A. Hyde had died, his sons continued to conduct the business following the principles of integrity laid down by their father. The editor said these were "pretty troublous times," but assured his readers that by being good Christians seven days a week and by "raising our children in the light of Christ's teachings, and training them to appreciate the spiritual things above the material, the common good above the individual," America might survive the "propaganda of race, class, or social hatreds" that was threatening to tear it apart. He concluded that to be a good patriot, one must first be a good Christian. "If the teachings of Jesus Christ were adopted . . . all the troubles that the world is facing would be done away with." If only it were that easy. A. A. Hyde thought it was.[30]

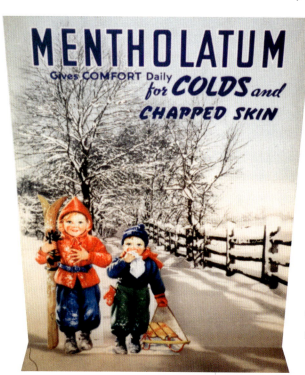

"Winter 'Sports'"
This is the award-winning window display from 1938.

The decade ended with unemployment still high and 58 percent of Americans convinced that the United States would eventually be drawn into the war that Britain and France had recently declared against Germany.[31]

Omi Mission Factory

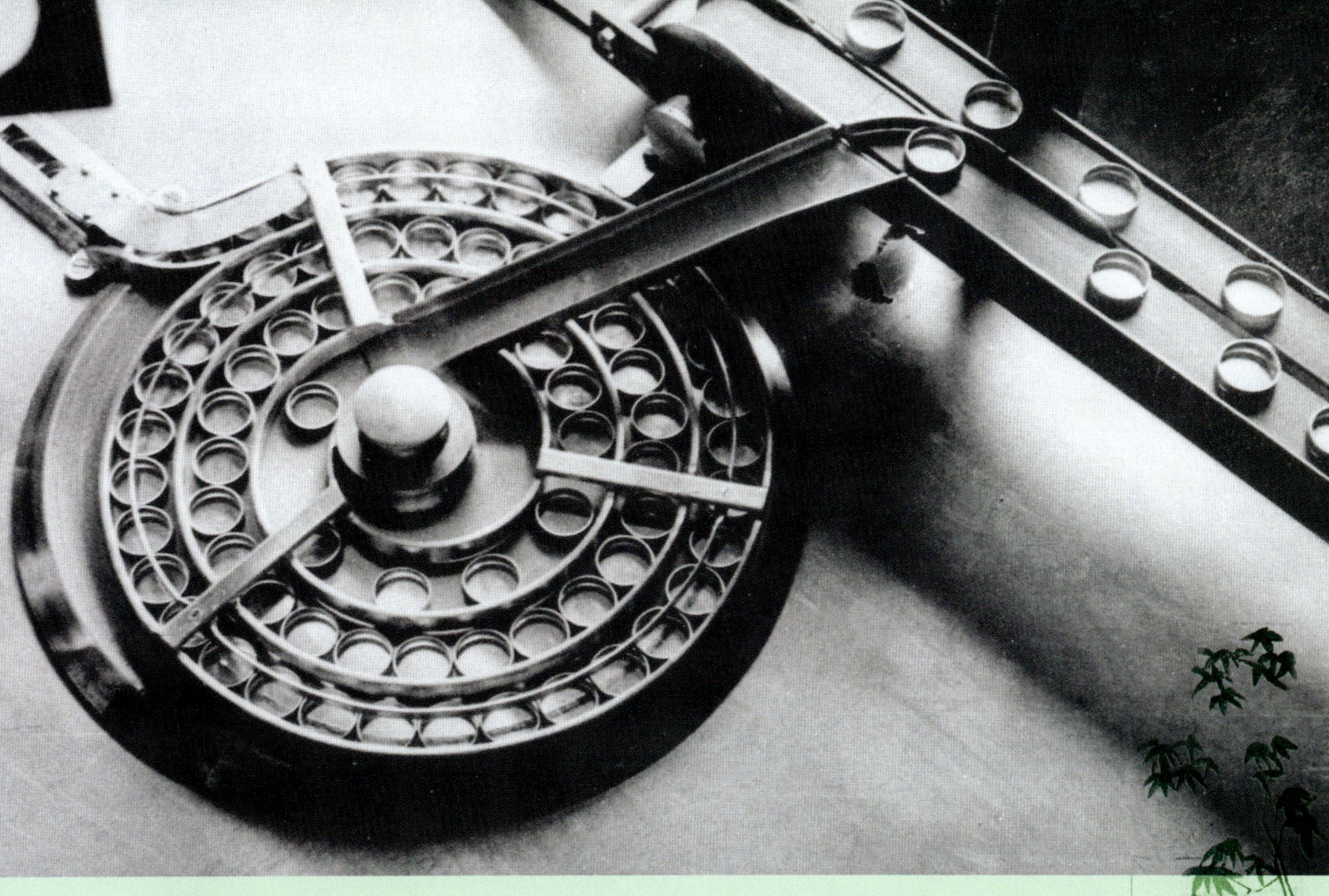

"Warm Plate" Machinery
In the new Omi factory, this spiral feeder warmed empty tins before filling.

From the very beginning Japan has played an important role in the Mentholatum story. Japan provided the all-important menthol, and for a short time the product was even called "the great Japanese salve." After Japan opened its borders to Western trade, Mentholatum was among the first to enter, and it has remained a beloved household product there ever since. The successful marketing of Mentholatum in Japan led to the company eventually building a local factory, which resulted in a long and thriving business relationship. In the world today, Japan has become Mentholatum's largest consumer market. The purchase of Mentholatum by a Japanese company in 1988 was therefore a logical next step.

The story of Mentholatum in Japan begins with a young missionary named William Merrell Vories (1880–1964). Vories was born in Leavenworth, Kansas, and lived there until the age of six. Due to William's poor health, his family moved to Flagstaff, Arizona. When he was sixteen, they moved again to Denver, Colorado, where he attended high school and later graduated from Colorado College at Colorado Springs in 1904. While at college, William became a Student Volunteer for Foreign Missions and dreamed of eventually becoming a missionary himself. He got his chance after graduation when one of the international secretaries of the YMCA asked him to go to Japan and teach English to students in the province of Omi. William departed San Francisco on January 10, 1905, aboard the square-rigged steamer SS *China*, bound for Tokyo, a nineteen-day passage.

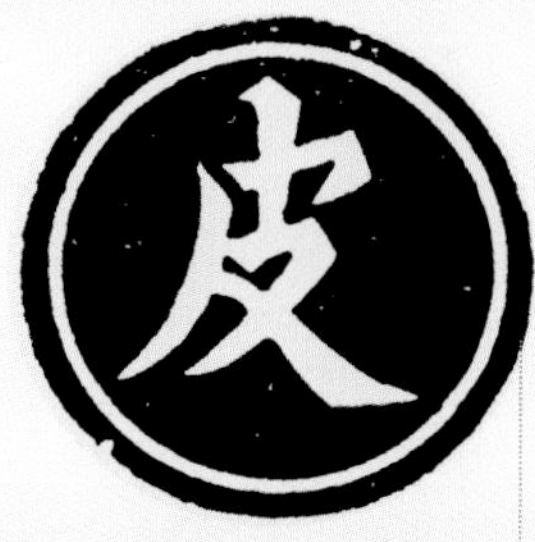

A. A. Hyde's Mark

Hyde used this character on his personal stationery. It is the word *kawa*, meaning skin or hide.

Omi-Hachiman is located on the main island of Honshu, about forty-five miles northeast of Osaka and the same distance due west of Nagoya. Originally the site of Hachiman Castle (1585), which guarded the ancient north-south trade route, the village eventually became a commercial trading center and the home of a large number of wealthy merchant families. Their prosperous town was built in the center of a picturesque mountain valley on the eastern shore of the forty-mile-long Lake Biwa, Japan's largest lake. The merchants wanted their sons to learn English, the language of international business, but were frustrated to find that the only English teachers willing to move to Japan were Christian missionaries. They turned to the International YMCA for help, and an agreement was reached to hire a "Y" missionary on the one stipulation that religion not be discussed during school hours.

Fiftieth Anniversary

This attractive wood-block print adorns a folder commemorating the fiftieth anniversary of the founding of the Omi Brotherhood in 1905. They consider the arrival of Vories the year of their founding. The text states: "The income from the sale of Mentholatum in Japan has been the most important financial resource in support of the Christian work of the Omi Brotherhood." Also of interest, the Mentholatum department sold more than ten million packages in 1954.

William Vories was told when he arrived at the national YMCA office in Tokyo that Omi was a conservative Buddhist "stronghold" isolated by a ring of mountains and that up until that point it had been a "neglected portion of the unevangelized world." Omi would be "virgin soil" for the earnest young missionary who didn't speak a word of Japanese. He described a "long lonely journey on the slow narrow-gauge train" before being "set down upon a forsaken-looking station-platform, in the midst of a wide plain." William was greeted by a cold northeast wind and darkening February sky, and he couldn't help suffering feelings of solitude, inadequacy, and homesickness. He had an overwhelming urge to run away, but as Vories later wrote, he was thankful he had spent all his money getting there and had "no means of escape." He would eventually fall in love with Japan and spend the rest of his life there.

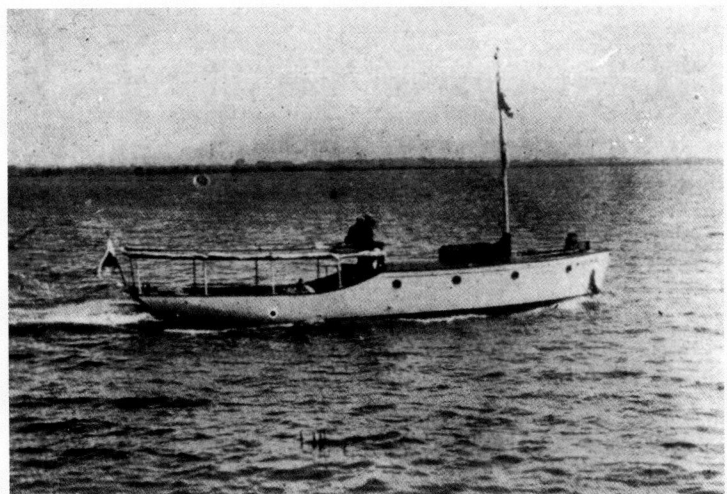

▲ The *Galilee Maru* on Lake Biwa

Young Vories taught English at the Shiga Prefectural Commercial School during the day and conducted Bible studies at his home at night. But he was constantly at odds with the merchant fathers, and within two years Vories was let go by the school. That didn't stop him, for he began working in the YMCA architect's office in Sanjo, Kyoto, and continued to serve the growing number of followers. Eventually he was able to open both a church and YMCA facility in the center of town with financial contributions from Christian Japanese and the YMCA. He continued to face opposition from non-Christian students and Buddhist priests. As is often the case, his most ardent detractors eventually became his most dedicated supporters.

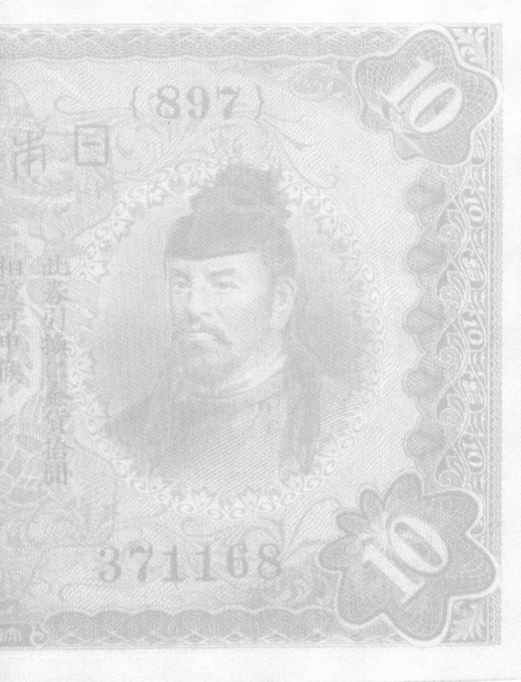

▲ 10 yen currency in use before WWII

In 1910, Vories recruited Etsuzo Yoshida and Lester Chapin, an American, to join him in a new architectural partnership. The success at Omi Mission attracted the attention of Alex Hyde, who was touring in Japan. Alex saw that they needed money and passed the word on to his father. In 1913, A. A. Hyde offered Vories two ideas. The first was to help in the Mission's effort to spread the Gospel to other communities along the shores of Lake Biwa; for this, he donated an American-built motor launch, which they named the *Galilee Maru*, and the construction of its boathouse. Second, he suggested the idea of selling Mentholatum to raise general funds for the Mission. In 1918, Omi Mission built a tuberculosis sanitarium, which is today the Vories Memorial Hospital. The architectural office

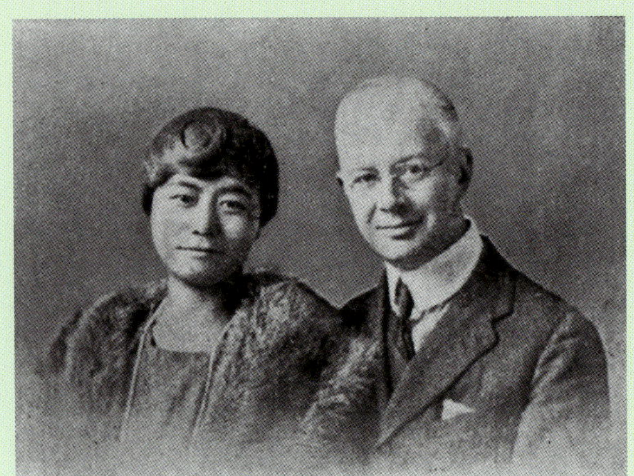

▲ Maki and William Merrell Vories c. 1925

grew to employ as many as thirty architects (c. 1930) who produced designs for hundreds of modern buildings throughout Japan. The office became the number one source of income for the Mission.

In 1919, the thirty-eight-year-old Vories married thirty-five-year-old Makiko "Maki" Hitotsuyanagi, the daughter of the Viscount Suenori Hitotsuyanagi. The viscount was the former daimyo of Ono, "ruler of one of the principalities into which feudal Japan was divided until the Restoration in 1868." Maki was the first member of Japanese nobility to give up her rank and nationality to marry a foreigner. In 1920, the Mission created the Omi Sales Company, Ltd., partly out of an ongoing need to import building materials and furnishings for their architectural clients, and mainly as a means of demonstrating Christian business principles among Japanese businessmen. The sales company became the Mission's number two revenue producer when A. A. Hyde gave them a license to represent all Mentholatum imported to Japan.[1] Mentholatum had been one of the first commercial Western products allowed to be marketed in Japan. It was now distributed exclusively through Christian organizations from one end of the empire to the other and came to be known in rural areas as the "Jesus medicine." Churches sold Mentholatum to raise funds, and students sold it to earn their school tuition. The Mission's newsletter, *The Mustard Seed*, announced that several million jars were sold in 1931 alone.

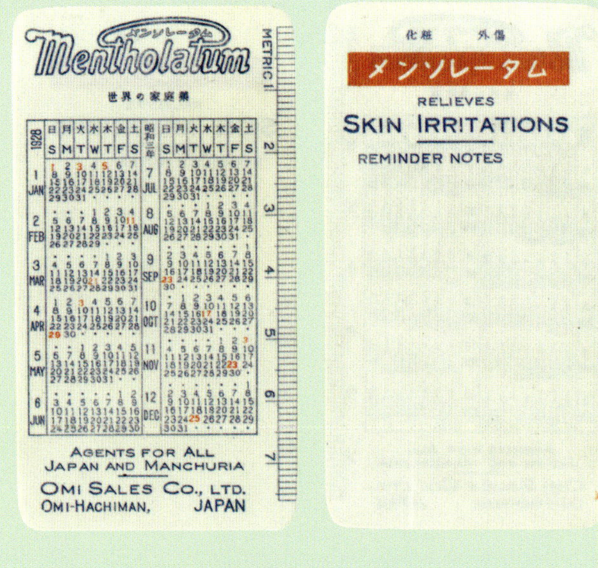

1928 Pocket Calendar

Space for reminder notes appeared on back.

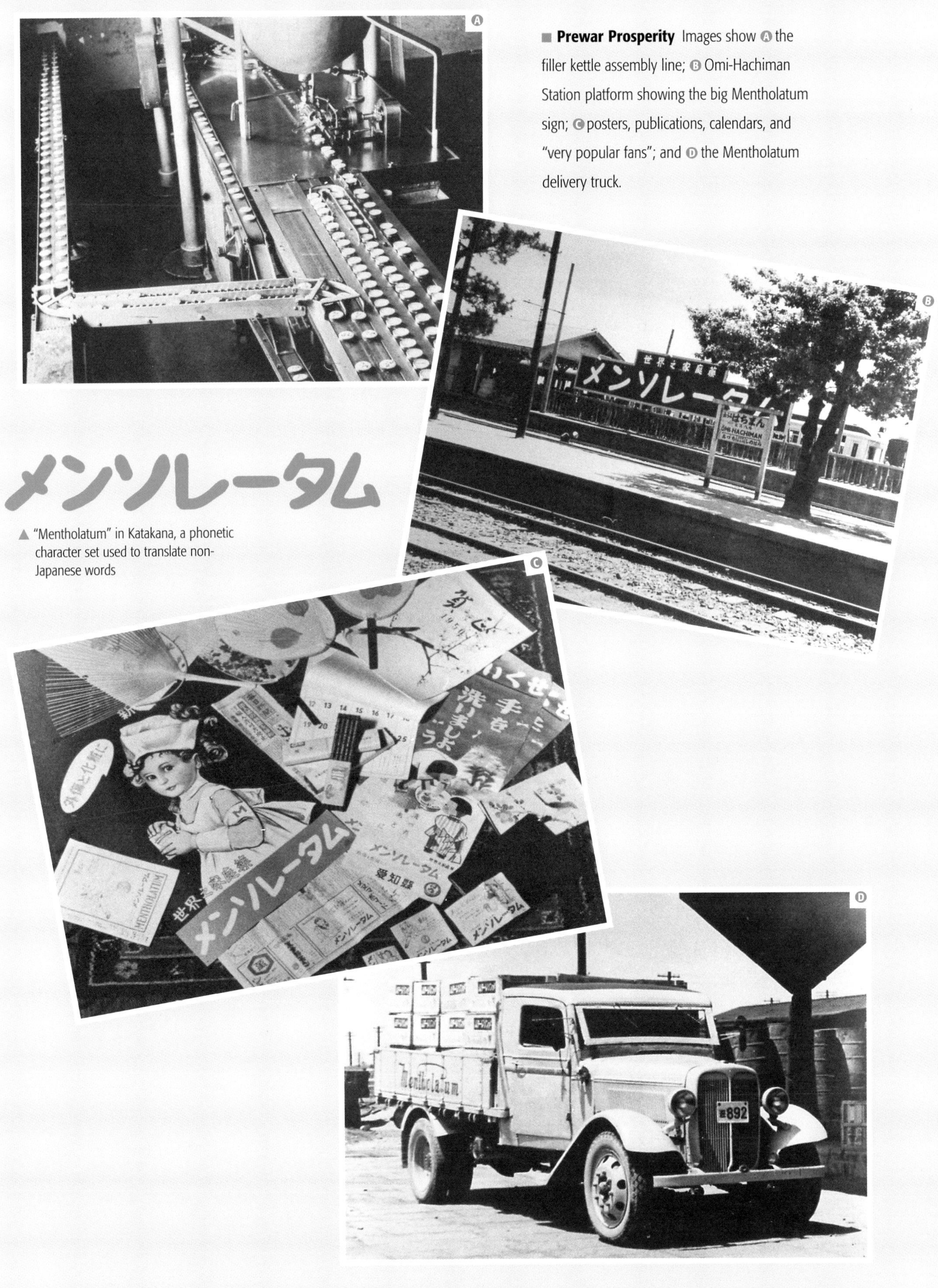

■ **Prewar Prosperity** Images show Ⓐ the filler kettle assembly line; Ⓑ Omi-Hachiman Station platform showing the big Mentholatum sign; Ⓒ posters, publications, calendars, and "very popular fans"; and Ⓓ the Mentholatum delivery truck.

メンソレータム

▲ "Mentholatum" in Katakana, a phonetic character set used to translate non-Japanese words

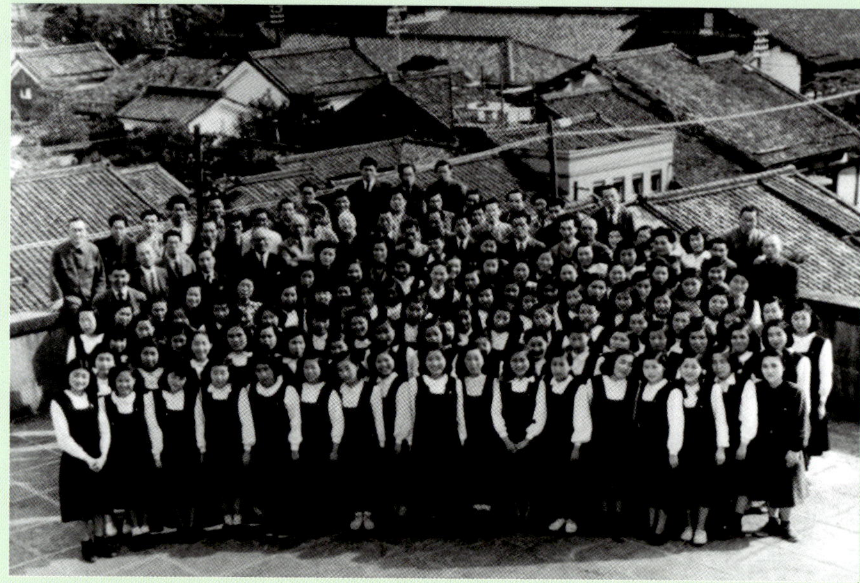

Factory Workers

The "Entire Staff of the Mentholatum Department" is the title of this picture. Many of the young women in the photograph were also students at the Omi Mission High School.

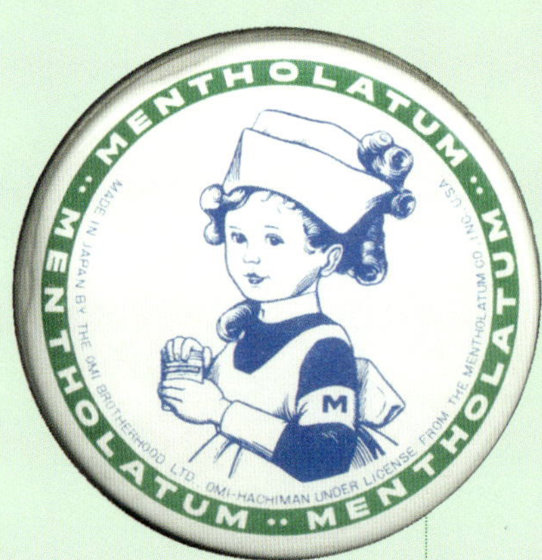

Little Nurse®

She always faced left in Japan and right in the West.

A. A. Hyde felt that there was no reason to continue spending extra money to ship Mentholatum across the Pacific when it could be manufactured locally. In 1933, he donated 100,000 yen to build a factory in Omi-Hachiman. In 1934, the Mission was renamed the Omi Kyodaisha, or Omi Brotherhood. The Brotherhood went on to build a library (1940), a kindergarten through twelfth-grade school (1947), and an evangelical publishing house (Kohan Press). Vories's continued good work won the support of the merchant leaders. During periods of anti-Western sentiment, Vories was singled out as the exception, at one point being chosen by the press as one of the only two Americans who should be allowed to stay in Japan, the other being U.S. Ambassador Cyrus Woods.

To avoid deportation at the start of World War II, the blue-eyed Vories became a naturalized Japanese citizen and changed his name to Hitotsuyanagi Mereru. After the war, he played an important role in discussions between General Douglas MacArthur and the Japanese reconstruction government.[2] Up until his death in 1964 at age eighty-three, Hitotsuyanagi Mereru had received many honorary awards and medals for his lifelong friendship and service to the people of Japan. He was buried in Koshunnen. The modern cities of Omi-Hachiman and Leavenworth, Kansas, became sister cities in 1997. The Vories family house at 1044 Fifth Avenue in Leavenworth is visited annually by Japanese tourists to this day.

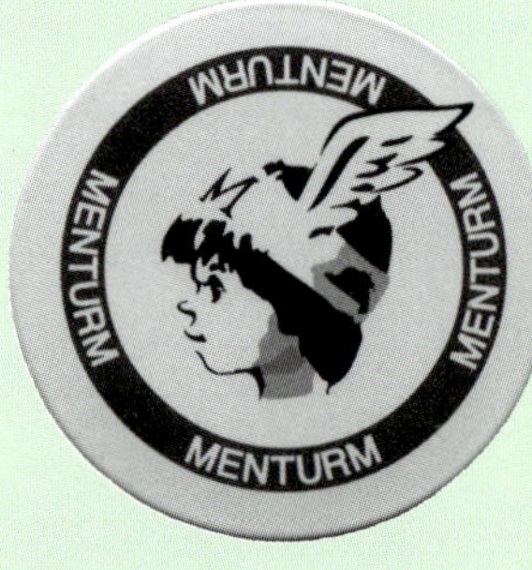

Menturm®

In 1974, the Mentholatum Company decided not to renew its contract with the Omi Brotherhood, and the resulting loss of income caused the Brotherhood to go bankrupt. Recovery was achieved by finding new supporters and continuing to manufacture the same products under the new trademark name Menturm. A new logo was designed similar to Little Nurse, and by 1980 the company began to pay dividends to its investors.

Modernity's Test

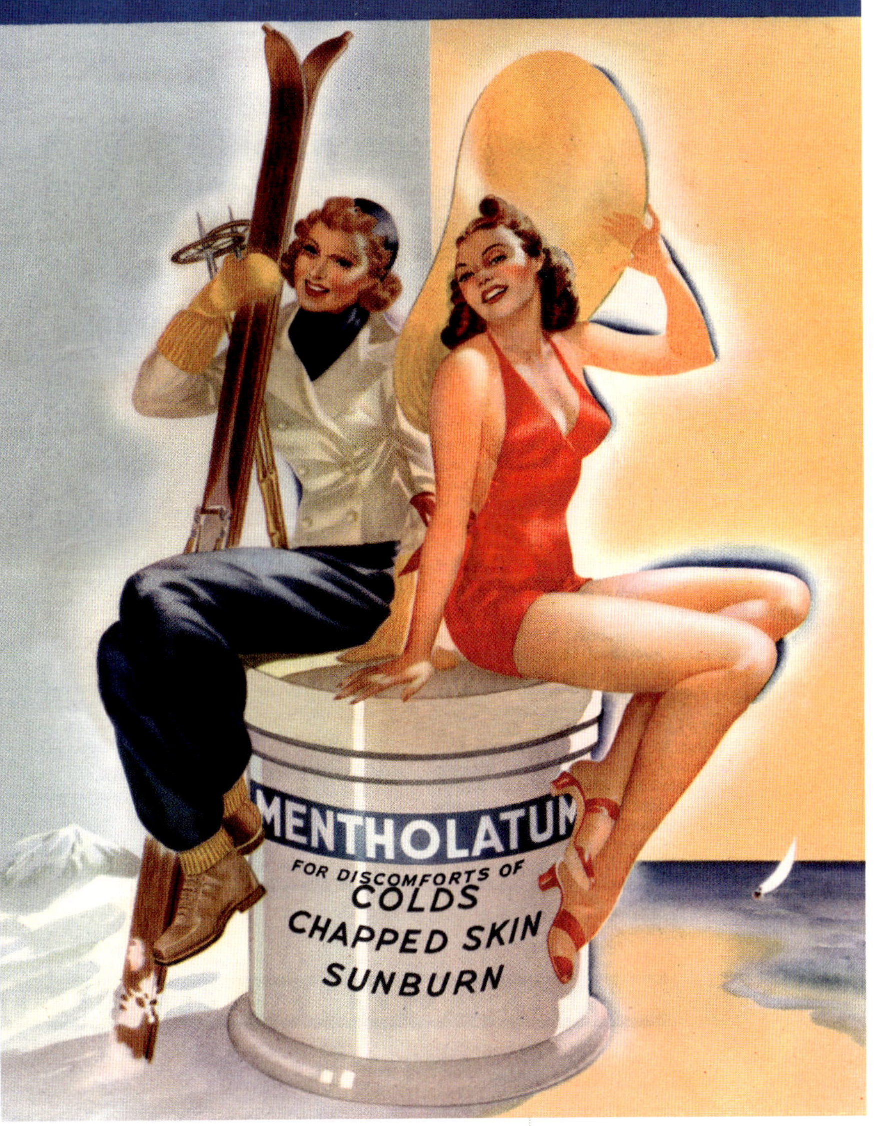

1940 Color Insert

12,500,000 packages were sold that year.

After ten lean and often desperate years of economic hardship, Americans were looking forward to a brighter future. But ominous clouds of war were darkening the horizon. Japanese aggression in the distant Pacific and the recent Axis invasion of Europe, Russia, and North Africa could no longer be ignored. Political and economic forces were pushing the reluctant nation toward global war just as the Mentholatum Company was facing its most critical challenge. Modern developments in various sectors of the marketplace had been converging, and the rules of the game were about to change. The company sidestepped modernity's test when war was declared in 1941, and the nation turned its attention to national defense.

World War II (1941–1945) created the expected shortages of raw materials and a disruption of international trade. Mentholatum's London factory would endure the German blitz, while on the other side of the world the company's relationship with Japan would be abruptly severed. The Hyde brothers watched helplessly as their missionary friends and business partners in faraway countries became engulfed in the fighting. The two North Amer-

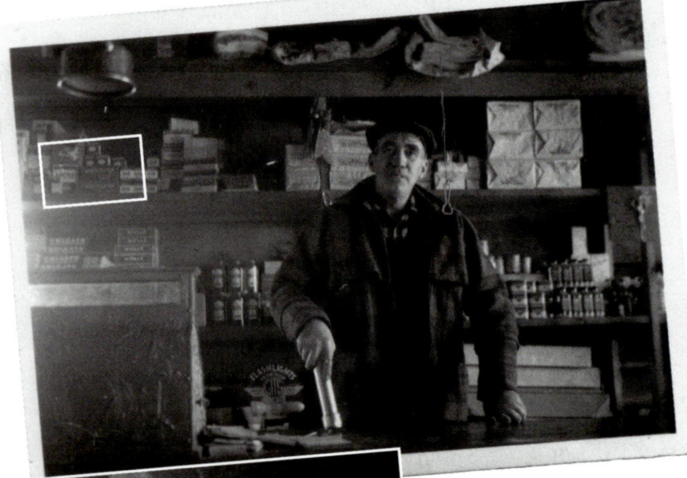

ican plants did their best to continue manufacturing with limited materials and at the same time give their support to the war effort. Throughout the intervening years of conflict and austerity, modernity waited patiently in the background. At the end of the war, a new world order was established by the victors, and America began to enjoy a boom in consumerism and prosperity. The nation's transition from an agricultural economy into an industrial economy was manifest. Around the world, factories were being retooled for peacetime production or rebuilt from the rubble, and it was the perfect opportunity to improve outdated systems. When people could once again dream of the future, that is when modernity stepped forward to show them the way.

Country Store Cold Supplies

This period photo of a 1940s country store on closer inspection reveals a well-stocked supply of the top-three cold rubs on the market. Listed from left to right on the shelf (and representing market share) are Vicks VapoRub, Mentholatum, and Musterole.

The World War II decade represents a massive paradigm shift in our view of the world. Many aspects of everyday life changed quickly and dramatically. Before the war we had dynamite; after the war, we had unleashed the atomic bomb. Changes in the area of medicine were just as big. Doctors entered the war using crude sulfa drugs to fight off bacterial infection and exited using penicillin. The rate at which scientists were isolating the chemicals within plants capable of therapeutic action, and then synthesizing them in their labs, was accelerating. Menthol was rapidly surpassed by stronger anesthetics and antiseptics.[1]

Fundamental changes in the way drugs were merchandised were also taking place. The old system was being pushed aside to make room for a new market dedicated to mass production and consumption. Mentholatum's friendly little salve was a product of simpler times when menthol was the strongest thing going. It had been a time when druggists could develop a personal relationship with their customers. Now the druggist's role was becoming corporate and impersonal. The limitless opportunities that had characterized Mentholatum's pioneer days were replaced by federal regulations and a glut of mimic brands. The inventive and moralistic course A. A. Hyde once charted for market success was losing speed while rivals were picking up the pace. Advertising had become more complicated

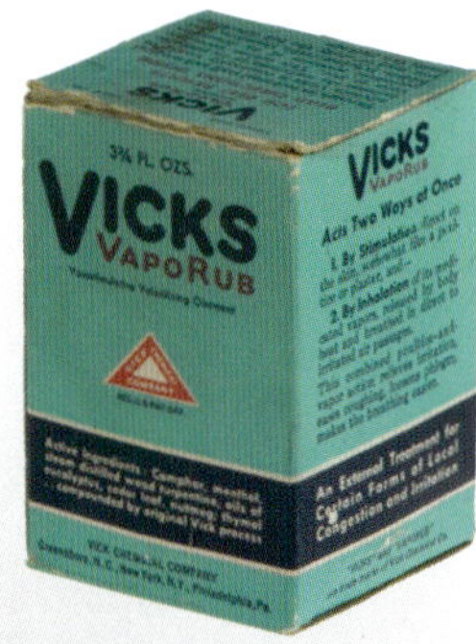

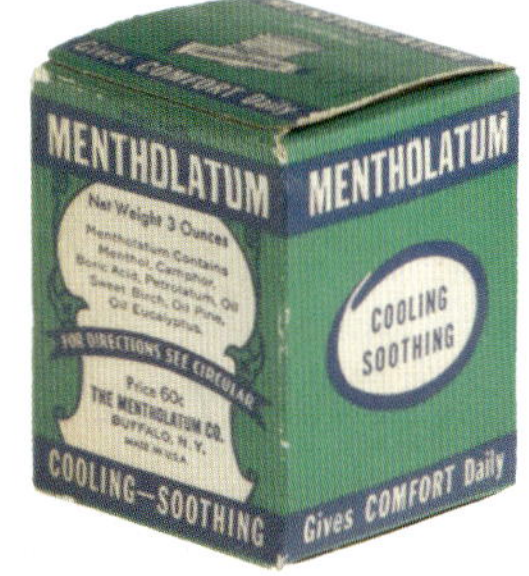

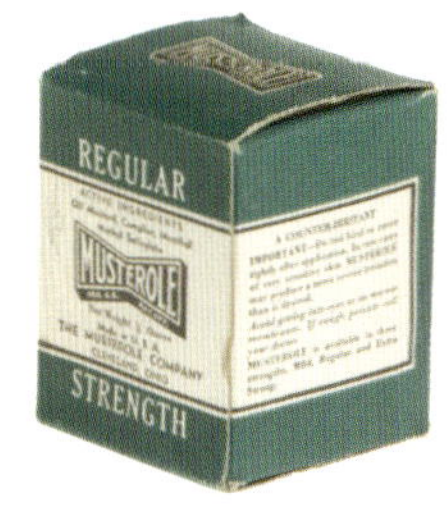

and expensive between the advent of radio in the early 1920s and the growing popularity of television during the 1940s. The resolve of Mentholatum's aging managers was also going to be tested during the postwar years. Would they be reactive and spend their energy on damage control, or would they be pro-active and carve a niche in the modern marketplace?

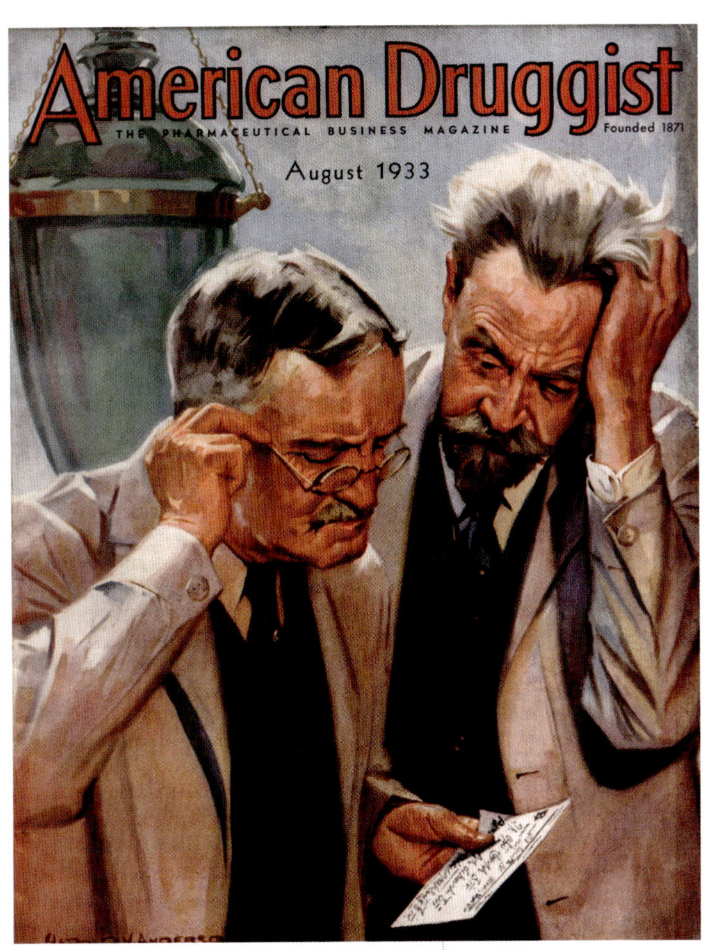

The Old Guard

American Druggist illustrated its cover each month with nostalgic scenes of the good old days and all too often kindly old druggists coping with the changes of modernization. Many of the young druggists who had helped Mentholatum when it was first starting out were retiring in the 1930s and swelling the ranks of the 40 Year Service Club. Scenes like this one painted by Harold Anderson in 1933, of two senior pharmacists pondering a doctor's scribbling on a prescription, dramatized that generation's long partnership with physicians and the pharmaceutical industry.

After the phenomenal successes the company enjoyed during the 1920s and its weathering of the Depression without crippling loss, Mentholatum had become an established institution with strong brand recognition. No longer a rebel at the gate, it was now one of the gatekeepers. But the symbiotic relationship it had nurtured with the retail druggists was diminishing in spite of its past investment. A change in *Menthology*'s tone suggested that its relationship with the druggists was changing from that of teacher to one of booster. After all, the retail drug business had matured and no longer needed the manufacturer's patronage. *Menthology*'s folksy sales tips and display ideas had obviously become passé.

The frontier environment that once nourished Mentholatum's rapid growth no longer existed. The drugstores, which had been the company's primary sales force for more than forty years, were preparing for a new role. Even the term "drugstore" had become archaic, reminiscent of a preprofessional time. By 1940, the preferred nomenclature was "pharmacy," derived from the Greek word meaning "drugs." In the early days, a new drugstore might be opened by a doctor who later sold it to a dedicated clerk. Or it was opened by a new pharmacy school graduate. Whatever route a druggist came by his training, pharmacy had always been considered a simple trade and part-time profession to be changed for another if business didn't go well. Pharmacists were generally the owners of drugstores. To stay in business they had to become merchants who were accustomed to selling more prepackaged remedies than they did custom-mixed prescriptions. But the nostrums on their shelves sold at very narrow margins, and therefore Mentholatum's generous profit schedule was clearly welcomed. However, by the 1940s druggists had grown to expect a 33⅓ percent markup on all packaged remedies, and Mentholatum's edge was lost.[2]

Drugstores in the Western territory where Mentholatum made its start were newly established businesses in newly chartered towns within soon-to-be or recently admitted states. Mentholatum's traveling agents met with proprietors who were, for the most part, "greenhorns" to the trade. The quarterly issues of *Menthology* gave them much appreciated suggestions for more effective ways to display and sell the product and a few new jokes to share with their neighborhood customers. But as the druggists "grew up," the company's mentoring relationship had to change. A factor to consider was that not all drugstores were alike. If the stores survived, they matured in different directions at different rates. They often became unique to their particular regions of the country, making industrywide standards hard to maintain. Although the wholesalers provided a buffer between the company and the multitudes, they too were not immune to change. The formation of wholesale trade associations helped to regulate the market, but the forces of change were always one step ahead.[3]

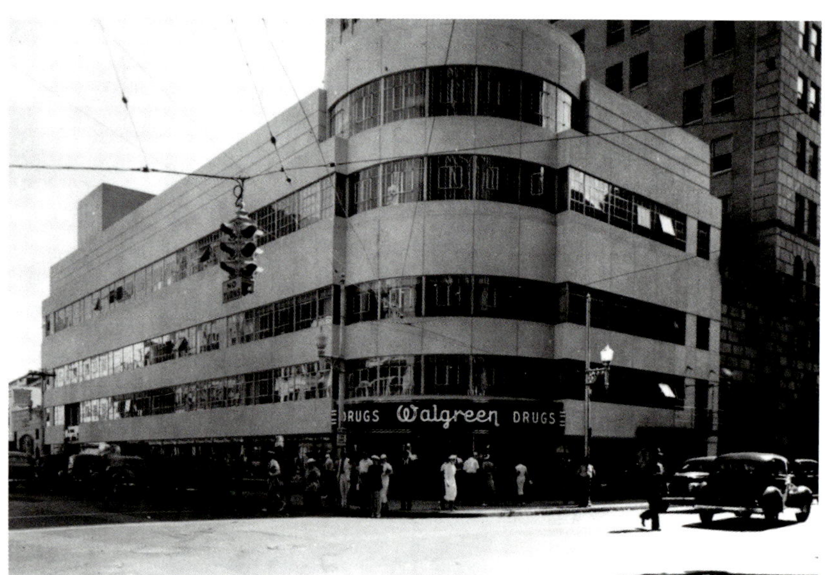

The Modern Corner Drugstore

Walgreen's superstore at 200 E. Flagler in Miami, Florida (c. 1947), boasted six floors of merchandise.

Chain Stores

The seeds that sprouted into the radical market transformations of the 1940s were sown at the turn of the century when Charles R. Walgreen and Louis K. Liggett created "chain" stores. The chains first thrived in urban areas where volumes were high and cut-rate pricing was popular. Walgreen and Liggett steadily redesigned the retail drug business, so that by the time the Miller-Tydings Act was passed in 1937 regulating fair trade, they had moved beyond price cutting by adopting alternative profit strategies. Charles R. Walgreen (1873–1939), a Chicago pharmacist, opened his first drugstore in 1901, then acquired another and another until his company had nine "units" in 1916, twenty-nine in 1922, and 413 by 1947. Along the way, Walgreen incorporated so many new sidelines into his business that by 1937 pharmaceuticals had become just one of many departments within his self-termed "gigantic stores." By the

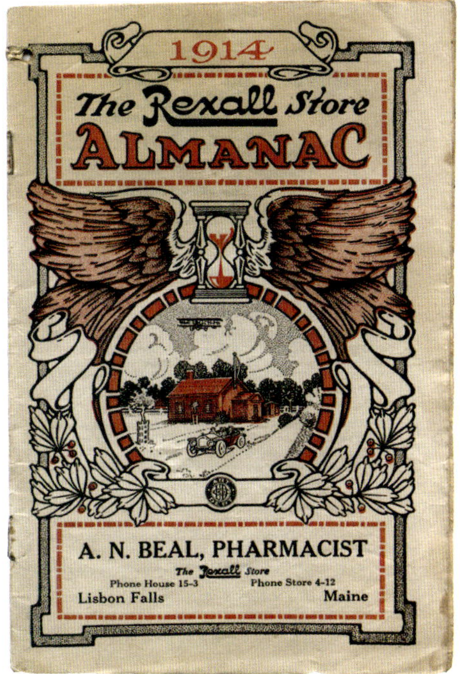

Rexall Brand

The Rexall brand was registered in 1914.

early 1940s, his son Charles Jr. was testing concepts of mass merchandising and self-service that would lead to the "superstores" that were built in the 1950s.[4]

Louis Liggett and his partners created the United Drug Company in 1903 to manufacture a line of generic remedies. Prior to the founding of United Drug, Liggett, a pharmacist, had spent several years operating a central "buying agency" that supplied retail drugstores. Based on this experience and his partners' financing, he planned to buy up a number of drugstores that United Drug Company could stock with its own line of products. Eventually, United Drug Company came to own forty-five drugstores in 1916; it owned 672 by 1930. As the story goes, an office boy suggested they name their products "Rexal," and Liggett added another "l" to better evoke the idea of "Rx to all." The Federal Trademark record shows that United Drug Company, a New Jersey Corporation, filed for the registration of "REXALL" on November 20, 1908, and claimed that its "first commerce date" and "first use date" was January 28, 1903. When Liggett's Rexall brand was finally registered on June 30, 1914, it was placed on dozens of pharmaceuticals, for example, "soothing-syrups, tooth powders, pastes, and washes, foot-powders, eye-washes, . . . laxatives and cathartics, . . . remedies for nervous disorders, general debility, and weakness, gargles and remedies for catarrh, bronchial, throat, and lung troubles and asthma, hoarseness and affections of mucous membranes of the mouth, nose, and throat, . . ." and many more.[5]

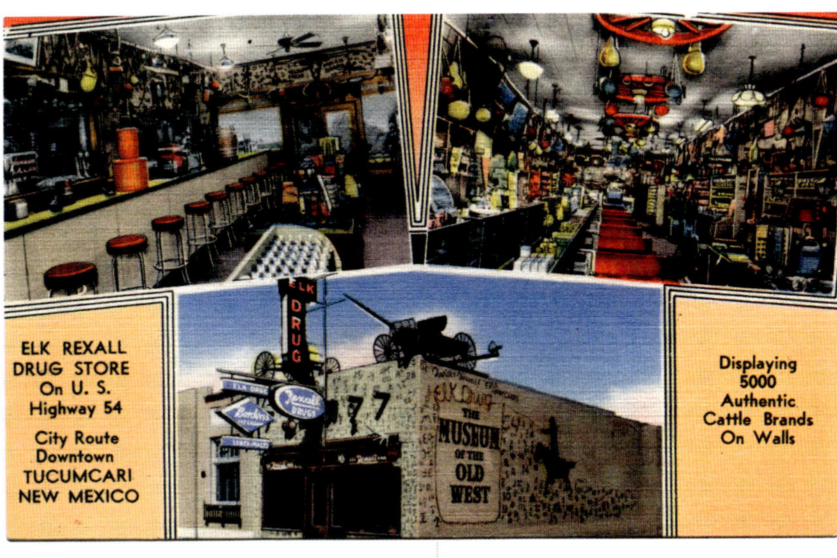

Independent Rexall Retailer (Est. 1906)

Pharmaceuticals were not the only featured items at some stores that adopted the Rexall name but maintained their unique personality.

A "Rexall Premium Catalogue" was published in 1915 and was presumably used to encourage salesmen to sell the Rexall line outside of the drugstore chain. It read: "Now You can get the things you have longed for at Half Cost. . . . You pay one-half cash. . . . Your coupons pay the other half." This sales system was no different from the one employed by companies like Watkin's and Rawleigh's, which also offered premiums to recruit door-to-door salesmen. (Watkin's

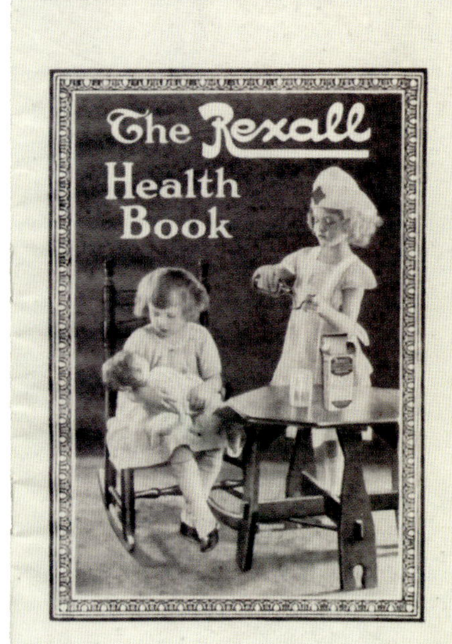

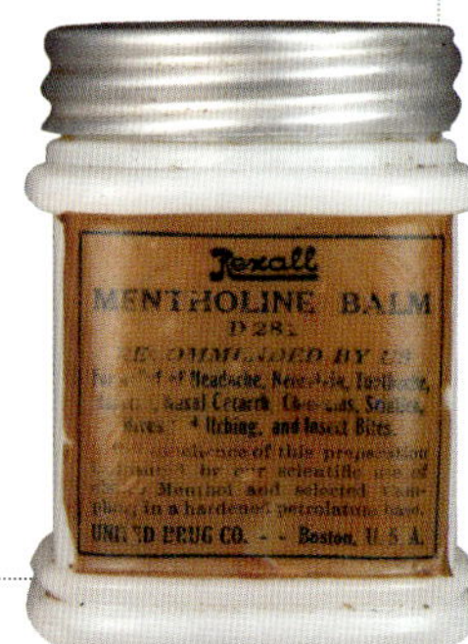

The Rexall Way

These are Rexall's version of Little Nurse and a copy of the familiar opal jar of menthol balm.

mimicked Mentholatum with its Menthol Camphor Ointment, and Rawleigh's mimicked it with Rawleigh's Medicated Ointment and Rawleigh's Vapor Balm.) Louis Liggett's big innovation, however, was to offer his line of pharmaceuticals and toiletries to independent druggists on a franchise basis. Participants contracted to "purchase at least minimum amounts of Rexall products in exchange for special discounts, local and national advertising advantages and a distinctive window sign." Eventually, independent retailers began adding Rexall to the name of their drugstores. By 1950, there were twelve thousand franchise units and 559 Rexall-owned drugstores. Rexall manufactured several items that mimicked Mentholatum, such as Rexall Catarrh Jelly, Rexall Bronchial Salve, Rexall Mentholine Balm, Rexall Vapure Inhalant (trademarked in 1928), and more recently Rex Mentho. Even a 1926 styled brochure titled "The Rexall Health Book" presented on its cover the image of a little girl dressed up as a nurse!

While the chains expanded, independents found other ways to increase their profits. Some formed cooperatives, and others organized buying clubs to combine orders and qualify for volume discounts from the manufacturers. Cooperatives could also share common advertising costs. These creative schemes to cut costs were often the work of commercial interests that were purchasing drugstores and trying to make them profitable. And, although independents still outnumbered corporate owners during the 1940s, the dollar-volume ratio was growing disproportionately in favor of the chains. Of the 52,809 drugstores in 1947, only 4,655, or 9 percent, were chains, yet the chains took in 24 percent of all sales.[6]

The fight over fair trade was continuous. Manufacturers felt they had the right to lock down retail prices, chain stores believed they had the right to discount retail prices, small independents wanted the right to make a living under the shadow of the giants, and consumers demanded the right to get the most competitive price possible. To control its retail price, Mentholatum required its wholesalers to sign a contract that prohibited them from selling to anyone who used Mentholatum products as a "loss leader." (A loss leader is the sale of one product at below cost—at a loss—to attract customers into the store.) Mentholatum also wanted its product sold in as many stores as possible, large and small, so it sold at discount rates to "rack jobbers" who supplied small quantities to the independents. The rack jobbers, who belonged to a national association, took only 10 to 12 percent and passed the rest of the discount on so that the little guys could enjoy a reasonable profit margin.[7]

Menthol Is Replaced by Stronger Drugs

The next big adjustment was caused by a new class of packaged prescription drugs that quickly pushed remedies off their top market position. Mentholatum and its rivals were unilaterally shoved aside as this whole new class of packaged drugs entered the market. This remarkable development began at the turn of the century when medical science as we know it was just emerging. Germany was the leader in synthetic organic chemistry at the time and dominated production of synthetic drugs. After Germany's defeat in World War I, its technology was taken as a spoil of war and used to advance the American drug industry. Drug manufacturing laboratories like Parke-Davis and Co.; Eli Lilly and Co.; and Abbott Laboratories, which had traditionally supplied nonproprietary chemicals to pharmacists, benefited from this transfer and began to diversify with new factory-made medicinal products. As research scientists synthesized ever more effective and complex medicines, the industry rose to the challenge and manufactured them. A partnership soon developed between scientific researchers and chemical manufacturers that transformed them into the modern pharmaceutical industry we have today.[8]

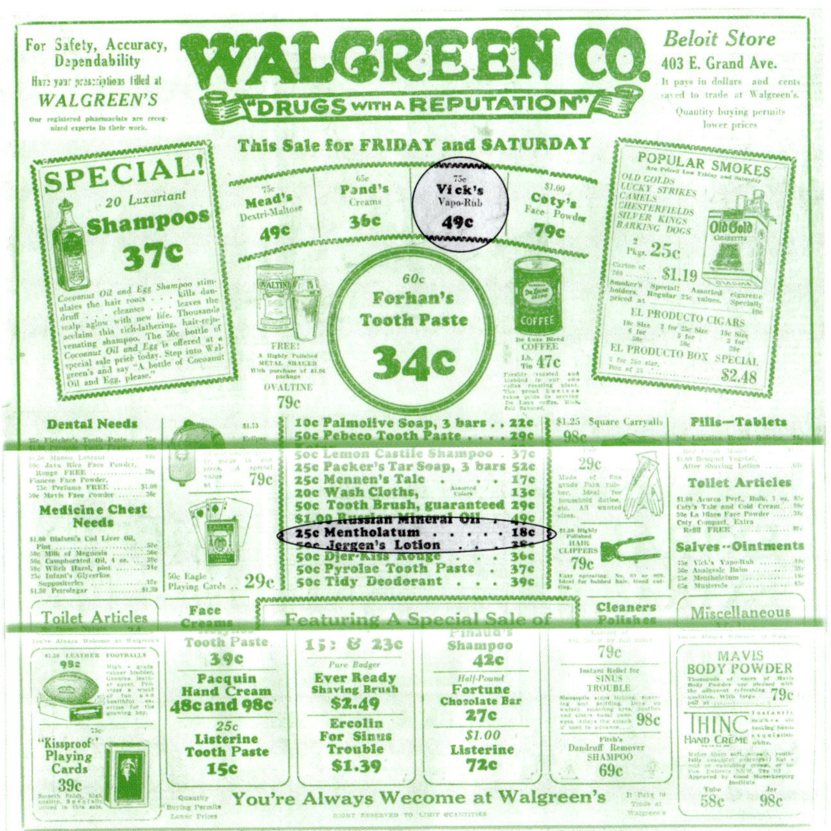

Fair or Unfair Trade?

This 1929 ad page from the *Beloit Daily News* offers a 75¢ jar of Vicks for 49¢ and a 25¢ jar of Mentholatum for 18¢. This sort of price cutting led to passage of the Miller-Tydings National Fair Trade Act in 1937 allowing manufacturers to regulate the minimum discount price for their products.

The new synthetic drugs required a doctor's prescription, but in every other respect they looked like patent remedies. Ironically, they could truly be called "patent" drugs, under the modern use of the term, because for the first time they were actually patented! Like the nostrums, they needed brand names and package designs. And though they were not going to be sold directly to the public, advertising would still be necessary to attract the doctor's attention and encourage him or her to write prescriptions. The pharmaceutical companies naturally followed the marketing model established by the packaged remedy industry. This commercialization of new synthetic drugs influenced a shift away from traditional scientific nomenclature and led toward the more familiar system of trademark naming. Pharmacists were already accustomed to selling packaged remedies, and they were not doing much compounding and mixing, so they had no trouble accepting these changes to their business. When doctors discovered it was easier to write out prescriptions using brand names, prescription orders to the pharmacist tripled between 1940 and 1955. Now, physicians rather than druggists were handing out free samples.[9]

It looked like institutionalized medicine was going to replace the age-old tradition of self-medication and home remedies, and it certainly threatened extinction of the apothecary's art in the Western world. The age of the pharmacist as keeper and purveyor of manufactured and packaged medicines had begun. In short order, remedies were reduced to second-class status. The modern pharmacist turned his attention toward the exciting new drugs, while Mentholatum was placed among its rivals off to the side on a crowded shelf. As this trend developed, *Menthology* became less relevant and was therefore discontinued in 1944.

The last transformation to affect the company came in the area of advertising. It is legend that A. A. Hyde refused to buy advertising in the early years. Not until his sons came to manage the company did Mentholatum begin to advertise in magazines (c. 1912). Print advertising was the standard until radio began to demonstrate its effectiveness as a new advertising medium during the 1920s. In a loose comparison of national advertising expenditures, representing all industries between the years 1927 and 1934, the trend toward radio can be illustrated. The National Broadcasting Company (NBC) reported in a 1935 survey that expenditures for newspaper advertising in 1927 were 48 times greater and

Rival Cold Rubs

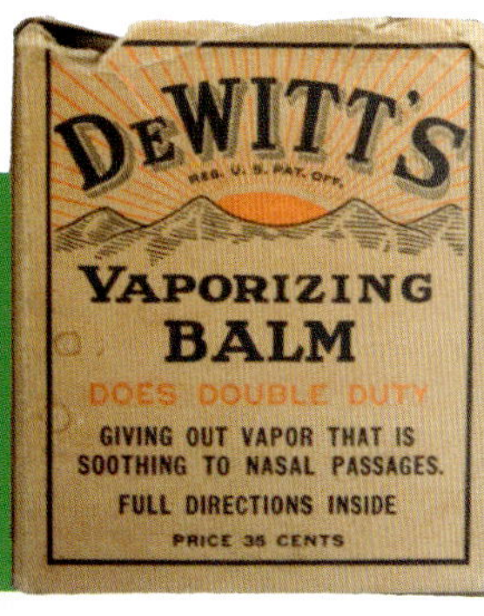

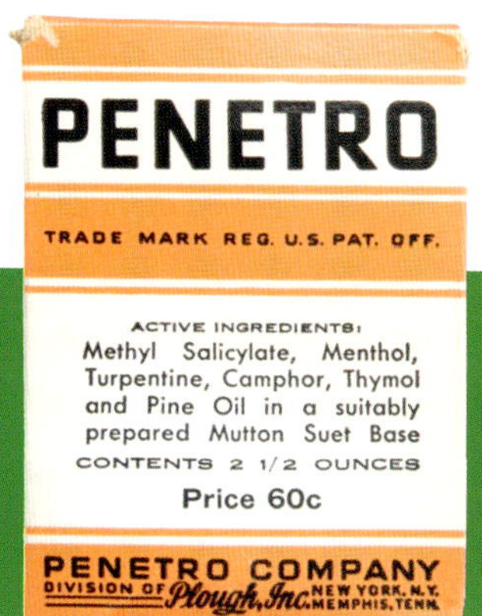

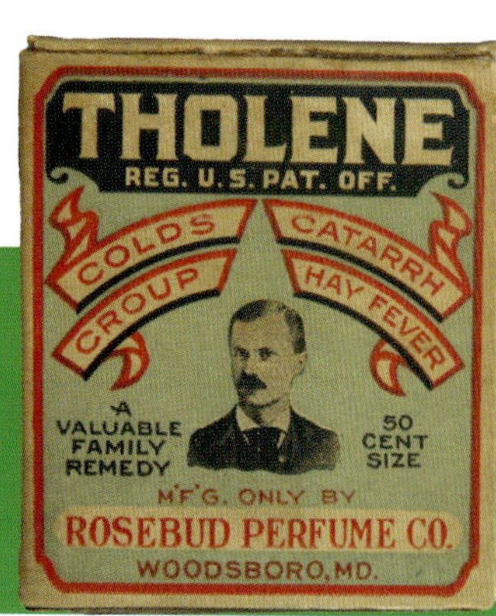

magazine advertising 46 times greater than radio expenditures. However, by 1934, newspapers were only 2.8 times and magazines only 2.65 times greater. After the stock market crash in 1929, advertising fell off in both print mediums while radio continued to climb steadily. It is not known how much money Mentholatum spent on advertising at the time, but a list of expenditures published in *Variety* provides an interesting comparison of its largest rivals using network radio (CBS and NBC) in 1935:

Humphrey's Homeopathic Medicine Co.	$33,124
Pinex Co.	$82,200
United Drug Co. (Rexall)	$151,018
Plough, Inc. (Penetro)	$210,000
Vicks Chemical Co.	$333,854

Although Humphrey's, Plough, and Rexall represent a wide range of products, it is sobering to compare their total expenditures to those of Vicks. Rival brands that appeared opposite Mentholatum in 1935 magazine ads included Pineoleum, Musterole, Vapo-Cresolene, and, of course, Vicks. Vicks ads were typically large, in color, and placed toward the front of the magazines, ahead of its competitors. The earliest documentation of Mentholatum's use of radio advertising is found in the fall 1942 issue of *Menthology*, although Albert Hyde said they were doing some radio when he started there in 1939.[10]

The last advertising campaign that was announced in *Menthology* included popular women's and farm magazines,

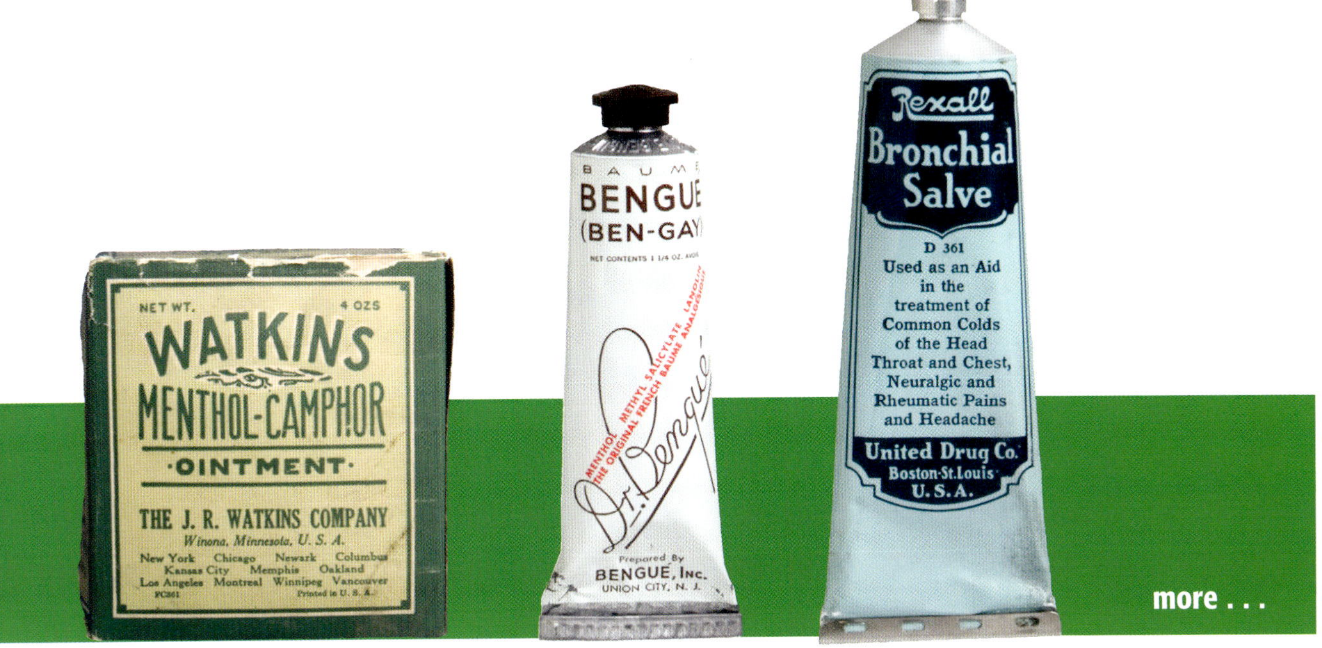

2,320 newspapers, and 70 radio stations. Radio spots were planned for National Health Week, from October 6 to 16, 1944:

> *. . . with such personalities and programs as Alois Havrilla, Cedric Foster, Martin Agronsky, Larry Smith,—"Early Birds," "Happy Home" with Carolyn Ellis, and the famous "What's Doin', Ladies?" on a West Coast network . . . "spots" . . . will reach millions of listeners with Mentholatum sales messages, linked with a government war message.*[11]

Mentholatum's use of magazine advertising dropped off after the war, and space in newspapers was limited to the economical "one percent club," or sections in the paper where only 1 percent of readership was guaranteed.[12]

The Wilmington Detour (1937–1945)

Two years after the death of its founder, Mentholatum reincorporated in the state of Delaware. George A. Hyde, who had remained in Wichita, was charged with moving the corporate office from Wichita to Wilmington, Delaware. Useful machinery was dismantled and shipped to Buffalo, and the old factory was put up for sale. George took with him several of the old and faithful office employees. Margaret Saxe came as George's secretary. It is not known exactly why the Hyde brothers bought land in Wilmington to build a new factory (which never materialized). The obvious motive was to incorporate in Delaware for the tax advantages, but why they were compelled to move the office there instead of to Buffalo is a mystery. George Hyde was a reluctant participant due to a chronic heart condition that limited his activities. George settled his family in Newark, a small university town twenty miles from Wilmington. George's son, John M. Hyde,

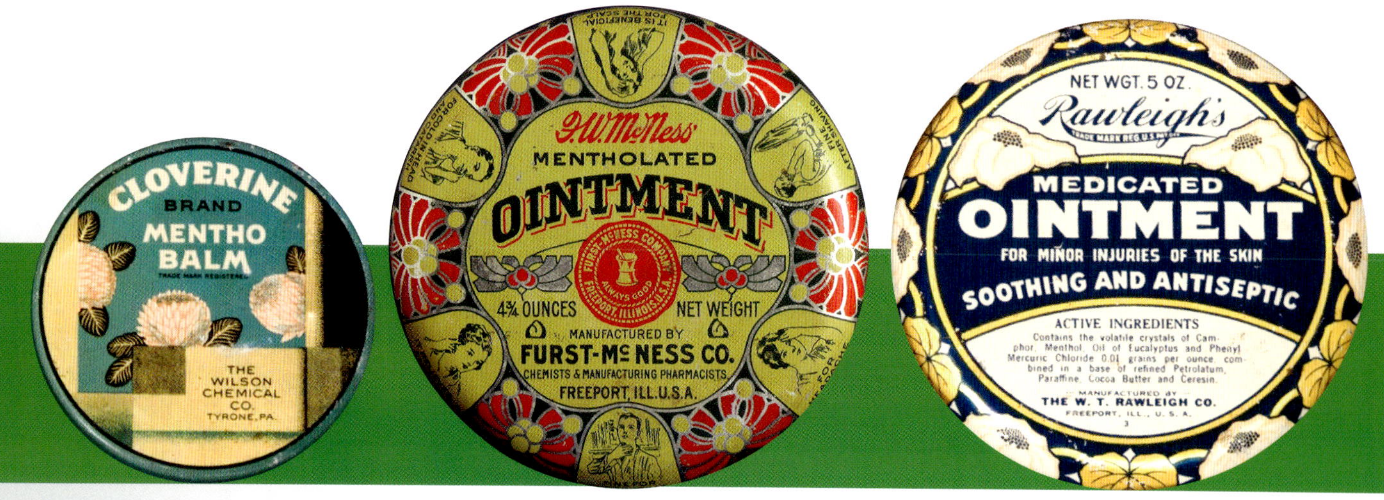

attended a private day school in Wilmington and traveled back and forth with his dad in the Mentholatum Company car pool (because of gas rationing). John recalled walking to the office after school to wait for the ride home. To help pass time at the office, he looked through the files and listened to the older women, who had "spent their lives working for the company," tell stories of the "old days" in Wichita. In 1944, George Hyde died from heart failure, and his brothers decided to close down the Wilmington office and move the operation to Buffalo.[13]

In the words of John Hyde:

> *When time came to close down the Wilmington office and unneeded files, inventory, records were being tossed, these women said to me: "Johnnie Mike [my nickname as a child], you should keep some of these records of the Company because some day you may come to work for it and should know some of its history." I was 14 years old, paid no attention except—luckily—to take what they gave me, put it in the car, and store it someplace at home. As luck would have it, that "collection" followed us as we moved from house to house and was supplemented with material from my father's files and from items sent to the family home in Lee, Massachusetts, at the time the Wichita office was closed, but I was still growing up, going to college and then the Navy, back to college—and again, the collection stayed intact largely through inertia. I certainly took no interest in preserving it.*

That is how much of the company's earliest history survived two floods, one office move, and two generations of benign neglect. As an adult, John Hyde took a more active interest in the safety of the archives, which he will leave to the Special Collections section of the University Libraries at Wichita State University.[14]

The officers of the company in 1941 were Edward K. Hyde, president; Paul H. Hyde, executive vice president; George A. Hyde, vice president; and Charles H. Hyde, vice president. Jim Devlin was the vice president of advertising. Albert Taylor "Bert" Hyde, the son of A.A.'s eldest son, Albert Todd Hyde, was given the exalted title of assistant advertising manager after he joined the company in 1939. Albert grew up in Carmel, California, and while a student at Stanford University he worked a few summers on the Mint Ranch. He graduated from Stanford in the class of 1937. Bert, as family members called him, would eventually become the president of the company before his fortieth birthday in 1955.

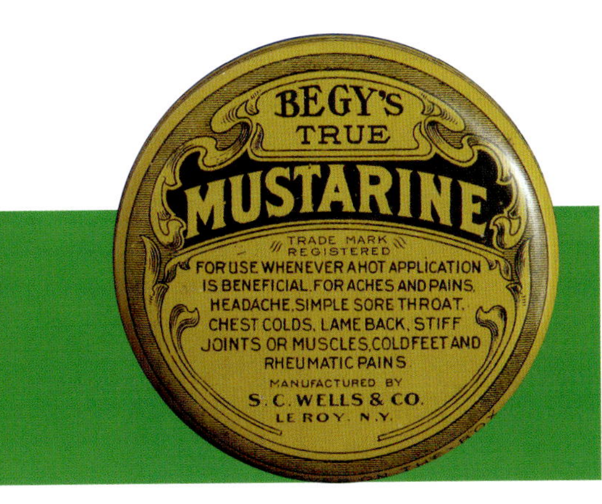

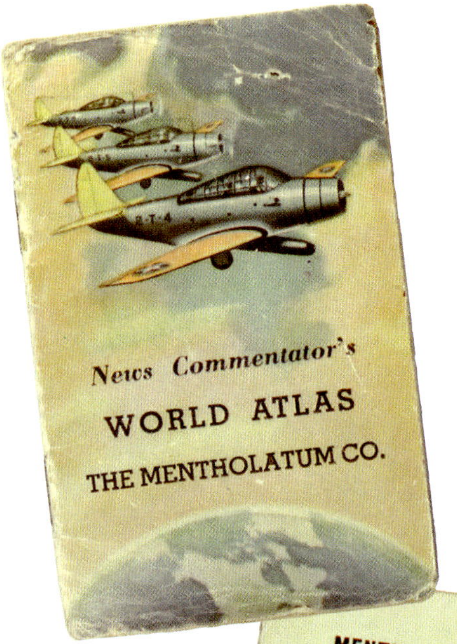

Menthology claimed the company produced twenty-five million packages a year (worldwide). Prices in 1941 were:

Tubes: travel size, 10¢; one-ounce size, 30¢
Jars: one-ounce size, 30¢; three-ounce size, 60¢
Brushless Shave: 35¢

These prices remained the same until sometime between January 1948 and April 1949, when they were raised to 35¢ for one ounce and 75¢ for three ounces. Before the war, a one-ounce jar cost more than three times a loaf of bread (8.1¢). After the war, prices for goods rose dramatically. Even so, by 1950 the one-ounce jar had dropped to less than three times the cost of a loaf (14.3¢). During the war, the one-ounce jar of Mentholatum was roughly equivalent to the cost of a five-pound bag of flour, or half a gallon of milk delivered, or one pound of coffee. In comparison, the same food items in 1895 were half the value of a one-ounce jar.[15]

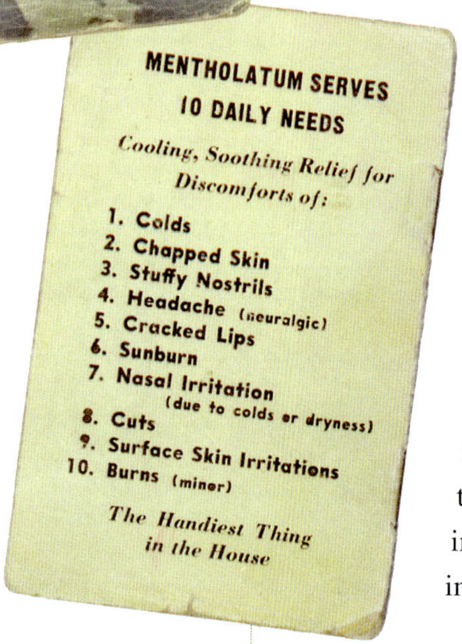

Pocket Atlas

This atlas was useful to follow the progress of the war.

War Stories

In the spring of 1940, the Slough plant was training employee squads for firefighting and decontamination in the event of either incendiary or gas bomb attacks. In June 1941 the plant was commandeered by the British government to be used for packing bacon, and Mentholatum was given five days to vacate to a nearby facility. Eventually, managing director T. W. D. "Billy" Turner returned to the United States with his family for the duration of the war as manufacturing was interrupted due to the extreme material shortages in Britain.[16]

In 1942, the company issued an "All-Purpose, Year-Round" display to help conserve paper for the war effort. In the spring issue of *Menthology*, Fred C. Mink, from Cassville, Wisconsin, submitted a paper-conservation idea to the "Sales Suggestion" column that signaled the eventual demise of a merchandising tradition. During checkout, he suggested putting items like sanitary napkins into a "No. 16" plain paper bag so that the customer would not be embarrassed to carry it home. Up to this time, druggists were tying everything up in white wrapping paper, which apparently made it easy for other people to recognize the "tell tale" dimensions of the sanitary napkin box. Mink said, "The size of this bag allows the inclusion of

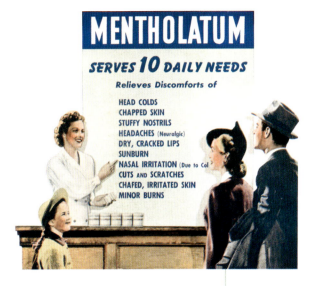

The All-Purpose Display

This year-round display replaced seasonal variations when paper was in short supply during the war years.

many other items at the same time . . . we find that the men do not object to carrying a box home in this manner."[17]

The company skipped the summer issue of *Menthology* due to a threatened paper shortage. Instead, it used the money it would have spent to purchase a Red Cross field ambulance and a U.S.O. mobile canteen unit, which were both donated to the war effort. Publication was reduced to two issues in 1943. Only one issue was printed in the fall of 1944, and that turned out to be the last. During the war years, *Menthology* was dedicated to reminding the druggists to push war bonds and support blood drives, and the cover art focused entirely on patriotic themes.[18]

The price of menthol before the war was a steady $2.50 a pound. During the war, it shot up as high as $14 on the world market. The Japanese manufacturers of menthol routed sales and shipments through Brazil to keep trade with the United States open. Mentholatum had established a practice of always keeping a two- or three-year supply of menthol on hand, a lesson it learned after the First World War. At one point during the war, opal glass jars became scarce, and the company had to substitute clear glass. This revision turned out fine because the white paper label covered most of the jar anyway.[19]

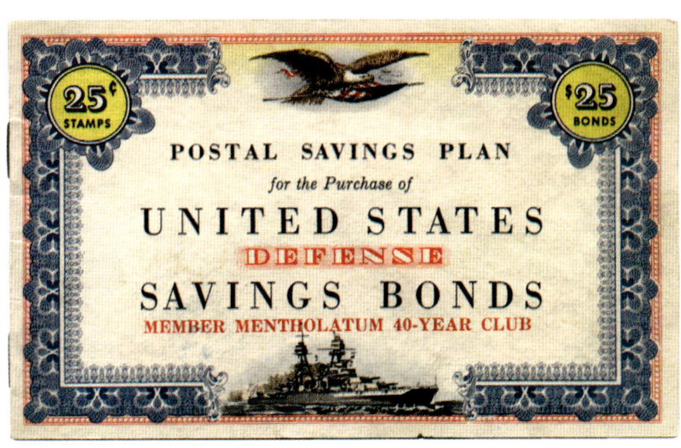

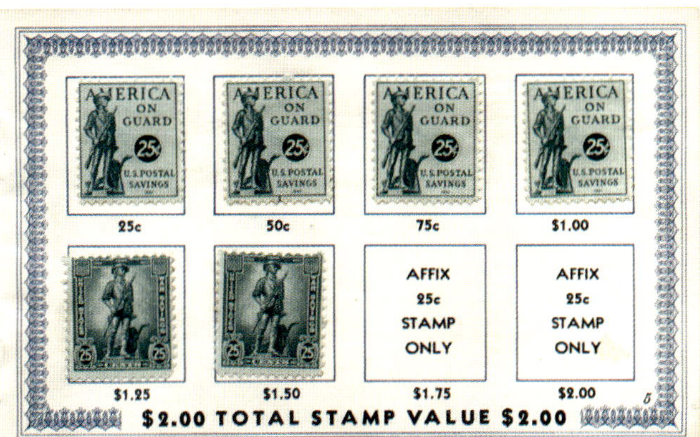

Patriotic Gift

War bonds were given to new members of the 40 Year Service Club sometime during the war.

Albert Hyde's (1915–2003) first job in advertising included ordering drugstore bags, or "delivery envelopes," from the printer. Each year, the small flat bags were printed with the latest Mentholatum ad in a bulk run of 100,000 and then stored at the printer's warehouse. When requests came in from the drugstores for a free supply of bags, the printer would customize each order with the individual store's name and send it out directly. When Albert placed the order in 1941 for the next year's supply of envelopes, he accidentally typed 1,000,000. The printer ordered the paper, printed the envelopes, and stored them before the uncles discovered Albert's error. Albert was sure he was going to be "canned." Then war was declared and paper was put on ration. Needless to say, Albert's mistake ensured that

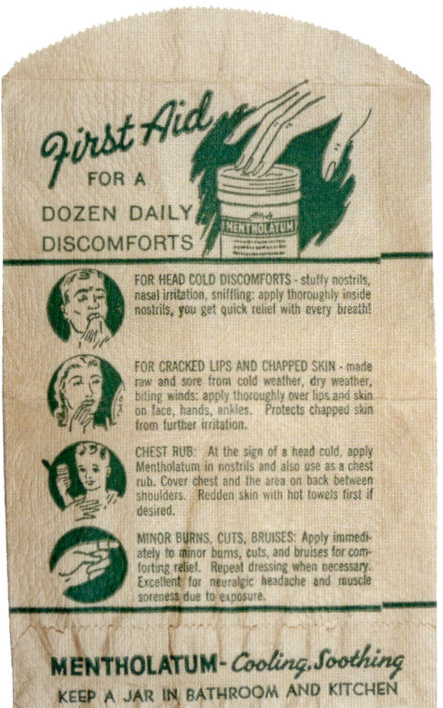

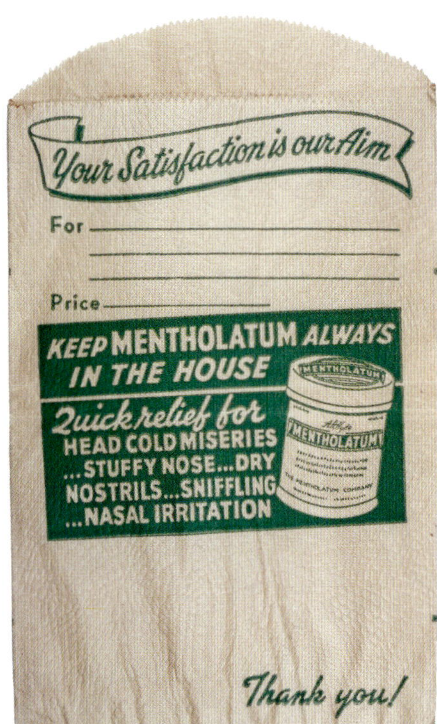

1942 Delivery Envelope

This is a likey candidate for Albert's one million envelope order. Evidence includes the jar design and the color of the ink. Albert remembered that the bags were printed in green.

Mentholatum was the only company to provide the coveted drugstore bags throughout the duration of the war.[20]

During the war, the Omi-Hachiman factory supplied Mentholatum to Japanese troops. Soldiers were given the same Little Nurse tins (with her profile facing left) that were used by civilians before the war. It upset U.S. Marines to find these recognizable tins in the possession of dead or captured Japanese soldiers. The company received many letters from vets during and after the war complaining that Mentholatum had supplied the enemy. They were careful to respond to each letter with an explanation of how the tins had come into the possession of the Japanese and assured the vets that Mentholatum factories in Allied countries had never aided the enemy. Although Mentholatum has been found in U.S. Army–issue first-aid kits at auction, the company did not have military contracts during the war. Mentholatum was for sale in the PX, so the kits must have been customized by the soldiers who carried them.[21]

Solutions

Albert Hyde was the first of the A. A. Hyde grandsons to work for the company when he started in 1939. He left to serve in the war and returned in 1946 when he was joined by four of his cousins. George H. Hyde, son of Edward K. "E. K." Hyde, worked in foreign trade under his father's supervision. Theodore "Ted" A. Hyde, son of Charles H. Hyde, worked in sales. Edward K. Hyde, son of Paul H. Hyde, joined his dad in manufacturing. Arthur H. Hyde, son of George A. Hyde, was the youngest and came to the company later. The five cousins eventually assumed the management and ran Mentholatum until its sale and their subsequent retirement in 1988.

The Hyde cousins brought with them youthful energy just when the company needed it the most. The 1950s were the "golden age" for many retail businesses, particularly the new self-service drugstores. Out-of-state corporations typically bought out the druggist/owner and replaced him with a manager whose primary interest was the bottom line. To the Hyde cousins, this appeared to be a natural progression. They had not experienced the days when Mentholatum relied on a personal recommendation from the druggist. They took it for granted that Mentholatum boxes would sit on a crowded shelf next to dozens of other boxes for the customers to pick through for themselves. So, it was clear to them that they needed to focus on making their box stand out and speak for itself. Mentholatum and Vicks VapoRub

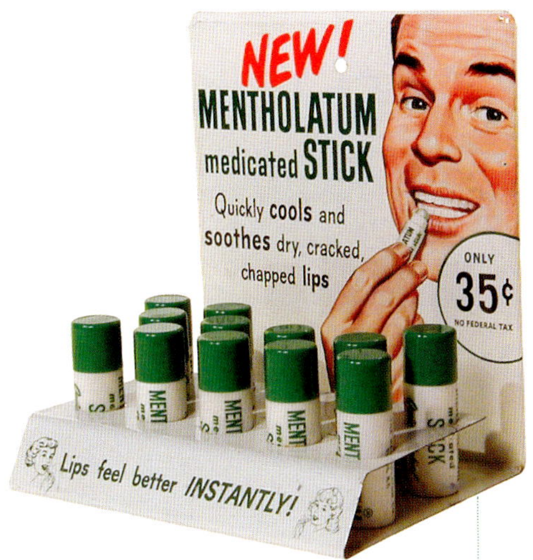

New Medicated Stick

From January 1952: "Use this new, small, metal display on drug, tobacco and cosmetic counters. Place this attractive 4-color metal display in your busy areas. It is the standard packing case for each dozen Mentholatum Medicated Sticks (14 to a dozen). 5½″ high, it needs only 4″ × 5″ counter space (equivalent to two packs of king-size cigarettes)." Stick shown actual size.

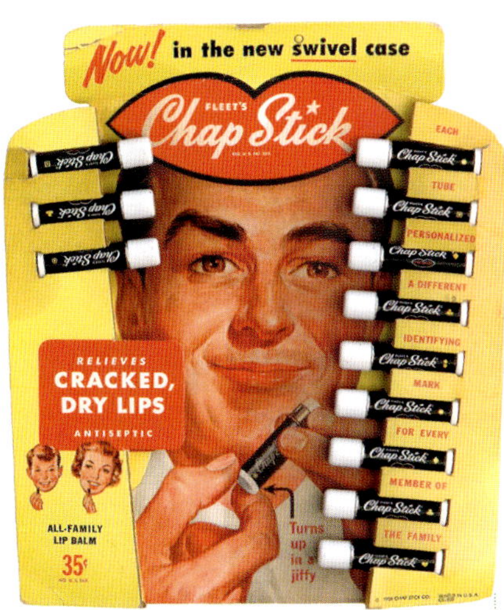

Winning Brand

In 1956 Chap Stick took control of the lip balm market with their new metal swivel case. "Turns up in a jiffy."

were already the Coke and Pepsi of the cold remedy or, as they now called it, "chest rub" business. This allowed the cousin managers to avoid working as hard on brand recognition as their fathers and grandfather had. Their mission now was to modernize and narrow the gap between Mentholatum and Vicks.

Market ranking for chest rubs since the 1920s had roughly been number one—Vicks VapoRub, number two—Mentholatum, and number three—Musterole. During the 1930s, Musterole began to lose third position to a French brand named Ben-Gay. "Baume Bengué" was a menthol salve invented by a French pharmacist named Jules Bengué in 1896 and first marketed in the United States in 1898. It was given the phonetic spelling "Ben-Gay" for the benefit of English speakers sometime after 1922 and before 1939. By 1950, Ben-Gay was clearly number three and closing the gap behind Mentholatum.[22]

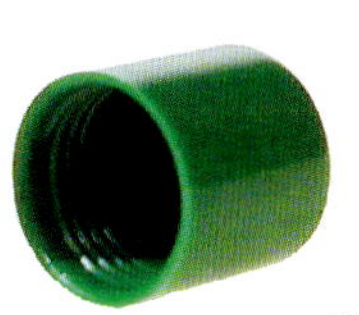

Mentholatum responded to the changing drug market with creativity and hard work. It modernized its image with new packaging and advertising designs. It diversified by adding new products like Medicated Stick and Deep Heat. And it moved into a new market arena, the food trade, which would eventually make up 40 percent of its overall sales.[23]

Medicated Stick came on the market in 1948. Its container design was inspired by the cosmetic lipstick tube, which in turn was a derivation of the old Camphor Ice tin with the push-up bottom. The small "pocket-sized" tube (1/10 ounce) was made of plastic and had a "screw-on cap [that] keeps out dust, lint, tobacco." The earliest trademark application named it "Lip Balms" and listed the first commerce date as November 1948. Then "MENTHOLATUM medicated STICK" appeared in 1952 with the introduction of a display offer to druggists. Medicated Sticks were shipped in quantities of fourteen set up in a metal countertop display stand. On the back side of the stand was printed "Important Notice. A shortage of metal may force us to discontinue this attractive, convenient display rack. Please save it for future use in case conditions make it necessary to ship Medicated Sticks in cardboard stands or in bulk." This was probably due to the Korean War (1950–1953). Medicated Stick sold for 35¢, or "33¢ if no Federal Tax." The machinery that filled the Medicated Stick was expensive and complicated to operate. Moreover, it was so efficient that the company did not need to run it very often. Subsequently, smaller brands that could not afford their own machines contracted the work to Mentholatum. The company was happy to do this even though the smaller brands often ended up competing with Mentholatum on retailers' shelves. Mentholatum didn't mind, however, because these contracts brought additional revenue, and the work kept the machinery in operation longer and their workers employed.[24]

The trend in advertising art after the war was becoming increasingly geometric and impersonal. Mentholatum was challenged to conform to modern standards and at the same time find a unique new image. Newspaper advertising picked up between 1948 and 1953, when they began a color cartoon ad called "Cold Demons" that was placed in the Sunday funny pages. This format was similar to the Ben-Gay series "Peter Pain" that had been running from the early 1940s. The cartoon ads put an end to Mentholatum's membership in the 1 percent club. National radio and television also became more important advertising media once druggists and clerks were no longer introducing the product to new customers. Mentholatum's advertising budget necessarily became the single largest expense.

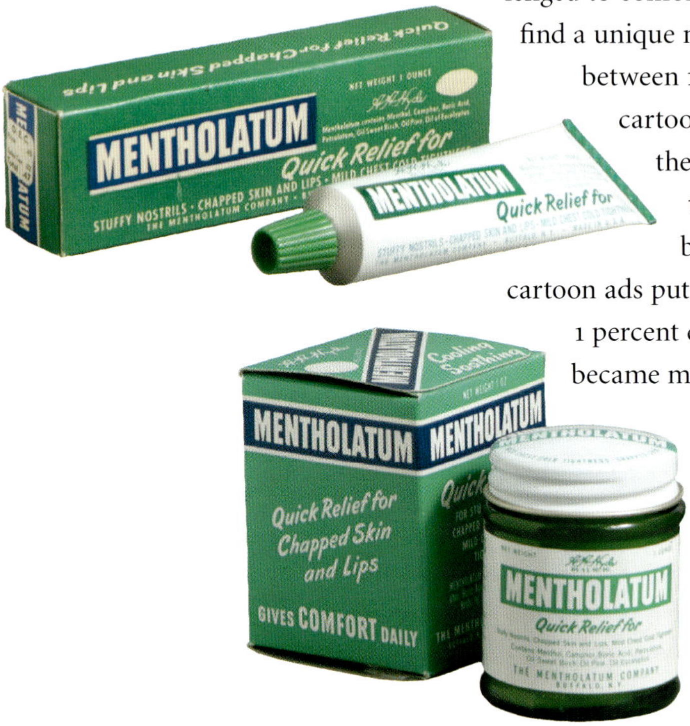

New product packaging was required to catch the attention of the customer by standing apart from rivals placed next to it on the shelf. Early versions of the new package designs were introduced in the late 1940s. The trademark scroll on the label was replaced with a minimal band. The curvilinear framing on box side panels was removed, as was the swirl logo. A. A. Hyde's signature was retained on labels late into the 1950s. The most dramatic change came in January 1955 when the white "opal" jars were replaced by emerald green glass.[25]

The most profitable innovation the company made came shortly after the war, when a rack jobber placed a small display of Mentholatum in a grocery store to see what would happen. When the initial supply sold out, the store manager asked the jobber for more and Mentholatum made its entry into a new, untapped market. Food retailers were used to selling at much smaller margins than drug retailers were. Grocers liked the 33⅓ percent markup on drugs compared to their traditional 1 percent on food. Jobbers across the country began placing racks in grocery stores, stocked only with the top-selling remedies in each category. Overnight, the jobbers' little three-by-four-foot racks became the grocers' biggest profit maker.

Because Mentholatum got in on the ground floor, it was virtually impossible for its rivals to break in. Soon grocers were asking the jobbers to install larger racks so they could add other nonfood products like toys, stationery supplies, and toothbrushes. Eventually the big grocery chains dropped the rack jobbers and began ordering stock directly from the manufacturers. Eliminating the jobber's cut meant that Mentholatum made money coming and going. Grocery stores had entered the same cycle of diversification initiated by drugstores fifty years earlier. Although the food market was more lucrative for Mentholatum, it imposed tighter requirements for participation. Shelf space in the grocery stores was limited to the top brand names in each category. Also, store managers did not include nonfood products in their local advertising specials. But as long as Mentholatum remained a top-selling chest rub, it was guaranteed shelf space.[26]

Entry into the food market for new, untested products was also difficult. The Hyde cousins wanted a stronger product for sore muscles that they could market to workers and athletes. In 1953 the research department produced Deep Heat Mentholatum Rub. It was proven in six test markets before being launched nationwide starting on October 11, 1954, and backed by the largest advertising campaign in Mentholatum history. Mentholatum spent one-third of its advertising budget entirely on Deep Heat so that it might achieve the coveted shelf position in the supermarkets. Ben-Gay became its primary competitor. The Deep Heat box was decorated with red, white, and blue graphics that simply "jumped off the shelf." On March 7, 1955, it was announced that Albert T. Hyde was elected the company's new president. Mentholatum had its young management team in place, a totally modernized logo and packaging designs, with several promising new products on the market and a few more on the drawing boards. Mentholatum had clearly passed the test.[27]

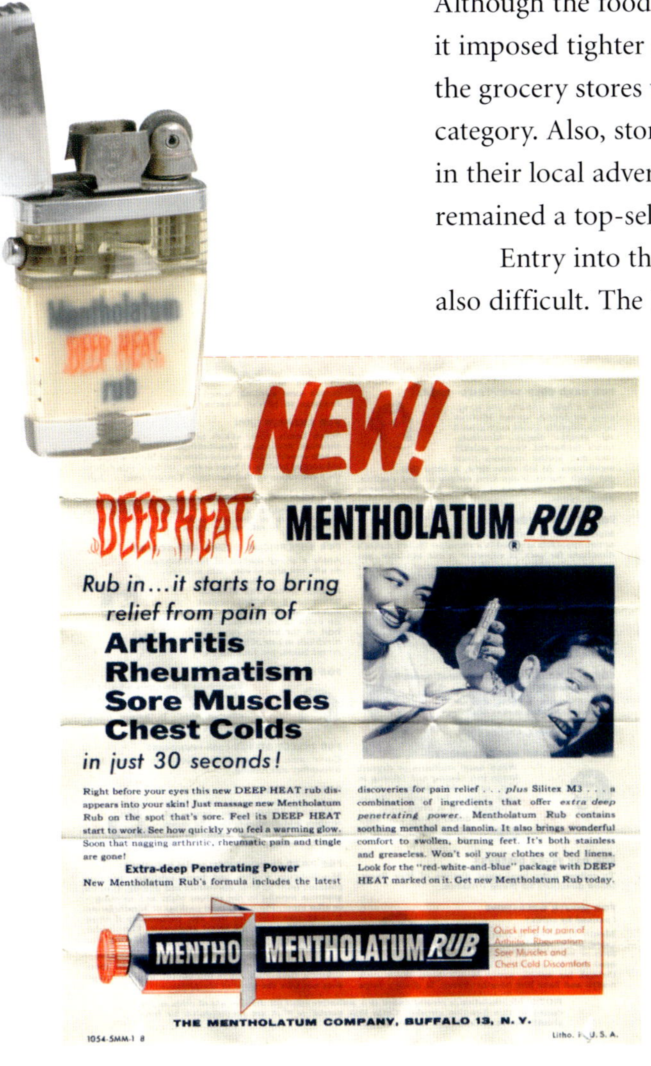

Epilogue

As the Hyde family tells the story, after Mentholatum's meteoric rise at the turn of the twentieth century, A.A. began buying up a number of smaller competitors that he thought might cause him trouble later on. One of his sons investigated a regional company in North Carolina named Vicks and suggested they buy it. A.A. said, "Nothing's going to happen with it—it's not worth the money." Then, during the influenza pandemic of 1917–18, sales of Vicks VapoRub went from $900,000 to $2.9 million in two years! Overnight, it became a national player, and by 1932 it was expanding its product line.

The irony in this tale certainly isn't lost on the Hyde family. It is told in the same manner a fisherman might describe "the fish that got away," with a slight tone of resignation. Mentholatum did not successfully expand its product line until 1950. Deep Heating Rub held its own against Ben-Gay for many years, but Medicated Stick lost ground to Chap Stick for the coveted most-recognizable-brand-name position. Still, Mentholatum chose not to promote its new products beyond a certain point. Something seemed to hold it back during the next four decades. The company automated its factories, but it never grew beyond the old walls. The governor that kept Mentholatum from going over the speed limit turned out to be the family itself. As past president of the company Albert T. Hyde described it, "Dividends held the company back."

In addition to the dividend burden, company bylaws forbade using stock options to promote and retain top nonfamily executives. The company was ultimately faced with a problem that is typical of many older family-owned businesses. By the 1980s, there were no fourth-generation Hydes interested in running the company. The cousin directors were aging and tired, and the sale of the company seemed the best option.

During the 1980s, the Japanese economy was booming. Japanese businesses were flush with cash, and they were purchasing American assets. Therefore it was not surprising when Mentholatum was sold to a Japanese concern in 1988. To the few who knew something about the company's pedigree, it was entirely fitting that it go to the Japanese. After all, Japanese consumers were still in love with A. A. Hyde's friendly salve, and they had become Mentholatum's largest market.

Mentholatum is still popular today in developing countries where many medicines are not affordable. Unfortunately, it has become hard to find Mentholatum Ointment in American stores. A friend complained to me recently that she could not find it in her

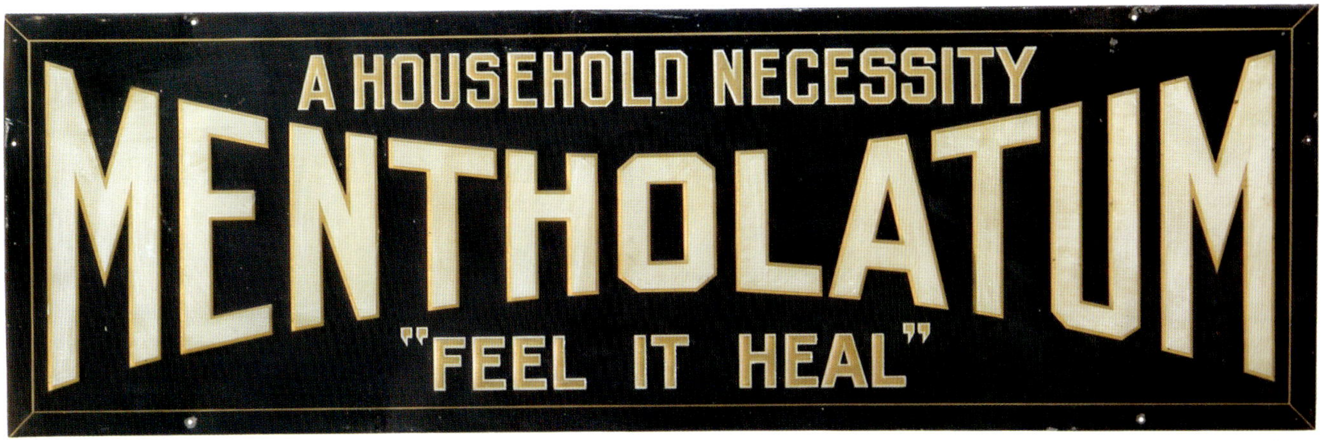

A HOUSEHOLD NECESSITY
MENTHOLATUM
"FEEL IT HEAL"

▲ "A Household Necessity" sign, 11¼"H × 35"W, embossed tin

neighborhood stores, so she now brings a supply back whenever she visits her parents in Japan.

The use of menthol in consumer products will certainly continue, but not at the levels it did during the first half of the twentieth century. It has been a long time since menthol was considered a miracle ingredient, yet marketers are still finding new uses for it, the latest being Vicks Mentholated Breathe Right® nasal strips.

The word *catarrh* has slipped into obscurity, and the science of hay fever has progressed light-years beyond "odors from grasses" to the understanding of endotoxins, pollen allergens, and histamines. Menthol and its volatile cousins are going to be challenged in the coming years by the new cyclic alpha-keto enamines, which are as much as thirty-five times stronger and possess no odor. As reported by David Bradley in *The Guardian* (November 14, 2001), these new compounds were found by German researchers among the chemicals that make up dark malt. They can be added to many other products that might benefit from a supercooling effect, like ice cream, chocolate, and even bottled water, without having their native taste and smell compromised by mint.

While most of America's Edwardian industrialists left behind mansions and granite monuments as testaments to their success, A. A. Hyde requested that Hillcrest be torn down after his death. A simple flat headstone marks his and Ida's grave site in Wichita's Maple Grove Cemetery. What he did leave behind was a lasting legacy of Christian philanthropy that has not yet been equaled by any of the three, going on four generations of Hyde descendants [nine children, thirty grandchildren, sixty-eight great-grandchildren, and eighty-six (and still counting) great-great-grandchildren]. He also left behind a friendly little salve that is still being manufactured today and a company whose 116-year history had almost been forgotten. I hope he wouldn't mind that I recovered and dusted off the first sixty-five years of that history for everyone to see—because making this book was a labor of honor and a balm for my soul.

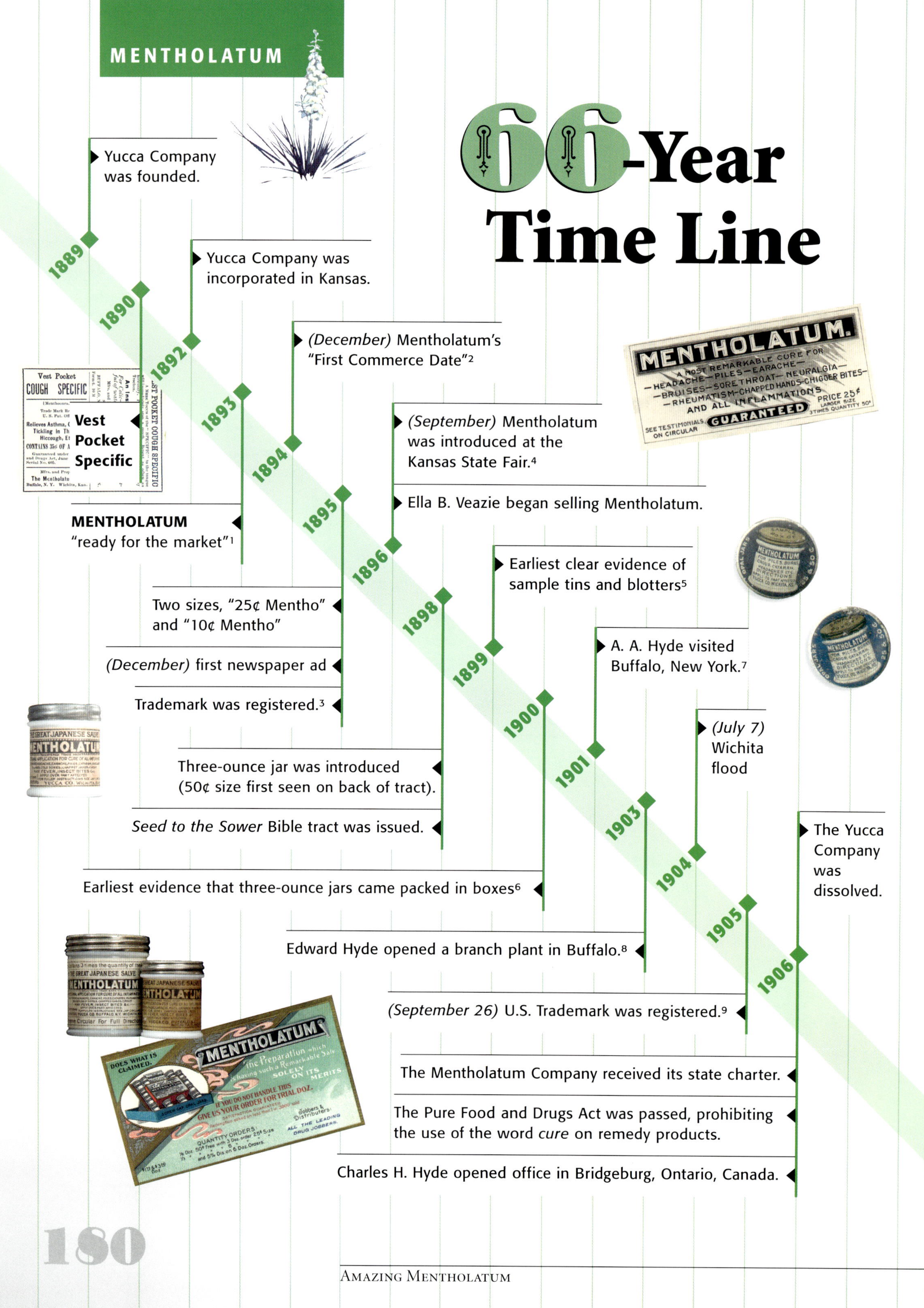

66-Year Time Line

1889
- Yucca Company was founded.

1890
- Yucca Company was incorporated in Kansas.

1892
- **Vest Pocket Specific**

1893
- **MENTHOLATUM** "ready for the market"[1]

1894
- *(December)* Mentholatum's "First Commerce Date"[2]

1895
- Two sizes, "25¢ Mentho" and "10¢ Mentho"
- *(December)* first newspaper ad
- Trademark was registered.[3]

1896
- *(September)* Mentholatum was introduced at the Kansas State Fair.[4]
- Ella B. Veazie began selling Mentholatum.

1898
- Three-ounce jar was introduced (50¢ size first seen on back of tract).
- *Seed to the Sower* Bible tract was issued.

1899
- Earliest clear evidence of sample tins and blotters[5]

1900
- Earliest evidence that three-ounce jars came packed in boxes[6]

1901
- A. A. Hyde visited Buffalo, New York.[7]

1903
- Edward Hyde opened a branch plant in Buffalo.[8]

1904
- *(July 7)* Wichita flood

1905
- *(September 26)* U.S. Trademark was registered.[9]

1906
- The Yucca Company was dissolved.
- The Mentholatum Company received its state charter.
- The Pure Food and Drugs Act was passed, prohibiting the use of the word *cure* on remedy products.
- Charles H. Hyde opened office in Bridgeburg, Ontario, Canada.

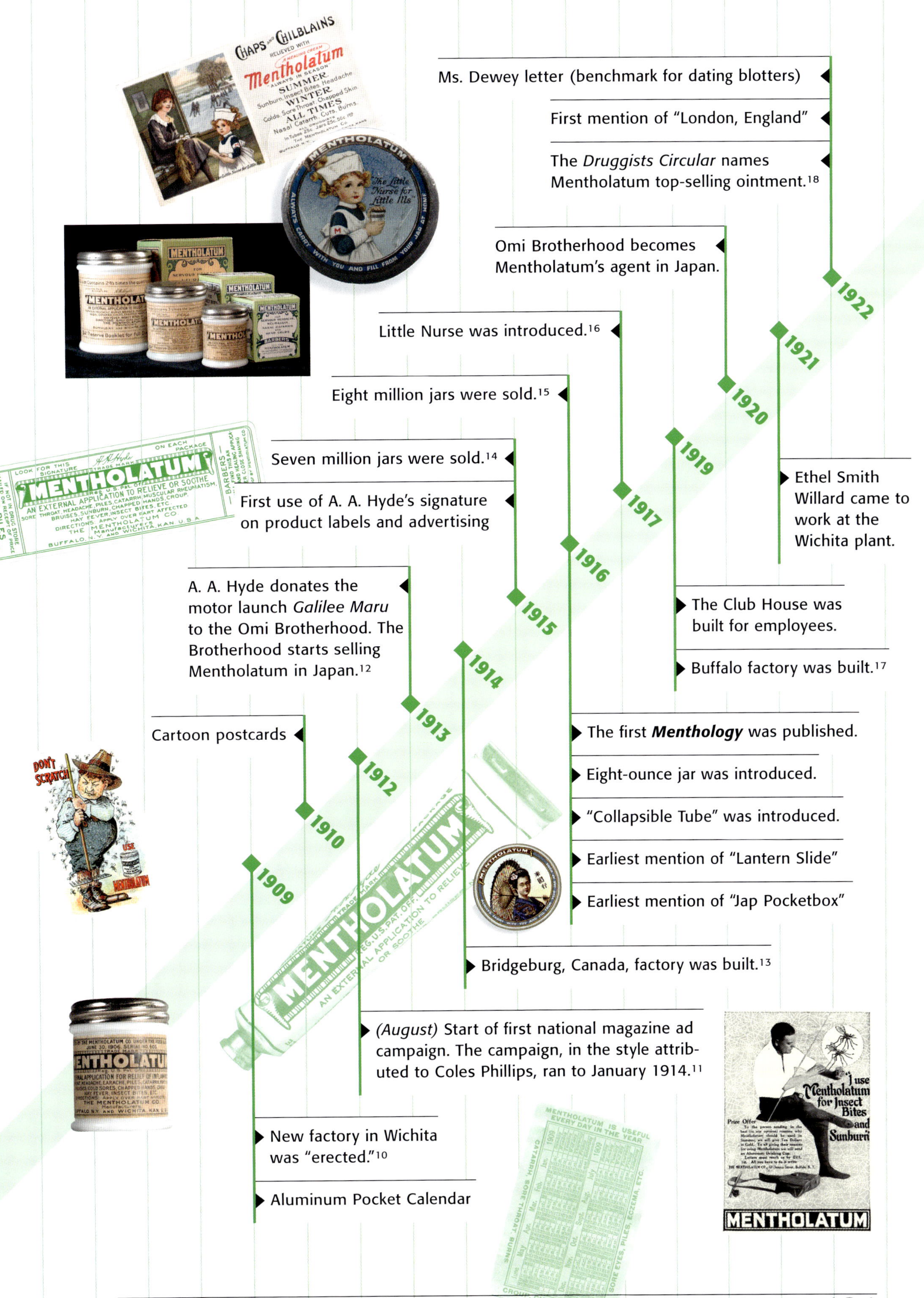

1909

New factory in Wichita was "erected."[10]

Aluminum Pocket Calendar

1910

Cartoon postcards

1912

(August) Start of first national magazine ad campaign. The campaign, in the style attributed to Coles Phillips, ran to January 1914.[11]

1913

A. A. Hyde donates the motor launch *Galilee Maru* to the Omi Brotherhood. The Brotherhood starts selling Mentholatum in Japan.[12]

1914

Bridgeburg, Canada, factory was built.[13]

1915

First use of A. A. Hyde's signature on product labels and advertising

Seven million jars were sold.[14]

1916

Eight million jars were sold.[15]

The first ***Menthology*** was published.

Eight-ounce jar was introduced.

"Collapsible Tube" was introduced.

Earliest mention of "Lantern Slide"

Earliest mention of "Jap Pocketbox"

1917

Little Nurse was introduced.[16]

1919

The Club House was built for employees.

Buffalo factory was built.[17]

1920

Omi Brotherhood becomes Mentholatum's agent in Japan.

1921

Ethel Smith Willard came to work at the Wichita plant.

1922

Ms. Dewey letter (benchmark for dating blotters)

First mention of "London, England"

The *Druggists Circular* names Mentholatum top-selling ointment.[18]

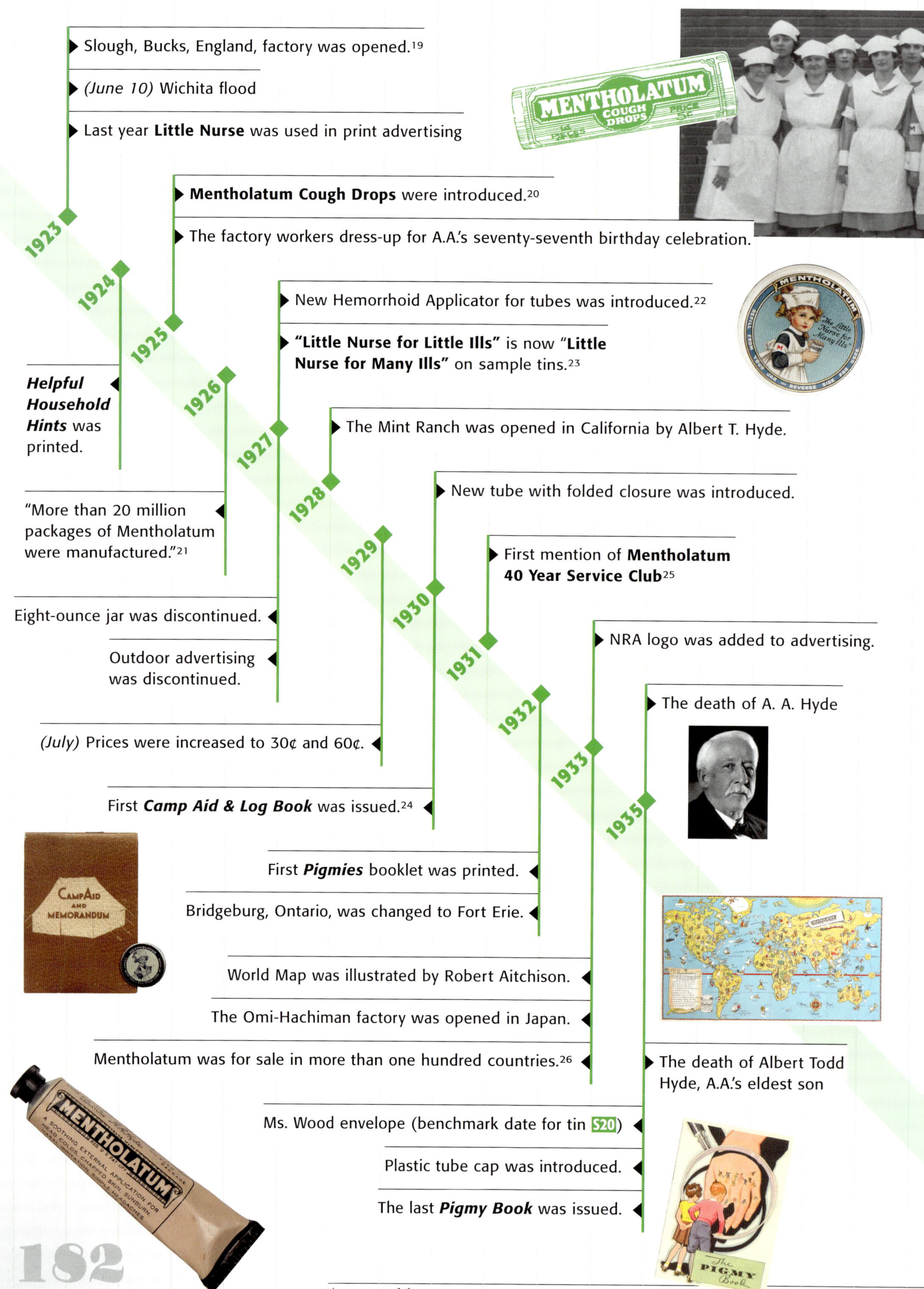

1923

- Slough, Bucks, England, factory was opened.[19]
- *(June 10)* Wichita flood
- Last year **Little Nurse** was used in print advertising

1924

- ***Helpful Household Hints*** was printed.

1925

- **Mentholatum Cough Drops** were introduced.[20]
- The factory workers dress-up for A.A.'s seventy-seventh birthday celebration.

1926

- "More than 20 million packages of Mentholatum were manufactured."[21]

1927

- New Hemorrhoid Applicator for tubes was introduced.[22]
- **"Little Nurse for Little Ills"** is now **"Little Nurse for Many Ills"** on sample tins.[23]
- Eight-ounce jar was discontinued.
- Outdoor advertising was discontinued.

1928

- The Mint Ranch was opened in California by Albert T. Hyde.

1929

- *(July)* Prices were increased to 30¢ and 60¢.

1930

- New tube with folded closure was introduced.
- First ***Camp Aid & Log Book*** was issued.[24]

1931

- First mention of **Mentholatum 40 Year Service Club**[25]

1932

- First ***Pigmies*** booklet was printed.
- Bridgeburg, Ontario, was changed to Fort Erie.

1933

- NRA logo was added to advertising.
- World Map was illustrated by Robert Aitchison.
- The Omi-Hachiman factory was opened in Japan.
- Mentholatum was for sale in more than one hundred countries.[26]

1935

- The death of A. A. Hyde
- The death of Albert Todd Hyde, A.A.'s eldest son
- Ms. Wood envelope (benchmark date for tin S20)
- Plastic tube cap was introduced.
- The last ***Pigmy Book*** was issued.

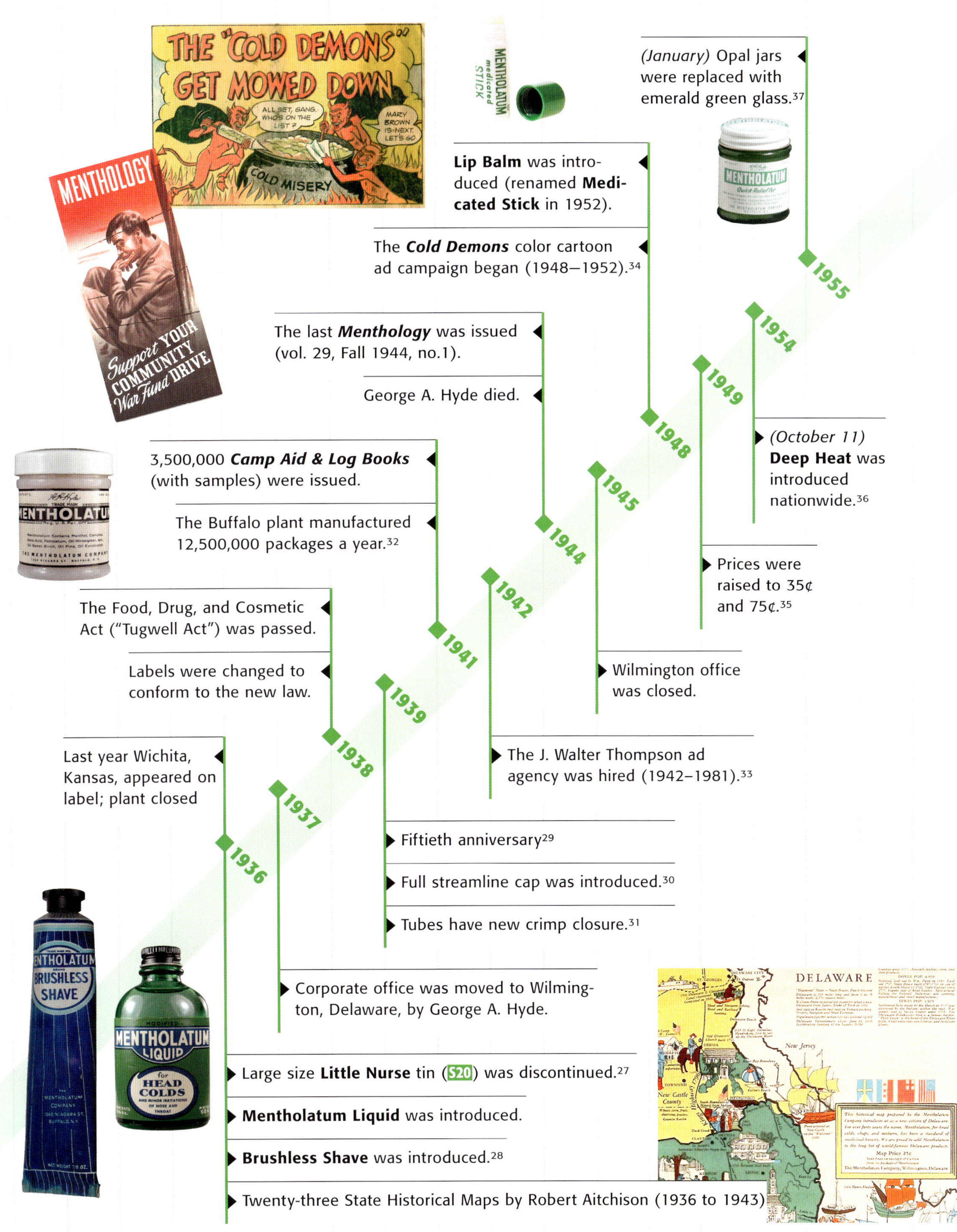

1936

- Last year Wichita, Kansas, appeared on label; plant closed
- Large size **Little Nurse** tin (S20) was discontinued.[27]
- **Mentholatum Liquid** was introduced.
- **Brushless Shave** was introduced.[28]
- Twenty-three State Historical Maps by Robert Aitchison (1936 to 1943)

1937

- Corporate office was moved to Wilmington, Delaware, by George A. Hyde.

1938

- The Food, Drug, and Cosmetic Act ("Tugwell Act") was passed.
- Labels were changed to conform to the new law.

1939

- Fiftieth anniversary[29]
- Full streamline cap was introduced.[30]
- Tubes have new crimp closure.[31]

1941

- 3,500,000 ***Camp Aid & Log Books*** (with samples) were issued.
- The Buffalo plant manufactured 12,500,000 packages a year.[32]

1942

- The J. Walter Thompson ad agency was hired (1942–1981).[33]

1944

- The last ***Menthology*** was issued (vol. 29, Fall 1944, no.1).
- George A. Hyde died.

1945

- Wilmington office was closed.

1948

- **Lip Balm** was introduced (renamed **Medicated Stick** in 1952).
- The ***Cold Demons*** color cartoon ad campaign began (1948–1952).[34]

1949

- Prices were raised to 35¢ and 75¢.[35]

1954

- *(October 11)* **Deep Heat** was introduced nationwide.[36]

1955

- *(January)* Opal jars were replaced with emerald green glass.[37]

The Competition

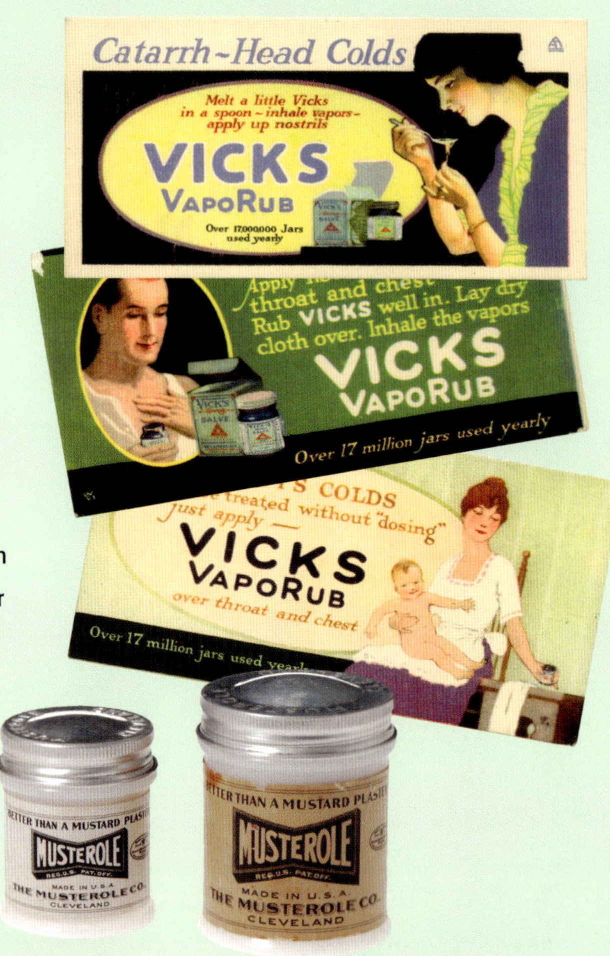

In 1932 *Fortune* made a thorough study of the business of colds. The article in its October issue detailed the obstacles facing a manufacturer of cold remedies competing in the crowded market of the day. It was estimated that there were between 70 and 142 different kinds of proprietary cold medicines on the average druggist's shelf and of these there were twenty-four inhalants, twenty cough syrups, and twenty rubs. Effective advertising during the cold season required a large part of a manufacturer's annual budget in order to distinguish his brand from the others. To quote the article, "Nowhere are sales and advertising more closely and immediately connected than in the cold business." Dealers posed a problem when they cut prices or joined the growing number of chains that manufactured imitation products and sold them at lower prices. Of the sixty thousand drugstores in 1932, about four thousand were owned by chains. Expensive window displays and special premiums weren't always enough to sway the ambitious drug clerk from mixing a pot of camphor, menthol, and Vaseline® and going into business for himself.[1]

An age-old grudge that placed another barrier between the manufacturer and his customer was the American Medical Association. The AMA had 96,000 of the country's 150,000 doctors as members, and although they still couldn't cure the common cold, they universally disapproved of people using patent remedies to self-medicate. Ironically, one government survey at the time revealed that out of 15,000 doctor's prescriptions written, 1,090 were actually for patent cough medicines.

Fortune ranked Vicks VapoRub the biggest-selling cold remedy in all categories, not to mention the largest cold rub. Mentholatum and Musterole followed in that order as its major competitors. Ben-Gay came in fourth in sales but was considered most popular with doctors. This ranking appears to have continued unchanged up through 1955, the end of the period covered by this book. Here are company profiles for Mentholatum's top-three competitors plus Asia's largest menthol rub, Tiger Balm. An alphabetical listing of thirty-five select menthol cold rubs that populated the market prior to 1955 follows.[2]

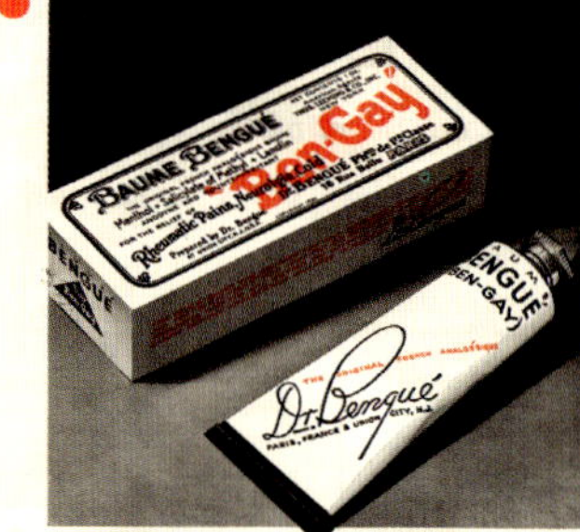

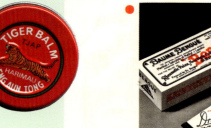

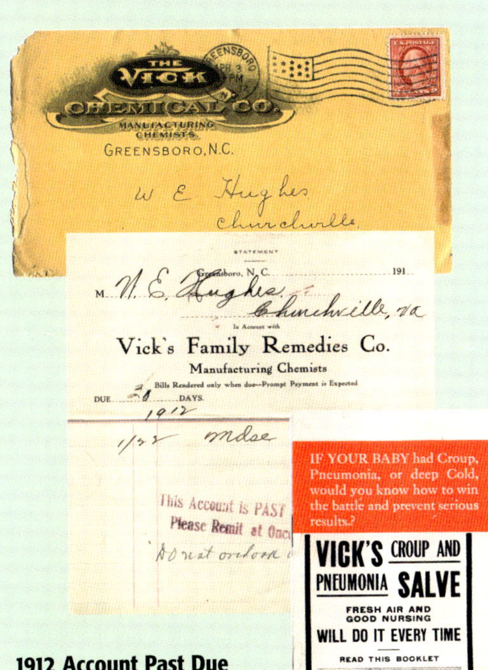

1912 Account Past Due

This document demonstrates frugal office management after the company changed its name from Vick's Family Remedies Company to the Vick Chemical Company because old stationery was still used. There was no appearance yet of the word *VapoRub*.

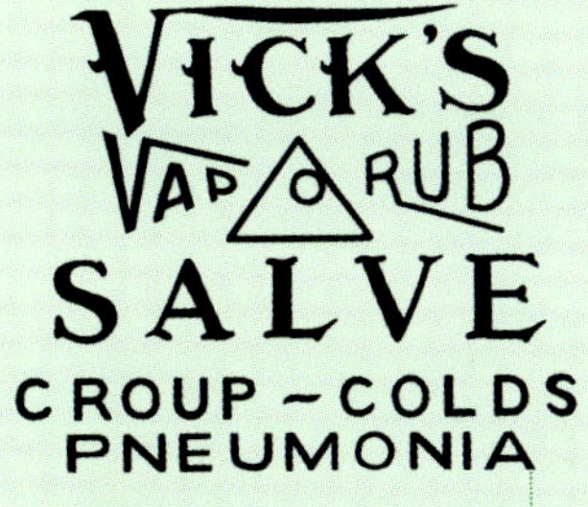

Early VapoRub Logo

This logo was seen on shipping crates after WWI.

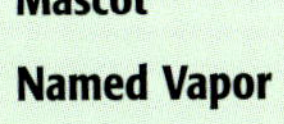

Mascot Named Vapor

Vicks' mascot was placed in drugstores and general stores throughout the South during the early 1920s.

VICKS VapoRub®

The story of Mentholatum's number one competitor starts in 1891, when pharmacist Lunsford Richardson (1854–1919) sold his small drugstore in Selma, North Carolina, and with partner John Ferris bought the larger Porter and Tate Drugstore located at 121 South Elm Street in Greensboro, North Carolina. By 1894, Richardson had added to his pharmaceutical business a line of twenty-one premixed doctors' remedies for customers who could not afford to see a doctor for a prescription. Among the remedies was one he called Richardson's Croup and Pneumonia Cure Salve, which contained menthol, camphor, thymol, eucalyptus, cedarleaf, nutmeg, and turpentine oils, mixed in a petrolatum base.[3]

In 1898, the forty-four-year-old druggist sold his interest in the drugstore and began commercial production of the twenty-one remedies plus standard drugs under the name Lundsford Richardson Wholesale Drug Company. In 1905 he sold the wholesale business and continued manufacturing his original twenty-one-product line as Vick's Family Remedies Co., Manufacturing Chemists. According to Smith Richardson's history, his father was first inspired to use Vicks by the popular *Vicks Illustrated Monthly Magazine* and thought it would be an easy name for his backwoods clientele to remember. It also happened to be the name of his brother-in-law, Dr. Joshua Vick. His Vick's products were marketed to drugstores and general stores within the twenty-county territory surrounding Greensboro. Yearly sales were modest, competition was stiff, and after several years Lunsford could see no prospect of ever expanding beyond the Greensboro territory. In 1907, his eldest son, Smith Richardson (1885–1972) joined the company and took charge of sales. Smith made changes that improved profitability by phasing out manufacture of all twenty products and convincing his father to focus everything on the Vick's Croup and Pneumonia Salve. Because he had little money to advertise, Smith expanded their territory by giving out free jars of the salve as incentives to new customers. It was a plan that paid off, and by 1910 sales had doubled.[4]

There were now seven traveling salesmen hired by the company each driving a Model T with a ladder strapped on the side for putting signs up on trees and barns along the back roads of Virginia, South Carolina, Alabama, and Tennessee. The company mascot was "Your bodyguard," a Vicks box with arms, legs, head, and the word *Vapor* on its face. The author has in his collection an envelope from the Vick Chemical Company, Manufacturing Chemists date stamped April 3, 1912, with an illustration of a box of Vick's Croup and Pneumonia Salve printed on the back which contained a

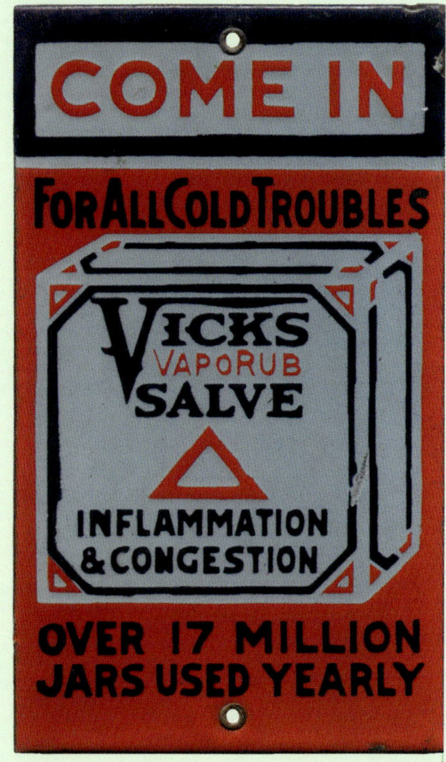

Porcelain Enamel Door Push–Early 1920s

This example was salvaged from the doors of a general store in east Texas.

booklet of testimonials. The booklet is titled "Vick's Croup and Pneumonia Salve," and inside there is one testimonial dated 1909. When Smith named the salve Vicks "VapoRub" he decided to protect it and filed with the trademark office on July 18, 1913. He claimed that January 1, 1911, was its first use date (contrary to the evidence) and received a trademark on April 6, 1915. VapoRub claimed to be "An Auxiliary Treatment for Certain Forms of Inflammation and Congestion." It was a "Medicinal Salve for use in such ailments as Croup, Colds, Pneumonia, Catarrh, Tonsillitis, Bronchitis, Sore Throat, Whooping Cough, Asthma, Burns, Bruises, Sprains, Neuralgia, Eczema, Itching Humors, Itching Piles, Boils, and Rheumatic Pains." Its ingredients were menthol, camphor, eucalyptus, oil of thyme, nutmeg oil, oil of turpentine, and petrolatum.[5]

Vicks remained a regional southeastern operation until 1913, when it began to expand its sales effort north of the Mason-Dixon Line. Vicks salesmen worked the Midwest from 1913 to 1916, then the New England states from 1917 to 1920. In 1915, Vicks stopped giving out free jars when it introduced its first sample tin to druggists in St. Louis. The western states were introduced to Vicks in a "sample-by-mail" campaign that shipped eight freight-car loads of sample tins to the population of thirty-one million in a fifty-day blitz. During WWI, the influenza pandemic caused sales to jump from $613,000 in 1917, to $2,940,000 in 1919. (See pages 76 and 77 for details.) To meet the increased demand for blue glass jars the company contracted with Hazel-Atlas Glass Company, the supplier of Mentholatum jars. In 1919, the slogan "Over 17 Million Jars Used Yearly" was added to advertising for the first time. Just as Vicks was becoming a national player, the founder, Lunsford Richardson died and Smith became president of the company.[6]

▲ 1915 sample tin

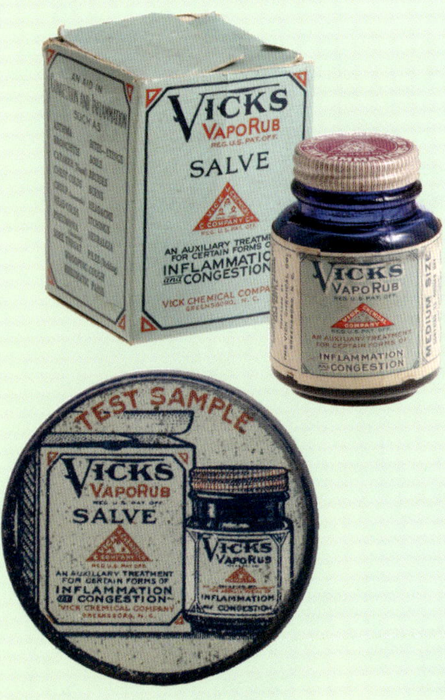

▲ 1920s box, jar, and sample tin

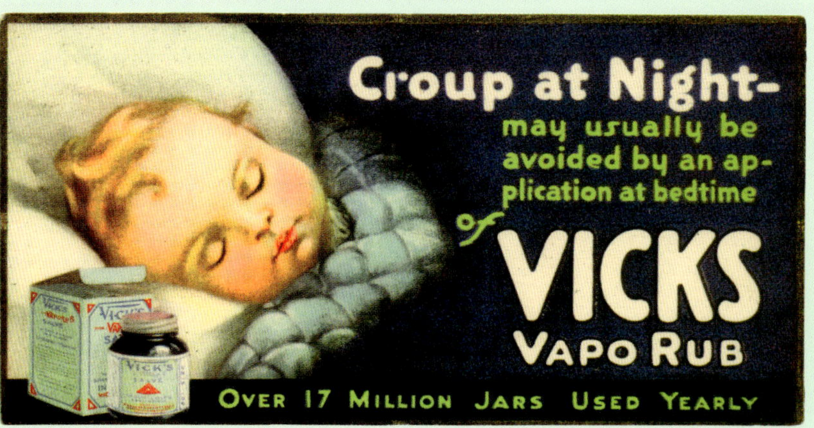

▲ Chromolitho blotter–early 1920s

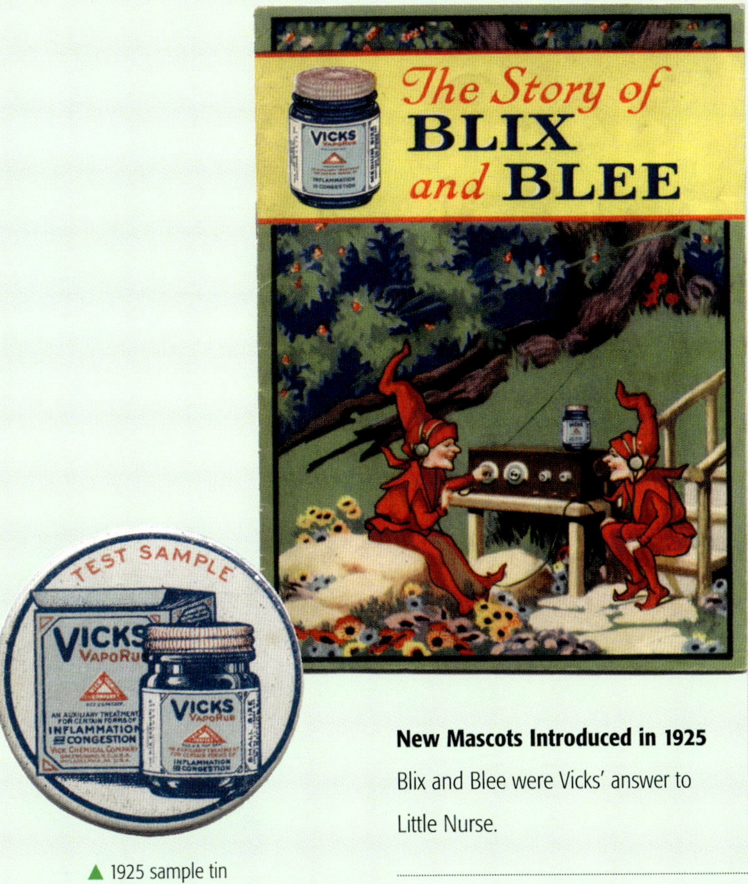

New Mascots Introduced in 1925

Blix and Blee were Vicks' answer to Little Nurse.

▲ 1925 sample tin

With the money earned during the epidemic, Vicks was able to afford to advertise in national magazines for the first time. Smith put a Dixie spin on his company's history in a full-page color ad in January 1921 (see page 77). Vicks continued to use the slogan "Over 17 Million Jars Used Yearly" each year for the next decade, and whenever sales surpassed that number they crossed out the 17 and added the higher number above it. Colorful new ink blotters were given to druggists to hand out to their best customers. The retail prices per jar were 30¢, 60¢, and $1.20. The apostrophe was dropped from Vick's by 1924. Sometime in the mid-twenties, a new factory was opened in Philadelphia, Pennsylvania. In 1925, two elf mascots appeared in a booklet titled *The Story of Blix and Blee*, which remained available for more than five years for children who mailed their 4¢ in stamps to Greensboro to cover the handling and postage.[7]

VICKS
VAPORUB
OVER 17 MILLION JARS USED YEARLY

A Modern-Looking Logo

This logo was first used in advertising c. 1921 and on packaging c. 1924.

The company went public in 1925 and sold one-quarter of its stock on the New York Stock Exchange for approximately $4,000,000. Between 1925 and 1929, while listed on the Big Board, it earned up to $10,392,000, of which $6,000,000 was distributed in dividends. In 1930, Drug, Inc. [a partnership of Sterling Products, Bristol-Myers, Life Savers, and the United Drug Company (Rexall)], merged with Vicks in an exchange of stock worth $38,000,000. Smith and little brother Lunsford, who joined the company in 1911, remained board chairman and president respectively. *Fortune* revealed that they enjoyed their wealth and leisure time, bought country homes, went fishing in Florida, and went hunting in Canada.[8]

Fortune reported in 1932 that Vicks spent "well over $1,000,000 a year on advertising." Vicks sales slogan was now "Over 26,000,000 jars used yearly." After the merger, the new board of directors decided it was time to expand the Vicks product line, and a new products department was initiated. In the fall of 1931, the company introduced a "white, stainless form" of VapoRub. The original blend continued to be sold as Amber VapoRub. Jars of either form retailed for 35¢ and 75¢. Despite the Depression, total sales for

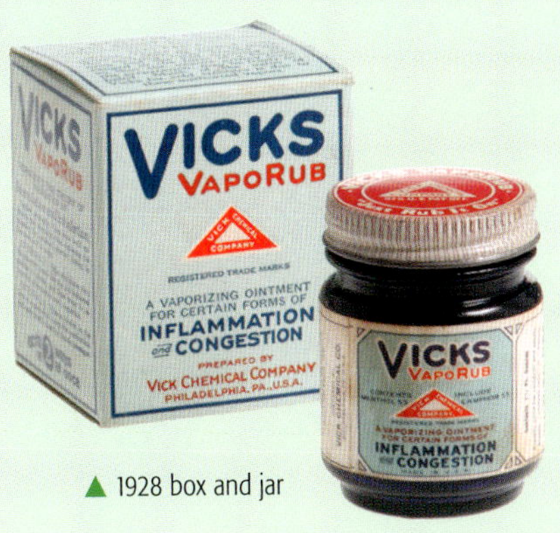

▲ 1928 box and jar

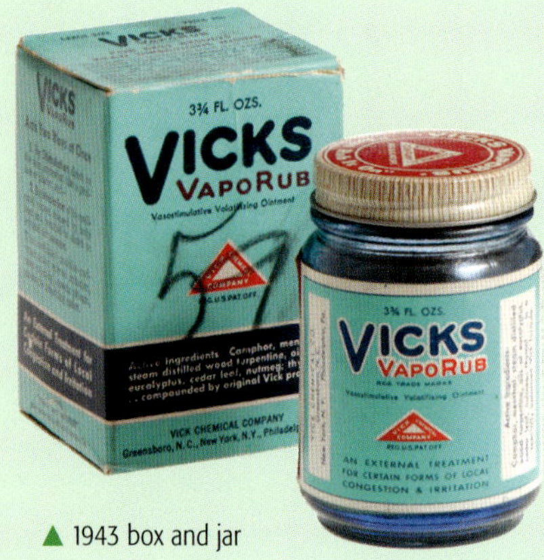

▲ 1943 box and jar

the year ending July 1, 1932, were up 34 percent. Due to the varied impact the Depression was having on each of the partners, the Drug, Inc., merger failed and the participating companies split apart in 1933.[9]

▲ 1935 sample tin

In 1934, the company filed an application to register its trademark VICK as Vick Chemical Company, (A Delaware Corporation), Philadelphia, Pennsylvania. The goods and services wording was upgraded to read, "A Medicinal Preparation Used in the Treatment or Prevention of Colds and Affections of the Throat and Nasal Passages." The first use and commerce date for VICK was entered as "June 12, 1911." The trademark was registered number 320752 on January 8, 1935. Vick Chemical Co. employed fewer than five hundred people, had factories located in Greensboro and Philadelphia, an international trade office in New York City, and four foreign offices. The English product was called "Vapour-Rub: A Vaporizing Ointment for Certain Forms of Inflammation and Congestion." In the summer of 1935, Smith Richardson testified before the House subcommittee working on what would later become the Food, Drug, and Cosmetic Act of 1938. He told the committee that he had "modified his labeling under Food and Drug Administration pressure rather than risk multiple seizures for implying, during an epidemic [1918], that his ointment might prevent pneumonia and the flu." In 1938, Vicks acquired the William S. Merrell Company, which was founded in 1828 and was then the oldest pharmaceutical company still operating in the United States. The merger became Richardson-Merrell, Inc., with its corporate offices in New York.[10]

▲ 1953 sample tin and box

By 1972, Richardson-Merrell, Inc., employed about fourteen thousand people worldwide, had fourteen factories in the United States and thirty abroad, and had forty-seven foreign offices. The company also manufactured thousands of products in the proprietary drug and other fields.

Richardson-Vicks, Inc., of Wilton, Connecticut, sold the Vicks brand to Procter & Gamble Company in 1985. The Vicks VapoRub® brand is still on the market today.

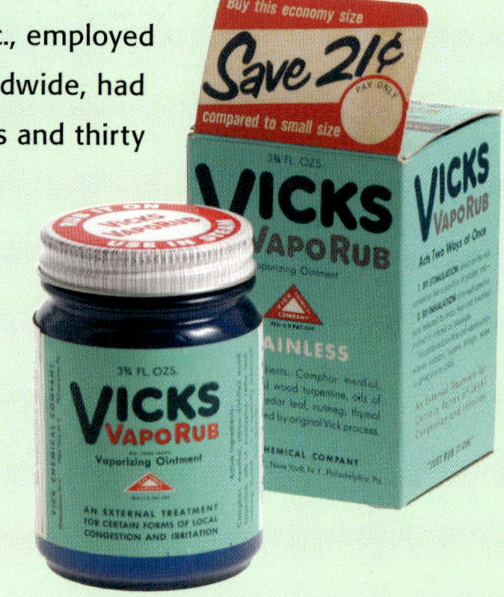

▲ 1958 box and jar

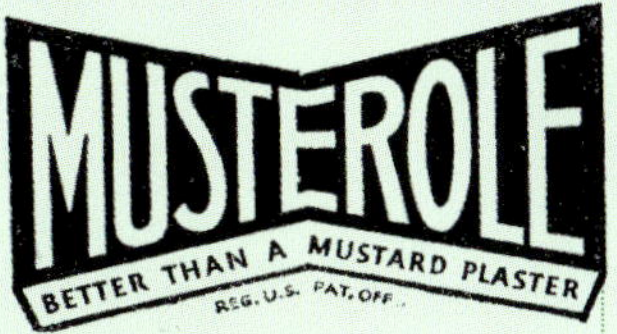

Bow Tie Logo

The text changed, but the distinctive bow tie remained unchanged throughout the eighty-four-year life of the product.

Musterole®

In 1905, A. L. McLaren, a pharmacist in Cleveland, Ohio, first formulated Musterole for his customers. In 1907, he and a local hardware merchant, George Miller, with other investors, incorporated the Musterole Company, which they ran full time. Sometime later they sold the company to another druggist, C. F. Buescher, who grew it into the third-largest cold rub in the country. World War I almost devastated the company when its supply of German-made synthetic oil of mustard was cut off. Buescher's chemists discovered how to produce their own oil, and the company survived the war. Musterole must have profited when people went on a buying spree for pneumonia cures during the influenza epidemic because by 1920, the company had earned enough to advertise in national magazines and expanded into markets worldwide. Musterole ads were frequently found in the same magazines in which Mentholatum advertised. Rarely did they appear in the same magazines used by Vicks for advertising.

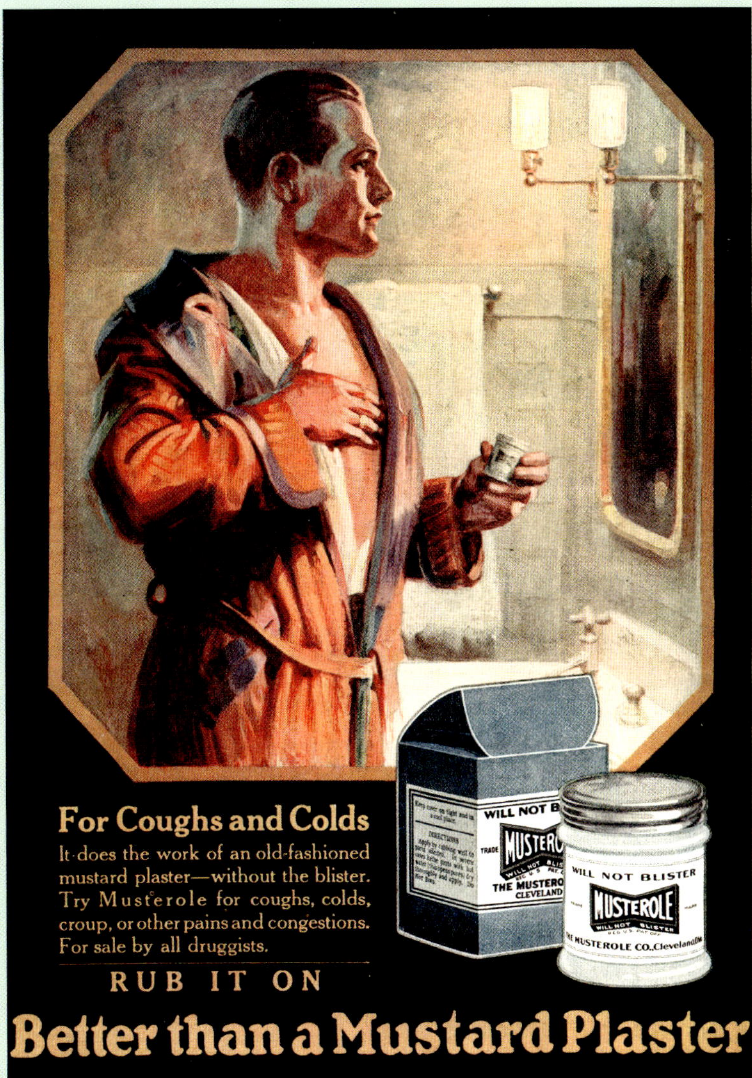

Colorful Introduction

Mentholatum kicked off its national advertising campaign (Little Nurse) with a big color ad in 1916. Musterole followed with two, first in 1919 and this ad in 1920. Vicks' big color ad came in 1921. Musterole continued to advertise in national magazines, limiting purchases to black-and-white art for the rest of its history.

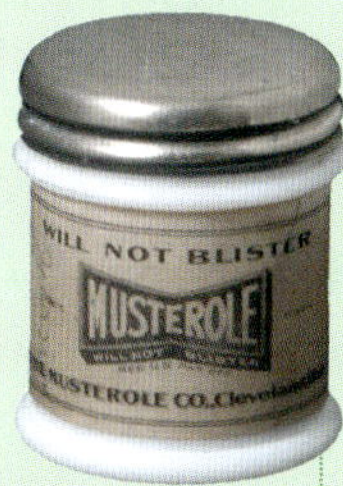

Familiar Style

In every way, this early 7/8-ounce Musterole jar is identical to a 1-ounce Mentholatum jar from the same period. It matches the jar illustrated in the 1920 color ad on this page. Sometime later the company added a larger 1¾-ounce jar.

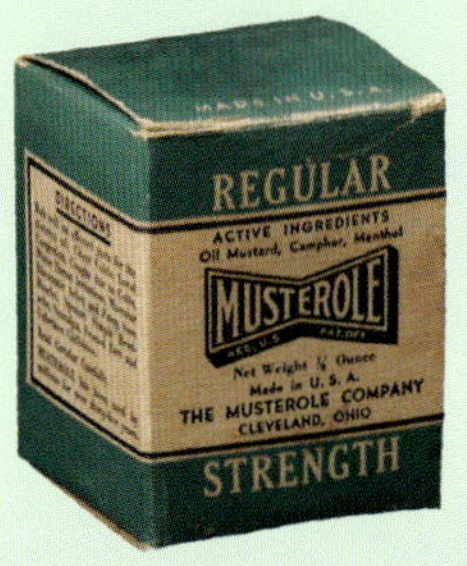

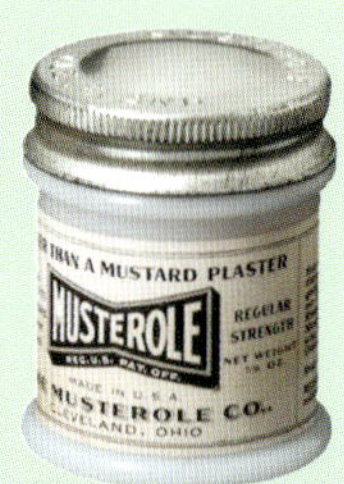

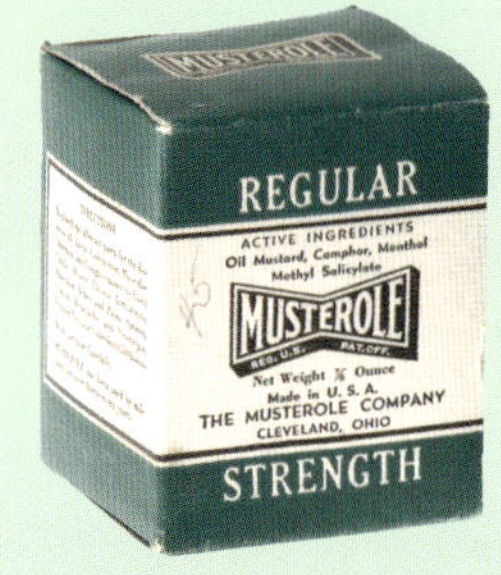

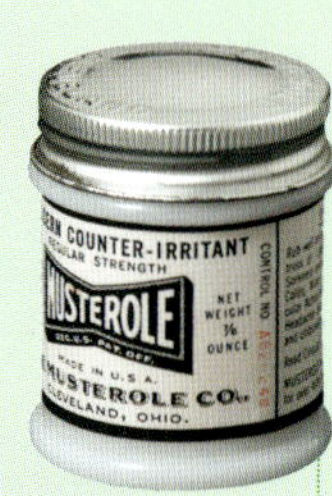

Evidence of a Change

Evidence that the slogan changed between 1941 and 1942 is illustrated by the box and jar on the left that are marked "1941" and "Better than a Mustard Plaster," and the box and jar on the right marked "1942" and "A Modern Counter-Irritant."

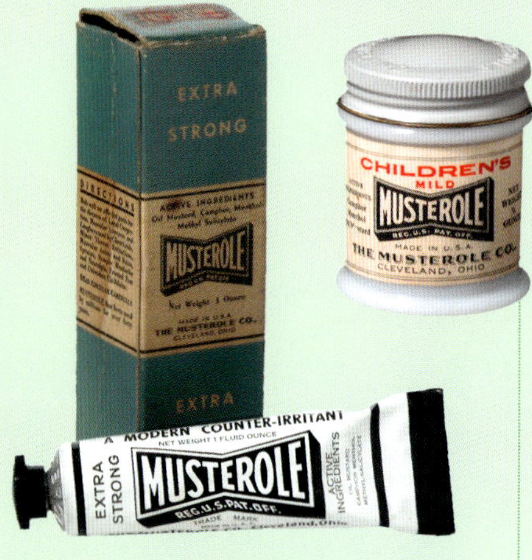

Additional Formulations for the 1940s

Extra Strong came in a tube. Childrens Mild came in a 7/8-ounce jar with a white-painted cap. Green glass replaced milk glass sometime in the mid-1950s.

During this time the slogan on the Musterole label was "Will Not Blister," an assurance for customers who had experienced a real mustard plaster. From the mid-1920s to 1941 the subtitle was changed to "Better than a Mustard Plaster," and after that it became "A Modern Counter-Irritant," to de-emphasize the outdated mustard plaster to a new generation of customers and put the emphasis on the effects of camphor and menthol. Its ingredients were oil of mustard, camphor, menthol, and lanolin in a petrolatum and paraffin base. There were three formulas: Extra Strong, which came in tubes only; and Regular Strength and Children's Mild, which were both packed in milk glass jars with distinctively embossed aluminum lids.

Buescher became a wealthy man and according to *Fortune* took frequent trips to Europe, owned a "thriving picture collection," and lived in a big house in Cleveland's Lakewood district. In the mid-1940s Musterole's magazine advertising featured the Dionne Quintuplets, as did other brand-name products like Carnation Evaporated Milk, Colgate Ribbon Dental Cream, Palmolive Soap, and Karo Syrup, to name a few. Consumers had followed with great affection the lives of the Dionne Quints since their births in 1934, and the few lucky advertisers that were sanctioned each year by the family's agent were sure to cash in on this goodwill. Musterole was acquired by Plough in 1956, and manufacturing was moved to Memphis, Tennessee. Schering-Plough, Inc., retired the Musterole brand c. 1990–91.[11]

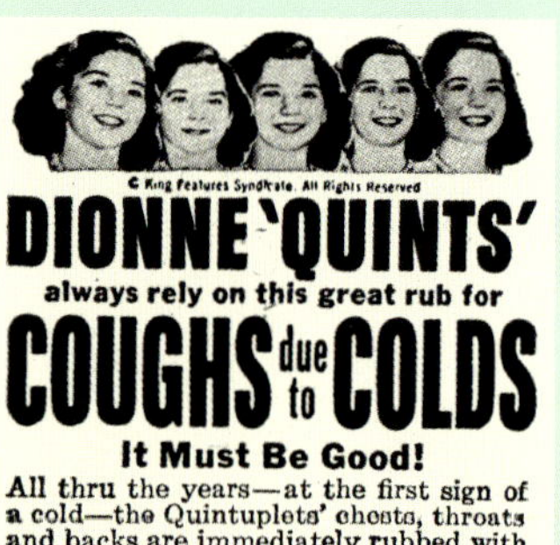

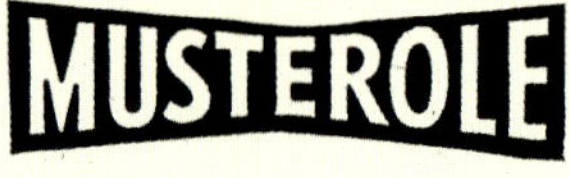

▲ Typical 1946 "Quints" ad

BENGUÉ

BAUME BENGUÉ

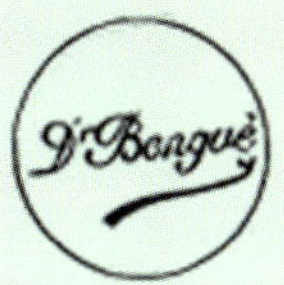

Ben-Gay®

Dr. Jules Bernard Bengué, a Paris physician and chemist who was in the business of manufacturing balsams, purgatives, pastilles, and anesthetics, created a lanolin-based menthol cream in 1891 that he named Baume Bengué Analgésique. The Baume was so popular that Dr. Bengué decided to market it in America too. In 1898, he set up a manufacturing plant in West Hoboken, New Jersey, and according to the trademark record his first product went on sale February 27, 1899. By 1907 he had registered three U.S. trademarks. Later, Thomas Leeming & Co., Inc., New York (founded in 1881), was the American agent printed on product packaging, but it is not known when this association began.[12]

By 1900 the product was called Baume Bengué, while an additional logo was added and its trademark (US66633, the signature within a circle logo) was registered. A French tin of *Dragees Bengué au Menthol* (a menthol candy cough drop with cocaine) has been found with this same logo indicating the doctor's continued interest in menthol and that the parent company sold a range of products that were not available in the American office. It is possible that the collapsible tube packaging was in use from the product's beginning in France. Though a relatively new technology in the 1890s, tin tubes were most commonly used by artists to hold their oil paint colors.[13]

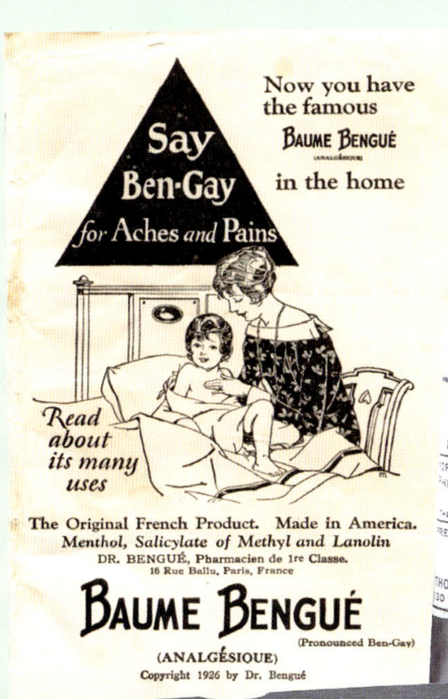

Say "Ben-Gay" in the 1920s

Packaging included simple paper label on a tin tube, sturdy two-part box with the old logo, and a family-friendly insert.

The British Medical Association reported in the *Journal of the American Medical Association*, December 14, 1912, that Dr. Bengué's Analgesic Balm contained 18 percent menthol, 20 percent methyl salicylate, 54 percent lanolin anhydrous, and 8 percent fat, "apparently lard." The estimated cost of the ingredients of a 50¢ tube was 2.5¢. *JAMA*'s editor wrote, "Evidently this imposingly named product is practically a lanolin ointment containing oil of wintergreen and menthol. . . . In this country (US), the exploiters find that space in cheap medical journals, reinforced by the aid of undiscriminating physicians, is a cheaper method of getting the stuff to the public."[14]

Thos. Leeming & Co. was having trouble selling the product with an imposing name to the general public. Despite Dr. Bengué's insistence that his French name sounded scientific, a change had to be made if the product was ever going to grow in market share. In 1922, to help Yankees pronounce the brand name, a phonetic spelling, "Ben-Gay," was added to packaging along with a solid triangle where reversed-out lettering, such as "Say Ben-Gay,"

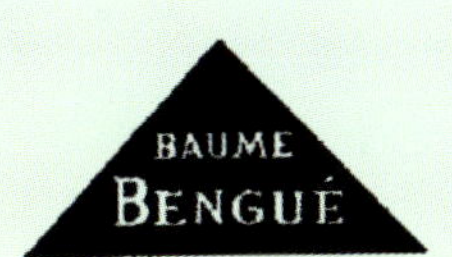

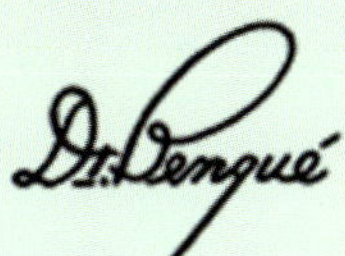

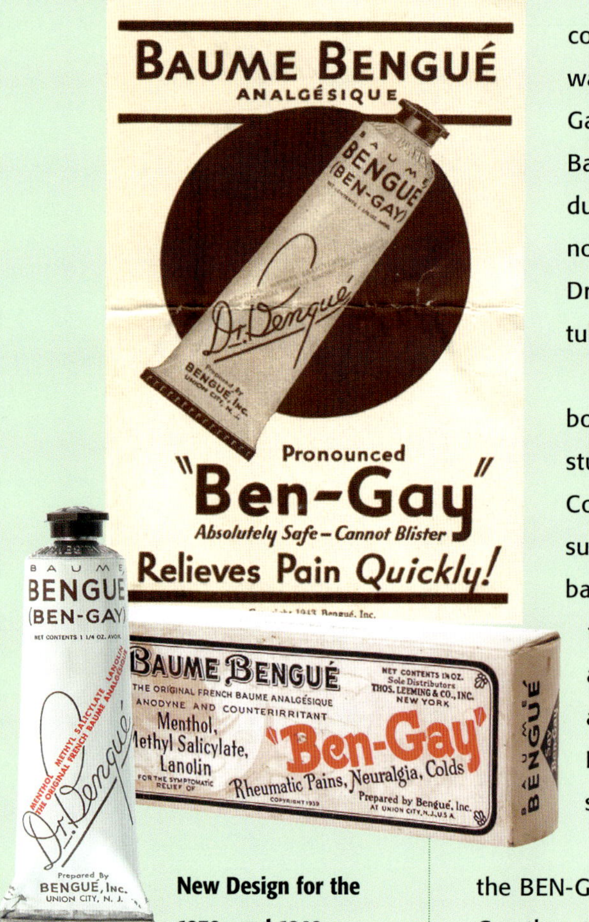

New Design for the 1930s and 1940s

In February 1933 new packaging designs were introduced, and in 1939 a new folded box replaced the traditional two-part box. The company described the new signature logo as "ultra-modern." See the announcement on page 184.

could be placed (US435135, US0565479). Manufacturing was now located in Union City, New Jersey. In 1933, "Ben-Gay" was printed large, in red ink across the traditional Baume Bengué box label, and a new tube design was introduced. The tube no longer had a bland paper label; it was now printed in three colors—cream, brown, and red—with Dr. Bengué's signature placed vertically the length of the tube, and it had a brown plastic cap (US510378).

In 1939, a new folded box replaced the old two-part box. There was also a Children's Mild Bengué. Dr. Bengué's stubborn use of the scientific title "Analgésique Anodyne and Counterirritant" and advertising in "cheap medical journals" succeeded in making doctors the product's core consumer base. The attractive new packaging improved marketing next to the top brands on the drugstore shelf. "Peter Pain" appeared in newspaper Sunday comics and magazine ads in the 1940s. Starting in 1954, Mentholatum Deep Heat became Ben-Gay's primary competition for the sports rub market.[15]

In 1967 the antique Baume Bengué was dropped from the BEN-GAY trademark (US840785) by new owner Charles Pfizer and Co., then that mark was transferred to Pfizer, Inc., in 1987. The current unhyphenated form, BenGay, was trademarked in 1998 (US2173169) by Pfizer, Inc., and the product is still on the market today.

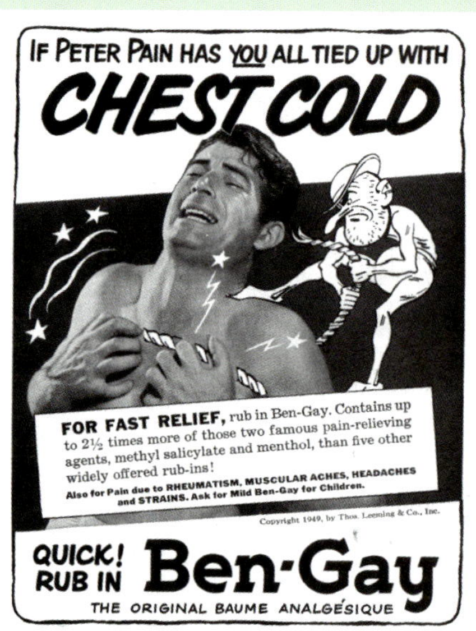

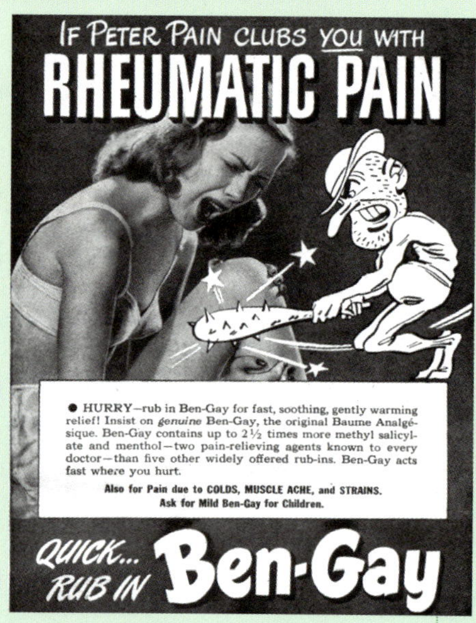

Ben-Gay vs. Peter Pain

"Peter Pain" appeared in newspaper Sunday comics throughout the 1940s and was also featured in these 1949 magazine ads.

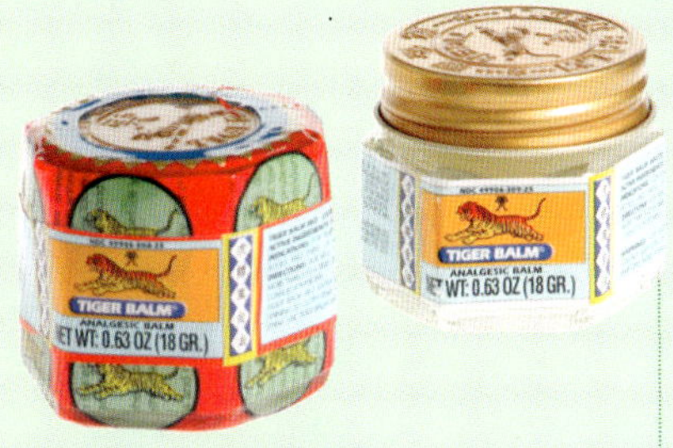

Modern Packaging

Shown above are a hexagonal jar of White Tiger Balm with gold-colored cap and Red Tiger Balm in wrappers.

Tiger Balm®

Very little is known of Mentholatum's marketing efforts in Asia beyond Japan and a few missions in China, but it is clear that Tiger Balm must have been a serious competitor. The story begins in 1908, when on his deathbed in Rangoon, Burma, the herbalist Aw Chu Kin passed on instructions about the future of the family business to his two sons, Aw Boon Haw (1882–1954) and Aw Boon Par (1888–1944). As the family legend is told, he passed on to his sons the secret formula for making his popular pain-relieving balm—a formula inspired by an ancient folk remedy created for a promiscuous Chinese emperor whose frequent exploits between the sheets had perpetuated a sore back. Knowing that legends and secrets were important marketing tools, Aw Chu Kin made his sons promise to hold the formula secret and give a portion of their income to charity.

The Aw brothers continued the pharmacy business after their father's death and improved the old formula, naming it Ban Kim Ewe (Ten Thousand Golden Oil), a panacea for all maladies. Boon Haw sold Ban Kim Ewe to local Chinese medicine shops and expanded its distribution throughout Burma. By adding cinnamon, the brothers created a second, "extra-potent," red balm. Today, the ingredients are camphor, menthol, cajeput oil, and clove oil in a petrolatum base. White Tiger Balm is scented with dementholized mint oil. Red Tiger Balm is scented with cassia oil, which is similar to cinnamon. After WWI, the brothers decided to use the anglicized version of Haw's name, "Tiger," as their trade name because it was synonymous in the East with vitality and strength. (Boon Par's name means Leopard.) Ban Kim Ewe became known as Tiger Balm. Boon Haw introduced Tiger Balm and Tiger-brand pharmaceutical products throughout Southeast Asia during the 1920s, driving a "tiger-shaped" car and distributing colorful enameled signs (see illustration) to participating druggists.

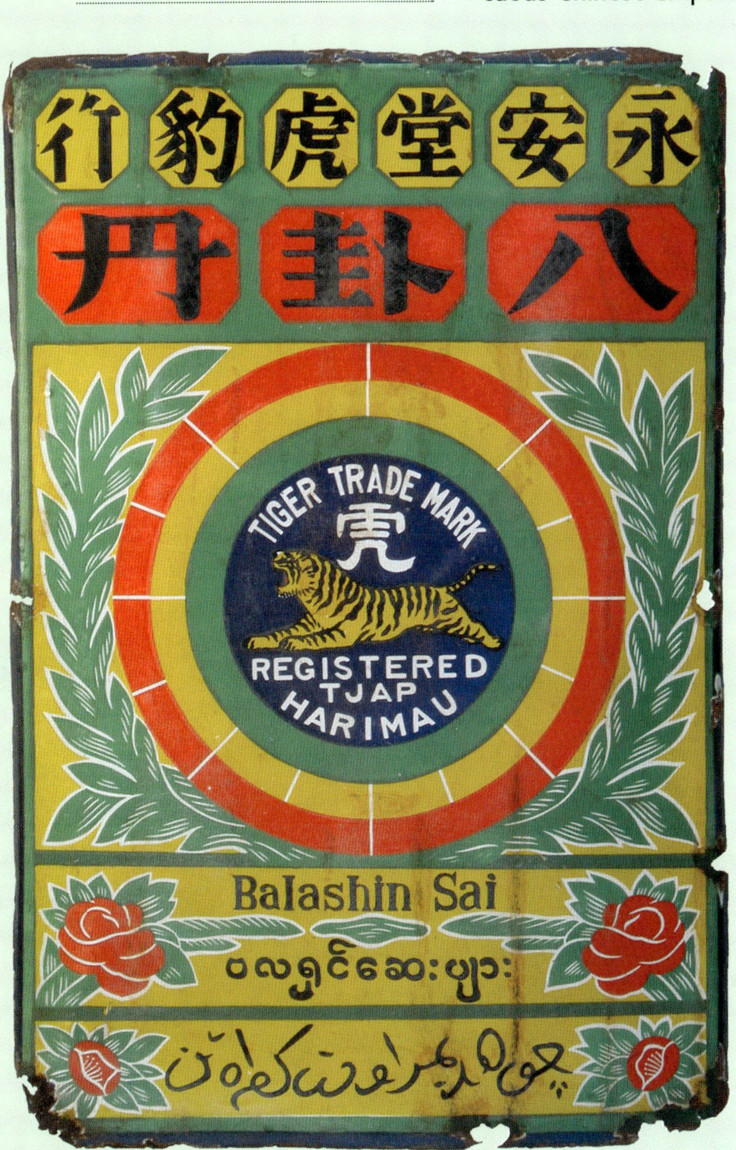

Tiger Brand Products

This brightly colored porcelain enamel store sign, c. late 1920s, is from Singapore.

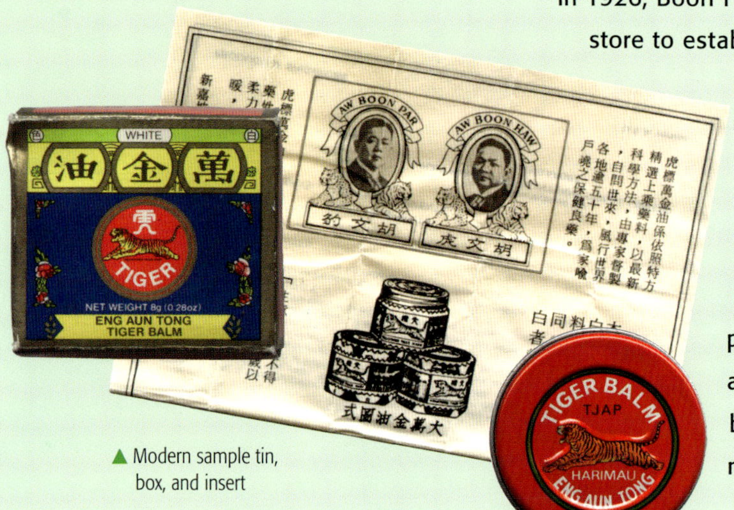

▲ Modern sample tin, box, and insert

In 1926, Boon Haw moved to Singapore and opened a second store to establish trade in Malaya and the East Indies. Boon Par remained in Rangoon. Known as the Haw Par Brothers, they eventually expanded their pharmaceutical empire to include banking, insurance, rubber plantations, and newspapers. And they never forgot their pledge to their father. The brothers were great philanthropists, donating to hospitals, schools, and nursing homes. Today, Tiger Balm is owned by Singapore's United Overseas Bank and is marketed in more than seventy countries.[16]

Competitor Menthol Cold Rubs

These products were on the market at various times between 1894 and 1955 and are followed by first use and commerce dates, where known.

1. Ben-Gay® (1891)
2. Cloverine® Brand Mentho Balm
3. Cushman's Mentho Balm
4. DeWitt's® Vaporizing Balm
5. Dr. Brigadell's Camphorole® Ointment (1912)
6. Kemp & Lane's Menthol Compound Cream
7. Kemp & Lane's Vaporizing Salve
8. MA-LE-NA® Ointment (1886)
9. McConnon's Compound Menthol-Camphor Ointment
10. McConnon's Mentholated Salve
11. McNess® Mentholated Ointment (1919)
12. McNess® Vaporole
13. Menthene
14. Mentholatum® (1894)
15. Mentho-Nova® (1913)
16. MIN-SO-LATE
17. Mustarine: Begy's True Mustarine
18. Musterole® (1905)
19. Penetro® (1914)
20. Rawleigh's® Medicated Ointment (1911)
21. Rawleigh's® Vapor Balm
22. Rexall® Bronchial Salve
23. Rexall® Catarrh Jelly [later Nasal Jelly]
24. Rexall® Mentholine Balm
25. Rexall® Rex-Mentho Brand Chest Rub
26. Tholene (1927) [later Smith's Mentholated Salve][17]
27. Tiger Balm®
28. Turpo® Vaporizing Ointment
29. UCA-Mentho
30. UCA Vapor Balm
31. Vaseline® Mentholated Petroleum Jelly
32. Vicks VapoRub® (1894)
33. Watkins® Menthol Camphor Ointment
34. Watkins® Vapor Balm
35. Watkins® Volatyle Salve

Information used for product descriptions was obtained from packaging and advertising literature found in the author's collection.
Trademark data when included is from CCH Trademark Research Corporation and the United States Patent and Trademark Office, Trademark Electronic Search System (TESS).

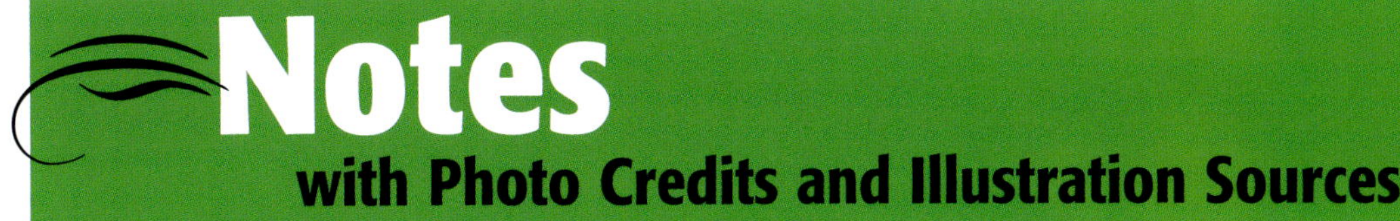

Chapter 1: Everything Goes in Wichita

NOTES

1 "Palmole Soap Factory," *Wichita Eagle* (July 21, 1891), p. 5. Ownership of the Palmole Soap Company changed hands several times between its founding c. 1886 and the 1891 owner, Charles Bros. of Evansville, Indiana. Richard M. Long, ed., *Wichita Century: A Pictorial History of Wichita, Kansas, 1870–1970* (The Wichita Historical Museum Association, Inc., 1969), pp. 24, 34, 35. The original survey by John A. Sroufe (July 3, 1871) called for a crossing of the Arkansas River at Douglas Avenue and for shipping pens to be erected next to the station at the east end of Douglas. Here the river runs north to south, and Douglas runs east and west. The Hon. J. R. Mead recalled that the first herds to reach Wichita in the spring of 1871 forded the river below where the bridge would later be built and followed the still-grass-covered Douglas Avenue east to Chisholm Creek and then on northward to the railhead in Abilene, Kansas. "All that summer and the next the stream of cattle, and trade, and traffic flowed in and through the streets of Wichita." Although the Sedgwick County Commissioners wanted the trail to cross at Kellogg Avenue to avoid the dust and noise, a private toll bridge was built at the Douglas Avenue crossing in 1872, which prolonged the route through town for a few more years. "Settlers and Texas cattle herd owners found it easier and quicker to pay the small toll." According to Sroufe's 1871 survey, the shipping pens were planned to be located east of Wichita on Douglas Avenue between present-day Broadway Avenue and Hydraulic Avenue. (See Long, p. 24.) Their final location, however, was southeast of town on N. A. English's addition adjacent to Kellogg Avenue. (See the 1873 Glover bird's-eye view map.) The *Wichita Eagle* announced that the "Wichita stock yards are now complete," on Friday, June 7, 1872. Perhaps the following statement in the *Wichita Eagle* (June 14, 1872), p. 2, has caused some confusion about the pens being located north of the city: "The old trail crossing, less than 100 yards below the bridge, where the outlet on the north side of the river leads the cattle straight to the stock yards . . ." Technically they crossed to the east side of the river and the straight line was in a southeast direction across the undeveloped town site. After the summer of 1872, the herds were held to crossing town on Douglas Avenue because newly built neighborhoods were blocking their way. Author's note: I have focused a great deal of attention on this portion of the trail because while doing my research in Wichita, I discovered a widespread misconception that somehow the stockyards were located north of town and therefore the cattle were driven up Main Street to reach them.

2 After fighting in the Civil War, A.A.'s oldest brother, George Hyde, went west and became the cashier at Clark & Co. in Leavenworth, Kansas. It was George who invited young Bert to come out from the family home in Lee, Massachusetts, and become his bookkeeper. Craig Miner, *Wichita: The Magic City* (Wichita-Sedgwick County Historical Museum Association, 1988), pp. 17, 63. Morris Kohn was twenty-eight years old when the New York Store opened in 1874. Craig Miner said that Sol Kohn later became the first Jewish mayor of Wichita. A. A. Hyde, *Diary* (Hyde Family Collection, book no. 3), pp. 21, 22. The Wichita Savings Bank would "have a capital of $100,000—50% of which only is expected to be called for and that in monthly installments of 10%." The First National Bank "are doing a rushing business and are reported to be making 50% on their capital of $50,000. It is a very close corporation and a great deal of dissatisfaction is expressed in regard to it and people seem very glad to know there is to be a rival institution."

3 Wayne Gard, *The Chisholm Trail* (Norman, OK: University of Oklahoma Press, 1954), pp. vi, vii, 85, 180, map on page 77; Long, p. 13.

4 Miner, pp. 17, 20; Gard, p. 183.

5 Hyde, *Diary* (book no. 3), p. 22; Long, pp. 33, 34. *Wichita Eagle* (June 5, 1873), p. 3, "The old keno room on the corner has now employed a brass band, which every afternoon discourses music from the balcony on Main Street."

6 A. A. Hyde, *Autobiographical Sketch of the Life of Albert Alexander Hyde* (Hyde Family Collection), pp. 1, 2. Hyde said the temporary bank was located on the "corner of the alley where the Schweiter building now [1930] stands." The *Wichita Eagle* wrote on Friday, July 19, 1872, p. 2, that it was "located first door south of Southern Hotel [east side of North Main]." (See photo of hotel in Long, p. 37.) The move to Eagle Block followed the bank's purchase of one-half of W. J. Hobson's interest for $6,000. A vault was erected in the corner front room, and Hyde took possession and opened the bank for business on Monday morning, September 2, 1872. *Wichita Eagle* (August 9, 1872), p. 3; (August 30, 1872), p. 3.

7 Gard, pp. 213–215; Hyde, *Autobiographical Sketch*, p. 2. Hyde described Keno Corner as "a big saloon, with gambling house over it." Walters's occupation was "looked upon with but little disfavor" in those days. Miner, pp. 21, 29. Keno Corner was on the northwest corner of Main and Douglas, the present site of the First National Bank. It served free meals to its gamblers and

was Wichita's major drinking and gambling establishment before it was closed by state prohibition in 1881.

8 Gard, p. 210; A. A. Hyde, *Diary* (book no. 3), p. 30; A. A. Hyde, *Autobiographical Sketch*, p. 2. "The bookkeeper of the bank, Johnnie Walters, and I furnished a room at the rear of the bank, opening on Main Street, and I lived there until I was married in 1875." "Todd and Royal, grocery jobbing firm, have commenced erection of two story brick business building, 25 by 130 feet, corner Main and 1st Street." *Wichita Eagle* (March 20, 1873), p. 3. "The number of buffalo hides bought at this point is simply enormous. Hays and Brother, C. M. Garrison, and Todd and Royal have been the largest buyers here this winter." *Wichita Beacon* (March 5, 1873), p. 5. Richard White, *"It's Your Misfortune and None of My Own": A History of the American West* (Norman, OK: University of Oklahoma Press, 1991), pp. 308, 309; *Wichita Eagle* (January 21, 1875). "Married—On Tuesday, January 19, 1875, by Rev. S. S. McCabe of Topeka, Mr. Albert A. Hyde and Miss Ida L. Todd, of Wichita. Both parties were favorites here, both parties having done well and our community is a unit in wishing them unbounded happiness and prosperity. We might adorn a notice of this worthy couple, but knowing their unostentatious dispositions, their matter of fact, sensible ideas of things, we desist. Wishing them in the meantime, however, truly from our hearts, A long and present [*sic*] voyage through life." The Todds' home was located on the corner of First and Broadway.

9 White, p. 221; Miner, p. 23. The ticks caused splenic fever, which was commonly called tick, Texas, or Spanish fever. Other factors that influenced the demise of the Chisholm Trail were the introduction of barbed wire fencing and lively competition from towns like Ellsworth and Dodge City. Gard, pp. 215, 236, 259; Long, p. 51.

10 Miner, pp. 27–29; *Annual Report of the Commissioner of Patents for the Year 1877* (Washington, D.C.: Government Printing Office, 1878), p. 103; Official Gazette, vol. 11, p. 570, no. 189,101, April 3, 1877, monthly vol. spec. 80, drg. 28. (Shown at right.)

11 Hyde, *Diary* (book no. 4), pp. 16, 17, 28, 35, 51. Hyde said, "We changed the Bank to a National on the first of November" (1882).

12 Long, p. 58, photographs on pp. 57, 58, 70; Miner, p. 50; White, p. 225.

13 Miner, pp. 51, 52; White, pp. 223–225.

14 Long, p. 58; Miner, pp. 56–58.

15 Hyde, *Autobiography*, p. 3. Hillcrest was located at 3728 East Second Street.

16 Long, p. 81; White, p. 230; Hyde, *Autobiographical Sketch*, pp. 3, 4. Hyde's younger sister, Mary Hyde, and Ida's aunt, Jane Todd (1818–1907)—Mary Hyde worked at the Yucca Company, while Aunt Jane helped Ida with the children.

17 "The Yucca Company," *Wichita Eagle* (May 17, 1890), p. 5.

18 Hyde, *Autobiographical Sketch*, pp. 4, 5; Miner, p. 88. The *Yucca Company Ledger Book* recorded income for 1892 at $6,400.78 and for 1893 at $10,000.25. *Menthology* (vol. 24, 1939, no. 1), insert, "Not until 1893, was it considered ready for the market."

PHOTO CREDITS/ILLUSTRATION SOURCES

Unless otherwise noted, all pictured items are from the author's collection or the Hyde family.

The Empire House (page 1) Wichita-Sedgwick County Historical Museum.

The Best Place to Cross (page 2) Wichita State University Libraries, Department of Special Collections.

New Terminus of the Chisholm Trail (page 3) Wichita-Sedgwick County Historical Museum.

Map (page 3) Based on "Map showing the Atchison, Topeka & Santa Fe Railroad and its Auxiliary Roads in the State of Kansas June 30th 1890" (G. W. & C. B. Colton & Co., New York).

The Eagle Block (page 5) Wichita-Sedgwick County Historical Museum.

Hyde's first house (page 6) Wichita Public Library.

A Period View of a Wichita Bank Interior c. 1887 (page 7) Wichita-Sedgwick County Historical Museum (Citizens Bank, built on the site of the old Keno Corner).

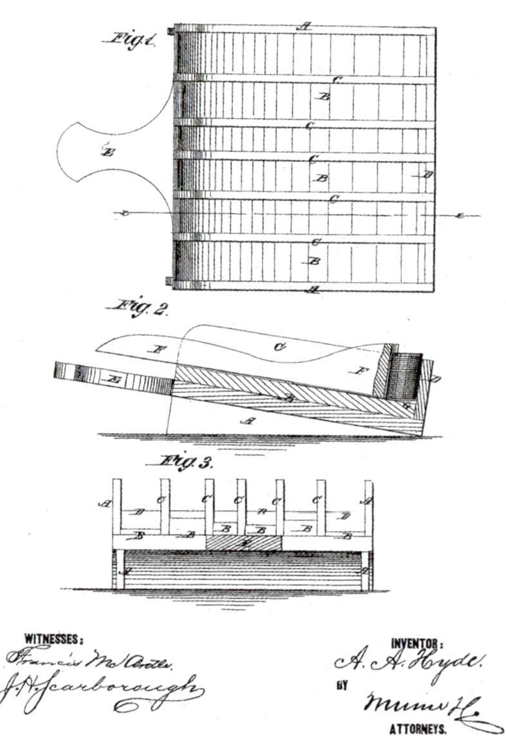

Chapter 2: MEN•THO•LA•TUM

NOTES

1 Hyde Collection, *Yucca Company Ledger Book* (inventory, July 14, 1893), p. 30. In addition to menthol and camphor, they stocked wintergreen, spearmint, sassafras, citronella, lavender, thyme, cedar of Lebanon, clove, and sandalwood oils, to name a few.

2 Ibid. (petrolatum estimates, December 1893), p. 30, a breakdown of material costs to repackage Vaseline in two-ounce corked bottles with a Petrolatum label; (inventory, March 31, 1894), p. 55, "67 Vaseline ($)2.01"; (inventory, July 20, 1899), p. 67, "100# Parafine [*sic*] ($)7.50, 100# Camphor ($)45, 80# Boraeic [*sic*] Acid ($)7.50, 22# Menthol ($)60." The large quantity of paraffin is interesting because there was no mention of petrolatum in the inventory. Note that camphor was 45¢ a pound and menthol was $2.73 a pound. The inventory also included "1/2 gro 4 oz. Vas ($)2.50," which would indicate they were still repackaging Vaseline in 1899. (Note: repackaging Vaseline seems to have been a common practice and considered no different from repackaging other petroleum products like paraffin and machine oil.)

3 *Prices Current of Drugs and Druggists' Sundries, Chemicals, Proprietary Medicines, Paints, Oils, Glass, Etc., Etc.* (Chicago: Lord, Owen & Co., Importers and Wholesale Druggists, 1885), pp. 93, 362.

4 Glenn Sonnedecker, Ph.D., *Kremers and Urdang's History of Pharmacy*, 4th ed. (Madison, WI: American Institute of the History of Pharmacy, 1986), p. 157; James Harvey Young, *The Toadstool Millionaires: A Social History of Patent Medicines in America Before Federal Regulation* (Princeton, NJ: Princeton University Press, 1961), pp. 9–10, 17–19, 32.

5 Sonnedecker, p. 155; Young, p. 8.

6 Laman A. Gray Sr., M.D., *The Life and Times of Ephraim McDowell* (Louisville, KY: Gheens Foundation, 1987), pp. 25, 53. McDowell performed the first successful abdominal surgery, when he removed an ovarian tumor from the abdomen of Jane Todd Crawford (related to Ida Todd Hyde) in 1809.

7 Sonnedecker, pp. 160, 161, 164.

8 Young, pp. 32, 38.

9 David Armstrong and Elizabeth Metzger Armstrong, *The Great American Medicine Show* (New York, NY: Prentice-Hall, 1991), pp. 7, 8.

10 Young, pp. 56, 69, 71.

11 Ibid., pp. 63–64, 68.

12 Hyde Collection, "The Great Japanese Salve," (box insert, c. 1903–1905).

13 Vince Staten, *Do Pharmacists Sell Farms?: A Trip Inside the Corner Drugstore* (New York: Simon & Schuster, 1998), p. 34; Sonnedecker, p. 325. Wholesale catalogs alone represented 2,700 items and sizes in 1880, 38,000 in 1916, and 60,000 in 1933. Young, p. 103.

14 Hyde Collection (card sent to druggists, c. 1902); Young (from the *Druggists Circular*, January 1901), p. 103.

15 Young, pp. 108–109; American Medical Association web page (www.ama-assn.org, Timelines, 1847 to 1899). One of the pernicious medical journals was *The Druggists Circular*, an advertising partner of Hyde's later on.

16 Sonnedecker, pp. 192–194, 207, 295.

17 Young, p. 210.

18 Ibid., pp. 208–210.

19 Ibid., pp. 205, 214, 215, 226, 239, 242.

20 Ibid., p. 244.

PHOTO CREDITS/ILLUSTRATION SOURCES

Unless otherwise noted, all pictured items are from the author's collection or the Hyde family. The Yucca Company Business Forms reside in the Hyde Collection in the Department of Special Collections at Wichita State University. (YBF = Yucca Company Business Forms, page, item number.)

A Brand Is Born (page 11) *Wichita Daily Eagle*, Sunday December 22, 1895.

Imported Menthol and Camphor (page 12) Hyde Collection YBF-1-4, YBF-1-2.

Menthol's Popularity (page 14) Lord, Owen & Co., Wholesale Druggists, Prices Current (Chicago, 1885), p. 362, 5¼″H × 7½″W.

Ponds trade cards (page 15) 3½″H × 5½″W.

Dr. McDowell's Apothecary Shop (page 16) McDowell House Museum, Inc. Restored by the Kentucky Pharmaceutical Association with help from the Eli Lilly Foundation and pharmacists from throughout the state. Charles Pfizer & Company, Inc., donated the Sydney Blumberg apothecary collection.

The Dreaded Scarificator (page 17) Lancet and case from McDowell House Museum, Inc.

Portable Remedies (page 18) Artist: Norman Price, Copyright 1939, Park, Davis & Company, Detroit, Michigan. *The Saturday Evening Post*, October 21, 1939, p. 65.

Mentholatum Cures All (page 20) Hyde Collection YBF-60-70A.

Hyde Speaks Out (page 20) Hyde Collection YBF-27-35.

An Honest Druggist or Bartender? (page 21) *Frank Leslie's Popular Monthly*, May 1889, p. i.

King Catarrh

NOTES

1 John M. Hyde, "A Balm in Gilead," *Kansas History* (vol. 9, no. 4, winter 1986/1987), p. 156; *The American Heritage Dictionary of the English Language* (Boston: Houghton Mifflin Company, 1973), p. 211. Old French *catarrhe*, from late Latin *catarrhus*, from Greek *katarrhous*, a flowing down, from *katarrhein*, to flow down: *kata-*, down + *rhein*, to flow. Clarence Meyer, *The Herbalist Almanac: A 50-Year Anthology* (Glenwood, IL: Meyerbooks, 1988), p. 53.

2 David Freeman Hawke, *Benjamin Rush: Revolutionary Gadfly* (Indianapolis: The Bobbs-Merrill Company, Inc., 1971), p. 397; George M. Beard, A.M., M.D., *Hay-Fever; or,*

Summer Catarrh: Its Nature and Treatment (New York: Harper & Brothers, Publishers, 1876), p. 11 (Beard cites: Bostock, "Medico-Chirurgical Transactions," vol. xii, 1828, p. 437); David Tyrrell and Michael Fielder, *Cold Wars: The Fight Against the Common Cold* (New York: Oxford University Press, 2002), p. 12.

3 Beard, pp. 13, 14 (Beard cites: Gream, *On the Use of Nux Vomica as a Remedy in Hay-Fever*, 1850; Hyde Salter, 1859; and Watson, *Lectures on the Principles and Practice of Physics,* 1857), 24, 27. Blackley's book was titled *Experimental Researches on the Cause and Nature of Catarrhus Æstivus (Hay-Fever, or Hay-Asthma)*, London, 1873. Blackley also suggested it be called "pollen fever."

4 Ibid., pp. 33, 87. Beard limited his research to mountain and seaside resorts and health spas.

5 Ibid., pp. iii, 143, 149, 158–169.

6 "Therapeutic Indications for Acute Nasal Catarrh," *Merck Manual of the Materia Medica* (New York: Merck & Co., 1899), p. 101; Beard, pp. vi, 180, 181.

7 George H. Patchen, M.D., "Chronic Nasal Catarrh; Its Cause and Radical Cure" (*Health Culture*, vol. XVIII, no. 2, February 1912, Whole No. 174), pp. 63–70.

8 Elmer Lee, M.D., editor, "Questions and Answers" (*Health Culture*, February 1912), p. 112. Dr. Lee is considered the father of colonics in America.

9 Jim Bennett, *Bernarr Macfadden*. (www.riverflow.com/macfadden/macfadden1.html) Eugene Sandow (1867–1925). Born Bernard McFadden (1868–1955). When Macfadden realized that publishing alone was going to make him rich, he came up with an idea for the first true-confession magazine called *True Story,* which hit the streets in 1919. *True Story* was a great success and urged him on to create a string of other magazines that included *True Detective*, *True Romances*, *Liberty*, and *Photoplay*, making him a tabloid tycoon.

10 Macfadden, Bernarr, *Colds, Coughs and Catarrh* (New York: Macfadden Publications, Inc., 1926), pp. 31, 38, 40, 53, 55, 56, 111.

11 Ibid., pp. 91–103, 124, 125. Robert Ernst, *Weakness Is a Crime: The Life of Bernarr Macfadden* (New York: Syracuse University Press, 1991).

12 J. H. Kellogg, M.D., *Man the Masterpiece* (Battle Creek, MI: Health Publishing Company, 1891), p. 553.

13 Sanford's Radical Cure for Catarrh, label, c. 1873 (Potter Drug & Chemical Corporation, Boston).

14 *Hazeltine's Pocket Book Almanac for 1894* (Warren, Pennsylvania: Hazeltine & Company).

15 *The Centaur Company Receipt Book*, 1879, p. 25 (author's collection).

16 *Marshall's Illustrated Almanac and Pocket Compendium,* 1904 (author's collection).

17 R. V. Pierce, M.D., *The People's Common Sense Medical Adviser in Plain English; or, Medicine Simplified*, 95th ed. (Buffalo, NY: The World's Dispensary Medical Association, 1924), p. 475.

18 Ibid., pp. 478, 479, 514, 515.

19 Pierce, pp. 480, 482; Gerald Carson, *One for a Man, Two for a Horse: A Pictorial History, Grave and Comic, of Patent Medicines* (Garden City, NY: Doubleday & Co., Inc., 1961), p. 71.

20 R. L. Alsaker, M.D., *Curing Catarrh Coughs and Colds* (New York: Grant Publishing Company, Inc., 1925), pp. 24, 28, 34, 41, 96, 97, 98.

21 Sir Christopher Andrewes, *The Common Cold* (New York: W. W. Norton & Company Inc., 1965), p. 51.

22 Andrewes, pp. 52, 53. Tyrrell and Fielder, pp. 17, 18, 19.

23 J. Barnard Gilmore, *In Cold Pursuit: Medical Intelligence Investigates the Common Cold* (Toronto: Stoddard Publishing Co., Lmtd., 1998), pp. 75, 76, 92. Latter day investigators who applied the wrong deffinition of catarrh were bound to miss Dr. Eric Marshall's meaning. Marshall used catarrh to describe hay fever symptoms that passed almost as soon as the men left the hut where the bale of clothing had been opened. Gilmore observed that when Marshall's report was published in Shackleton's book, "by implication, Marshall refers to these symptoms . . . as if they were colds" and from there the myth was created that colds do not occur in Antarctica unless germs are carried in from temperate climates. I suggest that Marshall implied nothing and that his use of "catarrh" was correct for 1908—it represented colds as well as hay fever inasmuch as they were both "catarrhal effections." In other parts of the report when the illness was clearly a head cold, he said it. Surrounded by rocks, ice, and water, it would have been hard to imagine hay fever was the culprit when sudden catarrhal symptoms developed and then dissipated in a day or two. He called it correctly.

24 Horatio C. Wood, "Sickroom Appliances: Atomizers" (*American Druggist*, July 1932), p. 40. The venturi principle is based on the work of Italian physicist G. B. Venturi (1746–1822).

25 Gilmore, pp. 36, 37, 138.

26 Andrewes, p. 52; Tyrrell and Fielder, p. 23; The Wellcome Trust, http://library.wellcome.ac.uk. Sir Christopher Howard Andrewes, Wilson Smith, and Sir Patrick Laidlaw isolated the first human influenza virus in 1933.

27 Andrewes, p. 173. Andrewes's landmark study was based on his work as the medical officer in charge of the Common Cold Research Unit at the Harvard Hospital in Salisbury, England, from 1946 to 1963 where a massive study was conducted with the help of 8,187 volunteers that were tested with cold virus and lived in dormitories at the complex during the course of their sickness.

PHOTO CREDITS/ILLUSTRATION SOURCES

Unless otherwise noted, all pictured items are from the author's collection or the Hyde family.

A Practical Remedy (page 31) "World's Dispensary and Family Medicine Depot" 1876 Pierce's Memorandum and Account Book (back cover); federal revenue stamp for income tax during and after the Civil War, Private Die Proprietary Stamp (printing cost paid by the company), rs 190b Scott US Specialized Catalog, 3½"H × 7½"W;

unopened bottle of Dr. Sage's Catarrh Remedy (see wax seal) and paper wrapper, c. 1906.

Tankard Inhaler (page 33) A similar example can be found in R. G. Hornsby, *Pewter of the Western World, 1600–1850* (Atglen, PA: Schiffer Publishing, 1983), p. 121, plate 294.

Hunter's Inhaler (page 33) N. B. Wolfe, M.D., *Inhalation: or, How to Cure Catarrh, Asthma, and Consumption* (Cincinnati: self-published, 1975), pp. 8, 9; Beverley Robinson, *A Practical Treatise on Nasal Catarrh and Allied Diseases* (New York: William Wood & Company, 1885), p. 28; Lord, Owen & Co., p. 204.

Cold Vapor (page 34) Robinson, p. 29.

Chapter 3: The Friendly Salve

NOTES

1 Robert B. Cialdini, "The Science of Persuasion" (*Scientific American*, February 2001), pp. 76–81.

2 *Menthology* (vol. 24, 1939, no. 1), insert.

3 "Little Biographies of Famous Products—Number Twenty-six" (*The Glass Packer*, October 1940), p. 600; *Menthology* (vol. 24, 1939, no. 1), insert. "Not until 1893, was it considered ready for the market" (quoted from both sources). *Bulletin of the United States Trade-Mark Association, Forty-Ninth Year* (vol. 31, New York, 1936). CCH Trademark Research Corporation, 1999.

4 Hyde, *Autobiographical Sketch*, p. 5; U.S. Department of Commerce, Bureau of the Census. *Historical Statistics of the United States: Colonial Times to 1970*, part 1 (Washington, DC: Government Printing Office, 1975), p. 213. In 1895, five pounds of flour cost 12¢, and ½ gallon of milk cost 13.6¢. *Yucca Company Ledger Book* (inventory, July 20, 1899), p. 67, "3½ gro 25(¢) Mentho ($)21"; (monthly book sales, 1894 to 1899), pp. 131, 132.

5 Hyde Collection YBF-40-52.

6 Hyde, "A Balm in Gilead," p. 158.

7 *Menthology* (vol. 2, 1917, no. 3), p. 3.

8 Hyde Collection YBF-26-34, *Salesman's Daily Letter* (c. 1900–1903).

9 Hyde, *Autobiographical Sketch*, p. 5; Hyde, *Diary* (book no. 3), p. 10.

10 Scott Eberle and Joseph A. Grand, *Second Looks: A Pictorial History of Buffalo and Erie County* (Virginia Beach, VA: Donning Company/Publishers, 1993).

11 Eberle and Grand, pp. 69, 129, 138–140; R. V. Pierce, *The People's Common Sense Medical Adviser in Plain English: or, Medicine Simplified*, 42nd ed. (Buffalo, NY: World's Dispensary Printing Office, 1895), pp. 944, 946. The first edition was printed in 1875.

12 Eberle and Grand, pp. 118, 119, 136.

13 Ibid., pp. 138–140.

14 Hyde, *Autobiographical Sketch*, p. 5; Hyde Collection, "The Great Japanese Salve" (box insert, c. 1903–1905).

15 CCH Trademark Research Corporation, 1999.

16 Author's collection, jars: no. 2, no. 13, no. 68.

PHOTO CREDITS/ILLUSTRATION SOURCES

Unless otherwise noted, all pictured items are from the author's collection or the Hyde family. The Yucca Company Business Forms reside in the Hyde Collection in the Department of Special Collections at Wichita State University. (YBF = Yucca Company Business Forms, page, item number.)

A First-Class Product (page 38) Drawing of Yucca Company building: *Wichita Eagle*, May 17, 1890, p. 5. Label: 3¼″H × 5¾″W from Hyde Collection YBF-15-22. Photo of Yucca Company building: Wichita-Sedgwick County Historical Museum. 3 oz. jar: Dorsey Museum.

Priming the Pump (page 39) Tin manufacturing information in caption found in Zimmerman, vol. II, p. 6. Envelope in Hyde Collection YBF-16-24A.

Dr. Ella B. Veazie (page 41) *Menthology* (vol. 24, 1939, no. 1), insert. Veazie testimonial verso "The Great Japanese Salve" circular, c. 1903.

Meyer Brothers (page 41) Business card: 2½″H × 3¾″W. Quote from pink trial dozen form c. 1900 (author's collection).

Shipping Mentholatum (page 42) Wichita-Sedgwick County Historical Museum; crate label, 3″H × 6½″W, Hyde Collection YBF-3-7A.

Mentholatum's First Decade of Earnings (page 43) Yucca Co. Ledger Book; Lewis quote: Miner, p. 88; "The Best Thing on Earth" logo: Hyde Collection YBF-48-58.

Cash Back for Sales (page 44) 3¾″H × 7¼″W perforated, Hyde Collection YBF-15-23.

Display Instructions (page 44) 3¼″H × 3¼″W, Hyde Collection YBF-2-6A.

Medicine Time Indicator and Protective Envelope (page 45) 3¼″H × 3¼″W, Hyde Collection YBF-47-57. Indicator: author's collection.

Return Postcard (private mailing card) (page 45) 1898, 3¼″H × 5⅜″W, YBF-16-25A.

Return Postcard (opal jars card) (page 45) YBF-16-25B.

Parker Fountain Pen (page 45) Printer's code 500-8-04, 7¼″H × 3⅜″W, printed in red and blue ink on pink colored bank safety paper, YBF-54-64A.

Spreading the Word (page 46) 16 pages, light blue paper cover, 6″H × 3¼″W.

Write Plain (page 46) refund slip, 7½″H × 3½″W, printed in red and blue on blue card, Hyde Collection YBF-29-39.

Mentholatum Nouveau (page 47) 5¼″H × 1⅞″W, six color plus embossed gold tone on coated card stock.

"A Spa for the Nervous & Careworn" (page 48) Pierce, 42nd edition, p. 922. Eberle and Grand, p. 139.

World's Dispensary Medical Association (page 49) Pierce, 42nd edition, pp. 938, 940, 949.

Working Man's Watch Fob (page 51) Copper- and silver-colored metal disk with Japanese lantern motif, "Nothing Better After Shaving and for Any Inflammation" on verso, 1½″DIA, "Duplicate Fobs 25¢." Original leather strap is rare to find. 4″ length with brass buckle. Courtesy of Houston Barclay. Also: two dragon motif, "Our Best Salve Your Money Back If Not Satisfied" on verso.

The Great Flood (page 52) *The Flood At Wichita, Kansas July 7, 1904.* Souvenir book (Wichita Engraving Co., 1904) 9″H × 7″W.

Touring the 1904 Wichita Flood (page 52) Wichita-Sedgwick County Historical Museum.

Rare Menthocura Bottle and Box (page 53) Courtesy John Hyde.

After Shaving barber shop thermometer (page 53) This handsome wood thermometer stands 21″ high and is 5 1/4″ wide and 3/4″ thick. It is painted in four colors: blue/gray border, cream base, red stripes, and black type. Instructions are provided on the back, in one version pasted on a paper label and in another branded directly into the wood.

After Shaving direction card (page 53) 3 1/2″H × 5 1/2″W. Hyde Collection YBF-20-29.

Chapter 4: "Live Druggists Are the Best"

NOTES

1 Jane Baker, "Home Remedies" (The Gobbler, 1993, www.netsync.net/users/jwilson/fd_06_Remedies.html).

2 Joyce Reinhardt Larson, "Interview with Helmuth Herbert Huber" (www.lib.ndsu.nodak.edu/gerrus/interviews/huber.html).

3 Joyce Gibson Roach, "The News from Horned Toad, Texas: Feeling Puny? Reach for the Mentholatum" (Virtual Texan, November 9, 1997, www.virtualtexan.com/writers/joyce/toad9.htm); Hyde Collection "The Great Japanese Salve," (box insert, c. 1903–1905).

4 Lois Gordon and Alan Gordon, *The Columbia Chronicles of American Life, 1910–1992* (New York: Columbia University Press, 1995), pp. 3, 98, 350.

5 *Menthology* (vol. 1, 1916, no. 2).

6 U.S. Department of Commerce, Bureau of the Census, p. 11.

7 Harold Thomas Hyde, *A. A. Hyde: The Mentholatum Company as Remembered by His Grand Nephew, March 9, 1993* (Hyde Family Reunion, Estes Park, CO, 1993).

8 Harold Thomas Hyde.

9 Hyde Collection YBF-72-83 "Form 5. 20M. 11-06" and YBF-72-82 "Form 13. 25M. 12-06."

10 "The Mentholatum Company of Canada" (Canada Heirloom Series, http://collections.ic.gc.ca/heirloom_series/volume4/404-405.htm); "Railway Industrial Park" (The Economic Development Corporation of Fort Erie, 2000, www.forterie.on.ca/edc/industrial/railwaypark.html); John Robbins, "Mentholatum factory closing doors for good," *The Standard* (St. Catharine's, Ontario), February 20, 2004, Business, p. C8. The building now houses the Fort Erie Multicultural Center.

11 *Menthology* (vol. 12, 1927, no. 3), p. 8; (vol. 16, 1931, no. 4), back inside cover; "Fort Erie, Ontario" (The Economic Development Corporation of Fort Erie, 2000, www.forterie.on.ca).

12 "U.G. Charles" (Skyways, The KSGen Web Project, http://skyways.lib.ks.us/genweb/archives/1918ks/bioc/charleug.html). Revised architectural plans courtesy of the current owner, the Spice Merchant and Schmidt Allen Pott Architects, 1994. Calculations of square footage do not include the basement areas in the front and back of the building.

13 *Menthology* (vol. 1, 1916, no. 2), back cover.

14 "Attacks Wichita Factory, United States Attorney Files Charges That Mentholatum Is Offered as Cure in Cases It Cannot Cure," *Wichita Eagle* (April 23, 1915).

15 "Federal Grand Jury," *Wichita Eagle* (September 27, 1915).

16 James Harvey Young, *The Medical Messiahs: A Social History of Health Quackery in Twentieth-Century America* (Princeton, NJ: Princeton University Press, 1967), pp. 41, 42.

17 Ibid., pp. 45, 48, 49.

18 Smith Richardson, *The Early History and Management Philosophy of Richardson-Merrell* (1975) pp. 47, 50, 52, 53. Richardson provided dates for each phase of the Vicks sales campaign; he even remembers how many sample tins were shipped and how many days it took to do it, yet he couldn't tell us the date they mailed the sample tins to the western states. He wrote, "the Post Office Department issued a new regulation providing that mail would be delivered to the residents of towns and to the rural free delivery boxes surrounding them without the necessity of naming the individual to whom the letter or parcel was to be delivered. It was a simple matter to find out from the local post offices the number of people receiving mail in each area." The USPS has written a book on its own history and even has a Web site with a time line, and nowhere does it mention when this regulation was written. A map is provided in the book that shows each territory Vicks moved into, and the dates are listed. The caption reads, "This map traces the Vick expansion, largely completed by 1920, throughout the United States." Richardson wrote that the effect on sales by giving sample tins directly to the customers on a large scale was learned in New England and that the lesson learned there informed their approach to the western states. I would conclude that the boxcar mailing took place c. 1917–1920. Otherwise, the date remains unknown.

19 Martin M. Kaplan and Robert G. Webster, "The Epidemiology of Influenza," (*Scientific American*, December 1977), pp. 88, 89. *American Experience*, Influenza 1918. www.pbs.org/wgbh/amex/influenza/timeline/index.html.

20 Young, p. 52.

21 C. Howard Hopkins, *20th Century Ecumenical Statesman John R. Mott 1865–1955: A Biography* (Grand Rapids, MI: William B. Eerdmans Publishing Company, 1979), p. 387; Hyde, "A Balm in Gilead," p. 158.

22 *Menthology* (vol. 1, 1916, no. 1), back cover; (vol. 1, 1916, no. 2), inside front cover; (vol. 12, 1927, no. 4), p. 7.

23 Ibid. (vol. 24, 1939, no. 2), p. 10; (vol. 4, 1919, no. 4), p. 8. Details of Walt Mason's life were provided by the Lyon County Historical Archives in Emporia, Kansas.

24 Ibid. (vol. 2, 1917, no. 2), pp. 4, 5, 6.

25 Ibid. (vol. 2, 1917, no. 3), p. 1; (vol. 3, 1918, no. 3), p. 1; Albert T. Hyde, phone interview, May 24, 2001: "Due to shortages of materials in World War II, and I suppose World War I, they used whatever they could find."

26 "Butterick: Our History" (New York: Butterick Publishing Company, www.butterick.com/bhc/pages/articles/histpgs/about.html).

27 *Menthology* (vol. 2, 1917, no. 4), p. 2.

28 Ibid. (vol. 2, 1917, no. 4), inside back cover; 1927 insert from a sample tin and box, titled "Health and Beauty Hints."

29 Morton Salt History (www.mortonsalt.com/mile/girlmile.htm).

30 Young, *The Medical Messiahs*, pp. 113, 117; *FTC v. Block & Co.*, 1 *FTC Decisions* 154 (1918). Violation of section 5 of the act of September 26, 1914. Docket No. 38—June 6, 1918.

31 *Menthology* (vol. 3, 1918, no. 2), pp. 1, 5; (vol. 4, 1919, no. 3), p. 3.

32 Ibid. (vol. 3, 1918, no. 3), p. 4.

33 Gordon and Gordon, p. 86; *Menthology* (vol. 4, 1919, no. 1), p. 3; (vol. 4, 1919, no. 2), p. 2.

PHOTO CREDITS/ILLUSTRATION SOURCES

Unless otherwise noted, all pictured items are from the author's collection or the Hyde family. The Yucca Company Business Forms reside in the Hyde Collection in the Department of Special Collections at Wichita State University. (YBF = Yucca Company Business Forms, page, item number.)

Shelley's Drugstore in 1910 (page 58) Wichita-Sedgwick County Historical Museum. Fancy glass candy globe came from a period drugstore in Pueblo, Colorado.

Match Strike (page 59) Three-color lithographed tin match strike, 4¾″H × 3⅜″W.

Aluminum Novelty (page 60) 3½″H × 5″W. Printed two sides. Scalloped die-cut edges and embossed corner embellishments.

First Advertising Postcard (page 61) 3½″H × 5½″W, chromolith.

Aluminum Calendar/Memo Pad (page 61) 3½″H × 2¼″W, printed two sides.

1912 Postcard (page 62) 3¼″H × 5½″W, chromolith.

Art Nouveau Counter Card (page 63) 3½″H × 5½″W, printed across base of front panel: PAT. 1910, STECHER LITHOGRAPHIC CO. ROCHESTER, N.Y. (See Catalog page C119, Window Displays, Posters, and Signs.)

Pharmacist's Spatula (page 63) Two variations. Serif lettering (pictured below) with a period (.) placed at the end of "MENTHOLATUM," acid etched on full tang blade, brass riveted hardwood scales with concave chamfer at the blade end of handle similar in style to the ferrule on spatulas made by J. Russell & Co., Green River Works. Box lettering (pictured above) acid etched on full tang blade, brass riveted hardwood scales with chamfered bevel at pommel end and rounded at blade end of handle.

Advertising Had No Limits (page 66) Dr. Pierce's Family Medicine trade card, 3¾″H × 2⅜″W, color, c. 1871. Dr. Pierce magazine ad, 1888.

A Nurturing Influence (page 67) Seven-color lithograph. 17¾″H × 11¾″W. Printed on lightweight press board. In addition to the two large chips missing at the corners, an unknown portion of the bottom has also been cut off and is missing from this example.

Japanese "Hang" (page 68) Dorsey Museum. 36″H × 16½″W. Jack Melton at the Dorsey Museum gave the Hyde photograph a date of c. 1910–12.

Mother's Little Helper (page 68) 13¾″H × 9½″W (at base). Die-cut cardboard, easel-back, countertop display. Printed by Hays Litho Co., Buffalo, New York. The 1912 copyright date is printed on the lower right corner. A full-size widow display is in the collection of the Wichita-Sedgewick County Historical Museum.

Temperature Signaled the Cold and Hay Fever Seasons (page 69) "Pure Drugs" 27″H × 7″W × ⅝″D. "Sanitary Barber Shop" 19″H × 6″W × ⅝″D. High-fired porcelain enamel on steel.

What Happened? (page 69) Mentholatum Plaster 8¾″H × 6″W, Hyde Collection YBF-77-90.

Souvenir Postcard c. 1917 (page 71) 3½″H × 5½″W. A similar card was seen at auction with the following postal cancellation: "International Wheat Show October 1–13, 1917 Wichita, Kansas." The card was listed No. 114 in *Peerless Princess of the Plains: Postcard Views of Early Wichita*, Two Rivers Publishing Co., 1976.

Milestone Ad (page 72) *The Delineator*, July 1916, p. 24. 16″H × 10¾″W (full page).

First Vicks Sample Tin (page 76) 1¼″ diameter.

Vicks Was a Salve on a Mission (page 76) Vick's Croup and Pneumonia Salve booklet, eight pages, 6″H × 3″W, 1912.

Bragging Rights (page 77) Vicks VapoRub ad, *Pictorial Review*, January 1921, 15⅝″H × 10¾″W.

Felt Drugstore Pennant (page 82) Duane Shrader.

Butterick Trio (page 82) Cover art from *The Delineator*, July 1918, 16″H × 11¼″W, the Butterick Publishing Company, New York; fashions from page 57.

Limited-Edition Desk Calendar (page 84) 6⅜″H × 3⅜″W.

Little Nurse Aids the Troops (page 86) *The Delineator*, February 1918, 7⅛″H × 4½″W.

MENTHOLATUM

The Ointment with the largest Profit.

SALES LAST YEAR OVER 7 MILLION JARS.

THE MENTHOLATUM CO., 329 HIGH HOLBORN, LONDON, W.C.

The Chemist & Druggist Text Book (London, England, 1917), p. 278

Mighty Menthol

NOTES

1 *The Merck Index: An Encyclopedia of Chemicals, Drugs, and Biologicals, 12th edition* (Merck & Co., Inc., 1996), p. 5882. *Herbal Drugs and Phytopharmaceuticals*, English edition edited by Norman Grainger Bisset (Stuttgart, Germany: Medpharm Scientific Publishers, 1994).

2 *Menthology* (vol. 12, 1927, no. 3), p. 6. Vicks Circular in author's collection.

3 Clarence Meyer, *The Herbalist Almanac, A 50-Year Anthology* (Glenwood, IL: Meyerbooks, 1988), pp. 19, 21.

4 *Menthology* (vol. 12, 1927, no. 3), p. 6; (vol. 14, 1929, no. 3), p. 3, 4. The author of this report, John N. Davies, thought the flowering plant was cut. Other sources disagree and say that the plant should be cut before budding occurs.

5 Jonathan Rose, "Japan's Century of Rapid Progress: From Isolation to Leading Economy," *Scholastic* (vol. 119, April 6, 1987), p. 16. The shoguns had permitted a few Dutch and Chinese merchants to enter.

6 S. Casket, "Menthol," *The Druggists Circular and Chemical Gazette* (vol. XXX, June 1886), p. 138. Sonnedecker, Appendix 7, p. 455. M. J. Dumas, *Memoire sur les Substances vegetales qui se rapprochent du Camphre, et sur quelques huiles essentielles* (Paris: Annales de Chimie et de Physique, 1832), pp. 232, 233. Jean Baptiste Dumas (1800–1884) was one of the founders of physical chemistry.

7 S. Casket, p. 138; A. Oppenheim, Ph.D., "On the Camphor of Peppermint," *The Journal of The Chemical Society of London* (vol. XV, 1862), p. 29.

8 S. Casket, p. 138; Sonnedecker, Appendix 7, p. 457.

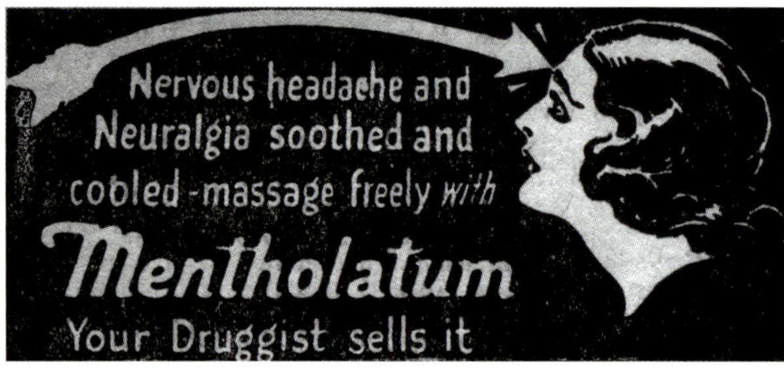

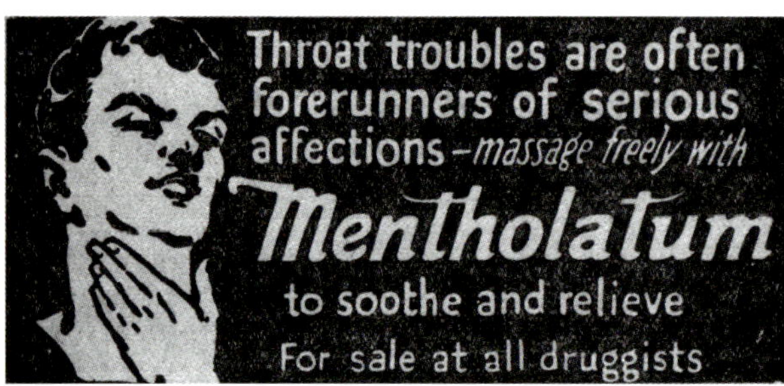

Grier's Almanac (Atlanta, GA: Grier's Almanac Publishing Co., 1925).

9 Product Matrix – Camphor (www.epa.gov); Rx.comPDR for Herbal Medicines (www.rx.com/reference/natural/Camphor.html), p. 751.

10 C. L. Coffin, "Menthol Cones," *The Druggists Circular and Chemical Gazette* (vol. XXX, July 1886), p. 147.

11 *Menthology* (vol. 5, 1920, no. 2), p. 2; (vol. 14, 1929, no. 3), pp. 3, 4; (vol. 14, 1929, no. 4), pp. 2, 3. In the July 1910 issue of *Druggists Circular* the price of menthol listed on page 50 was $3 per pound, indicating Japan's prior record of steady pricing.

12 Albert and his family lived at the "Stone House" in Carmel, eighty miles west of the Mint Ranch. The stone house is today a bed-and-breakfast.

13 The story of the Mint Ranch was assembled from interviews with Robert Mitchell and Albert Hyde. Boelens Aroma Chemical Information Service (BACIS), the Netherlands, "The BACIS Archives: Peppermint Oils and Menthol" (www.xs4all.nl/~bacis/pom96121.html, January 28, 2002); Rajshree Agro Chem, Delhi, India, Knowledge Base: Natural Menthol (www.mentholworld.com/kbase.htm, January 28, 2002); Encyclopedia Britannica, Yahoo! Reference: The Britannica Concise, Menthol, Optical Isomers (http://education.yahoo.com, January 28, 2002); Leffingwell & Associates. Menthol - Page 1 (Background & Organoleptic Properties) (www.leffingwell.com/menthol1/menthol1.htm, January 28, 2002); George Stuart Clark IV, Cameron & Stuart Inc., Easton, Maryland, "Menthol: An Aroma Chemical Profile," *Perfumer & Flavorist* (vol. 23, September/October 1998, Allured Publishing Corp.), pp. 33–46.

14 William Howard Taft, Chairman of the Editorial Board, *Service with Fighting Men: An Account of the Work of the American Young Men's Christian Associations in the World War*. vol. I (New York: Associated Press, 1922), pp. 556, 561. The YMCA provided the services now filled by the USO and established Post Exchanges and Canteens on every battlefield where U.S. soldiers were involved. (General Orders No. 33.)

15 "Process of Treating Cigarette Tobacco" (www.uspto.gov).

16 Lloyd "Spud" Hughes (http://goodhealth.freeservers.com/SPUD1.html).

17 George Stuart Clark IV, pp. 33–46.

PHOTO CREDITS/ILLUSTRATION SOURCES

Unless otherwise noted, all pictured items are from the author's collection or the Hyde family. The Yucca Company Business Forms reside in the Hyde Collection in the Department of Special Collections at Wichita State University. (YBF = Yucca Company Business Forms, page, item number.)

Mentha Arvensis (page 88) Original art for the book by Sarah Abigail Young © 2003. All rights reserved.

K. Kobayashi label (page 88) $4\frac{5}{8}$"H × $3\frac{1}{2}$"W, Hyde Collection YBF-1-3.

***Menthology* cover** (page 89) (vol. 11, 1926, no. 2).

Chemical structure of menthol (page 91) *The Merck Index: An Encyclopedia of Chemicals and Drugs*, Eighth edition (Rahway, NJ: Merck & Co., Inc., 1968), p. 653.

1876 Centennial Exhibition Opening Day (page 92) Photos courtesy of the Print & Picture Collection, Free Library of Philadelphia.

"Menthol Novelties" (page 93) From *McKesson & Robbins' Prices Current*, 1887, p. 160.

Eucalyptus (page 94) Chromolith by J. L. Goffart, Brusselles, artist J. R. Guillot. del., *Revue Horticole Journal D'Horticulture Pratique* (Paris: Librairie Agricole de la Maison Rustique, 1901).

Novelty Spelled Success for Ludens (page 95) Ludens novelty perpetual calendar, ad from cover shown, 2½"H × 3⅞"W, 1895 edition, 16 pages plus cover.

Where Is the Menthol? Vicks jars (page 95) Seventy-fifth Anniversary of Richardson-Merrell, Inc., commemorative tray.

***Menthology* cover** (page 96) (vol. 11, 1926, no. 4).

Distillation Plant (page 98) Hyde family photo "Our Still, A. T. H. Ranch."

A Casualty of War (page 99) *Association Men* (vol. XLIV, no. 3, November 1918), p. 188.

The Fifth-Largest Brand (page 100) ½-pound can: Manufactured by Rock City Tobacco Co. Lmtd. Factory No. 6 Port 13D for Philip Morris & Co. Ltd., Inc. (1936).
Package: The Axton-Fisher Tobacco Co. Louisville, Kentucky Factory #24 US Pat. No. 1555580.
Ads: "Big Show," February 1936 *Fortune* magazine, 5"H × 13⅕"W, b&w. "Like a Trooper," July 1929 *Literary Digest* (detail).

The House of Menthol (page 101) Sign in store window.

Chapter 5: Feel It Heal

NOTES

1 Material for the Ethel Smith Willard (1900–2001) story came from an interview conducted by the author on October 28, 2000. Other material came from the following: *Grandma Willard's Mentholatum Company* (Kim Marvin Mann, manuscript, 1998) and "Working for a Great Company, a Great Man," Newton Kansan Online (http://thekansan.com, 1999), Kansan Online Reminiscing. White, pp. 432, 433.

2 *Menthology* (vol. 5, 1920, no. 1), insert, article by John S. Capper reprinted from the *Chicago Tribune*; (vol. 5, 1920, no. 2), p. 4, article by Elbert Hubbard; (vol. 5, 1920, no. 4), pp. 7, 8.

3 Miner, pp. 122, 123, 124, 129.

4 *Menthology* (vol. 12, 1927, special issue), pp. 3, 9, 14.

5 Miner, p. 126.

6 "Mentholatum Plant Planned for Perfect Dispersion of Ingredients," *The Glass Packer* (October 1940), pp. 598–601; *Menthology* (vol. 26, 1941, no. 2), pp. 6, 7.

7 *Menthology* (vol. 5, 1920, no. 4), p. 4; (vol. 6, 1921, no. 1), p. 4; (vol. 6, 1921, no. 4), p. 4; (vol. 7, 1922, no. 1), p. 4.

8 *Collier's, The National Weekly* (February 4, 1922), pp. 26, 28; *Menthology* (vol. 7, 1922, no. 2), p. 6. "Best Selling Toilet Preparations: Retail Druggists in all Sections of the Country Tell What Are Their Best Selling Dentifrices, Cold Creams, Ointments, Rouges and Face Powders," *The Druggists Circular* (vol. LXVI, no. 1, New York, January 1922) pp. 13, 14. The other ointments listed were Unguentine, Poslam, Iodex, and Palmer's Skin Success. The article also reported that Musterole and VapoRub were in more demand in the "cold-in-the-chest" regions of the East and Middle West than in the South with its longer summer season. In 1932, *Fortune* named Vicks, Mentholatum, and Musterole the top-three-selling cold rubs on the market. "The Cold Business," *Fortune* (vol. VI, no. 4, October 1932), pp. 26–31, 88.

9 *Menthology* (vol. 7, 1922, no. 3), pp. 3, 6.

10 Ibid. (vol. 10, 1925, no. 2), p. 4; (vol. 11, 1926, no. 3), p. 3; (vol. 12, 1927, no. 2), pp. 4, 7.

11 *Menthology* (vol. 5, 1920, no. 3), p. 8; (vol. 6, 1921, no. 1), p. 2; (vol. 12, 1927, no. 4), p. 10.

12 Ibid. (vol. 8, 1923, no. 3), notice on back cover said, "This issue of MENTHOLOGY is addressed from an entirely new mailing list - Our old list having been destroyed when the storage basements of our Wichita Factory were flooded on June 10th, 1923. We hope this issue will reach all of our old customers. Alex Hyde, Editor."

13 Ibid. (vol. 9, 1924, no. 4) p. 7; (vol. 10, 1925, no. 1), p. 7; (vol. 12, 1927, no. 2), p. 6; (vol. 12, 1927, no. 4), p. 9.

14 Ibid. (vol. 10, 1925, no. 4), p. 7; (vol. 12, 1927, no. 4), pp. 7, 12; "The Cold Business," *Fortune*, p. 88.

15 Ibid. (vol. 17, 1932, no. 3), inside back cover; Robert J. Samuelson, "What We Learn from the 1920s," *Newsweek* (February 12, 2001), p. 33; statistics quoted from Frederick Lewis Allen, *Only Yesterday* (1931).

16 Richardson, p. 82.

PHOTO CREDITS/ILLUSTRATION SOURCES

Unless otherwise noted, all pictured items are from the author's collection or the Hyde family.

Display case (page 102) Mock-up by author of period product display.

Shaving (page 103) ½-lb. can manufactured in Bridgeburg plant with directions in French and English; excerpt from *Menthology* (vol. 7, 1922, no. 2), p. 4

The Dapper Salesman (page 104) Courtesy of Biff Henrich and the CEPA Archive Collection (http://cepa.buffnet.net/exhibits/EXHIBIT.19961997/historic/). This photo was identified in the exhibit as a western New York image. The steering wheel is on the left side of the cab, there is a Kodak sign in the window, and the salesman looks like an American, leading one to doubt the English origin of the shot. The author's friend in London says it is clearly British in origin.

Little Nurse poster (page 104) 28¾"H × 17½"W.

The Breathable Balm English Jar (page 104) see Jars, Caps, Labels, and Boxes, J40 Catalog page C15.

Coleman Lamp (page 105) Carl R. Tucker and Herb Ebendorf, *Coleman Collectors Guide 1903–1954* (Wichita, KS: self-published,1996), p. 27.

Coleman ad (page 105) *Delineator*, February 1920.

Slough, Bucks, England Plant (page 105) "Mentholatum's Success Story," *The Buffalo News Magazine*, August 6, 1978.

The Wichita Plant (page 107) Two photos courtesy of Kathlyn Schoof, Salina, Kansas.

The Wichita Plant Floor Plan (page 109) Based on architectural plans of the building courtesy of Robert A. Boewe, the Spice Merchant, and Schmidt Allen Pott Architects, Wichita, Kansas.

The Front-Office Staff in 1925 (page 110) Courtesy of Ethel Willard family.

Lifetime Employee (page 111) Courtesy of his son Richard H. Taylor, Dodge City, Kansas.

The Club House (page 111) The Club House was described on page 9 of the souvenir book of the seventy-seventh birthday of A. A. Hyde, March 2, 1925.

Employee Respect (page 111) Courtesy of Ethel Willard family.

Y-Camp Vacation (page 112) Three photos courtesy of Ethel Willard family.

The Buffalo Factory (pages 114–117) Sixteen photos: Hyde Collection.

Mimics (pages 118–119) Mentho-Nova, Mentho Nova Company, Towson, MD; Menthene, S-P Laboratories, Dallas, TX; Japanese Menthodine, Pfeiffer Chemical Company, St. Louis and Philadelphia; Mere Mentho Vapo, Central Specialty Products Co., Navarre, KS; Hy Pure Mentholeum Balm, Hy Pure Laboratories, Cincinnati, OH; Mintol Vapocream, "Special Notice for Treating Spanish Influenza," Home Relief Laboratory, Malden, MA; Perrigo's Menthol Balm, L. Perrigo Company, Mfg. Chemists, Allegan, MI.

Helpful Household Hints (page 119) 6½″H × 3½″W, twelve pages, McCormick-Armstrong Press, Wichita, KS.

The Sunburn Triptych (page 120) Sunburn window display 30″H × 51″W.

A Rare Roll (page 121) Photo of package of cough drops courtesy Edgar Simon, Owanka, South Dakota.

The Not-So-Little Nurses (page 124) Courtesy of Ethel Willard family.

Better than French Creams (page 125) 6⅜″H × 3⅜″W, one fold, four-color front, black ink verso.

The Front-Office Staff in March 1928 (page 125) Courtesy of Ethel Willard family.

1929 Products Roster (page 126) c. 1929 product insert, 8½″H × 5½″W, one fold, blue ink front, black ink verso.

China Rep (page 126) *Menthology* (vol. 14, no. 1, 1929), p. 7.

A. A. Hyde's Favorite Photo (page 127) 9½″H × 7½″W, black-and-white print with color tinting; poem from *Menthology* (vol. 15, Spring 1930, no. 2).

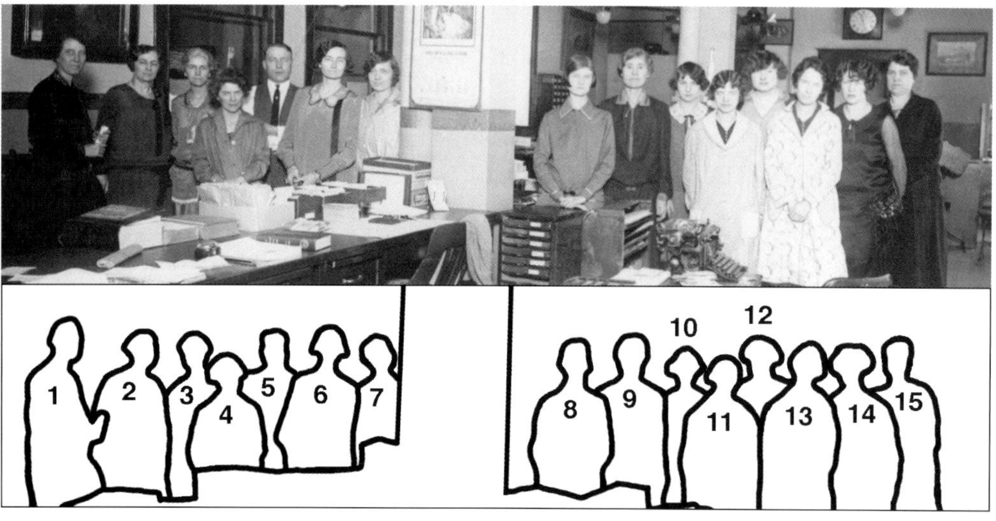

The Front-Office Staff of the Mentholatum Company, Wichita, Kansas, Factory (c. 1925)
1. Ida Dofflemyre; 2. Bess Martin; 3. Unknown; 4. Margaret Saxe; 5. A. J. Henson; 6. Clara Smith Fisher; 7. Ethel Smith; 8. Cecelia Schooley; 9. Unknown; 10. Aaron Reed; 11. Wilma Coffey; 12. Unknown; 13. Unknown; 14. Nell Satterfield; 15. Margaret Langowsky

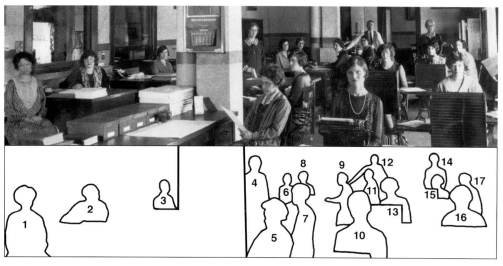

The Front-Office Staff of the Mentholatum Company, Wichita, Kansas, Factory (c. 1928)
1. Orpha Parks; 2. Aaron Reed; 3. Ethel Smith; 4. Bess Martin; 5. Margaret Saxe; 6. Unknown; 7. Mae Kissel (?); 8. Josephine Smith; 9. Ida Dofflemyre; 10. Cecelia Schooley; 11. Margaret Langowsky; 12. A. J. Henson; 13. Nell Satterfield; 14. Lela Hobson; 15. Earline Gaines; 16. Hattie Lou Howe; 17. Wilma Coffey

Chapter 6: Make the Passer-Buy

NOTES

1 Gordon and Gordon, pp. 211, 212, 220; *Menthology* (vol. 16, 1931, no. 4), inside front cover.

2 Contained in: *A Brief Extract of Governor Sweet's Remarks on the Life and Service of A. A. Hyde at the Meeting of the General Board of (the) National Council of the YMCA at the Shelton Hotel, Sunday, January 20, 1935*. Ms at the National YMCA Archives.

3 *Menthology* (vol. 17, 1932, no. 2), p. 10; (vol. 17, 1932, no. 4), pp. 4, 8.

4 Gordon and Gordon, pp. 194, 203, 238, 247; White, pp. 477–479; *Menthology* (vol. 21, 1936, no. 2), p. 6; (vol. 22, 1937, no. 2), p. 7. The company sent special reps into the devastated areas to help druggists destroy damaged stock and replace it with new.

5 *Menthology* (vol. 18, 1933, no. 2), p. 8; (vol. 19, 1934, no. 4), pp. 3, 6, 15, 20, 24, 26.

6 Ibid. (vol. 15, 1930, no. 3), pp. 2, 5; (vol. 15, 1930, no. 4), p. 7.

7 Ibid. (vol. 16, 1931, no. 2), inside front cover.

8 Ibid. (vol. 17, 1932, no. 2), p. 7.

9 Ibid. (vol. 18, 1933, no. 1), p. 6.

10 Ibid. (vol. 18, 1933, no. 4), pp. 6, 7.

11 Solomon H. Snyder, *Drugs and the Brain* (www.druglibrary.org/schaffer/cocaine/amphhis.htm) (www.narconon.org/druginfo/methamphetamine_hist.html).

12 *American Druggist* (July 1932), pp. 12, 92; (April 1932), p. 142.

13 *Menthology* (vol. 19, 1934, no. 1), p. 6, insert.

14 Young, *The Medical Messiahs*, pp. 158–161.

15 Ibid., pp. 160, 164–166.

16 Ibid., pp. 167–170, 175, 178, 188.

17 Ibid., pp. 184, 189, 190, 193, 194; *Menthology* (vol. 23, 1938, no. 3), p. 12.

18 Young, *The Medical Messiahs*, p. 311.

19 Gordon and Gordon, pp. 203, 212, 221; *Menthology* (vol. 15, 1930, no. 4), p. 8; (vol. 18, 1933, no. 3), pp. 7, 8; (vol. 20, 1935, no. 4), p. 7; (vol. 21, 1936, no. 3), p. 7; (vol. 24, 1939, no. 2), pp. 6, 7.

20 *Japan Commerce* (Tokyo: Japan Foreign Trade Federation, 1939 New York World's Fair). "Newark Retail Merchants Unite to Fight Jap Goods Threat," *American Druggist* (December 1935), p. 29.

21 *Menthology* (vol. 8, 1933, no. 2), p. 7; (vol. 20, 1935, no. 3), p. 12; (vol. 24, 1939, no. 3), pp. 6, 7. The Mentholatum agent in Colombia in 1945 was Cornelio Anzola, Apartado Aereo No. 37, Manizales, Colombia.

22 Gordon and Gordon, p. 265; *Menthology* (vol. 21, 1936, no. 1), pp. 6, 7; (vol. 22, 1937, no. 3), p. 7. Also spelled "Miller-Tidings." Sonnedecker, pp. 295, 296.

23 *Menthology* (vol. 20, 1935, no. 2), p. 13.

24 *Menthology*, (vol. 26, 1941, no. 2), p. 3; John Hyde, letter to the author, February 16, 2000.

25 *Menthology* (vol. 21, 1936, no. 1), inside back cover; (vol. 23, 1938, no. 2), p. 2; (vol. 26, 1941, no. 3), pp. 6, 7; Staten, pp. 96, 97.

26 *Menthology* (vol. 20, 1935, no. 1), pp. 6, 7; (vol. 21, 1936, no. 2), p. 12.

27 Walter A. Wells, "Why Catch Cold?" *The American Magazine* (November 1932), pp. 50, 97–99.

28 *Menthology* (vol. 7, 1922, no. 1), p. 4.

29 Ibid. (vol. 17, 1932, no. 2), inside back cover.

30 Ibid. (vol. 24, 1939, no. 1), pp. 4, 12.

31 Gordon and Gordon, pp. 275, 283.

PHOTO CREDITS/ILLUSTRATION SOURCES

Unless otherwise noted, all pictured items are from the author's collection or the Hyde family.

A. A. Hyde at His Desk (page 129) The earliest use of this image was in the souvenir book of his seventy-seventh birthday on March 2, 1925.

The Hydes (page 132) Sitting (left to right): George A. Hyde, youngest son; A. A. Hyde; Edward K. Hyde, second-oldest son. Standing (left to right): Paul H. Hyde, second-youngest son; Charles H. Hyde, third-youngest son; Albert T. Hyde, oldest son; Alexander Hyde, third-oldest son.

"Winter 'Sports'" (page 154) Courtesy Duane Shrader.

Omi Mission Factory

NOTES

1 The Mentholatum Company Web site history time line indicates: 1913 Vories acquired selling rights; 1920 Vories started importation and marketing. The Omi Brotherhood Company, Ltd., produced a historical time line which states under 1920, "Mr. Hyde offered to Mr. Vories the exclusive right to be the sales agent in Japan. Mr. Vories started the Omi Sales Co., Ltd. for Mentholatum in Japan."

2 "The Vories House," the Leavenworth County Historical Society (www.leavenworth-net.com/lchs/plaques.htm#vor). The Leavenworth Historical Society said that Vories's negotiations were between MacArthur and Emperor Hirohito and that he "is credited with Hirohito remaining as emperor after the occupation of U.S. Forces." The Japanese biography said that he "worked to arrange the discussions between Marshal MacArthur and Humimaro Konoe, the former Prime Minister." He was later thanked by Emperor Showa for making the arrangements. For more on Vories, see another biography that John Hyde brought to my attention: Grace Niles Fletcher, *The Bridge of Love* (New York: Dutton, 1967).

ADDITIONAL REFERENCES

William Merrell Vories, *A Mustard-Seed in Japan*, 5th ed. (Omi-Hachiman, Japan: Omi Mission, 1925): *Galilee Maru*, pp. 66, 67, 68; Mr. & Mrs. Vories, p. 70; Jesus Medicine, pp. 120, 121.

"William Merrell Vories," BIWALOBE Corporation (www.biwa.ne.jp/~v-c/englishversion/eindex.html).

PHOTO CREDITS/ILLUSTRATION SOURCES

Unless otherwise noted, all pictured items are from the author's collection or the Hyde family.

Fiftieth Anniversary (page 156) 7½″H × 5³⁄₁₆″W, two-color, three-fold over.

The *Galilee Maru* on Lake Biwa (page 157) Courtesy of Omi Brotherhood.

Maki and William Merrell Vories (page 158) Courtesy of Omi Brotherhood Co., Ltd.

Chapter 7: Modernity's Test

NOTES

1 Sonnedecker, pp. 50, 51.

2 Ibid., pp. 290, 291, 294, 297.

3 Albert T. Hyde, phone interview, May 30, 2001. Albert Hyde said there were two wholesale trade associations: the National Wholesale Drug Association and the Federal Wholesale Drug Association.

4 Sonnedecker, pp. 295, 299. Dan Jorndt, Chairman and CEO, *Walgreens Celebrating 100 Years*, Walgreen Co., 2001.

5 CCH Trademark Research Corporation, 1999; Sonnedecker, p. 299; Staten, pp. 35–37. Both Sonnedecker and Staten give 1907 for the founding of United Drug Company.

6 Sonnedecker, pp. 296, 297, 300–303.

7 Albert T. Hyde, phone interview, April 30, 2001, re: rack jobbers.

8 Sonnedecker, pp. 330–335. [Staten also provides the example of German-made Bayer Aspirin, which lost its trademark due to war reparations in the 1919 Treaty of Versailles (p. 50).]

9 Sonnedecker, pp. 297, 306, 315.

10 Peter Morell, *Poisons, Potions and Profits: The Antidote to Radio Advertising* (New York: Knight Publishers, Inc., 1937), pp. 261, 263, 264 (Morell cites: *Variety*, December 30, 1936); *The American Magazine* (January 1935), pp. 103, 123, 125, 129, 133; Albert T. Hyde, phone interview, May 30, 2001.

11 *Menthology* (vol. 29, 1944, no. 1), p. 9.

12 Albert T. Hyde, phone interview, May 24, 2001.

13 *Menthology* (vol. 23, 1937, no. 2), p. 1.

14 John Hyde, letter to the author, February 16, 2000.

15 *Menthology* (vol. 26, 1941, no. 3), p. 1; (vol. 26, 1941, nos. 2 & 3), p. 2; (vol. 26, 1941, no. 3), pp. 6, 7; *Life* magazine (January 26, 1948); *Esquire* magazine (April 1949); U.S. Department of Commerce, Bureau of the Census, p. 213. Five pounds of flour cost 26.4¢ in 1942 and 32.1¢ in 1945. One-half gallon of milk was 30¢ in 1942 and 31.2¢ in 1945. One pound of coffee cost 28.3¢ in 1942 and 30.5¢ in 1945.

16 *Menthology* (vol. 25, 1940, no. 1), pp. 6, 7; Albert T. Hyde, phone interview, May 30, 2001; "British Take U.S. Branch Plant," *New York Times* (June 10, 1941), p. 8.

17 *Menthology* (vol. 26, 1941, no. 1), pp. 6, 7, 9.

18 Ibid. (vol. 27, 1942, no. 2), pp. 6, 7.

19 Albert T. Hyde, phone interview, May 23, 2001.

20 Ibid., phone interview, May 24, 2001.

21 Ibid., phone interview, April 30, 2001, re: marines.

22 Staten, pp. 38, 39. The 1922 box label does not have "Ben-Gay" on it; the 1939 box label does.

23 Albert T. Hyde, phone interview, April 30, 2001. When Albert left in 1988, sales represented 60 percent from the drug business and 40 percent from the food business.

24 Albert T. Hyde, phone interview, April 30, 2001, re: stick packing machinery.

25 June Eastin, *Bottles West* (self-published, 1965), p. 6. Based on an interview with Edward K. Hyde II. Polystyrene jars were introduced in 1959.

26 Albert T. Hyde, phone interview, April 30, 2001, re: entry of retail food market.

27 Staten, p. 130; CCH Trademark Research Corporation. It was first labeled "Mentholatum Rub" (1953), then "Deep Heat Rub," then "Deep Heating Rub" (first commerce date October 5, 1960, trademark filing 1961, registered 1962), then "Deep Heating" (first commerce date October 1953, trademark filing September 24, 1973, registered August 6, 1974). September 1954 trade ad, J. Walter Thompson Collection, Hartman Center for Sales, Advertising & Marketing History, Duke University, Durham, NC. Albert T. Hyde, phone interview, April 30, 2001, re: Deep Heat. "Elected to Presidency of the Mentholatum Co.," *New York Times* (March 7, 1955), p. 36. "The directors of the Mentholatum Company have elected Albert Taylor Hyde as president, it was announced over the week-end." "Three other grandsons of the late A. A. Hyde are also with Mentholatum: Edward K. Hyde 2nd, Theodore A. Hyde, and George H. Hyde. They succeed their fathers, who became members of the advisory committee." "Added to the board are William Resor, a vice president of the J. Walter Thompson Company . . ." [Arthur joined later.]

PHOTO CREDITS/ILLUSTRATION SOURCES

Unless otherwise noted, all pictured items are from the author's collection or the Hyde family.

1940 Color Insert (page 161) Four-color litho courtesy Dorsey Museum; statistic found in *Menthology* (vol. 26, 1941, no. 2), p. 6.

The Old Guard (page 163) *American Druggist: The Pharmaceutical Business Magazine, Founded 1871*, vol. LXXXVIII, no. 2, August 1933. (New York: International Publications, Inc.) Cover Design by Harold N. Anderson.

The Modern Corner Drugtore (page 164) Black-and-white photo postcard, 3½″H × 5⅜″W.

Rexall Brand (page 165) 7¾″H × 5″W, 32 pages.

Independent Rexall Retailer (page 165) Color photo postcard, 3½″H × 5⅜″W, Le Deane Studio, Tucumcari, NM. Alfred McGarr Adv. Ser., P. O. Box 646, Albuquerque, NM.

The Rexall Way (page 166) 5¾″H × 3⅞″W, black ink, eight pages, stapled.

Rival Cold Rubs (pages 168–171) DeWitt's Vaporizing Balm, E. C. DeWitt & Co., Inc., Chicago, IL; Penetro, Penetro

Company, Division of Plough Inc., New York; Tholene, Rosebud Perfume Co., Woodsboro, MD; Watkins Menthol-Camphor Ointment, J. R. Watkins Co., Winona, MN; Bengue (Ben-gay), Bengue, Inc., Union City, NJ; Rexall Bronchial Salve, United Drug Company, Boston, St. Louis; Cloverine Mentho Balm, the Wilson Chemical Co., Tyrone, PA; McNess Mentholated Ointment, Furst-McNess Co., Freeport, IL; Rawleigh's Medicated Ointment, the W. T. Rawleigh Co., Freeport, IL; Begy's True Mustarine, S. C. Wells & Co., Le Roy, NY.

The All-Purpose Display (page 173) *Menthology* (vol. 27, 1942, no. 1).

New Medicated Stick (page 175) Quote from *Chain Store Age*, January 1952. J. Walter Thompson Advertising Agency Collection (Durham, NC: Duke University, Hartman Center for Sales, Advertising & Marketing History).

New packaging (page 176) 1 oz. box code "254-4MM-39" (1954); price tag on tube box reads "Price .45 Sales Tax .02 Total .47."

Ad lighter (page 177) "Vu-lighter" by Scripto, Vu-lighter Corporation, Atlanta, GA (Pat. No. 2529094).

Deep Heat ad (page 177) From back side of 1954 directions insert, large portion of 8½"H × 5½"W shown, blue and red ink.

Mentholatum 66-Year Time Line

NOTES

1 *Menthology* (vol. 24, 1939, no. 1), insert. There is also evidence in the 1893 inventory of all the right materials used to make Mentholatum.

2 CCH Trademark Research Corporation.

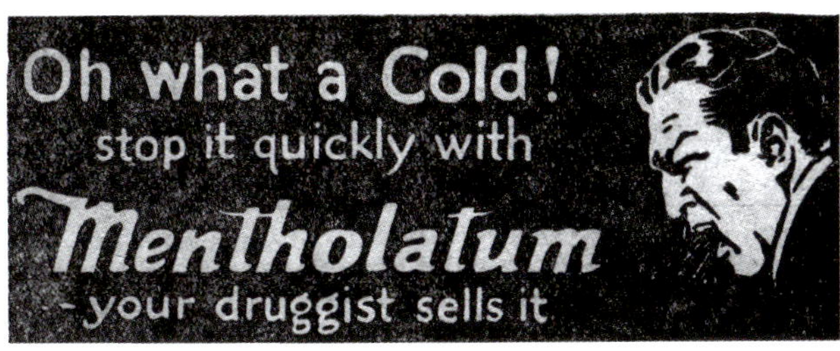

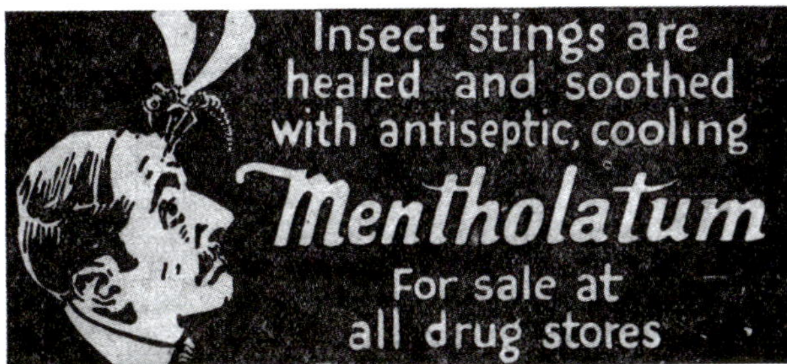

Grier's Almanac (Atlanta, GA: Grier's Almanac Publishing Co., 1925).

3 *Wichita Daily Eagle* (December 22, 1895). *Menthology* (vol. 24, 1939, no. 1), history insert. Yucca Company Ledger Book, p. 58. Specialties 1895.

4 *Wichita Daily Eagle* (September 27, 1896).

5 Yucca Company Ledger Book, p. 67. Inventory January 20, 1899. "10 gro 3/4 in tin boxs. 100 gro 3/8 in tin boxes." "Blotters." Only "Samples" are listed on inventories prior to this.

6 Hyde Collection, YBF-33-42. "50¢ jars contain 3 times quantity of 25¢ size and are packed in boxes." Yucca Company Ledger Book, p. 69. Inventory February 2, 1900. "150 - 50¢ Menth Bxs."

7 Hyde Autobiography, p. 5.

8 Hyde, *Autobiographical Sketch*, p. 5. *Menthology* (vol. 24, 1939, no. 1), history insert.

9 *Bulletin of the United States Trade-Mark Association, Forty-Ninth Year*, vol. 31 (New York: 1936).

10 *Menthology* (vol. 12, 1927, no. 3), p. 8.

11 *Cosmopolitan Magazine* (September 1912), p. 124.

12 Vories, *A Mustard-Seed in Japan*, pp. 66, 67.

13 *Menthology* (vol. 12, 1927, no. 3), p. 8. "Built in 1914."

14 Ibid. (vol. 1, 1916, no. 1), p. 1.

15 Ibid. (vol. 1, 1916, no. 3), inside back cover; (vol. 1, 1916, no. 4), inside back cover; (vol. 2, 1917, no. 2), p. 6. *The Delineator* (July 1916), p. 24. "Mail Coupon now for Free Sample or Jap Pocketbox."

16 *Menthology* (vol. 5, 1920, no. 2), p. 9, "was adopted in the early part of 1917."

17 Ibid. (vol. 12, 1927, no. 3), p. 9, "built in 1919."

18 *The Druggists Circular* (vol. LXVI, no. 1, New York, January 1922), pp. 13, 14; *Menthology* (vol. 7, Spring 1922, no. 1), p. 6.

19 *Menthology* (vol. 12, 1927, no. 3), p. 14, "under the direction of Mr. T.W. D. Turner."

20 Ibid. (vol. 10, 1925, no. 4), p. 7.

21 Ibid. (vol. 12, 1927, no. 3), p. 3.

22 Ibid. (vol. 12, 1927, no. 3), p. 13, advertising; (vol. 12, 1927, no. 4), pp. 7, 12, large jar, applicator.

23 Sample tin S20 found in box with insert titled "Health and Beauty Hints." Artwork corresponds with 1927 print advertising in *Woman's Home Companion* titled "Feel it Heal." Transition to "Many Ills" might have been as early as 1925, but the 1927 tin is the only hard evidence found so far.

24 *Menthology* (vol. 26, 1941, no. 2), p. 3, "For the eleventh year . . ."

25 Ibid. (vol. 16, 1931, no. 2), p. 6, in 1931, the club numbered 976 members.

26 National Recovery Administration, August 25, 1933. *Menthology* (vol. 18, 1933, no. 1), cover. Sample tin insert code #1033195-656M; (vol. 18, 1933, no. 3), pp. 6, 7.

27 Kathlyn Schoof said that the large tins were filled at the Wichita plant. The 1935 Woods letter contained a large tin mailed from the Wichita address. No large tins have been found with just the Buffalo or Wilmington address with the exception of the Canada tin.

28 *Menthology* (vol. 21, 1936, no. 1), inside back cover.

29 Ibid. (vol. 24, 1939, no. 1).

30 Wallace C. Mills, assignor to J. L. Clark Mfg., Co., Patent No. 2,186,728 Jan 9, 1940. *Menthology* (vol. 24, Summer 1939, no. 2), cover illustration.

31 *Good Housekeeping* (January, 1939), ad illustration. Crimping was probably in use much earlier, c. 1937.

32 *Menthology* (vol. 26, 1941, no. 2), pp. 3, 6.

33 J. Walter Thompson Advertising Agency Collection (Durham, NC: Duke University, Hartman Center for Sales, Advertising & Marketing History).

34 J. Walter Thompson Advertising Agency Collection (Durham, NC: Duke University, Hartman Center for Sales, Advertising & Marketing History). Survey of Center's collection compared with author's collection.

35 Prices published in the April 1949 *Esquire Magazine* ad. (See print advertising p. 381.)

36 J. Walter Thompson Collection, September 1954 trade ad.

37 June Eastin, *Bottles West*, 1965, p. 6. Based on an interview with Edward K. Hyde II. Polystyrene jars were introduced in 1959.

The Competition

NOTES

1 "The Cold Business," *Fortune*, pp. 26, 30, 31. Numbers of medicines quoted in the article were taken from *The American Druggist's Yearbook*.

2 "The Cold Business," *Fortune*, p. 88.

3 Richardson, pp. 16, 17. When Smith Richardson referred to the ingredients in his book, he called them "rubefacient," or substances that irritate the skin (p. 30). One of the young clerks in the store was a nephew of Dr. Porter, William Sydney Porter, who later became the famous short story writer "O. Henry" (p. 16). Leadership Greensboro. Porter-Richardson Drugstore (http://www.greensboro.com/gsotour/porter.htm). Product inserts tell different variations of the company history.

4 Richardson, pp. 16, 17, 19, 27, 29, 30, 34. The first use date for Vicks in the trademark record is 1894, 72292134; 0314174; 0386984; and others.

5 Richardson, pp. 29, 37, 39. VapoRub trademark US0103601. Some sources give 1907 for the first use of VapoRub, but the company's own trademark registration claims that 1911 was the first use date, and the date was repeated in subsequent claims. I have a Vick Chemical Co. envelope dated 1912 with an illustration of a box of Vick's Croup and Pneumonia Salve on the back. No mention of VapoRub. The envelope contained a Vick's Croup and Pneumonia Salve testimonial booklet dated c. 1909–1912 that has an illustration of the jar, and there is no mention of VapoRub. Smith Richardson wrote that it was his idea to change the company name from Vicks Family Remedies Co. to Vick Chemical Co. after he arrived in 1907 (p. 30). What confuses this is the 1934 trademark registration number 314175 claiming that the first use of the Vick Chemical Co. triangle was April 1, 1898. There are five more patents that support this (157235, 241960, 241961, and others). An undated product insert states that Lunsford founded the Vick Chemical Co. at age fifty-one. He was born in 1854, so that would be 1905. I have a Vick's Family Remedies Co. bill dated 1912, to make it more confusing.

6 Richardson, pp. 43, sample tins 50, 52, 57, 61. Gene and Cathy Florence, *The Hazel-Atlas Glass Identification and Value Guide* (Paducah, KY: Collector Books, 2005), p. 7.

7 1930 product insert.

8 Richardson, pp. 71, 74, 75; "The Cold Business," *Fortune*, pp. 26, 27.

9 Richardson, p. 76, 80, 81, 82; "The Cold Business," *Fortune*, p. 26. Based on an original 1938 invoice in the author's collection, wholesale prices for jars were 22¢ and 45¢.

10 CCH Trademark Research Corporation. Smith remembered that the corporate office was moved to New York in 1933. The trademark record shows that Philadelphia was the corporate address both in 1928 and 1934 (1928—US241961, 1934—US314174). Young, *The Medical Messiahs*, p. 178.

11 "The Cold Business," *Fortune*, p. 88; Danny Goodwin, *Famous Babies Sell Products on Radio* (www.old-time.com/commercials/famousbabies.html).

12 Determining when the Baume (*balm* in English) was invented is not perfectly clear. Several dates have been found. A claim printed on the company's 1939 packaging reads "invented in Paris by Dr. Bengue in 1896." Pfizer Products, Inc., the present owner of the brand, states on their BenGay Web page that it was "developed in the late 1800's." When Dr. Bengue filled out his first two U.S.

Daily Mail. Published by Associated Newspapers, Ltd., London: No. 14,688, May 29, 1943.

trademark applications he entered "1891" for the "First Use Date" (US519204, US564584). He was probably using French commerce dates. The first commerce dates for the first two logos support the product's arrival in 1898, and the "First Use Date" entered for the Baume Bengue logo was "1891." It appears that the 1939 packaging was mistaken about the 1896 founding date. If the patent record is correct, and "Baume Bengue" had existed in France as early as 1891, it places BenGay ahead of Mentholatum and Vicks in seniority as the first menthol cream and improves Pfizer's bragging rights by several years.

13 The first commerce date Bengué, Inc., entered for the Baume Bengué logo in the company's 1949 application was "1899" (US564584).

14 American Medical Association, *The Propaganda for Reform in Proprietary Medicines*. 8th ed. (New York). Reprinted from *Journal of the American Medical Association*, c. 1913.

15 "The Cold Business," *Fortune*, p. 88.

16 (www.huayinet.org/biography/biography_awboonhaw.htm); (www.brandchannel.com/features_profile.asp?pr_id=12); Robin D. Rusch, *Tiger Balm, Fit for an Emperor* (www.tigerbalm.co.uk/history.html).

17 Tholene was renamed in 1981 and its trademark abandoned by Rosebud Perfume Co., Inc., Woodsboro, MD.

PHOTO CREDITS/ILLUSTRATION SOURCES

Unless otherwise noted, all pictured items are from the author's collection or the Hyde family.

1912 Account Past Due (page 185) Envelope size: 3½″H × 6½″W, statement size: 5¾″H × 5½″W, booklet size: 6″H × 3″W.

Early VapoRub Logo (page 185) Smith Richardson, *The Early History and Management Philosophy of Richardson-Merrell*, pp. 68, 69. Art from the 1920 photo.

Mascot Named Vapor (page 185) Art found on flyer (c. 1924) titled "How to Treat Croup and Cold Troubles Externally."

Porcelain Enamel Door Push—Early 1920s (page 186) Three colors on steel plate, 6½″H × 3¾″W.

1915 Sample Tin (page 186) ⅜″H × 1¼″DIA.

1920s Box, Jar, and Sample Tin (page 186) Jar: 3¾ oz., box: 3½″H × 2¾″W × 2¾″D, tin: ¼″H × 1½″DIA.

Chromolitho Blotter—Early 1920s (page 186) This blotter and the three on page 184 are courtesy of Duane Shrader.

New Mascots Introduced in 1925 (page 187) Twelve-page chromolith booklet, 7″H × 5″W.

1925 Sample Tin (page 187) ¼″H × 1½″DIA.

1928 Box and Jar (page 187) Jar: 1½ oz., box: 2¾″H × 2¼″W × 2¼″D.

1943 Box and Jar (page 188) Jar: 3¾ oz., box: 3½″H × 2¼″W × 2¼″D.

1953 Sample Tin and Box (page 188) Tin: ½″H × 1½″DIA, box: 2″H × 2″W × 1″D.

1958 Box and Jar (page 188) Jar: 3¾ oz., box: 3½″H × 2¼″W × 2¼″D.

Familiar Style (page 189) "Will Not Blister" ⅞-ounce milk glass jar with tin screw cap and paper label: 2¼″H × 1¾″DIA, C. 1920.

Colorful Introduction (page 189) *Everybody's Magazine*, January 1920, 10½″H × 7″W.

Evidence of a Change (page 190) 1941 box: 2⅜″H × 1¾″W × 1¾″D, top lid reads "Made in U.S.A.," interior flap reads "New Carton Adopted July 1941." 1941 jar: ⅞-ounce milk glass, 2⅛″H × 1⅝″DIA, label reads old slogan with aluminum cap. 1942 box: bow tie logo replacing USA on top lid, interior flap reads "New Carton Adopted Dec. 1942." 1942 jar: same as 1941 except label reads new slogan, is stamped with a control number (a new feature), and has printed green banding on the top and bottom edges; the aluminum cap is sometimes painted white.

Additional Formulations for the 1940s (page 190) Tube: 4″H × 1¼″W, box: 4½″H × 1⅜″W × 1⅜″D, childrens jar: 2⅛″H × 1¾″DIA.

Typical 1946 "Quints" Ad (page 190) 3¼″H × 2″W, March 1946 *Woman's Day*.

Say "Ben-Gay" in the 1920s (page 191) Overlapping top box: 1¾″H × 4½″W × 1⅛″D. Minor variations to the box label design were made between 1922 and 1931. One-ounce tube: 4⅛″H × 1″W. One-color instruction sheet: 6″H × 16″W, folded to 4″W, remained unchanged during this period.

New Design for the 1930s and 1940s (page 192) Tube: 1¼ ounces, 4⅛″H × 1″W. Box: 1¾″H × 4⅜″W × 1″D. Insert: 6″H × 16″W, folded to 6″H × 4″W. New-packaging announcement on page 184: *American Druggist* (vol. LXXXVII, February 1933, no. 2), p. 2.

Ben-Gay vs. Peter Pain (page 192) 1949 Chest Cold ad (source unknown); Rheumatic Pain ad (January 1949 *Farm Journal*), 6″H × 4⅝″W.

Modern Packaging (page 193) Jar: .63 ounce, 1⅜″H × 1½″DIA.

Tiger Brand Products (page 193) Porcelain enamel and paint on steel with rounded edges, 35½″H × 23½″W.

Modern Sample Tin, Box, and Insert (page 194) Box: 1¾″H × 2″W × ¾″D, tin: ½″H × 1½″DIA, insert: 8″H × 5¾″W, shown folded to 4″H × 5¾″W.

Bibliography

Alsaker, R. L., M.D. *Curing Catarrh Coughs and Colds.* New York: Grant Publishing Company, Inc., 1925.

American Medical Association. *The Propaganda for Reform in Proprietary Medicines.* 5th ed., rev. to September 12, 1908. New York: Council on Pharmacy and Chemistry of the American Medical Association. Collected reprints from *The Journal of the American Medical Association*, 1908.

———. *The Propaganda for Reform in Proprietary Medicines.* 8th ed. New York: Reprinted from *The Journal of the American Medical Association*, c. 1913.

Andrewes, Sir Christopher. *The Common Cold.* New York: W. W. Norton & Company Inc., 1965.

Andrews, Theodora. *A Bibliography on Herbs, Herbal Medicine, "Natural" Foods, and Unconventional Medical Treatment.* Littleton, CO: Libraries Unlimited, Inc., 1982.

Armstrong, David, and Elizabeth Metzger Armstrong. *The Great American Medicine Show, Being an Illustrated History of Hucksters, Healers, Health Evangelists, and Heroes from Plymouth Rock to the Present.* New York: Prentice Hall, 1991.

Beard, George M., A.M., M.D. *Hay-Fever; or, Summer Catarrh: Its Nature and Treatment.* New York: Harper & Brothers, Publishers, 1876.

Carson, Gerald. *One for a Man, Two for a Horse: A Pictorial History, Grave and Comic, of Patent Medicines.* Garden City, NY: Doubleday & Co., Inc., 1961.

Chase, A. W., M.D. *Dr. Chase's Recipes; or, Information for Everybody: An Invaluable Collection of About Eight Hundred Practical Recipes.* 29th ed. Ann Arbor, MI: Published by the Author, 1866.

The Chemist & Druggist Text Book, 1917. London: The Chemist & Druggist, 1917.

Chord, Jack T. *The Window Display Manual.* Cincinnati: The Display Publishing Company, 1931.

Eberle, Scott, and Joseph A. Grand. *Second Looks: A Pictorial History of Buffalo and Erie County.* Virginia Beach, VA: The Donning Company/Publishers, 1993.

Eli Lilly & Company. *Hand Book of Pharmacy and Therapeutics.* 6th rev. Indianapolis: Eli Lilly & Company, 1919.

Florence, Gene and Cathy. *The Hazel-Atlas Glass Identification and Value Guide.* Paducah, KY: Collector Books, 2005.

Gard, Wayne. *The Chisholm Trail.* Norman, OK: University of Oklahoma Press, 1965.

Gordon, Lois, and Alan Gordon. *The Columbia Chronicles of American Life, 1910–1992.* New York: Columbia University Press, 1995.

Hawke, David Freeman. *Benjamin Rush: Revolutionary Gadfly.* Indianapolis: The Bobbs-Merrill Company, Inc., 1971.

Holbrook, Stewart H. *The Golden Age of Quackery.* New York: The MacMillan Company, 1959.

Hyde, John M. "A Balm in Gilead." *Kansas History* 9, no. 4 (Winter 1986/1987): 150–163.

Irving, George. *Master of Money: A. A. Hyde of Wichita.* New York: Fleming H. Revell Company, 1936.

Latson, W. R. C., M.D. *Catarrh: The Nature, Causation, Prevention and Cure of This Prevalent and Distressing Malady, with Chapters on Colds and Hay Fever.* New York: The Health-Culture Co., 1911.

Long, Richard, ed. *Wichita Century: A Pictorial History of Wichita, Kansas 1870–1970*. Wichita, KS: The Wichita Historical Museum Association, Inc., 1969.

Lord, Owen & Co., Importers and Wholesale Druggists. *1885 Prices Current of Drugs and Druggists' Sundries, Chemicals, Proprietary Medicines, Paints, Oils, Glass, Etc., Etc.* Chicago: C. H. Blakely & Co., Printers, 1885.

The Merck Index: An Encyclopedia of Chemicals, Drugs, and Biologicals. 12th ed. Whitehouse Station, NJ: Merck & Co., Inc., 1996.

Merck's 1899 Manual of the Materia Medica. facsimile. New York: Merck & Co., 1899.

Meyer, Clarence. *The Herbalist Almanac: A 50-Year Anthology*. Glenwood, IL: Meyerbooks, 1988.

Miner, Craig. *Wichita: The Magic City*. Wichita, KS: Wichita-Sedgwick County Historical Museum Association, 1988.

Morell, Peter. *Poisons, Potions and Profits: The Antidote to Radio Advertising*. New York: Knight Publishers, Inc., 1937.

Munsey, Cecil. *The Illustrated Guide to Collecting Bottles*. New York: Hawthorn Books, Inc., Publishers, 1970.

Opie, Robert. *Miller's Advertising Tins: A Collector's Guide*. London: Octopus Publishing Group Ltd., 1999.

Physician's Desk Reference. PDR for Herbal Medicines, 1st ed. Montvale, NJ: Medical Economics Company, 1998.

Robinson, Beverley, A.M., M.D. *A Practical Treatise on Nasal Catarrh and Allied Diseases*. New York: William Wood & Company, 1885.

Sonnedecker, Glenn, Ph.D. *Kremers and Urdang's History of Pharmacy*. 4th ed. Madison, WI: American Institute of the History of Pharmacy, 1986.

Staten, Vince. *Do Pharmacists Sell Farms?: A Trip Inside the Corner Drugstore*. New York: Simon & Schuster, 1998.

U.S. Department of Commerce, Bureau of the Census. *Historical Statistics of the United States: Colonial Times to 1970*. Part 1. Washington, D.C.: Government Printing Office, 1975.

Vories, William Merrell. *A Mustard-Seed in Japan*. 5th ed. Omi-Hachiman, Japan: Omi Mission, 1925.

White, Richard. *"It's Your Misfortune and None of My Own": A History of the American West*. Norman, OK: University of Oklahoma Press, 1991.

Young, James Harvey. *The Medical Messiahs: A Social History of Health Quackery in Twentieth-Century America*. Princeton, NJ: Princeton University Press, 1967.

———. *The Toadstool Millionaires: A Social History of Patent Medicines in America Before Federal Regulation*. Princeton, NJ: Princeton University Press, 1961.

Zimmerman, David. *Encyclopedia of Advertising Tins: Identification & Values*. Vol. II. Paducah, KY: Collector Books, 1999.

Index

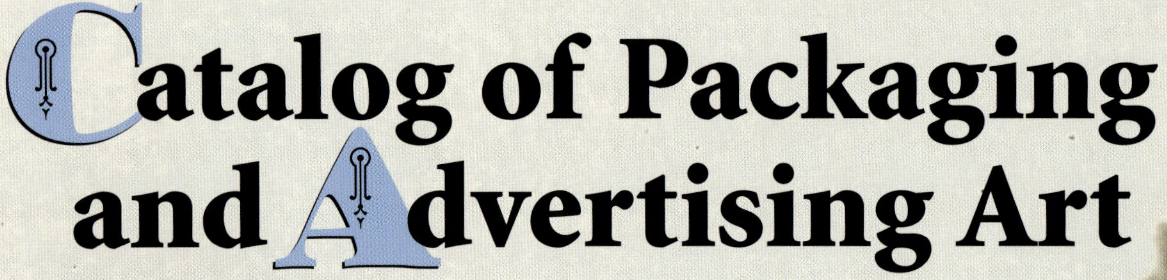

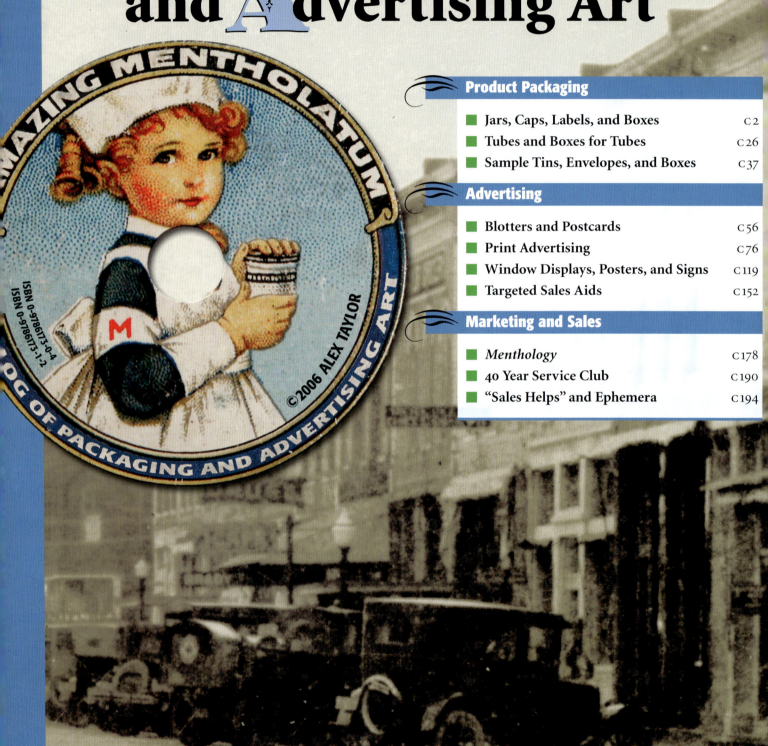

Catalog of Packaging and Advertising Art

MAZING MENTHOLATUM
M
ISBN 0-9786173-0-4
ISBN 0-9786173-1-2
©2006 ALEX TAYLOR
OG OF PACKAGING AND ADVERTISING ART

Product Packaging

Advertising

Marketing and Sales

This is a photo of 1928 Oswego, Kansas.

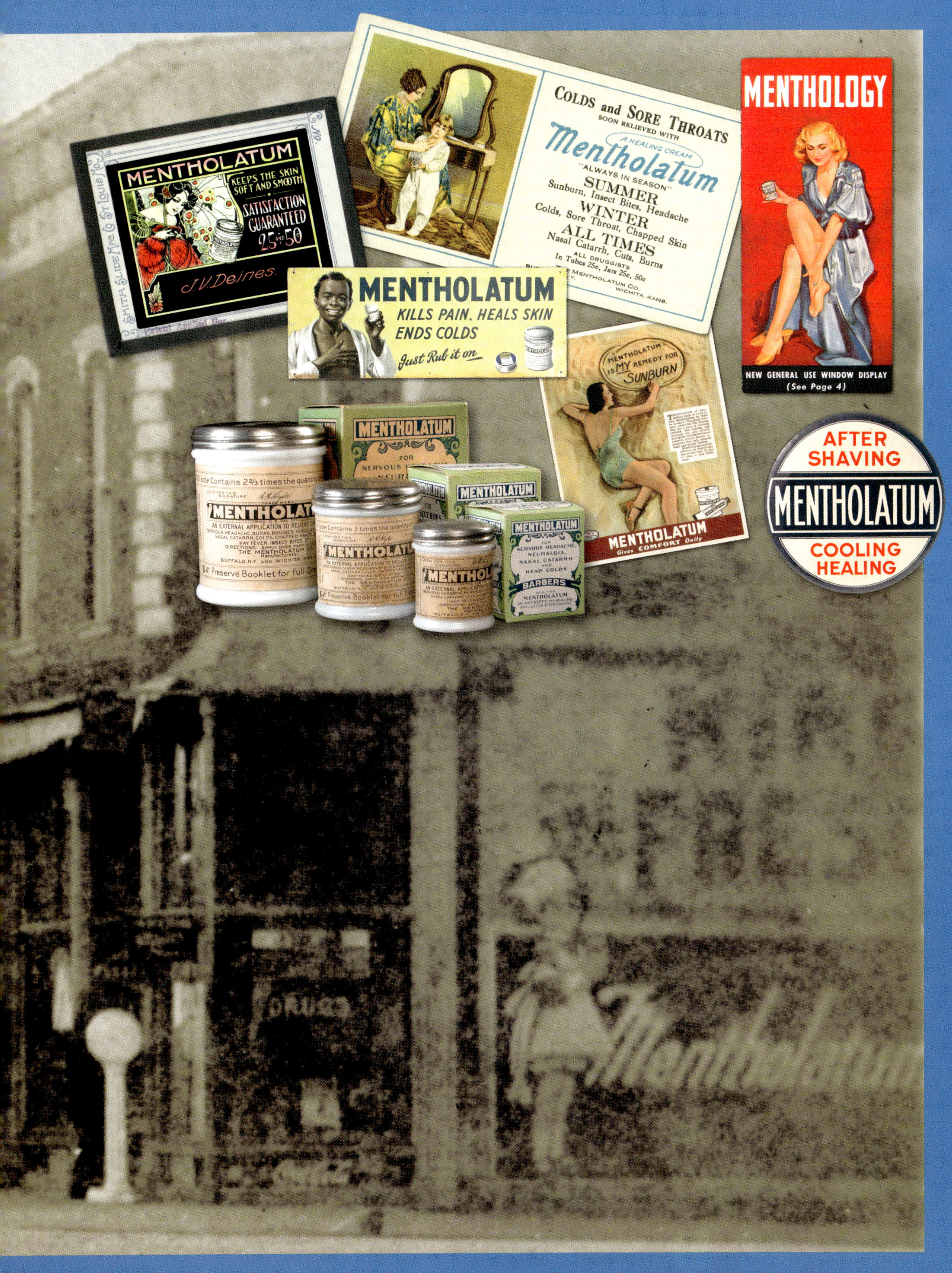

MENTHOLATUM
KEEPS THE SKIN SOFT AND SMOOTH
SATISFACTION GUARANTEED
25 AND 50
J.V. Deines
SMITH SLIDE MFG. CO. ST. LOUIS, MO.
Patent Applied For
COLDS and SORE THROATS
SOON RELIEVED WITH
Mentholatum
A HEALING CREAM
"ALWAYS IN SEASON"
SUMMER
Sunburn, Insect Bites, Headache
WINTER
Colds, Sore Throat, Chapped Skin
ALL TIMES
Nasal Catarrh, Cuts, Burns
ALL DRUGGISTS
In Tubes 25c, Jars 25c, 50c
THE MENTHOLATUM CO.
WICHITA, KANS.
MENTHOLOGY
NEW GENERAL USE WINDOW DISPLAY
(See Page 4)
MENTHOLATUM
KILLS PAIN, HEALS SKIN
ENDS COLDS
Just Rub it on
MENTHOLATUM IS MY REMEDY FOR SUNBURN
MENTHOLATUM
Gives COMFORT Daily
AFTER SHAVING
MENTHOLATUM
COOLING HEALING
MENTHOLATUM
MENTHOLATUM
FOR NERVOUS HEADACHE, NEURALGIA, NASAL CATARRH AND HEAD COLDS
BARBERS
Preserve Booklet for Full Directions
Mentholatum

This section shows the pages from the Acrobat PDF catalog in thumbnail form. Page numbers in the catalog are preceeded by the letter *C*.

The items in the catalog are numbered as follows:

- **J** for jars
- **JB** for jar boxes
- **T** for tubes
- **TB** for tube boxes
- **S** for sample tins
- **SE** for sample tin envelopes
- **SB** for sample tin boxes
- **B** for blotters
- **BS** for Spanish-language blotters
- **TC** for trade cards
- **P** for postcards

To view the catalog you will need Adobe Reader 3.0 or later. Download it free at www.adobe.com.

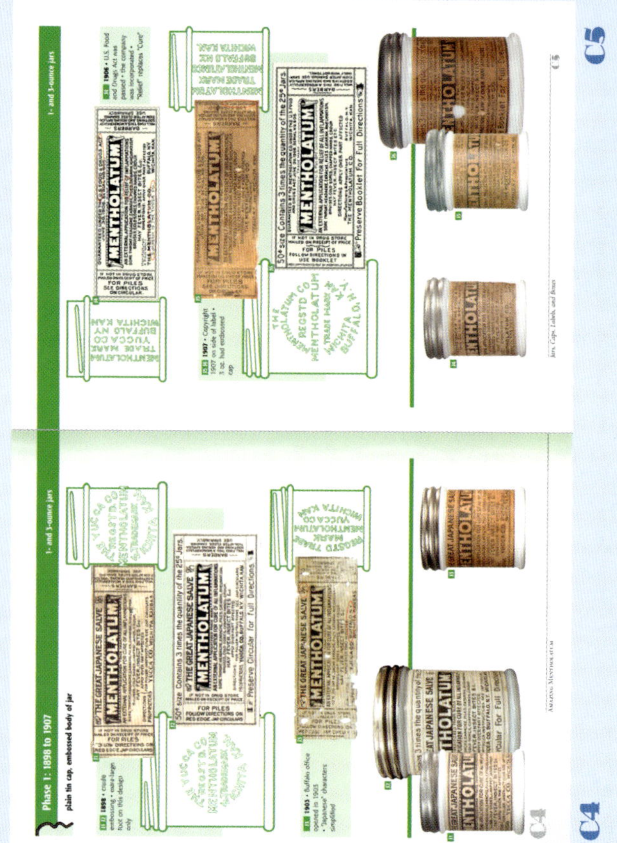

C5

C4

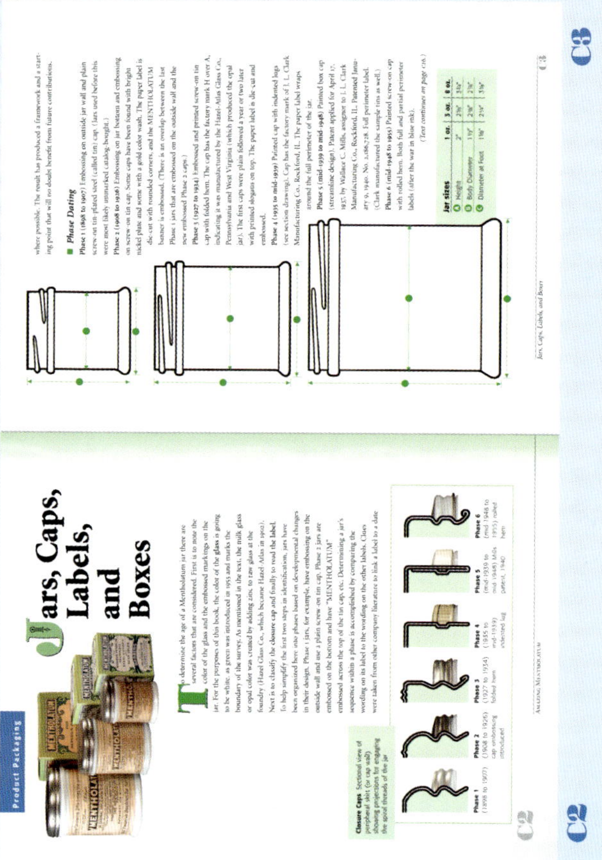

C3

C2

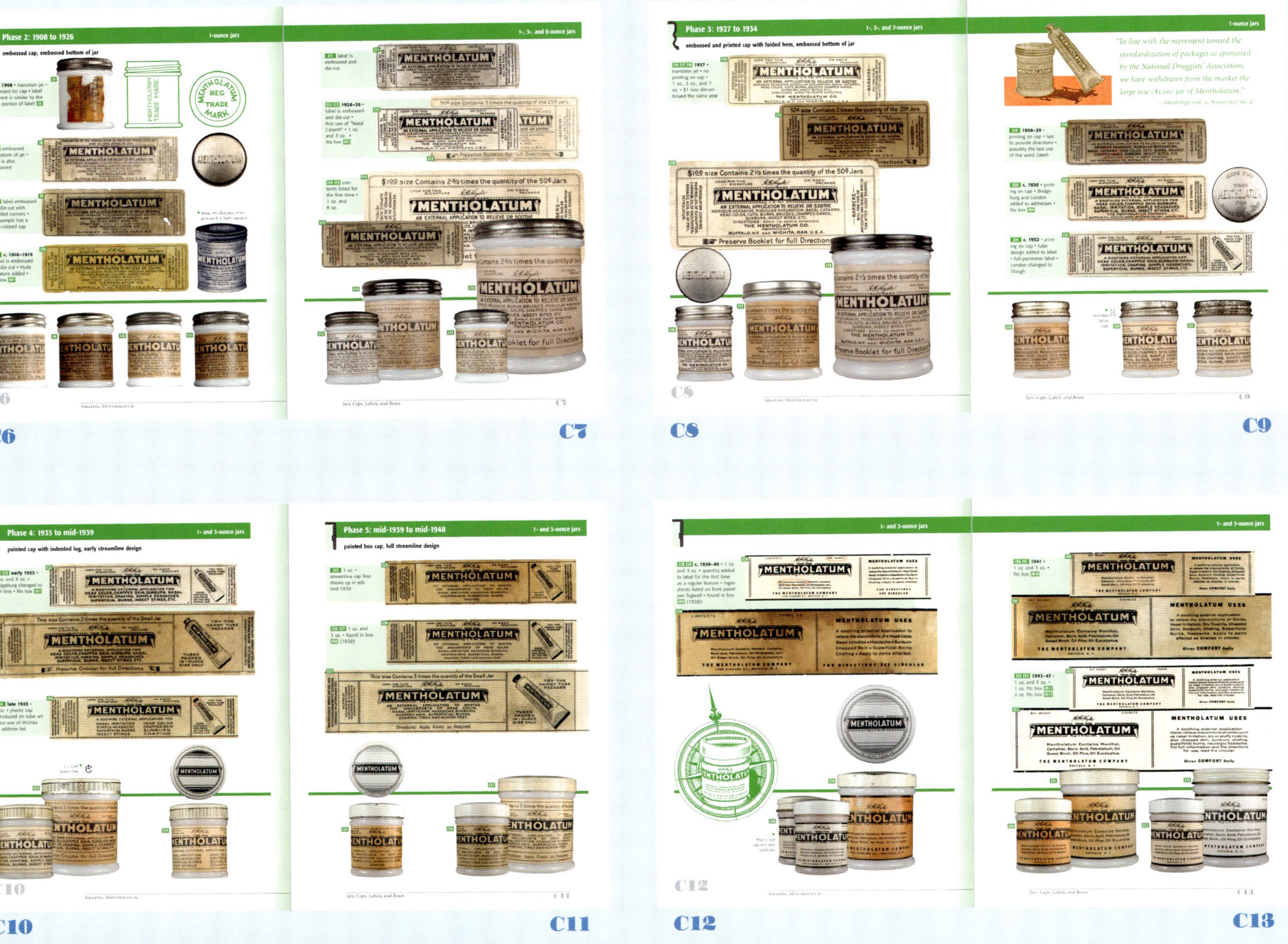
Phase 2: 1908 to 1926
1-ounce jars
embossed cap, embossed bottom of jar
1-, 3-, and 8-ounce jars
Phase 3: 1927 to 1934
1-, 3-, and 7-ounce jars
embossed and printed cap with folded hem, embossed bottom of jar
1-ounce jars
"In line with the movement toward the standardization of packages as sponsored by the National Druggists' Association, we have withdrawn from the market the large size ($1.00) jar of Mentholatum."
Phase 4: 1935 to mid-1939
1- and 3-ounce jars
painted cap with indented lug, early streamline design
Phase 5: mid-1939 to mid-1948
1- and 3-ounce jars
painted box cap, full streamline design
1- and 3-ounce jars
1- and 3-ounce jars
C6
C7
C8
C9
C10
C11
C12
C13

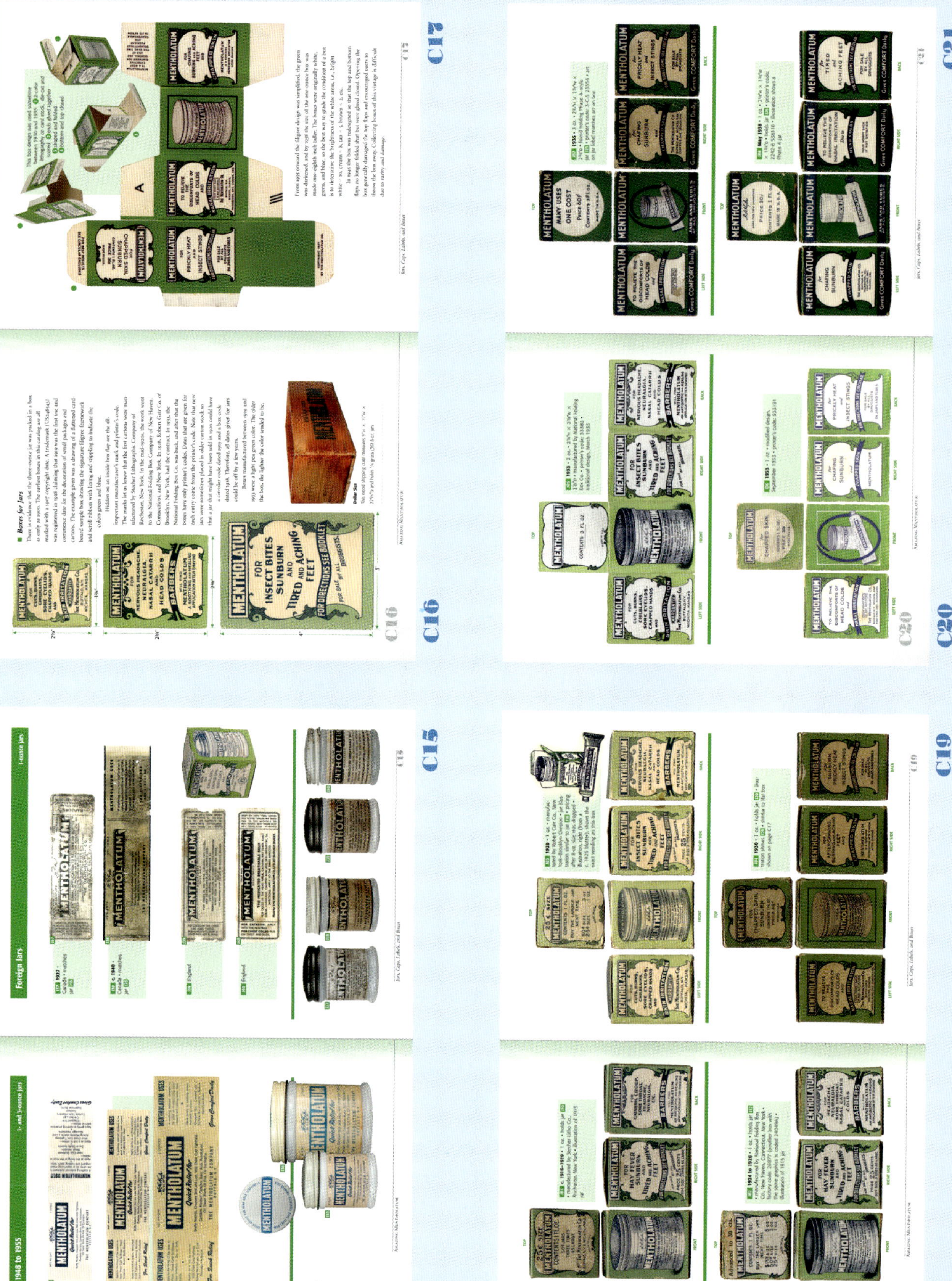

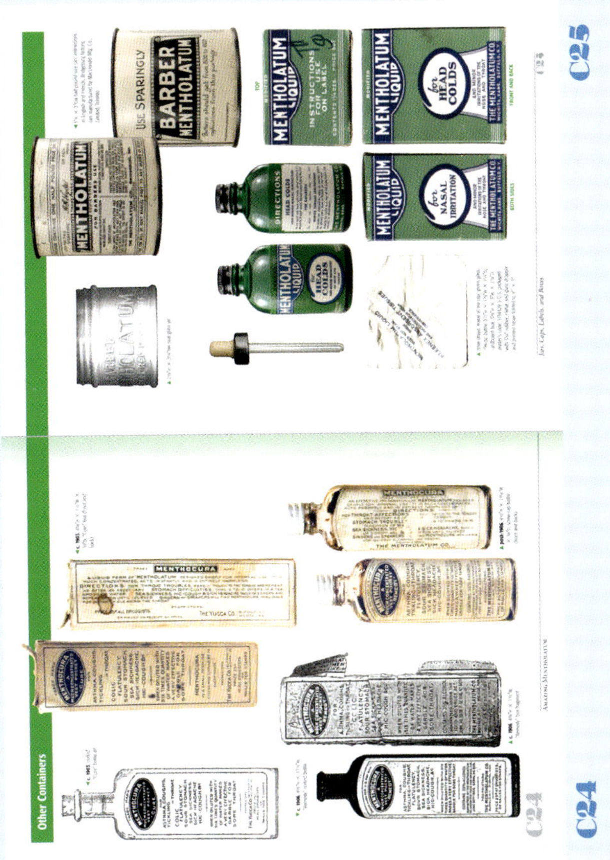

C24 C25

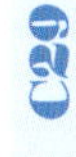

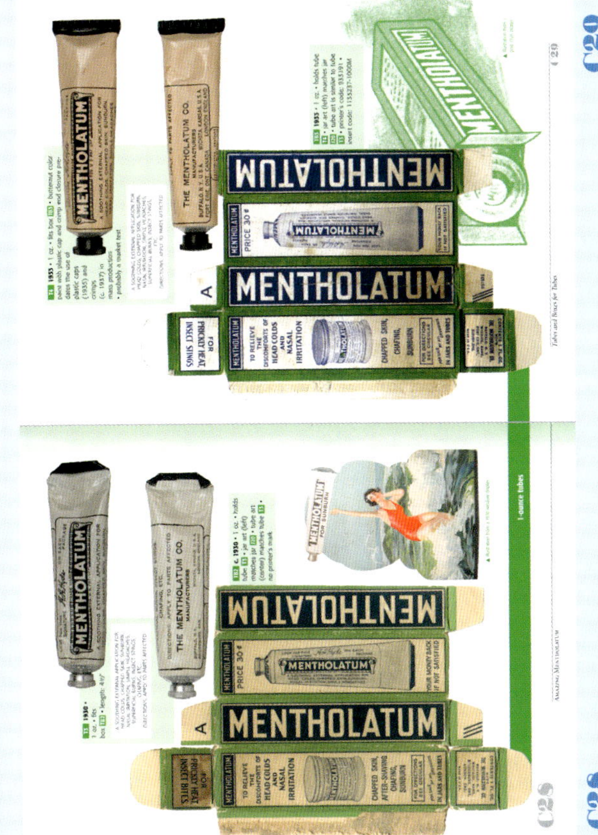

C28 C29

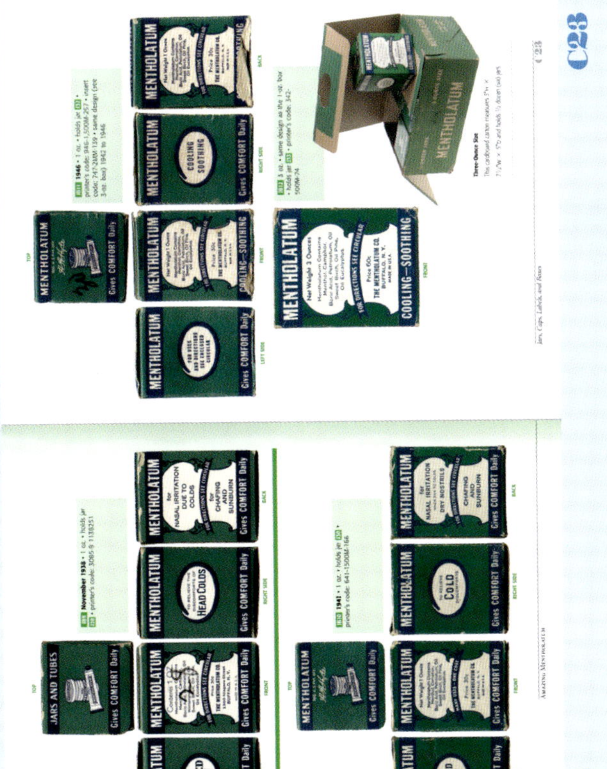

C22 C23

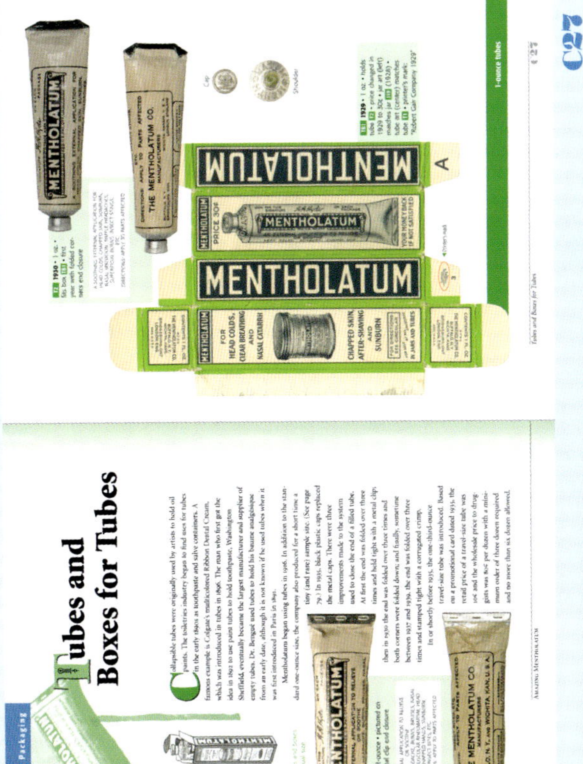

C26 C27

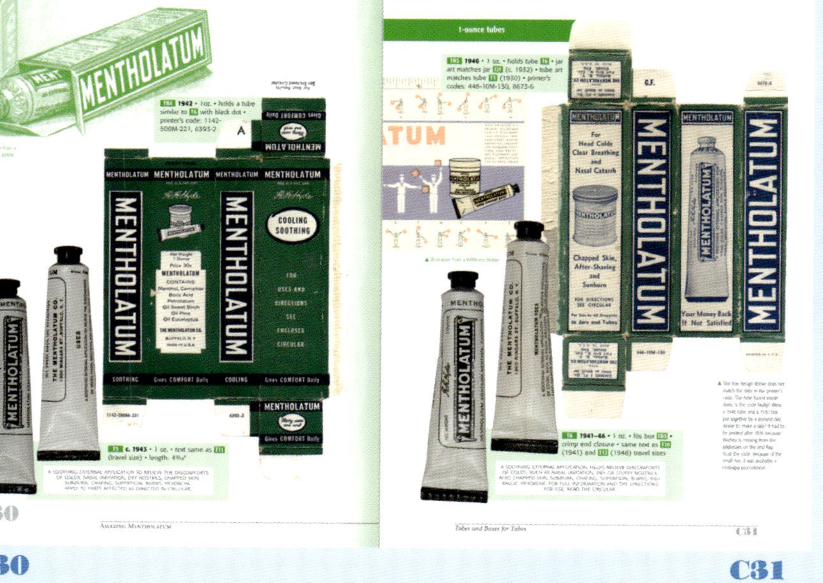

C30

C31

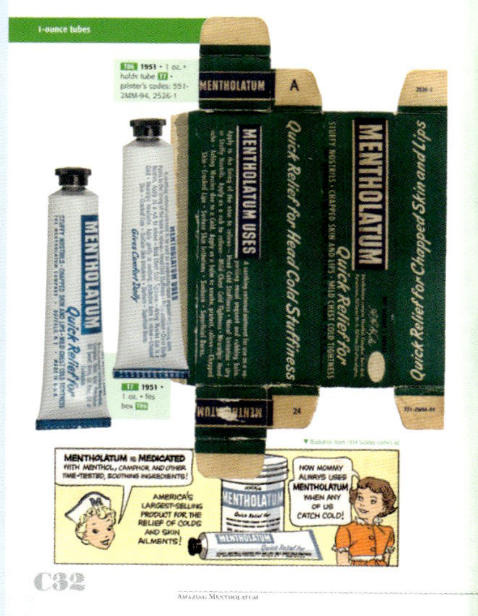

C32

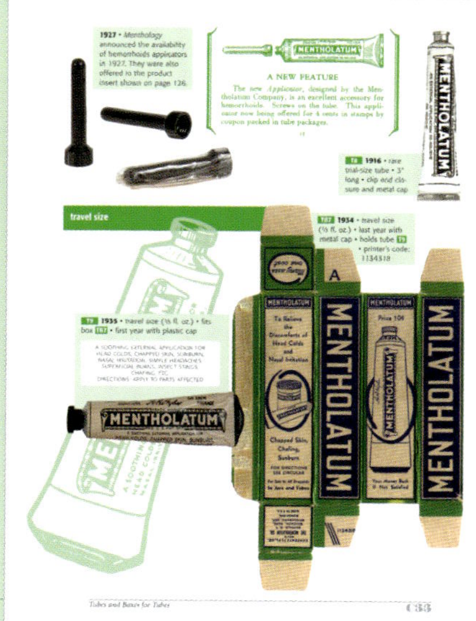

C33

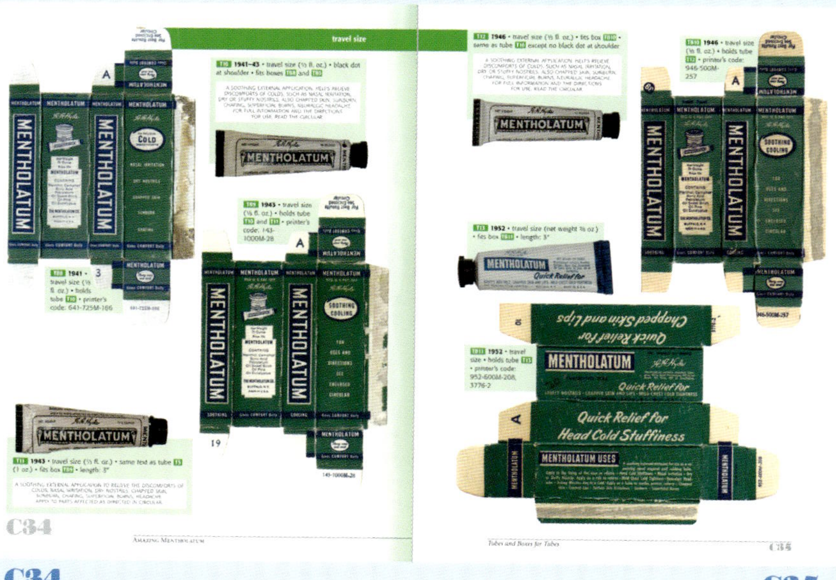

C34

C35

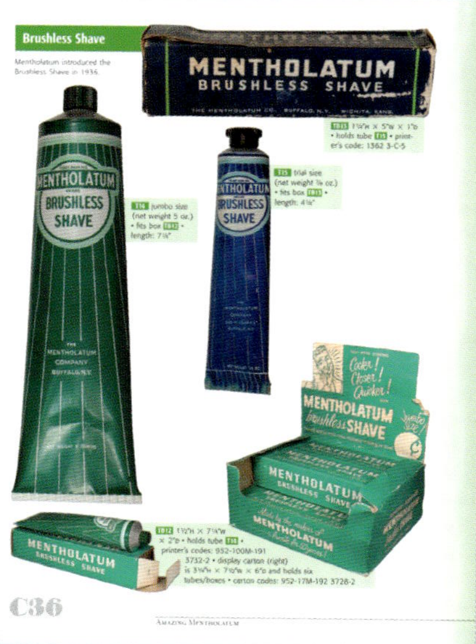

C36

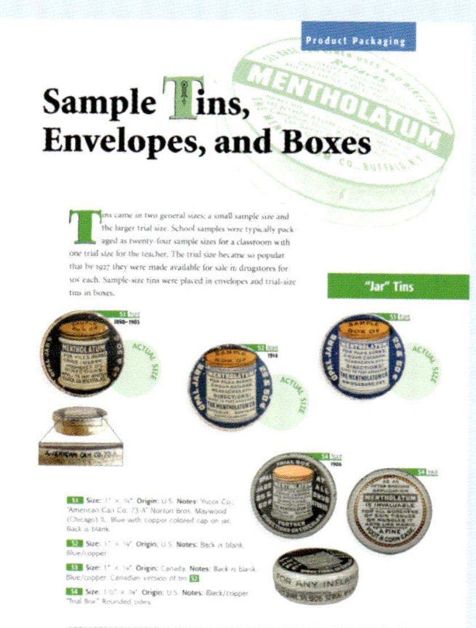

C37

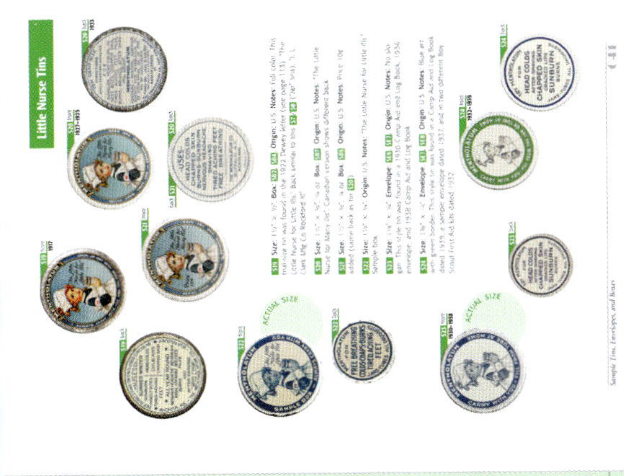
C41

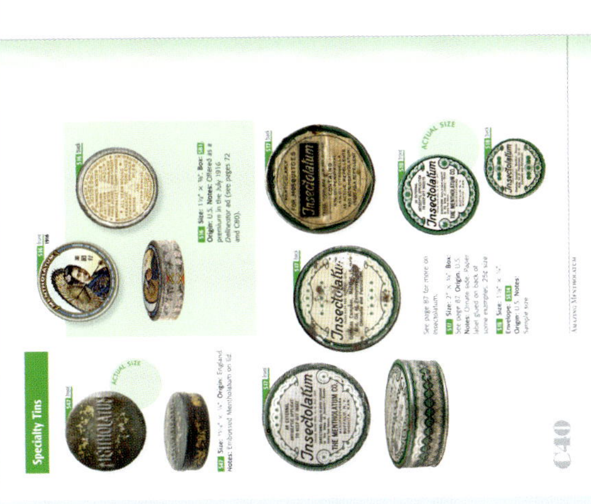
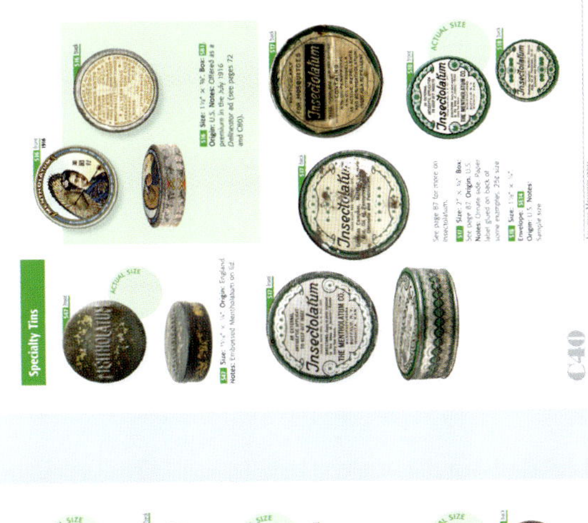
C40

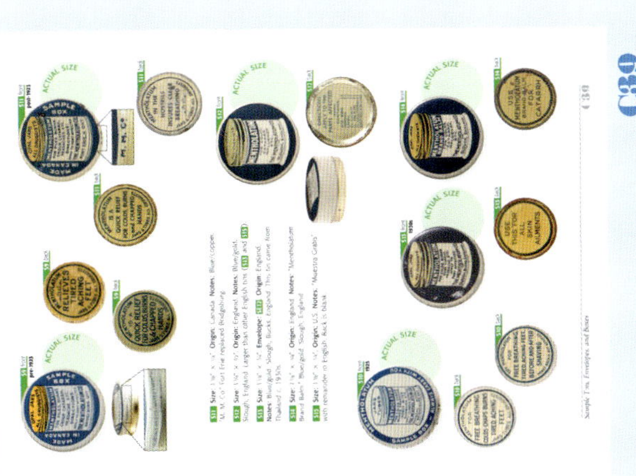
C39

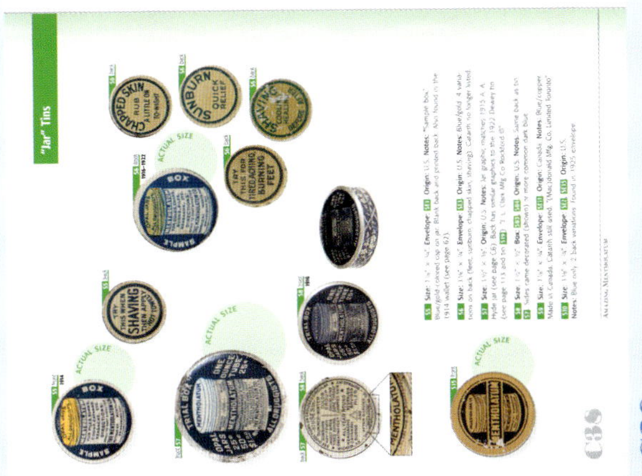
C38

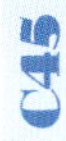
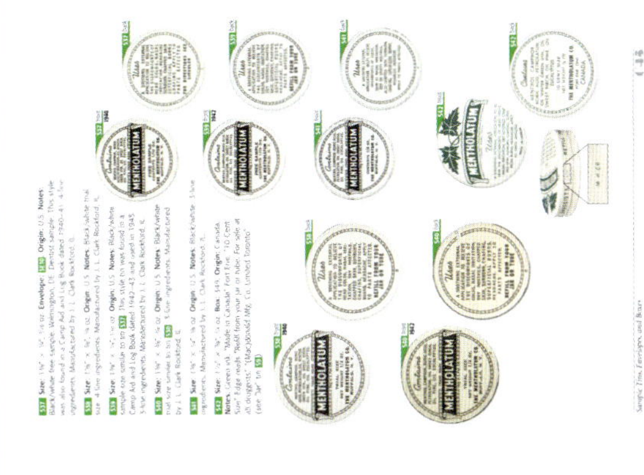
C45

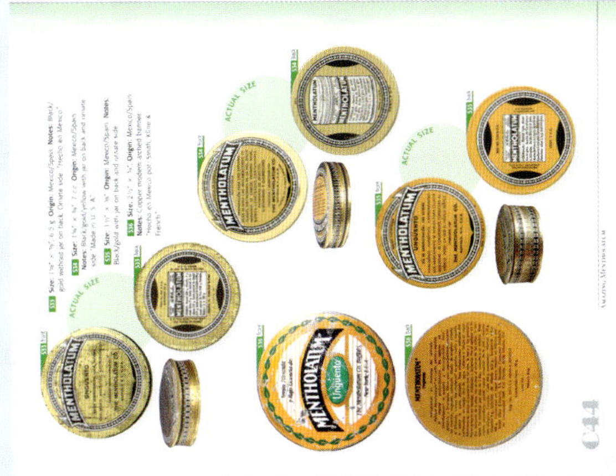
C44

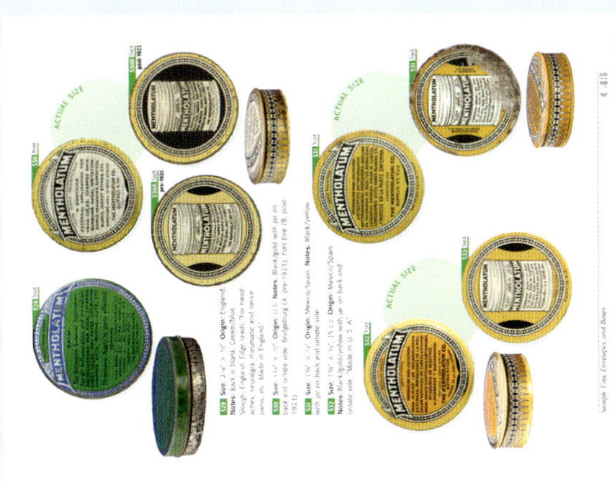
C43

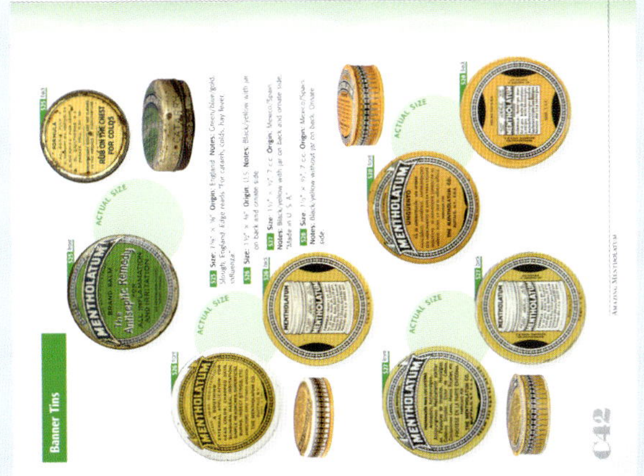
C42

C46

C47

C48

C49

C50

C51

C52

C53

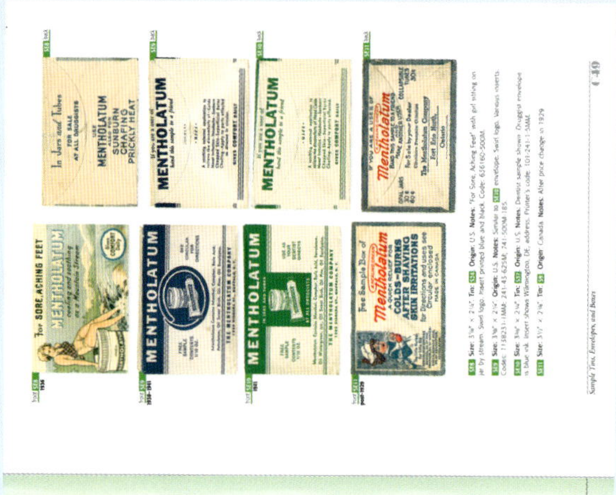

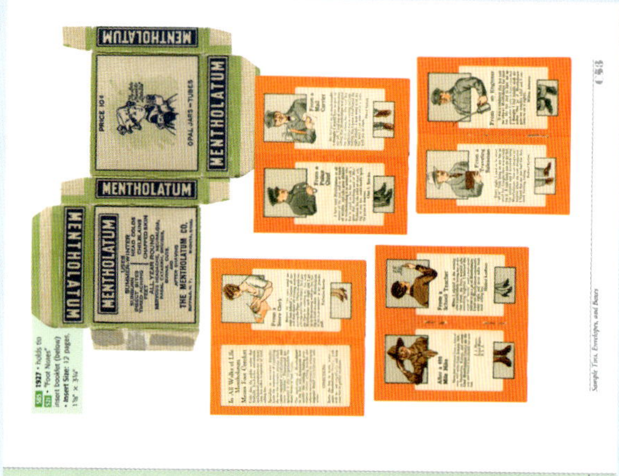

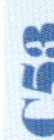

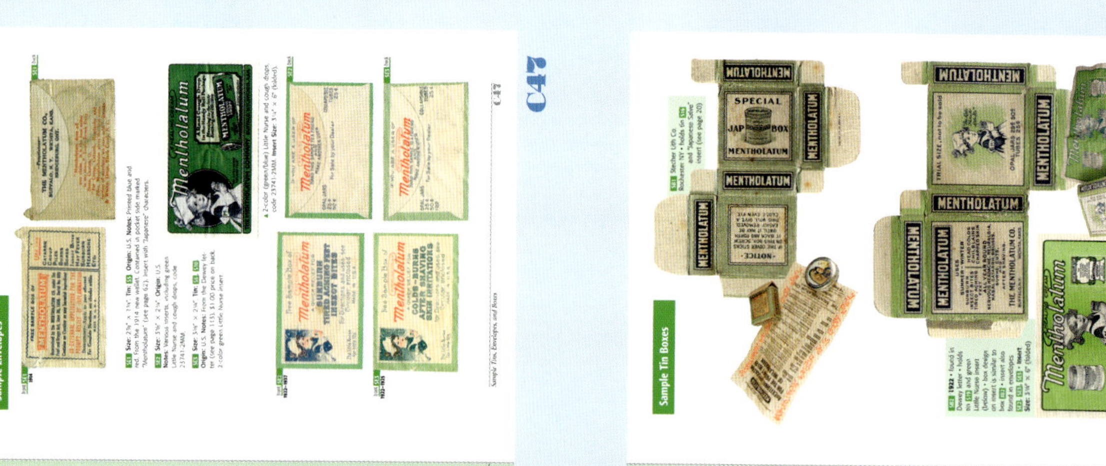

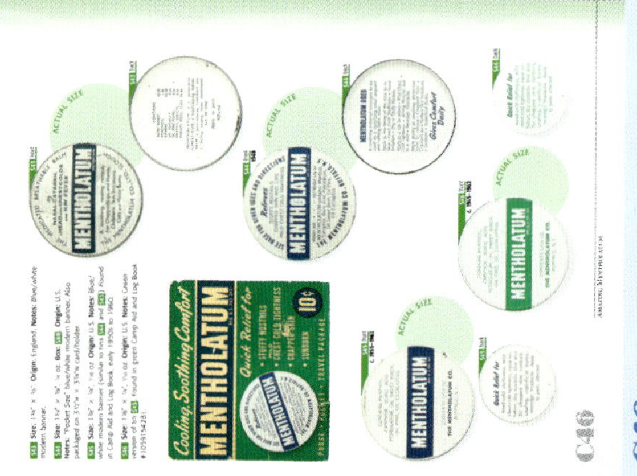

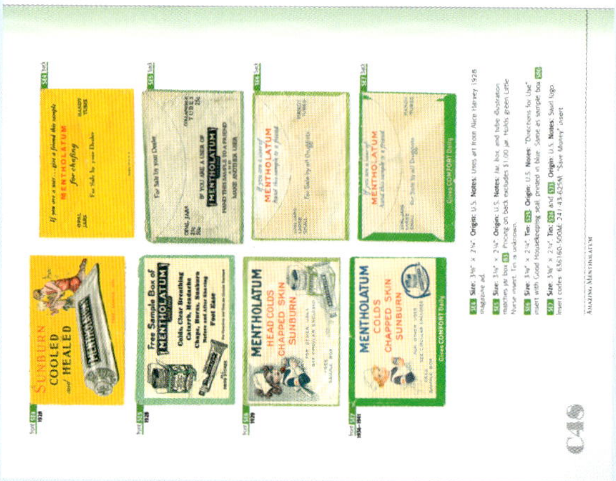

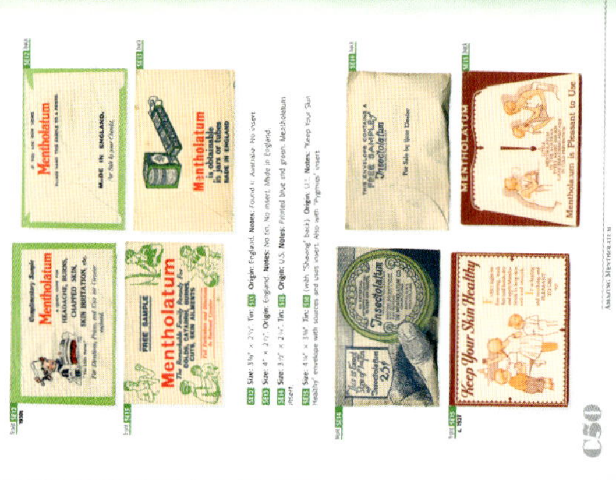

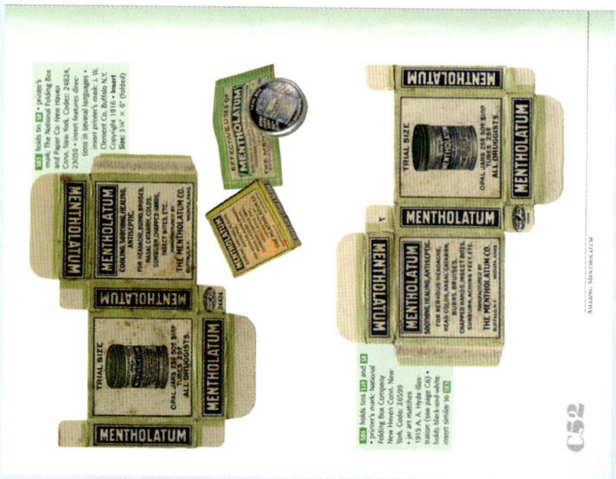

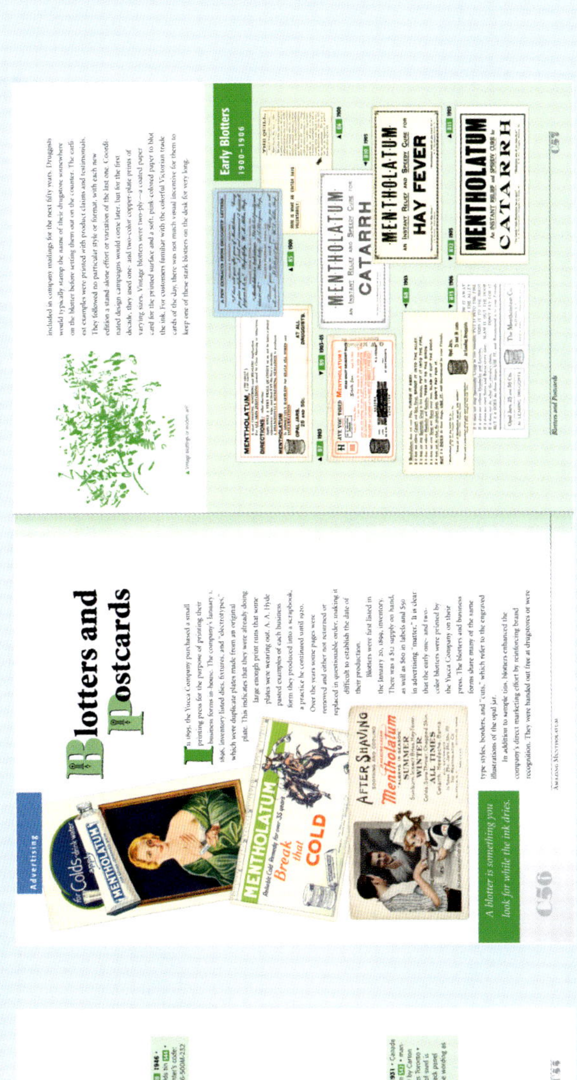

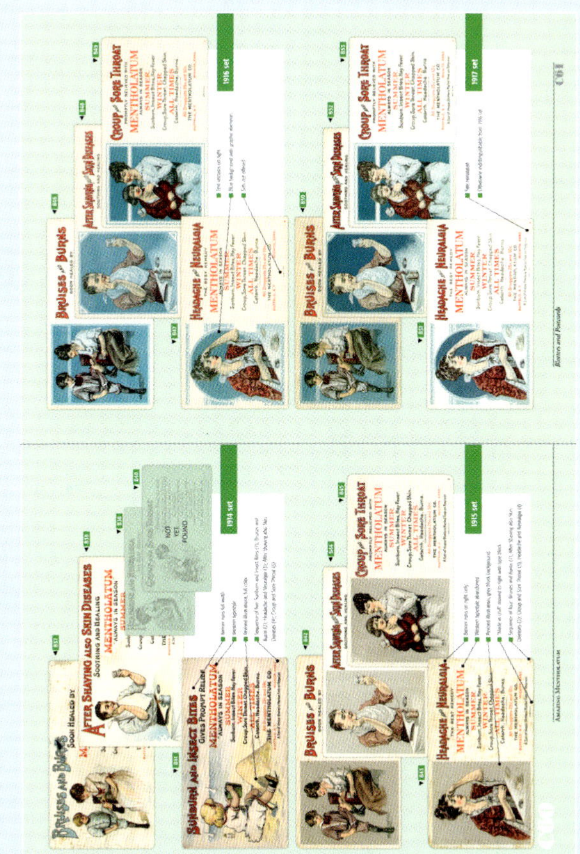

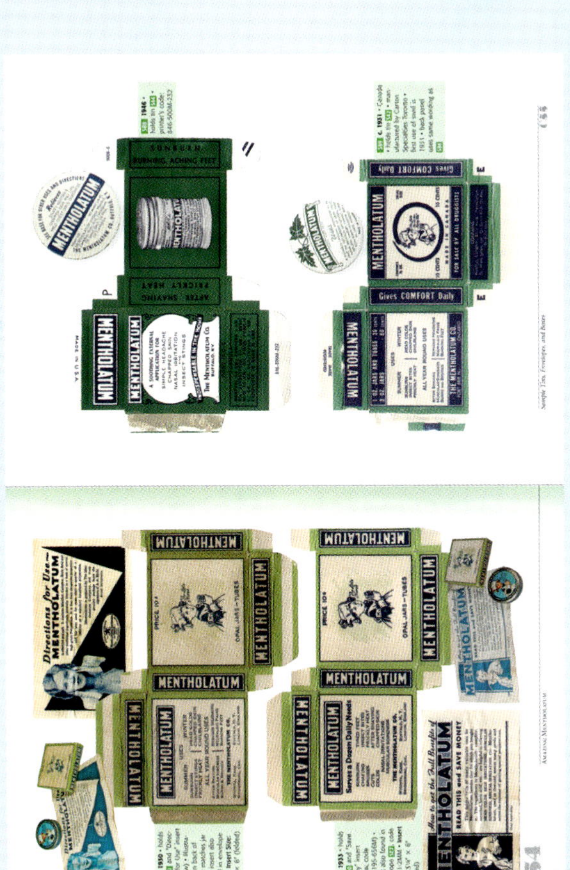

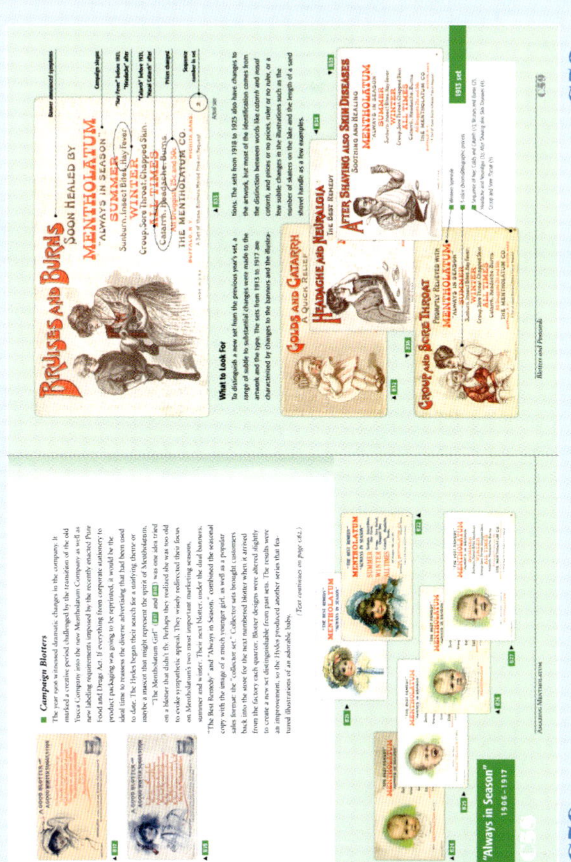

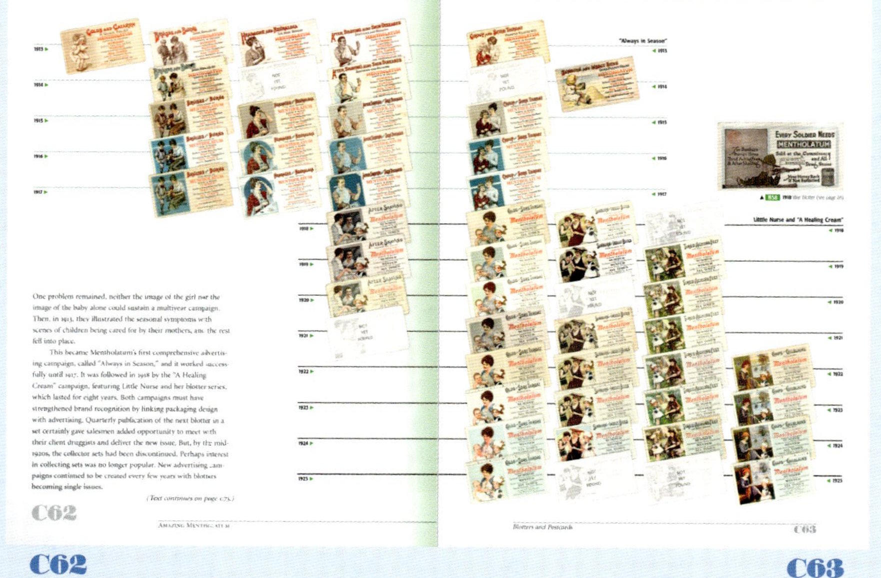

One problem remained, neither the image of the girl nor the image of the baby alone could sustain a multiyear campaign. Then, in 1913, they illustrated the seasonal symptoms with scenes of children being cared for by their mothers, and the rest fell into place.

This became Mentholatum's first comprehensive advertising campaign, called "Always in Season," and it worked successfully until 1917. It was followed in 1918 by the "A Healing Cream" campaign, featuring Little Nurse and her blotter series, which lasted for eight years. Both campaigns must have strengthened brand recognition by linking packaging design with advertising. Quarterly publication of the next blotter in a set certainly gave salesmen added opportunity to meet with their client druggists and deliver the new issue. But, by the mid-1920s, the collector sets had been discontinued. Perhaps interest in collecting sets was no longer popular. New advertising campaigns continued to be created every few years with blotters becoming single issues.

(Text continues on page c75.)

C62 C63

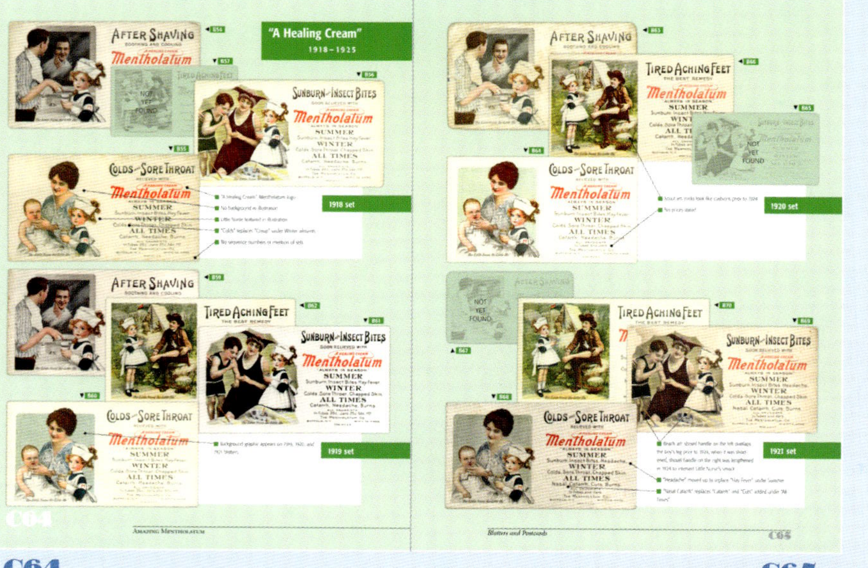

C64 C65

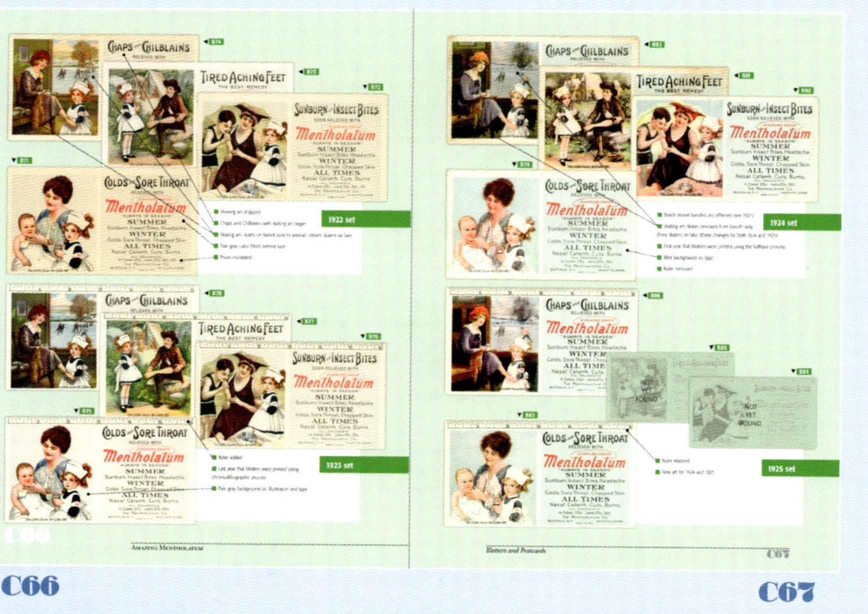

C66 C67

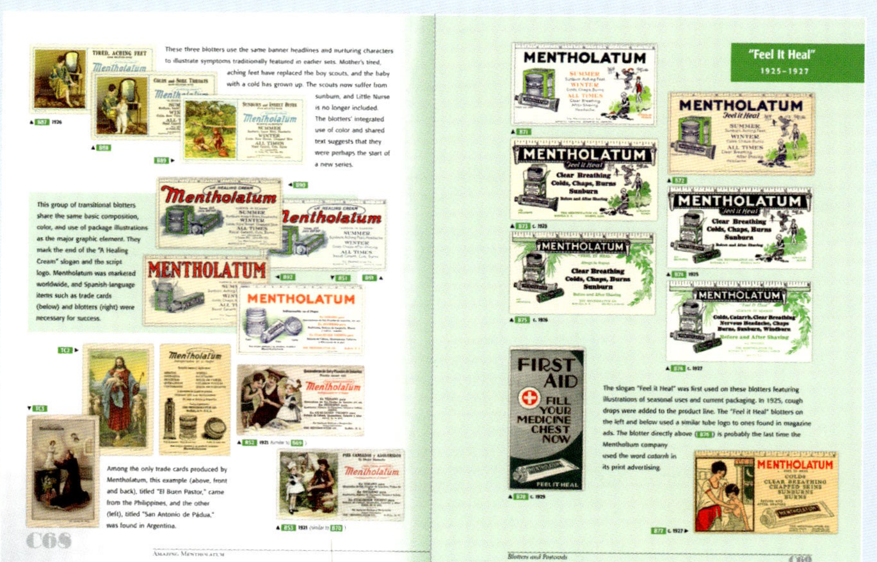

These three blotters use the same banner headlines and nurturing characters to illustrate symptoms traditionally featured in earlier sets. Mother's tired, aching feet have replaced the boy scouts, and the baby with a cold has grown up. The scouts now suffer from sunburn, and Little Nurse is no longer included. The blotters' integrated use of color and shared text suggests that they were perhaps the start of a new series.

This group of transitional blotters share the same basic composition, color, and use of package illustrations as the major graphic element. They mark the end of the "A Healing Cream" slogan and the script logo. Mentholatum was marketed worldwide, and Spanish-language items such as trade cards (below) and blotters (right) were necessary for success.

Among the only trade cards produced by Mentholatum, this example (above, front and back), titled "El Buen Pastor," came from the Philippines, and the other (left), titled "San Antonio de Pádua," was found in Argentina.

The slogan "Feel it Heal" was first used on these blotters featuring illustrations of seasonal uses and current packaging. In 1925, cough drops were added to the product line. The "Feel it Heal" blotters on the left and below used a similar tube logo to ones found in magazine ads. The blotter directly above (B76) is probably the last time the Mentholatum company used the word *catarrh* in its print advertising.

C68 C69

C70

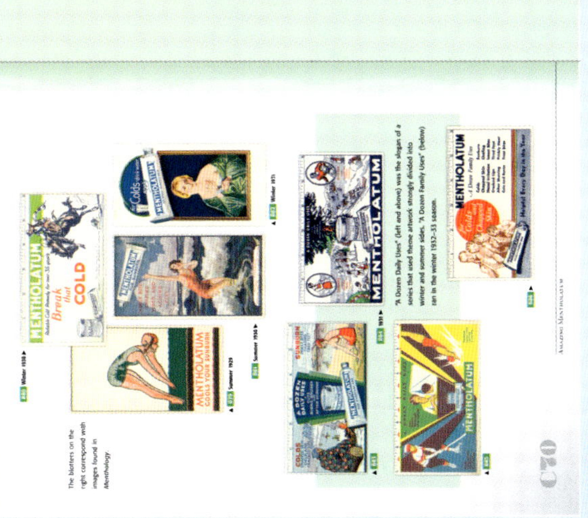

C71

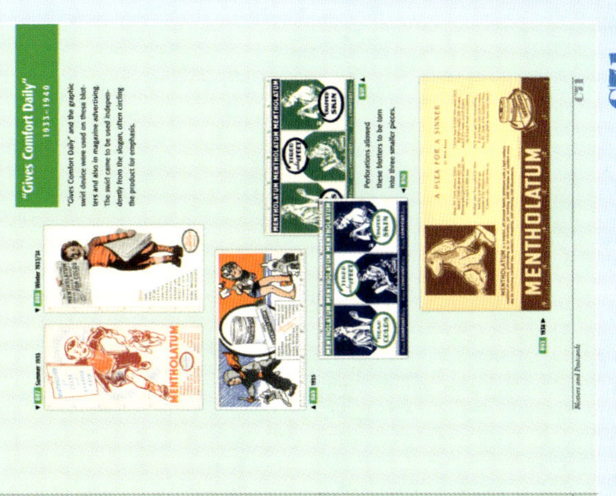

C72

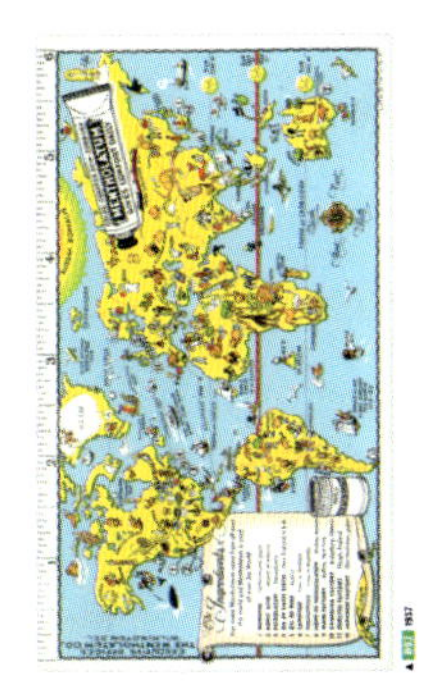

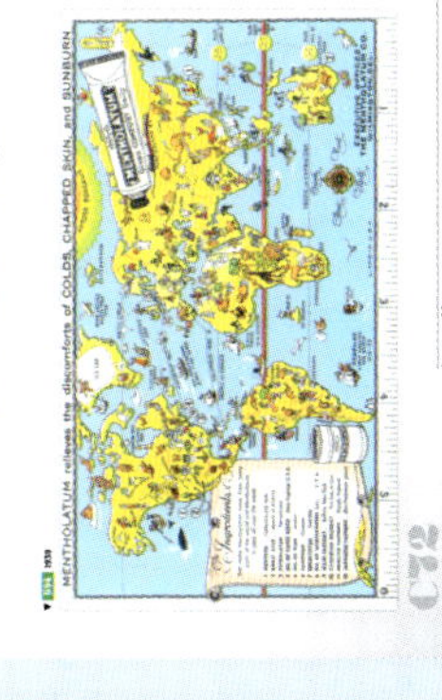

C73

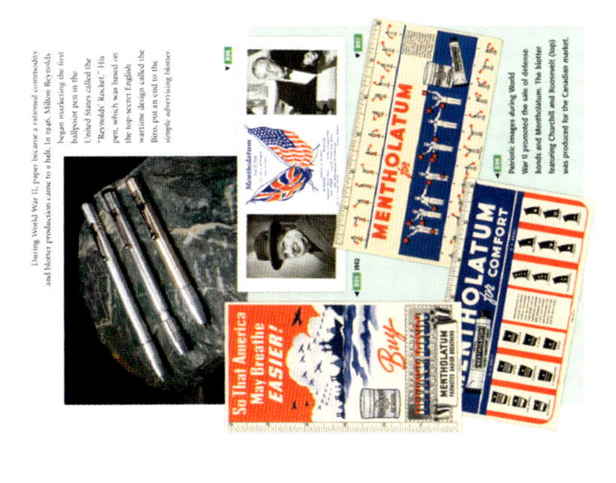

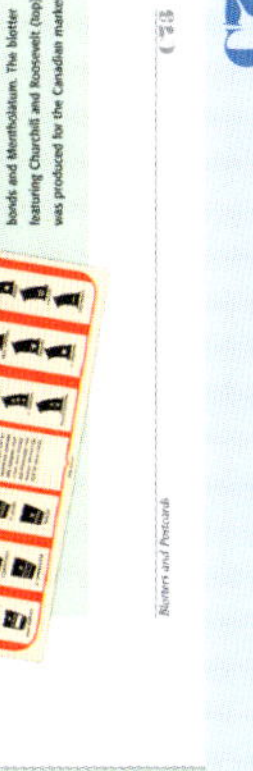

C74

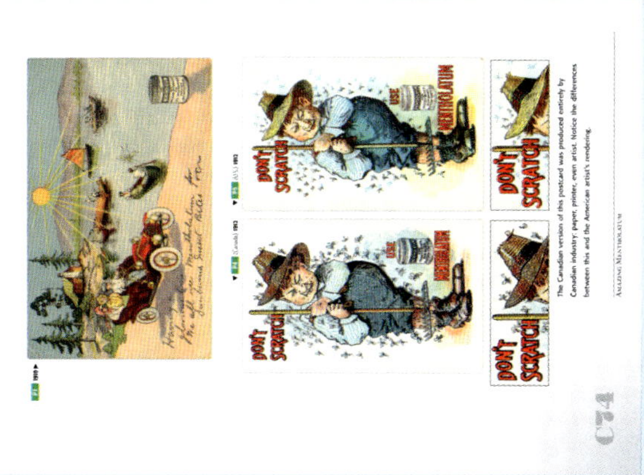

C75

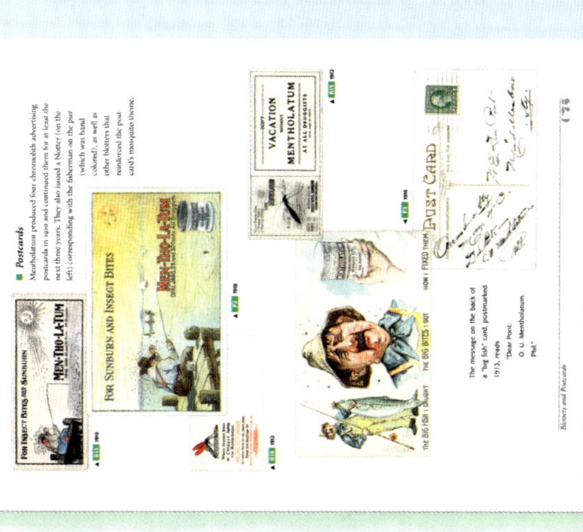

C76

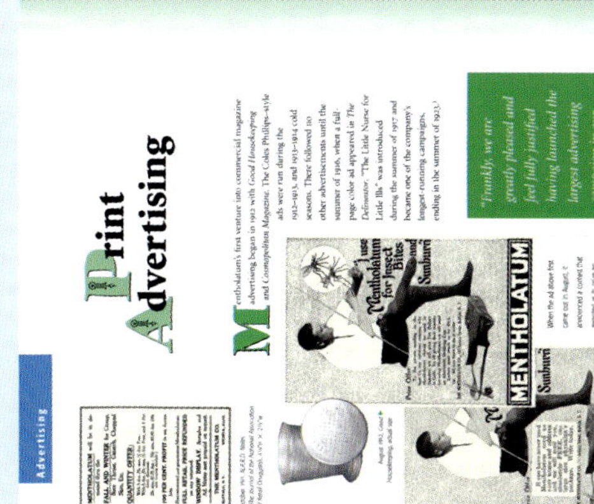

C77

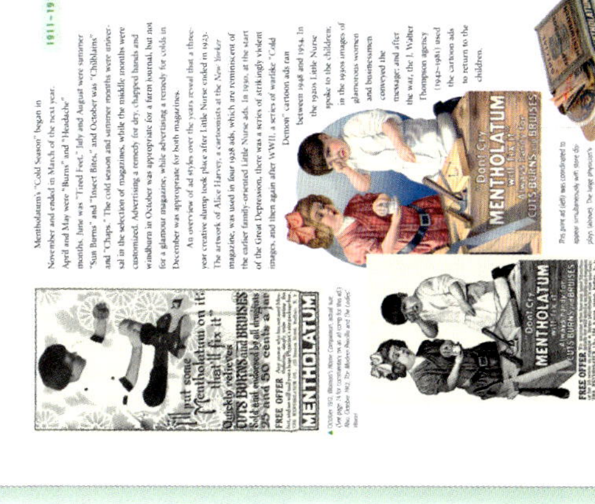

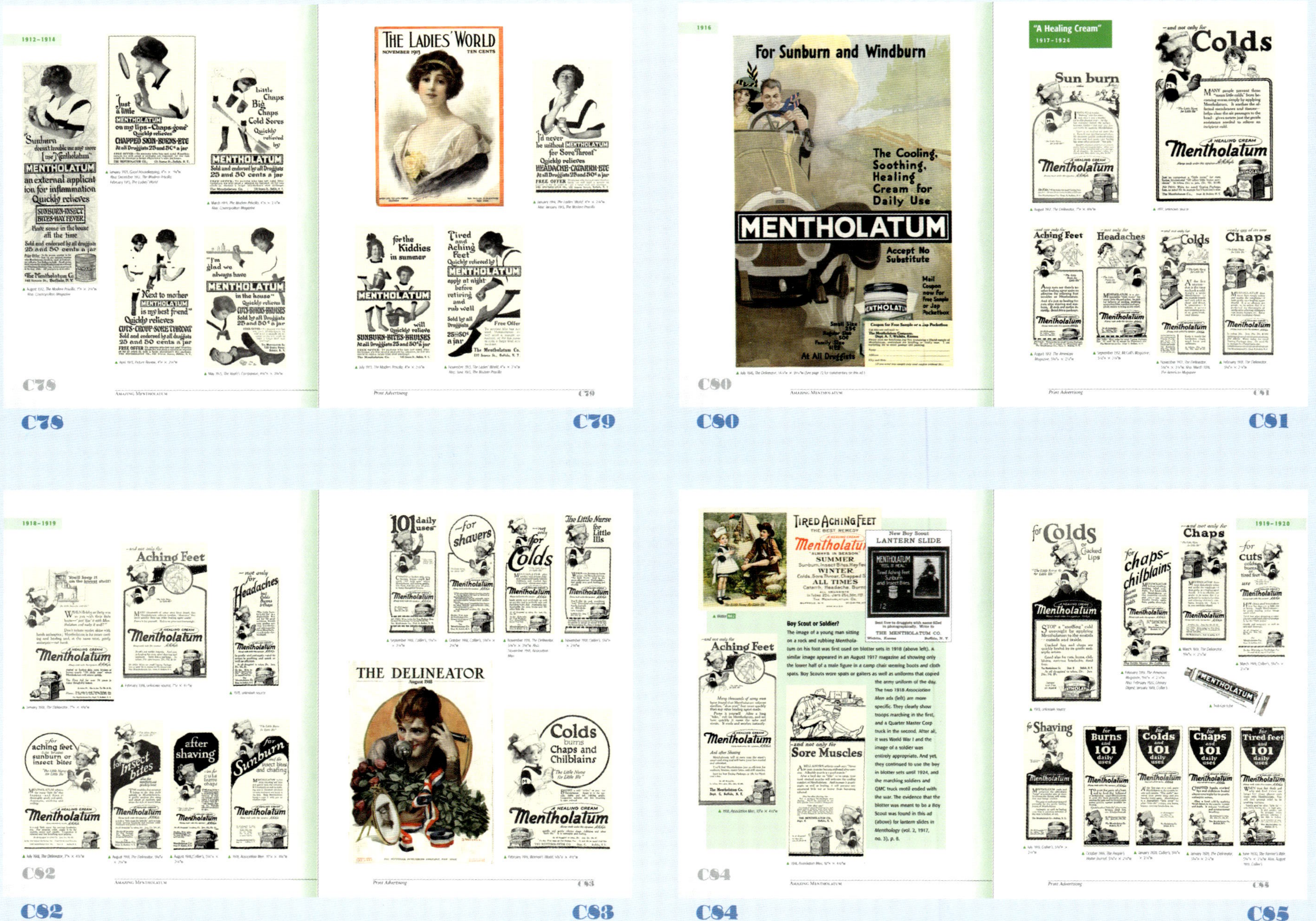

1912–1914
Sunburn
MENTHOLATUM
Just a little MENTHOLATUM
Little Chaps Big Chaps Cold Sores
MENTHOLATUM
Next to mother MENTHOLATUM is my best friend
I'm glad we always have MENTHOLATUM in the house
C78
THE LADIES' WORLD
NOVEMBER 1913
TEN CENTS
I'd never be without MENTHOLATUM for Sore Throat
for the Kiddies in summer
MENTHOLATUM
Tired and Aching Feet
MENTHOLATUM
C79
1916
For Sunburn and Windburn
The Cooling, Soothing, Healing Cream for Daily Use
MENTHOLATUM
Accept No Substitute
At All Druggists
C80
"A Healing Cream"
1917–1924
Sun burn
Colds
Mentholatum
Aching Feet
Headaches
Colds
Chaps
C81
1918–1919
Mentholatum
Aching Feet
Mentholatum
Headaches
aching feet sunburn or insect bites
Mentholatum
insect bites
after shaving
Sunburn
C82
101 daily uses
for shavers
for Colds
The Little Nurse for Little Ills
THE DELINEATOR
August 1918
Colds burns Chaps and Chilblains
Mentholatum
C83
TIRED ACHING FEET
THE BEST REMEDY
Mentholatum
SUMMER
WINTER
ALL TIMES
New Boy Scout
LANTERN SLIDE
THE MENTHOLATUM CO.
Boy Scout or Soldier?
The image of a young man sitting on a rock and rubbing Mentholatum on his foot was first used on blotter sets in 1918 (above left). A similar image appeared in an August 1917 magazine ad showing only the lower half of a male figure in a camp chair wearing boots and cloth spats. Boy Scouts wore spats or gaiters as well as uniforms that copied the army uniform of the day. The two 1918 *Association Men* ads (left) are more specific. They clearly show troops marching in the first, and a Quarter Master Corp truck in the second. After all, it was World War I and the image of a soldier was entirely appropriate. And yet, they continued to use the boy in blotter sets until 1924, and the marching soldiers and QMC truck motif ended with the war. The evidence that the blotter was meant to be a Boy Scout was found in this ad (above) for lantern slides in *Menthology* (vol. 2, 1917, no. 3), p. 8.
Aching Feet
Mentholatum
Sore Muscles
C84
1919–1920
for Colds or Cracked Lips
Mentholatum
for chaps-chilblains
Chaps
for cuts
for Shaving
Burns 101 daily uses
Colds 101 daily uses
Chaps 101 daily uses
Tired feet 101 daily uses
C85

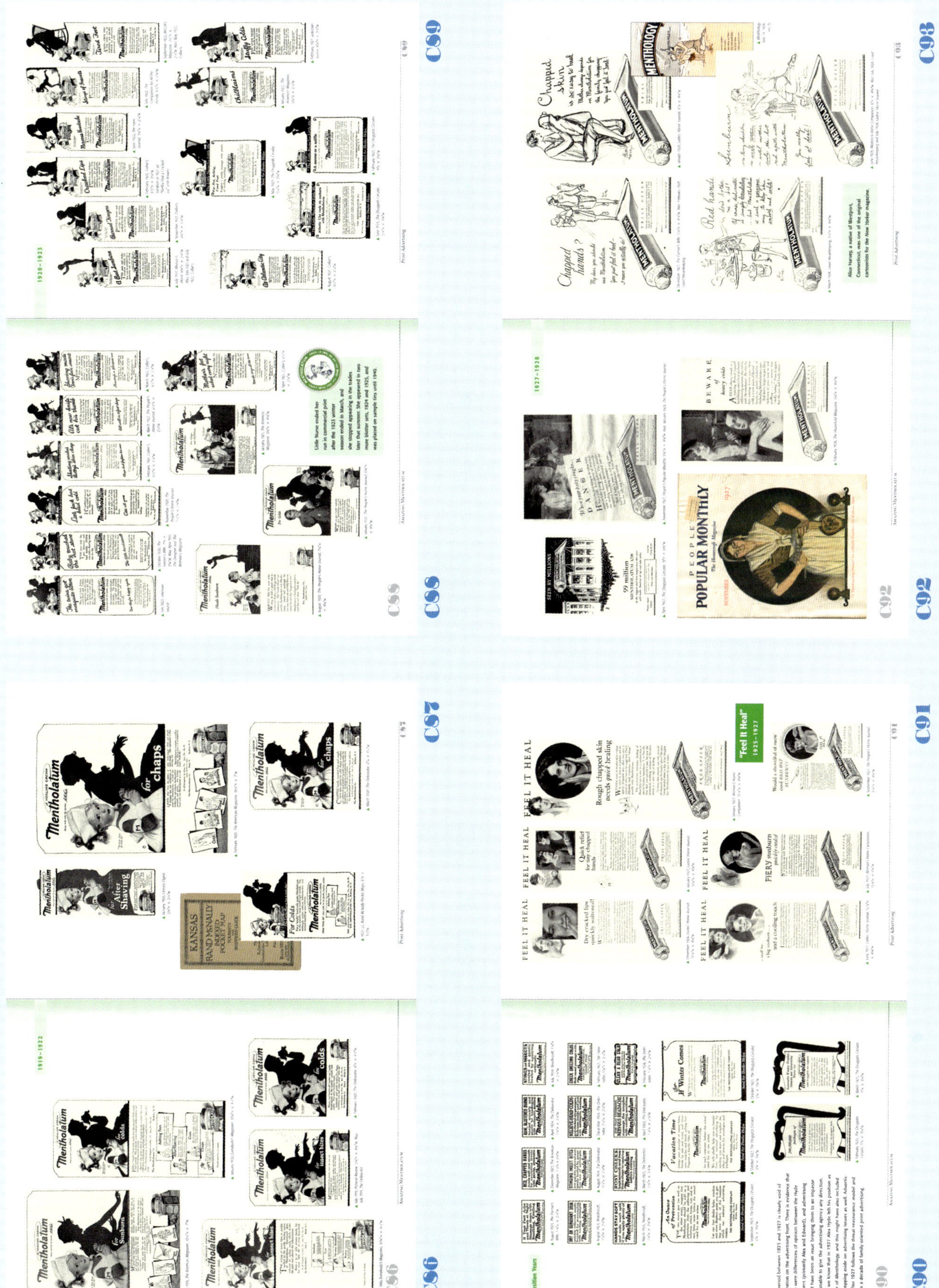

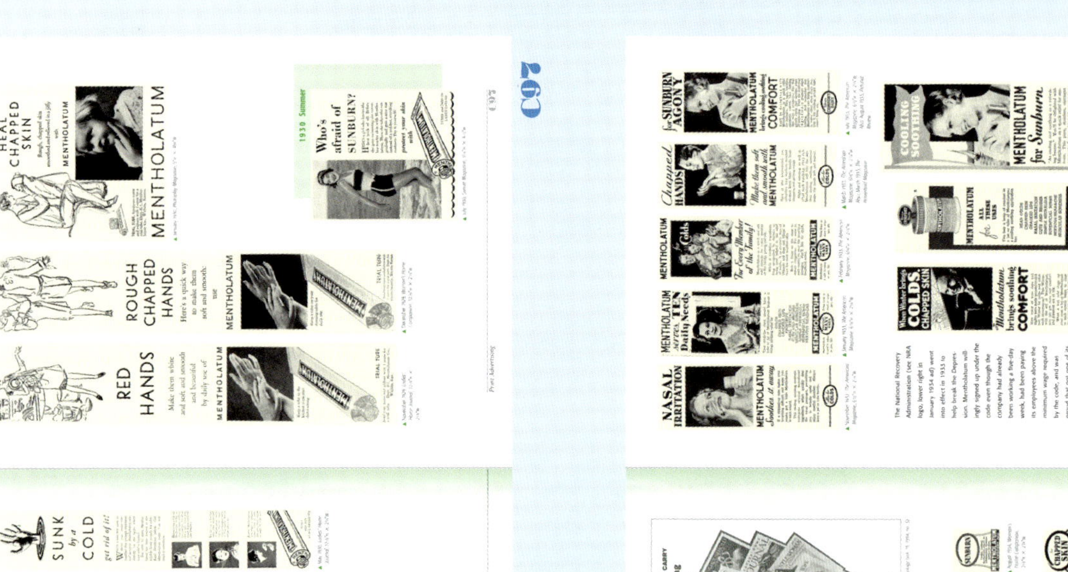

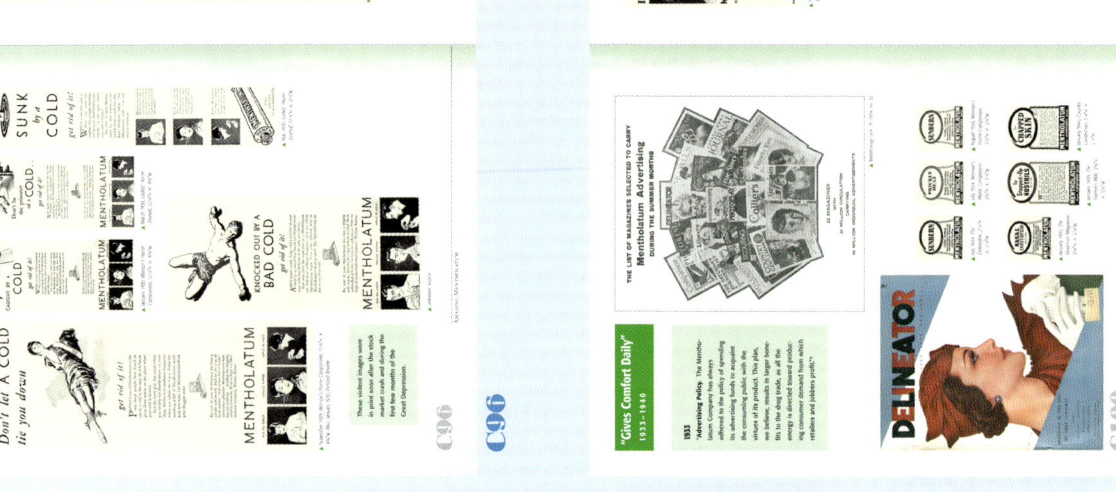

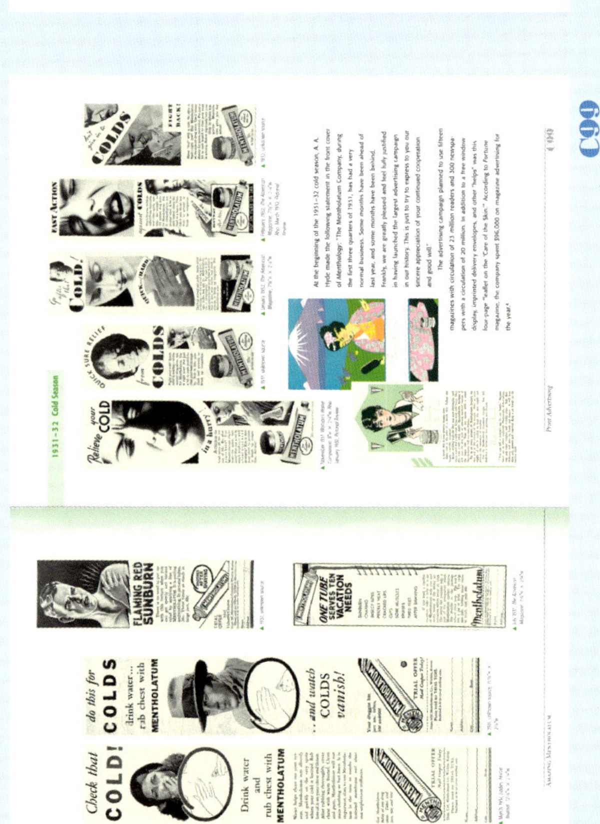

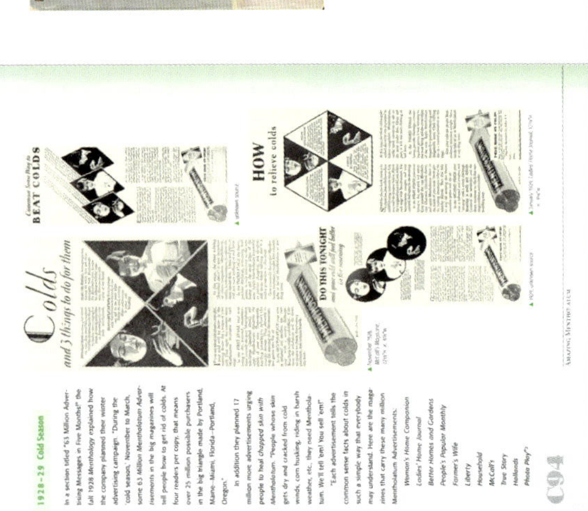

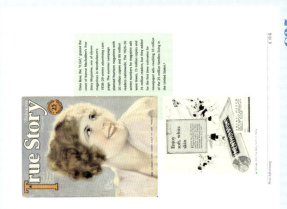

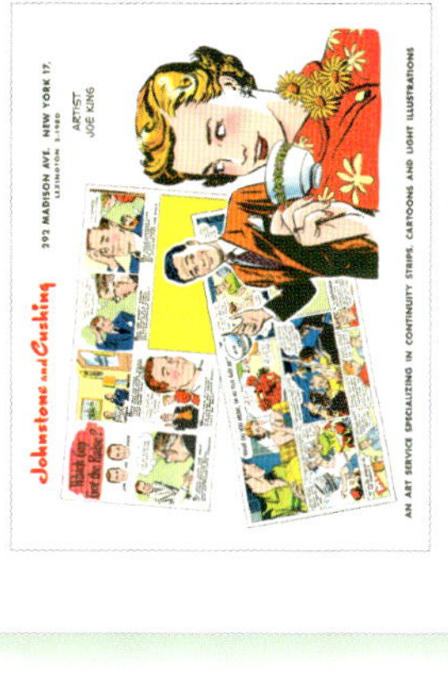

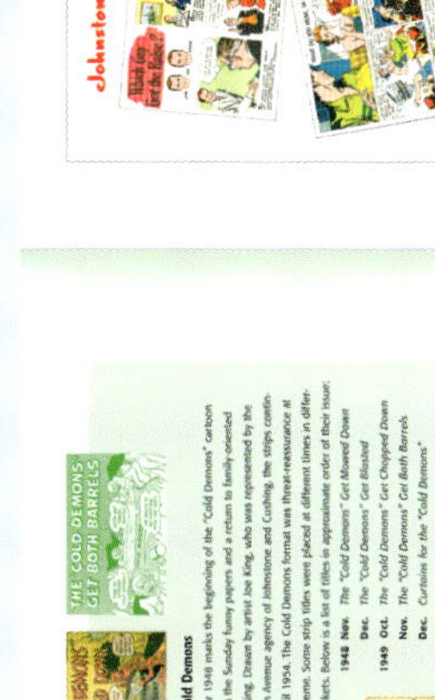

C105

C104

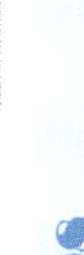

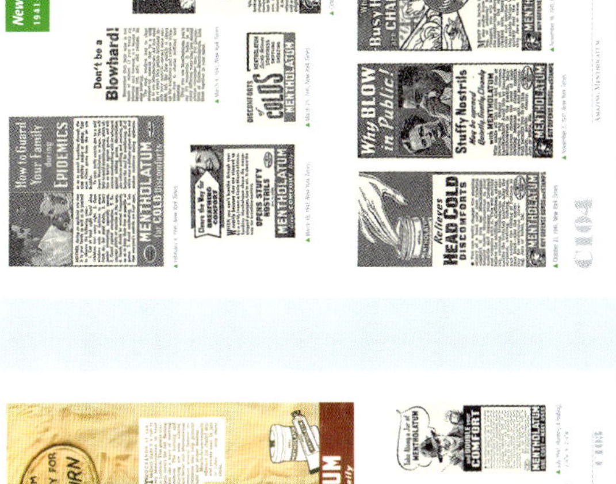

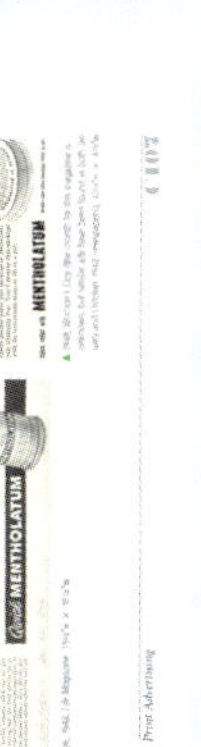

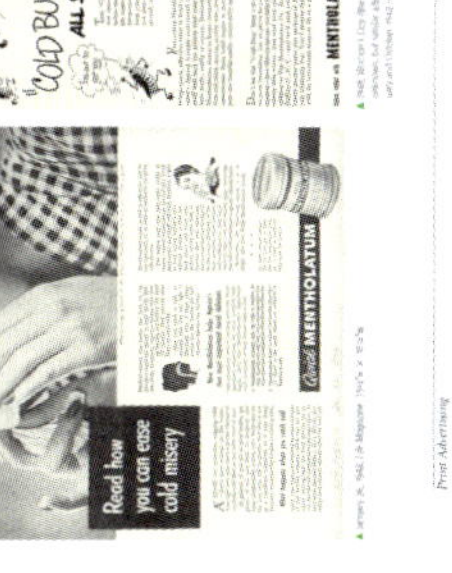

C109

C108

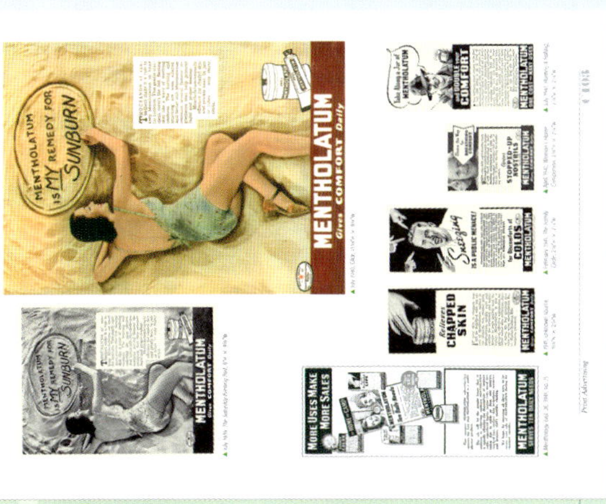

C103

C102

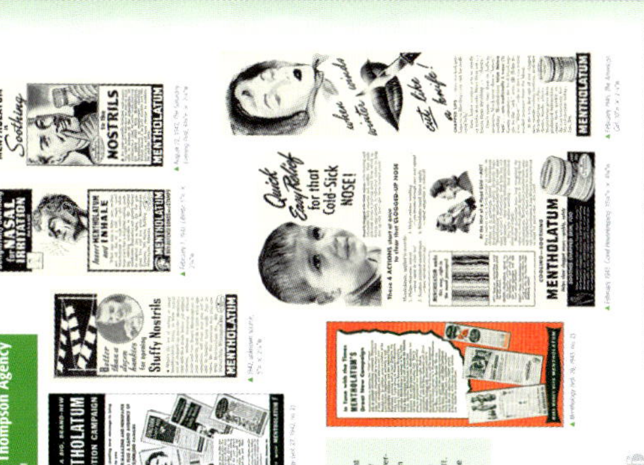

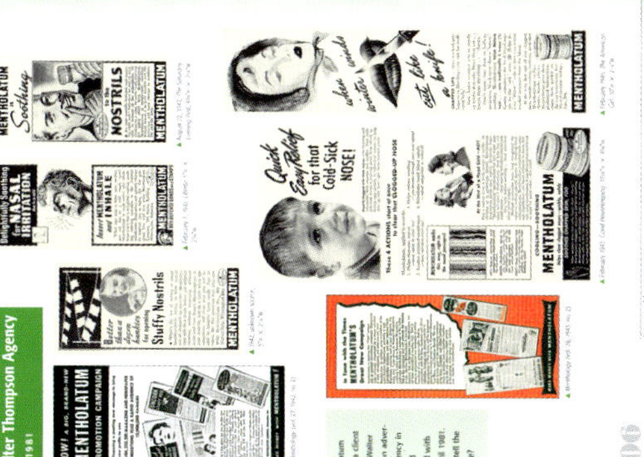

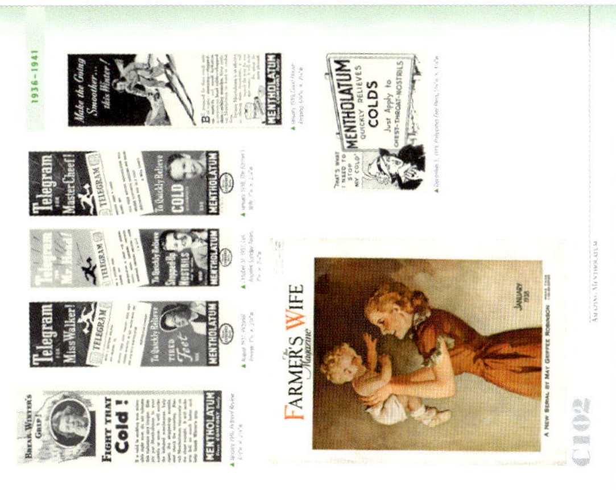

C107

C106

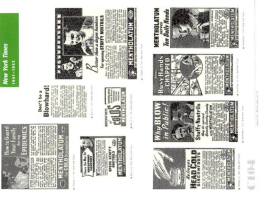

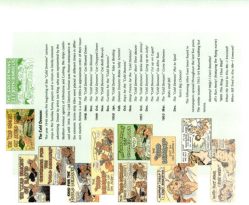

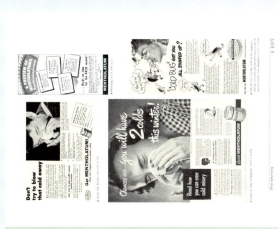

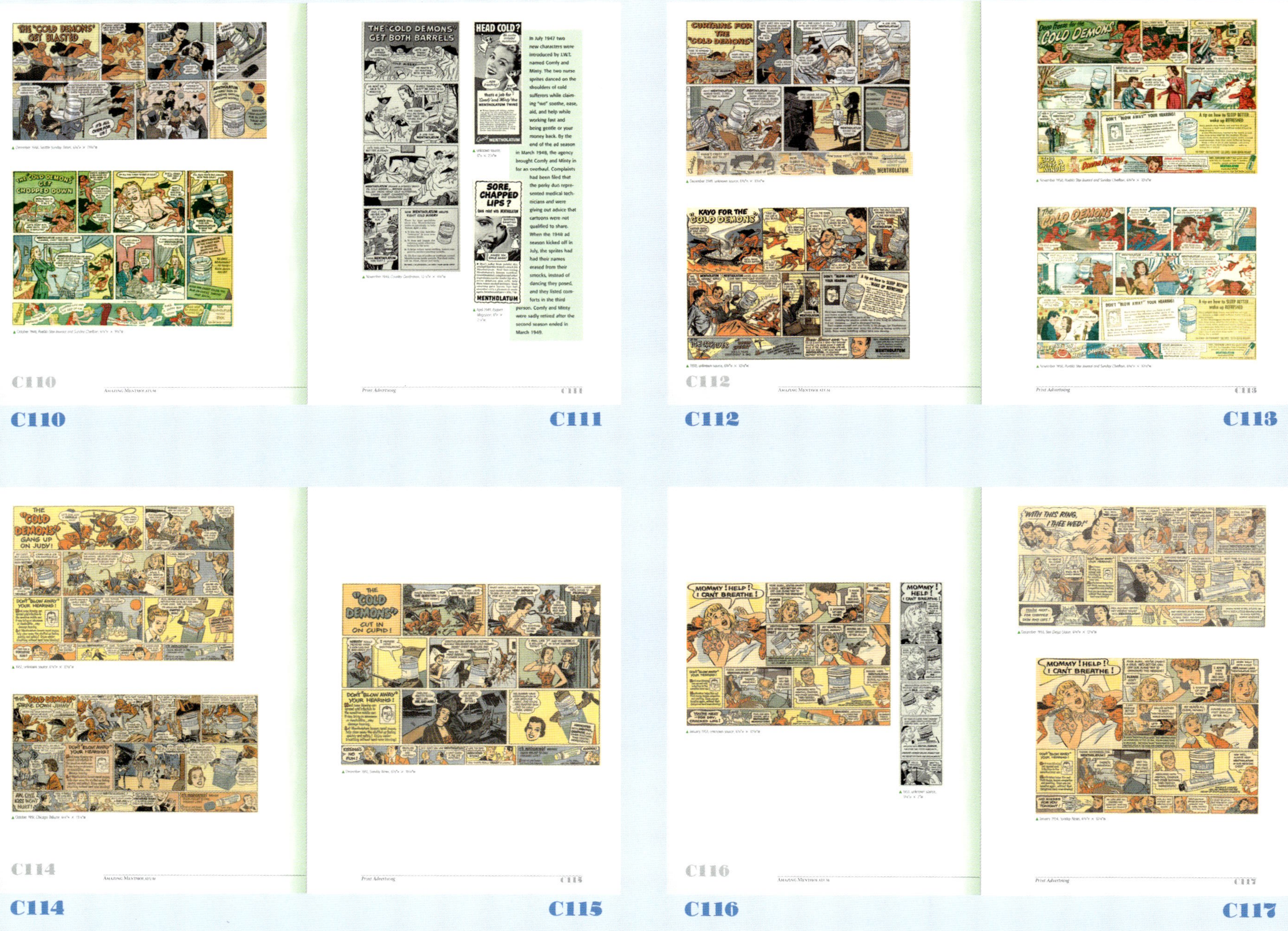

In July 1947 two new characters were introduced by J.W.T. named Comfy and Minty. The two nurse sprites danced on the shoulders of cold sufferers while claiming "we" soothe, ease, aid, and help while working fast and being gentle or your money back. By the end of the ad season in March 1948, the agency brought Comfy and Minty in for an overhaul. Complaints had been filed that the perky duo represented medical technicians and were giving out advice that cartoons were not qualified to share. When the 1948 ad season kicked off in July, the sprites had had their names erased from their smocks, instead of dancing they posed, and they listed comforts in the third person. Comfy and Minty were sadly retired after the second season ended in March 1949.

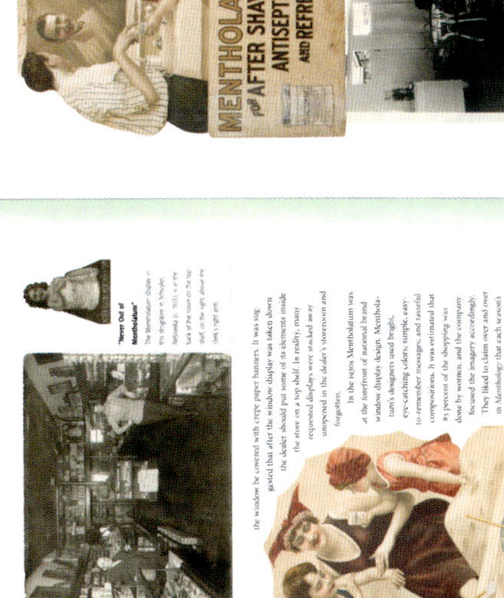
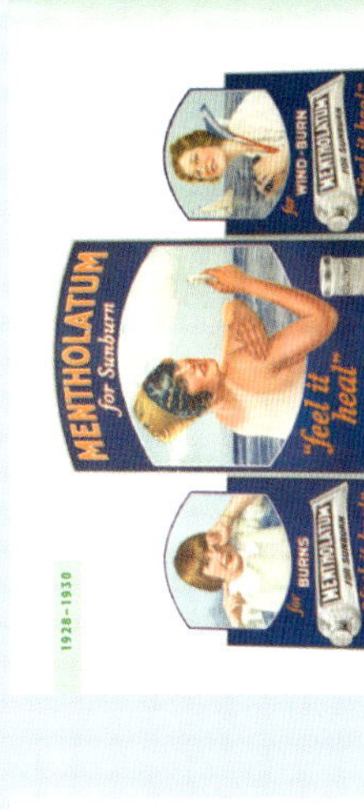
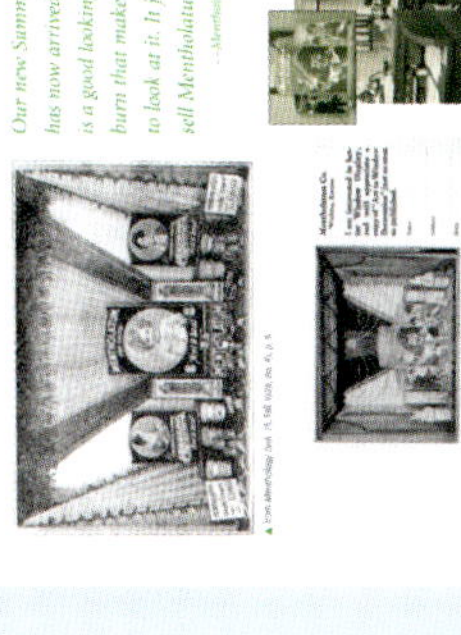
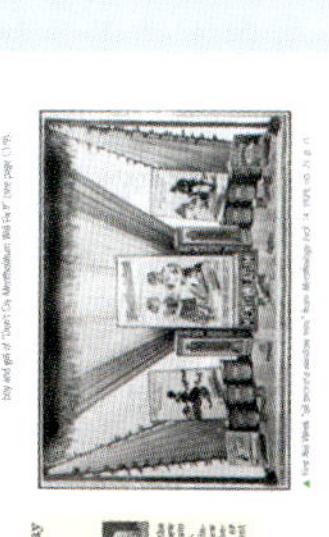
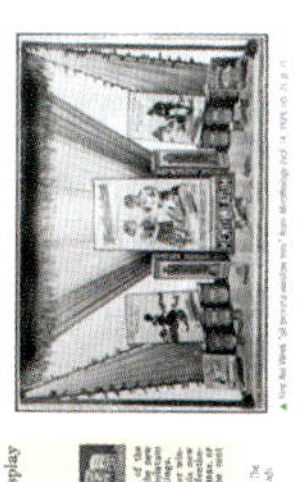
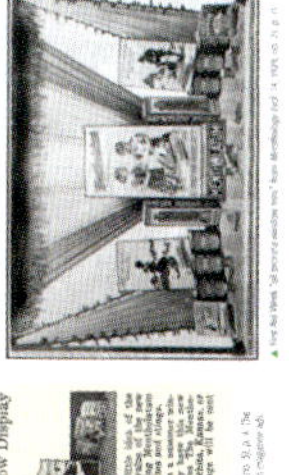
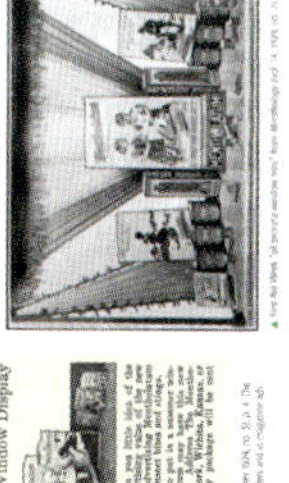
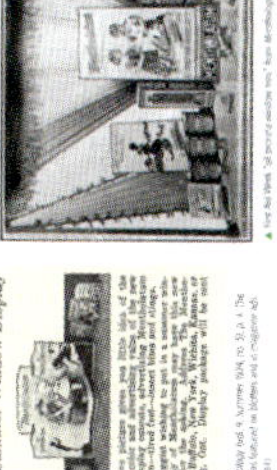
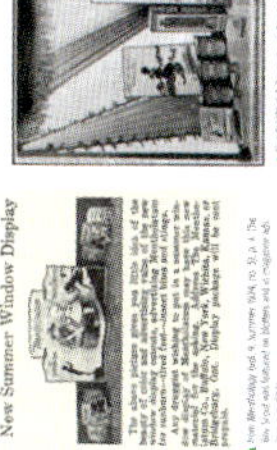
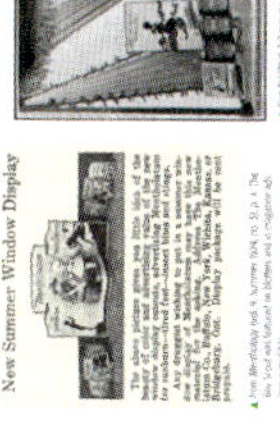
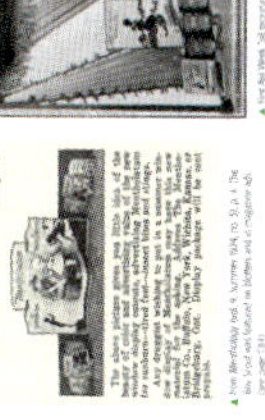
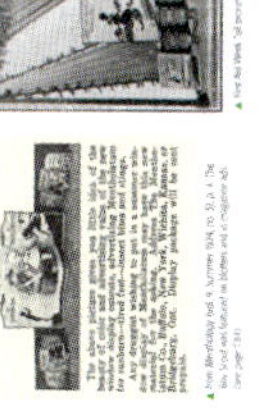
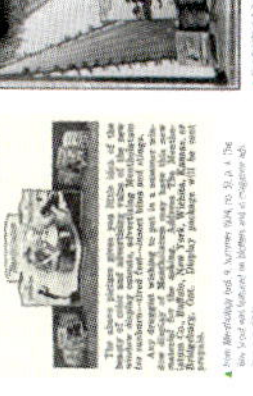
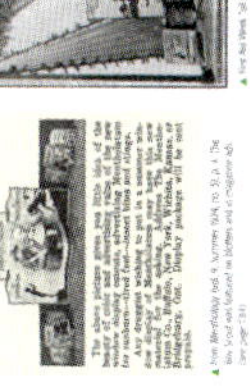
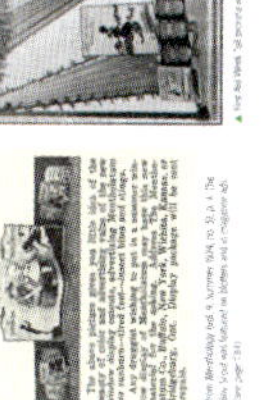
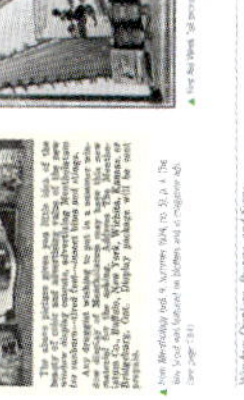
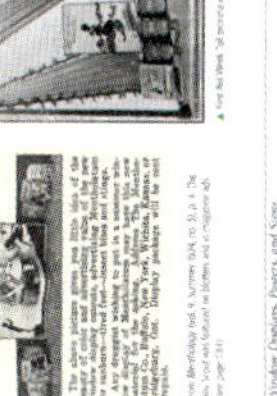
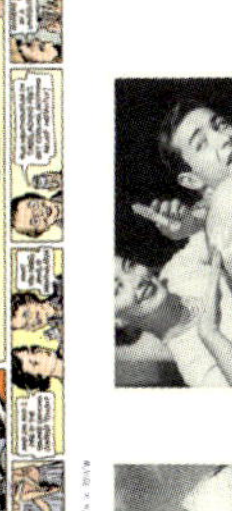
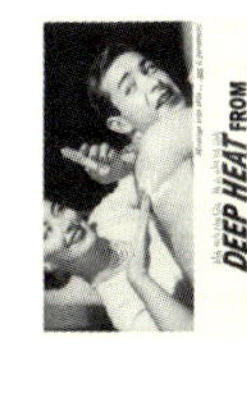
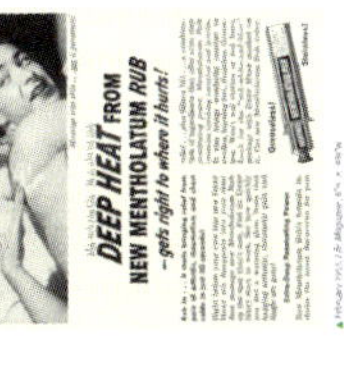
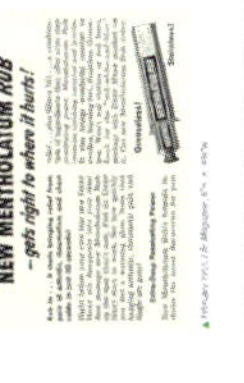
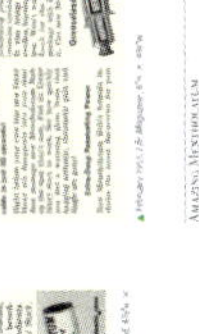

C121

C120

C119

C118

C125

C124

C123

C122

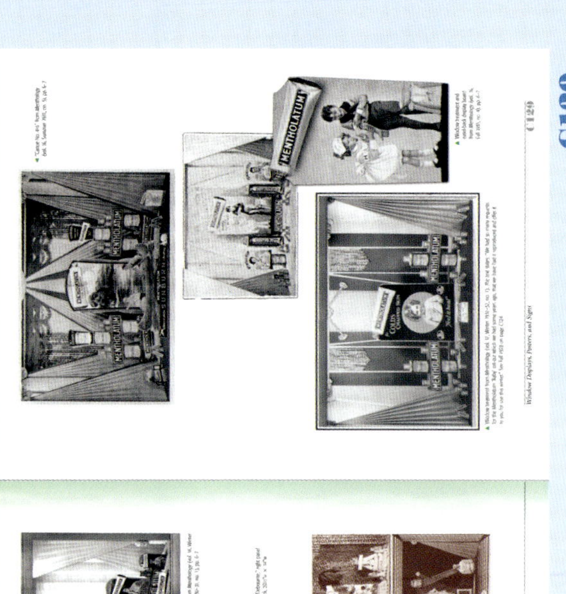

C129

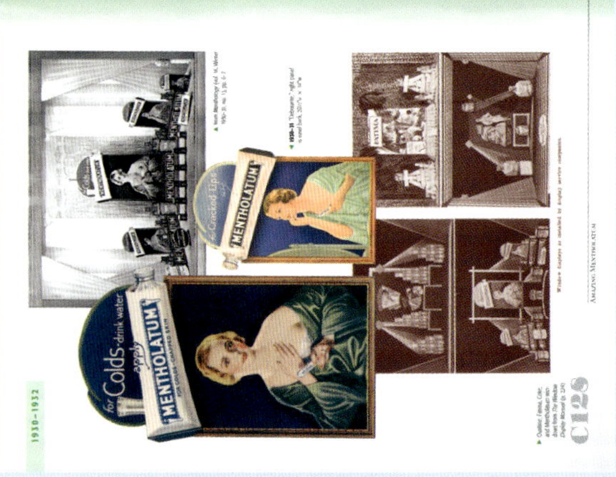

C128

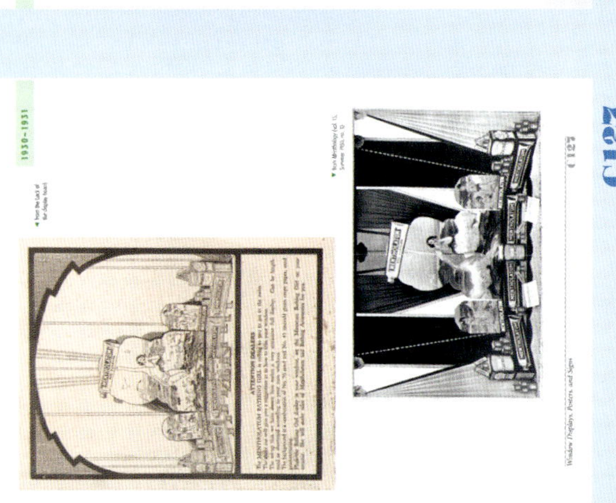

C127

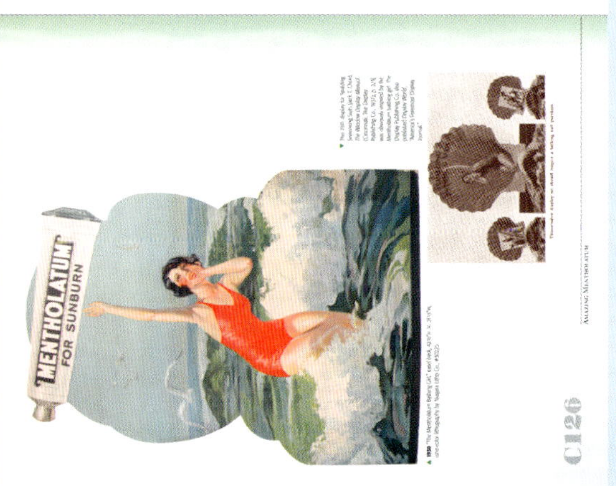

C126

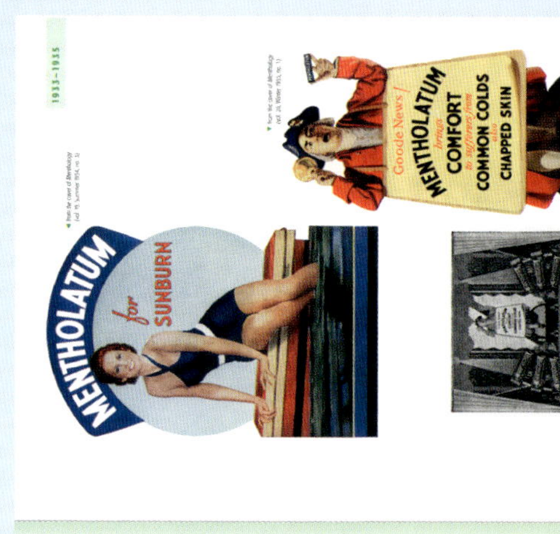

C133

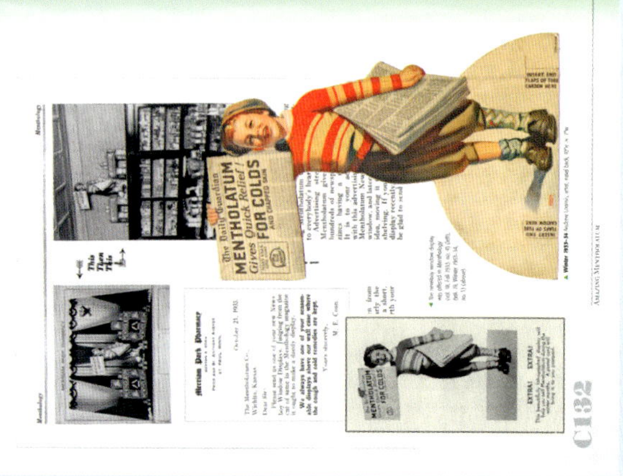

C132

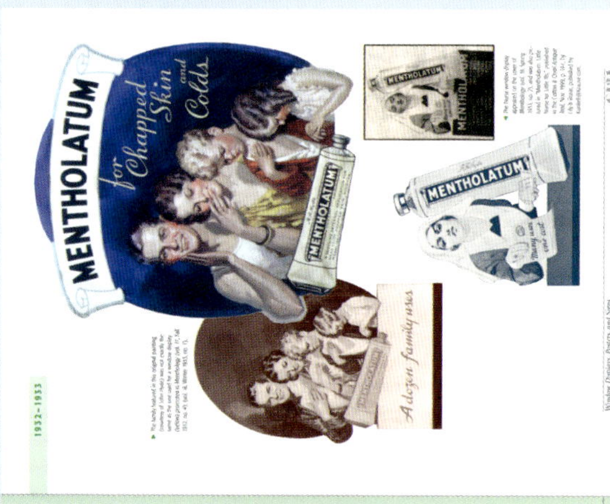

C131

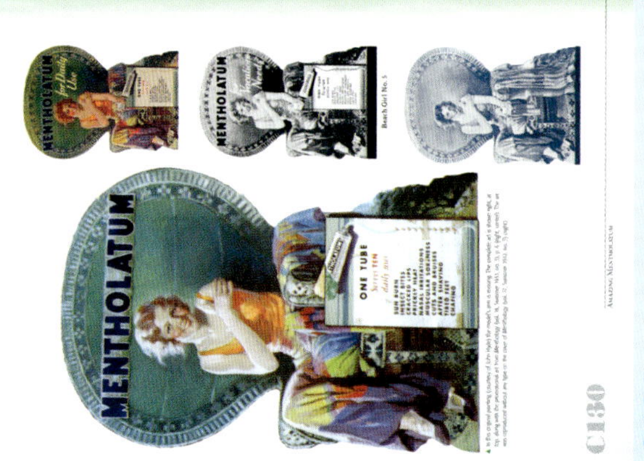

C130

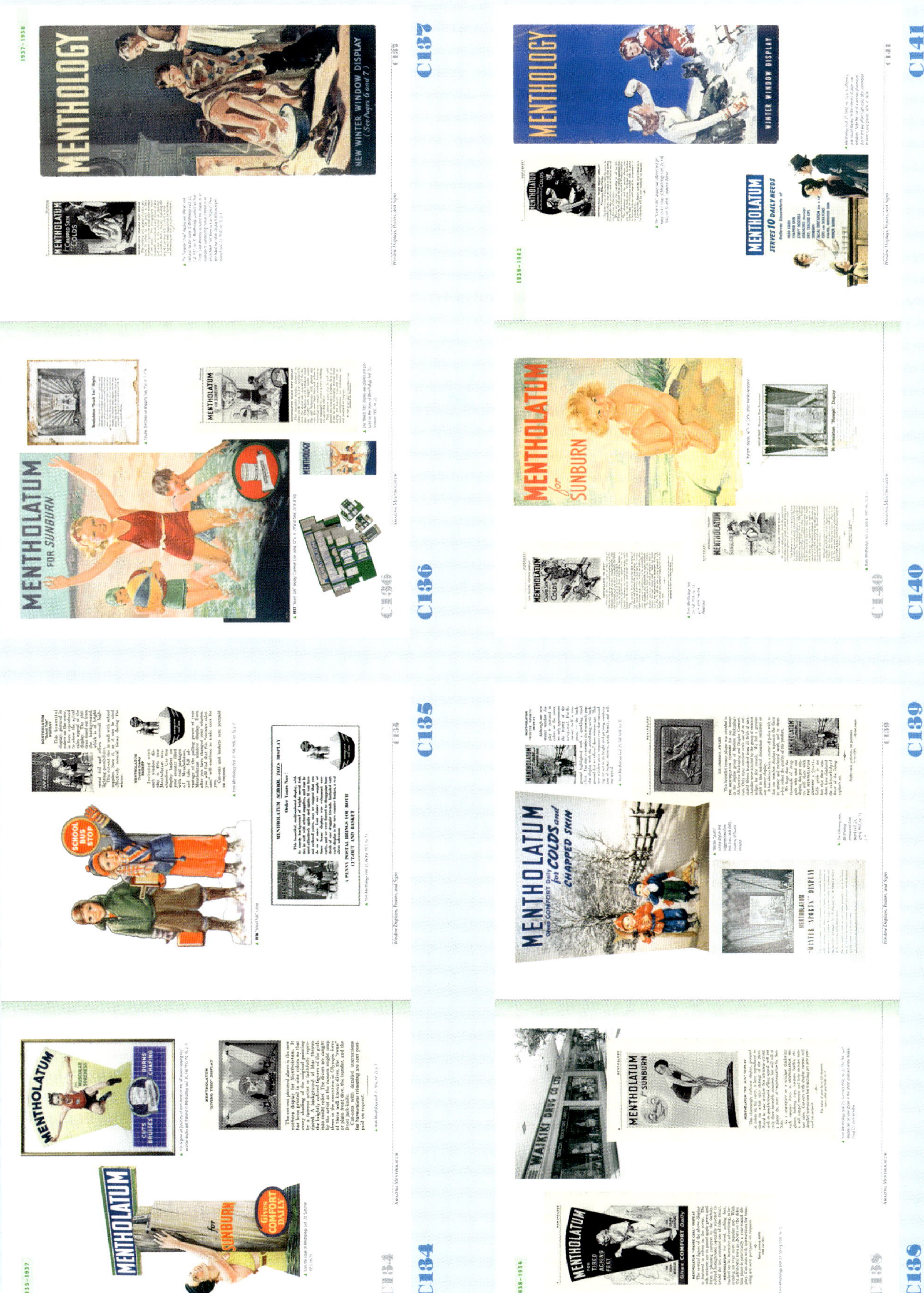
C134
C135
C136
C137
C138
C139
C140
C141

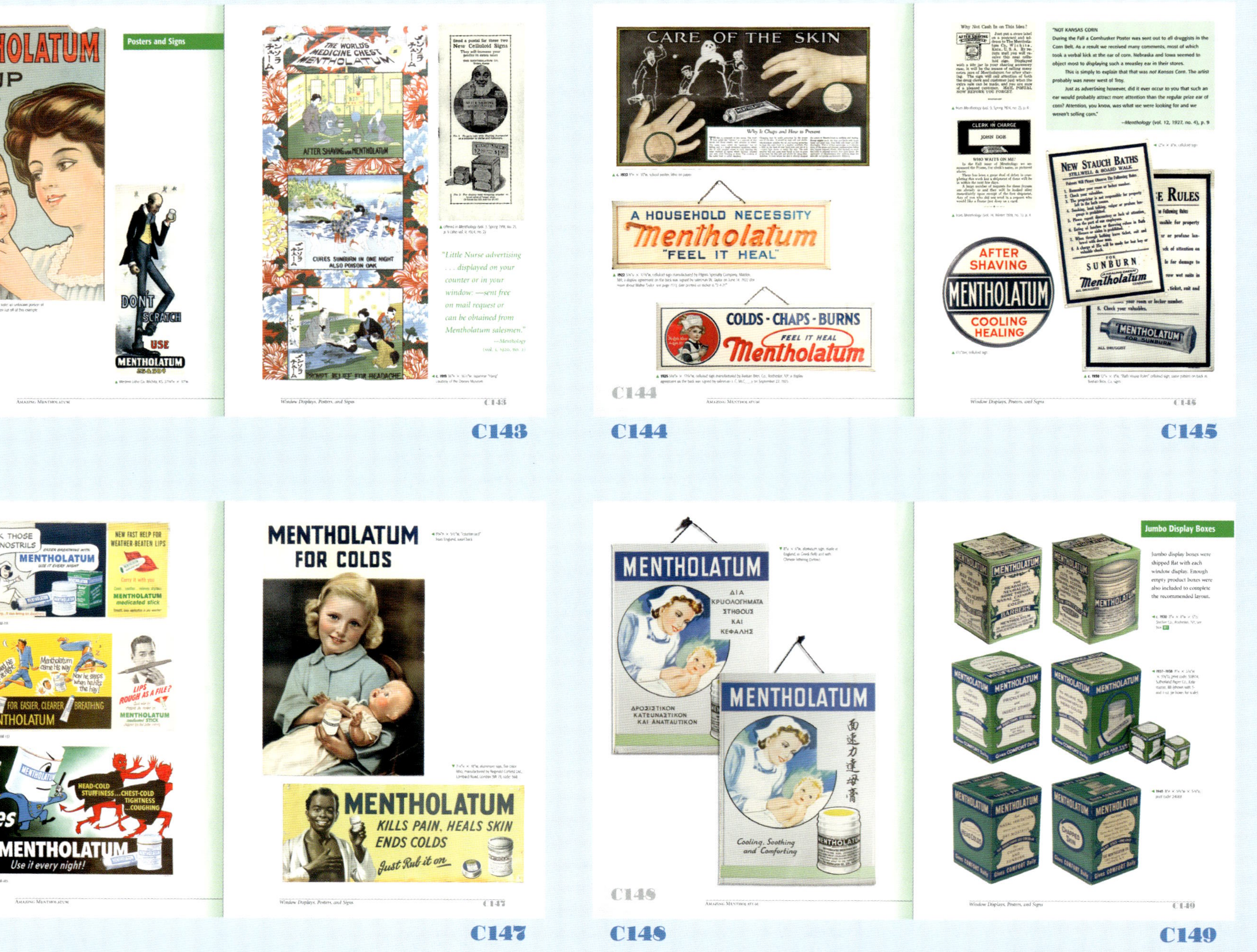
MENTHOLATUM
FOR CROUP AND SORE THROAT
Posters and Signs
DON'T SCRATCH
USE MENTHOLATUM
C142
THE WORLD'S MEDICINE CHEST MENTHOLATUM
AFTER SHAVING use MENTHOLATUM
CURES SUNBURN IN ONE NIGHT ALSO POISON OAK
PROMPT RELIEF FOR HEADACHE
"Little Nurse advertising . . . displayed on your counter or in your window: —sent free on mail request or can be obtained from Mentholatum salesmen."
C143
CARE OF THE SKIN
A HOUSEHOLD NECESSITY
Mentholatum
"FEEL IT HEAL"
COLDS - CHAPS - BURNS
FEEL IT HEAL
Mentholatum
C144
AFTER SHAVING
MENTHOLATUM
COOLING HEALING
NEW STAUCH BATHS
SUNBURN
Mentholatum
C145
UNCORK THOSE STUFFY NOSTRILS
MENTHOLATUM
NEW FAST HELP FOR WEATHER-BEATEN LIPS
USE IT EVERY NIGHT FOR EASIER, CLEARER BREATHING
MENTHOLATUM
LIPS ROUGH AS A FILE?
Chases Cold Miseries
HEAD-COLD STUFFINESS...CHEST-COLD TIGHTNESS ...COUGHING
MENTHOLATUM
Use it every night!
C146
MENTHOLATUM FOR COLDS
MENTHOLATUM
KILLS PAIN, HEALS SKIN
ENDS COLDS
Just Rub it on
C147
MENTHOLATUM
ΔΙΑ ΚΡΥΟΛΟΓΗΜΑΤΑ ΣΤΗΘΟΥΣ ΚΑΙ ΚΕΦΑΛΗΣ
MENTHOLATUM
Cooling, Soothing and Comforting
C148
Jumbo Display Boxes
Jumbo display boxes were shipped flat with each window display. Enough empty product boxes were also included to complete the recommended layout.
C149

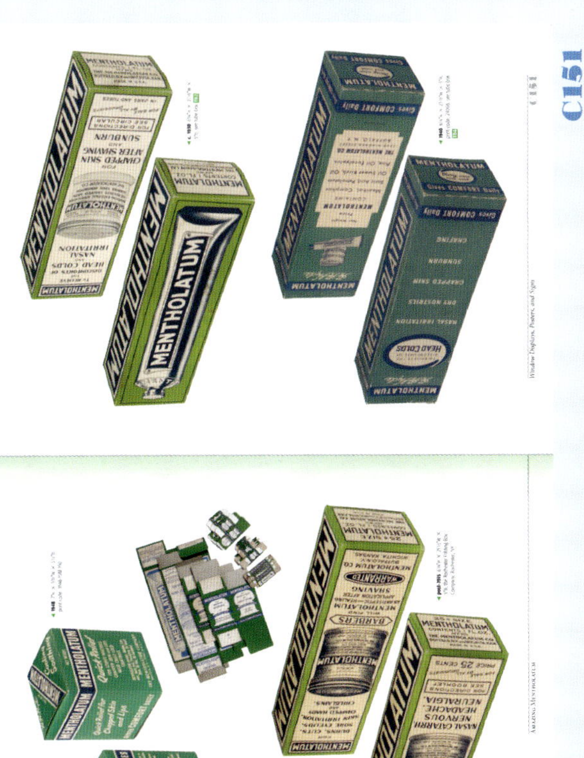

C150

C151

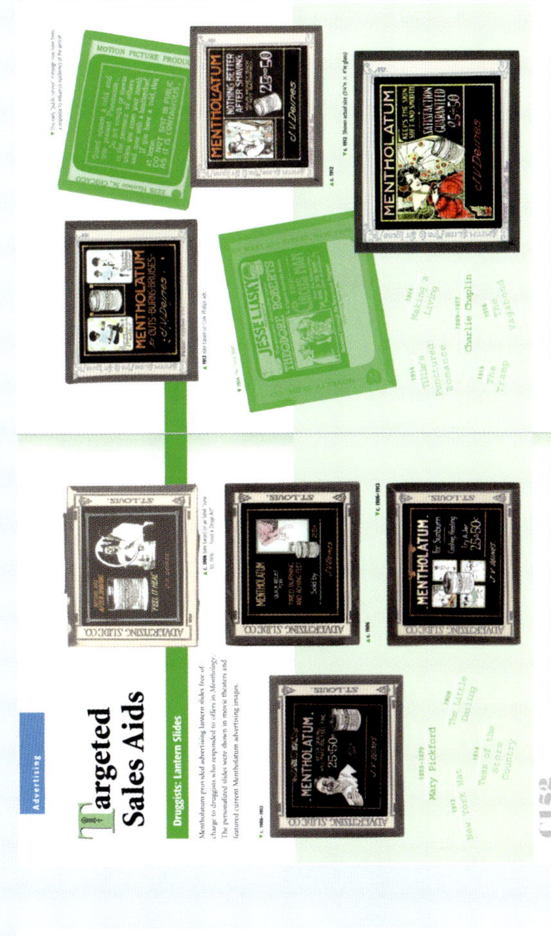

C152

C153

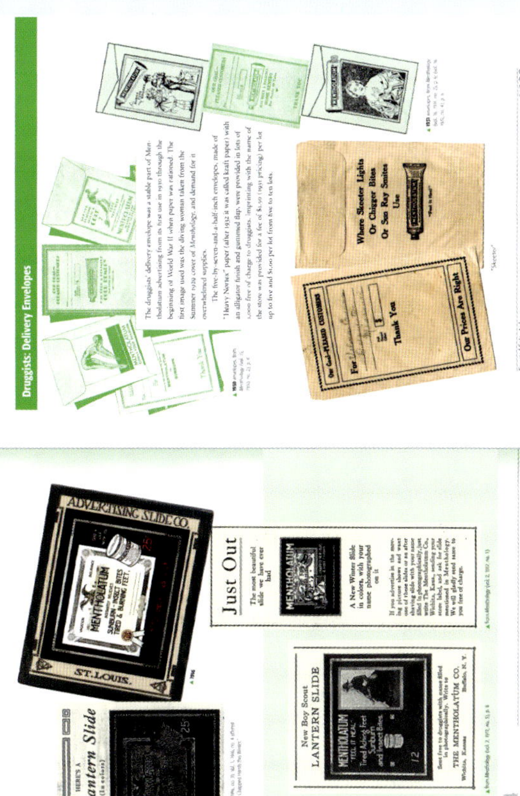

C154

C155

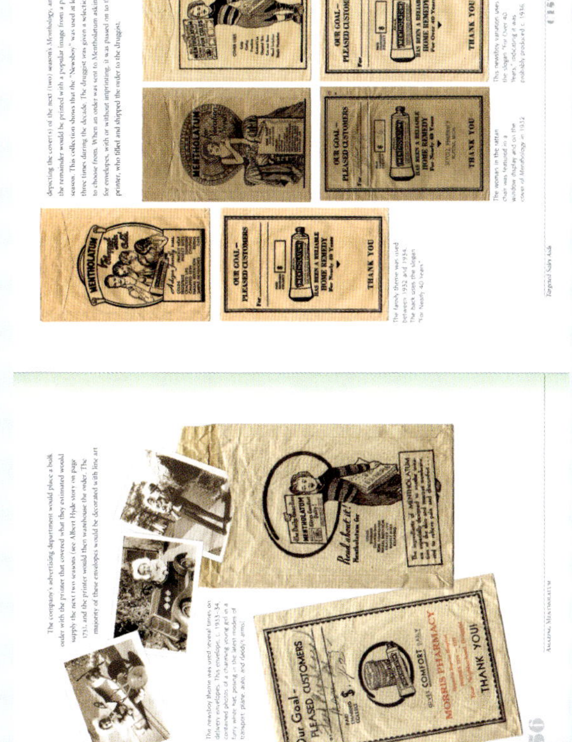

C156

C157

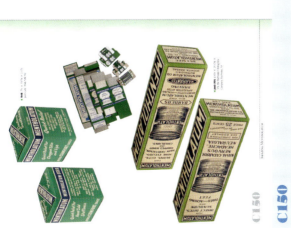

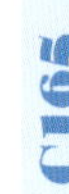

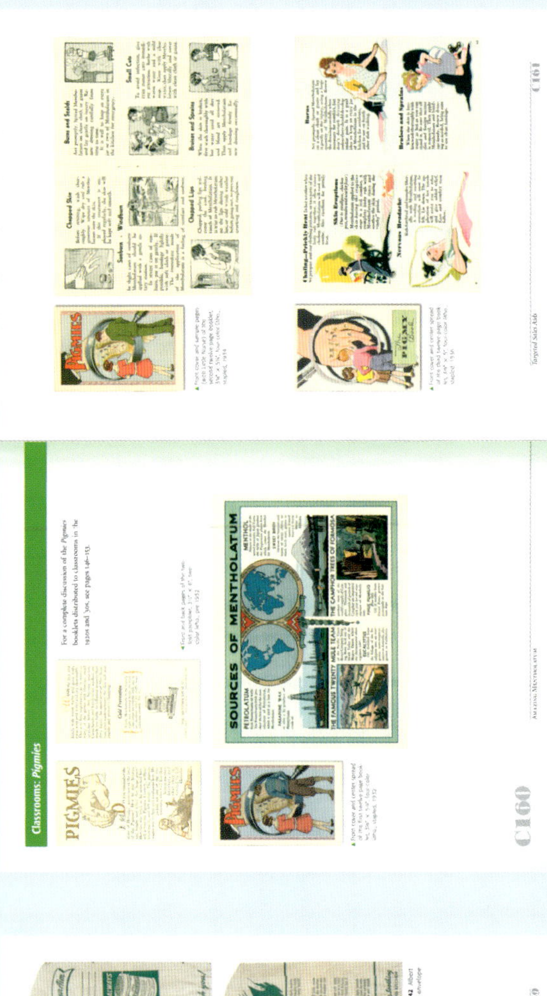

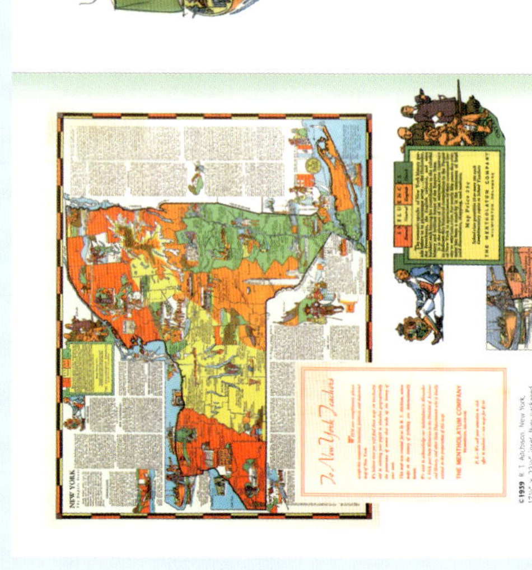

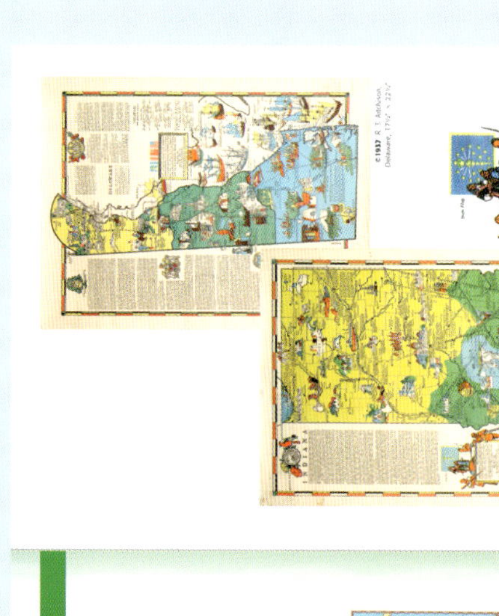

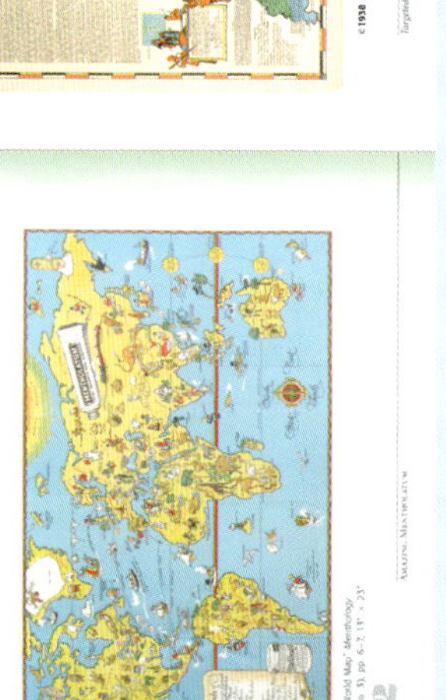

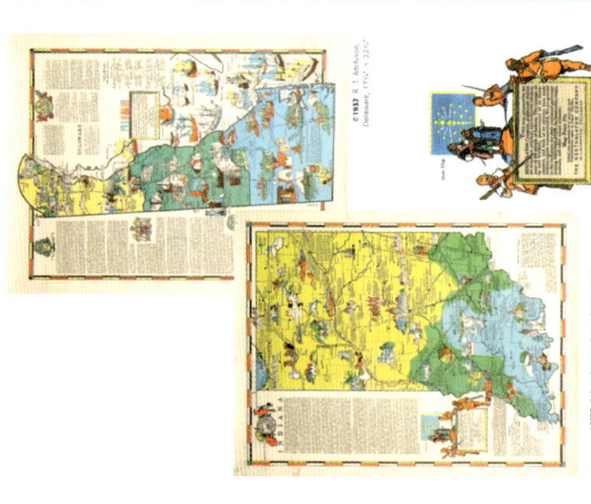

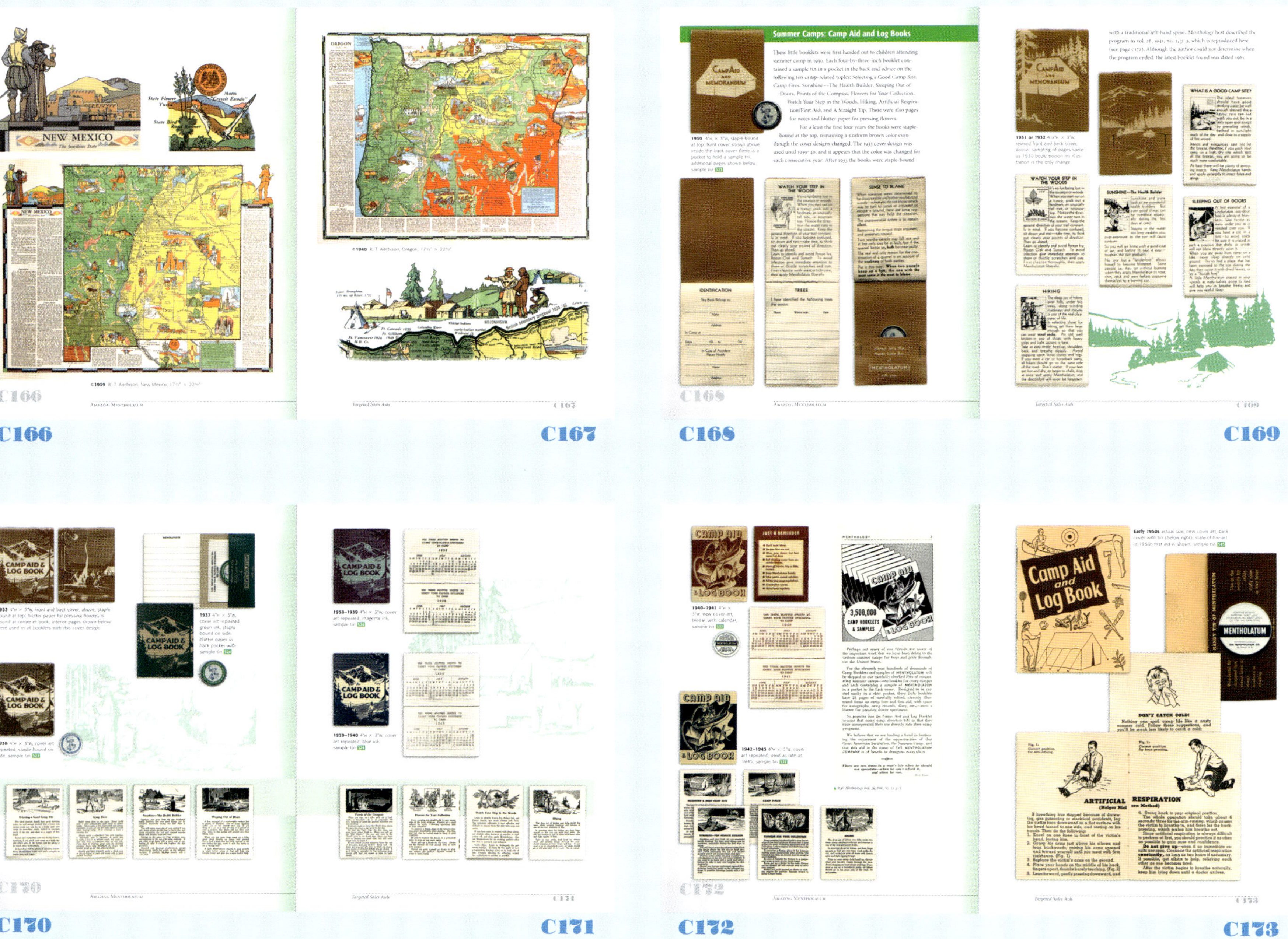
C166
C167
C168
Summer Camps: Camp Aid and Log Books
C169
C170
C171
C172
C173

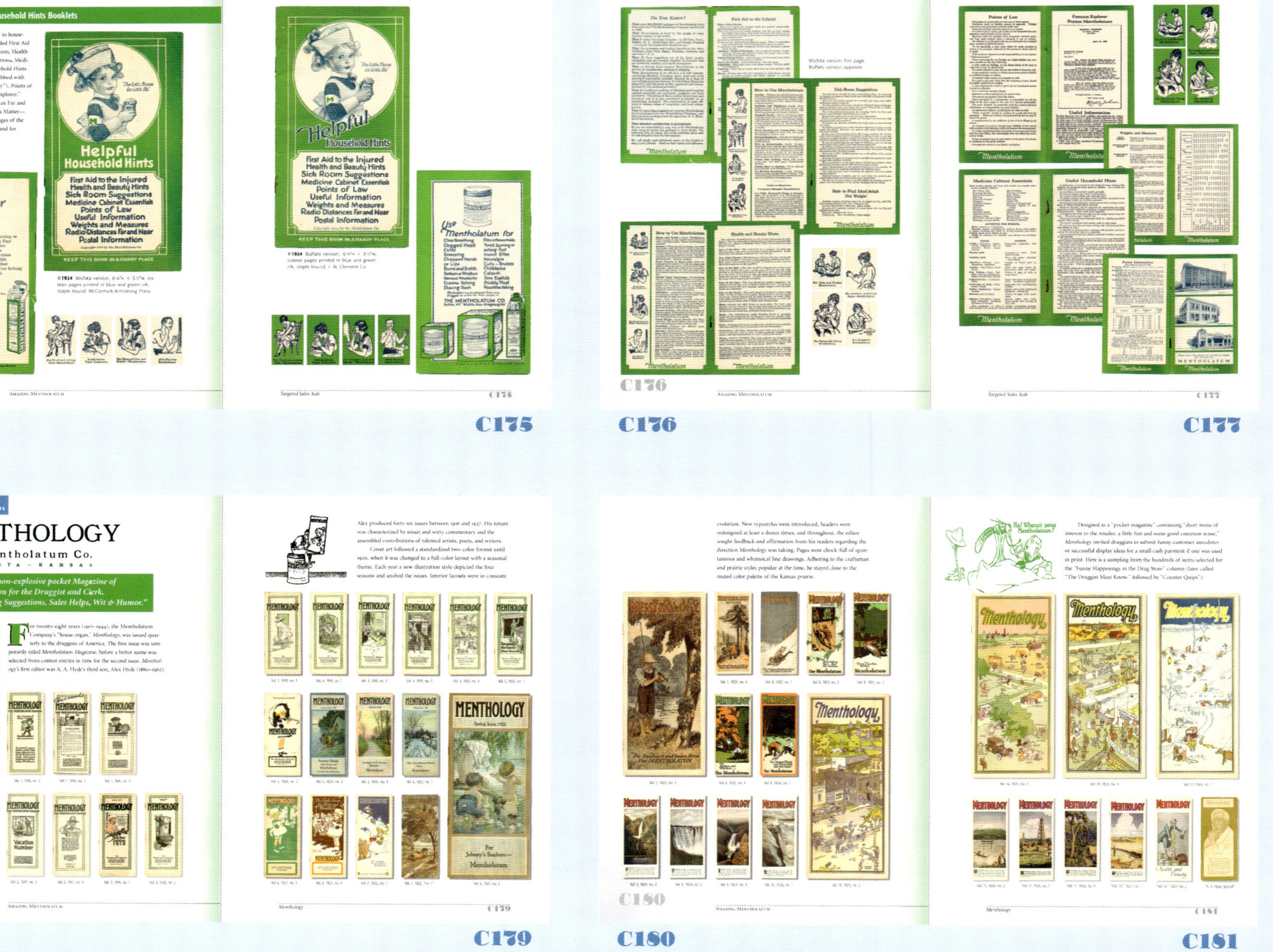

Housewives: Helpful Household Hints Booklets

These little booklets were handed out to housewives. The helpful information included First Aid to the Injured, How to use Mentholatum, Health and Beauty Hints, Sick-Room Suggestions, Medicine Cabinet Essentials, Useful Household Hints (such as "Grass stains having been rubbed with lard will then come out in the laundry"), Points of Law, a testimonial from a "Famous Explorer," Weights and Measures, Radio Distances Far and Near, Postal Information ("First Class Matter—Two cents per ounce"), as well as images of the "three big plants" supplying the demand for Mentholatum.

©1924 Wichita version, 6¼"H × 3⅝"W, sixteen pages printed in blue and green ink, staple bound. McCormick-Armstrong Press

©1924 Buffalo version, 6¼"H × 3½"W, sixteen pages printed in blue and green ink, staple bound, J. W. Clement Co.

Wichita version this page. Buffalo version opposite

C174 C175 C176 C177

Marketing and Sales

Menthology

The Mentholatum Co.
Wichita – Kansas

"A neutral non-explosive pocket Magazine of Ammunition for the Druggist and Clerk. Advertising Suggestions, Sales Helps, Wit & Humor."

For twenty-eight years (1916–1944), the Mentholatum Company's "house organ," *Menthology*, was issued quarterly to the druggists of America. The first issue was temporarily titled *Mentholatum Magazine*, before a better name was selected from contest entries in time for the second issue. *Menthology's* first editor was A. A. Hyde's third son, Alex Hyde (1880–1962).

Alex produced forty-six issues between 1916 and 1927. His tenure was characterized by smart and witty commentary and the assembled contributions of talented artists, poets, and writers.

Cover art followed a standardized two-color format until 1920, when it was changed to a full-color layout with a seasonal theme. Each year a new illustration style depicted the four seasons and unified the issues. Interior layouts were in constant evolution. New typestyles were introduced, headers were redesigned at least a dozen times, and throughout, the editor sought feedback and affirmation from his readers regarding the direction *Menthology* was taking. Pages were chock-full of spontaneous and whimsical line drawings. Adhering to the craftsman and prairie styles popular at the time, he stayed close to the muted color palette of the Kansas prairie.

Designed as a "pocket magazine" containing "short items of interest to the retailer, a little fun and some good common sense," *Menthology* invited druggists to submit funny customer anecdotes or successful display ideas for a small cash payment if one was used in print. Here is a sampling from the hundreds of items selected for the "Funny Happenings in the Drug Store" column (later called "The Druggist Must Know," followed by "Counter Quips"):

C178 C179 C180 C181

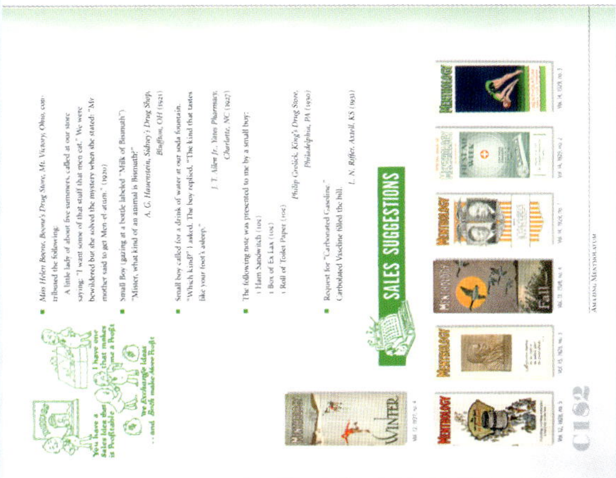

C182

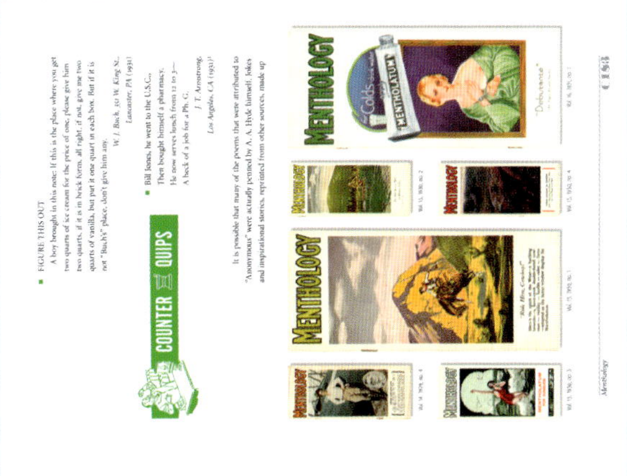

C183

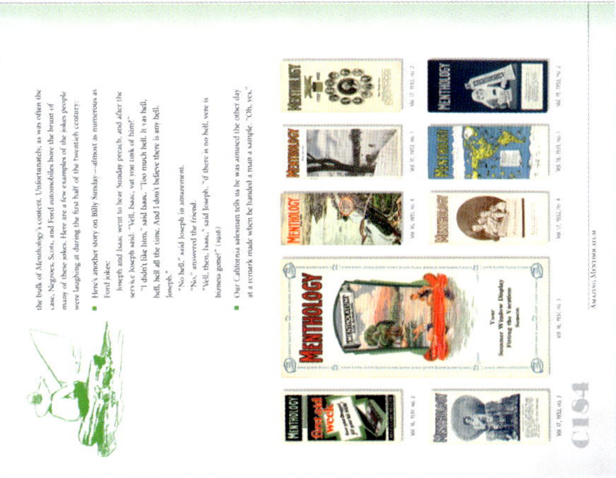

C184

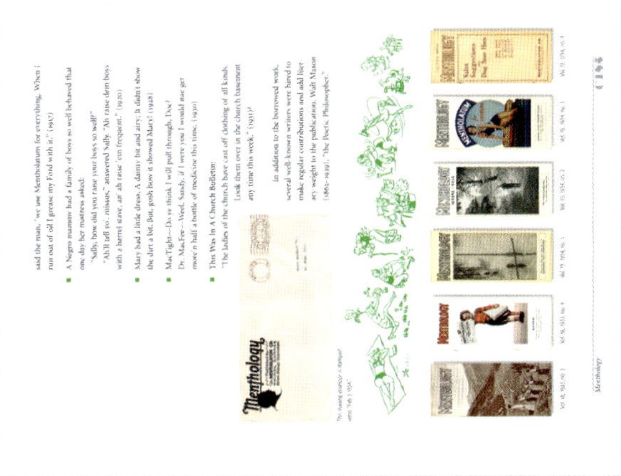

C185

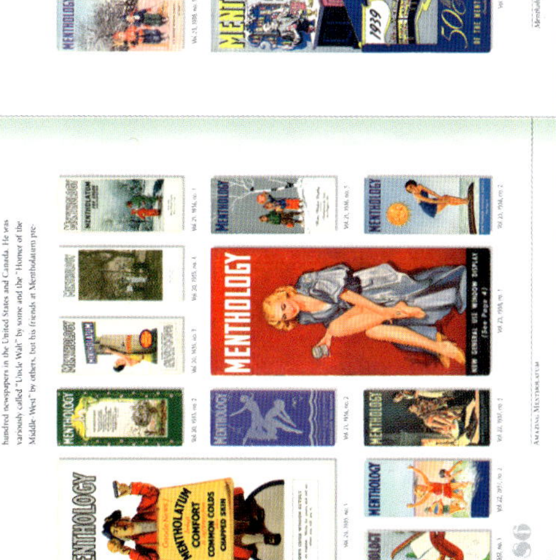

C186

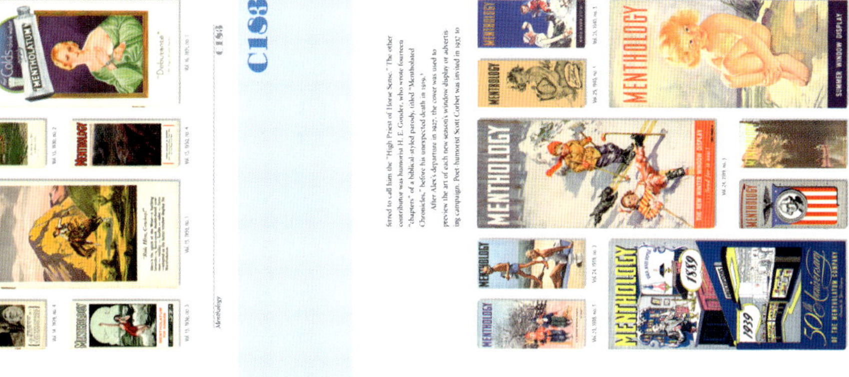

C187

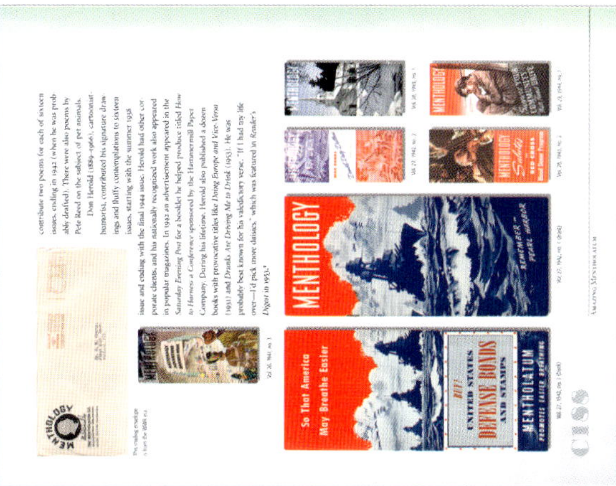

C188

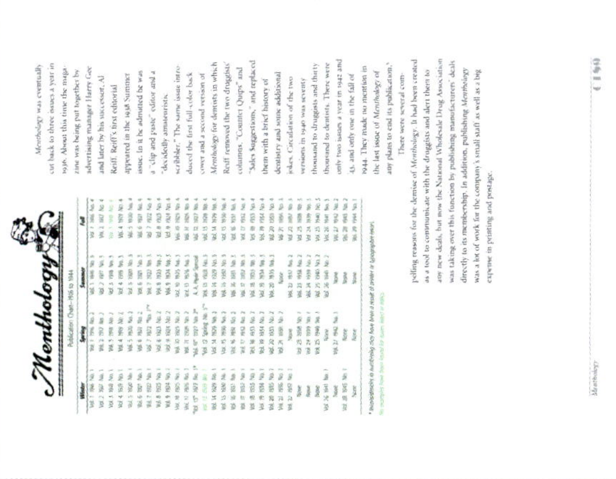

C189

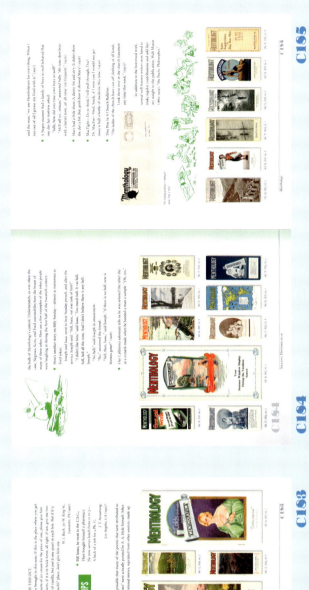

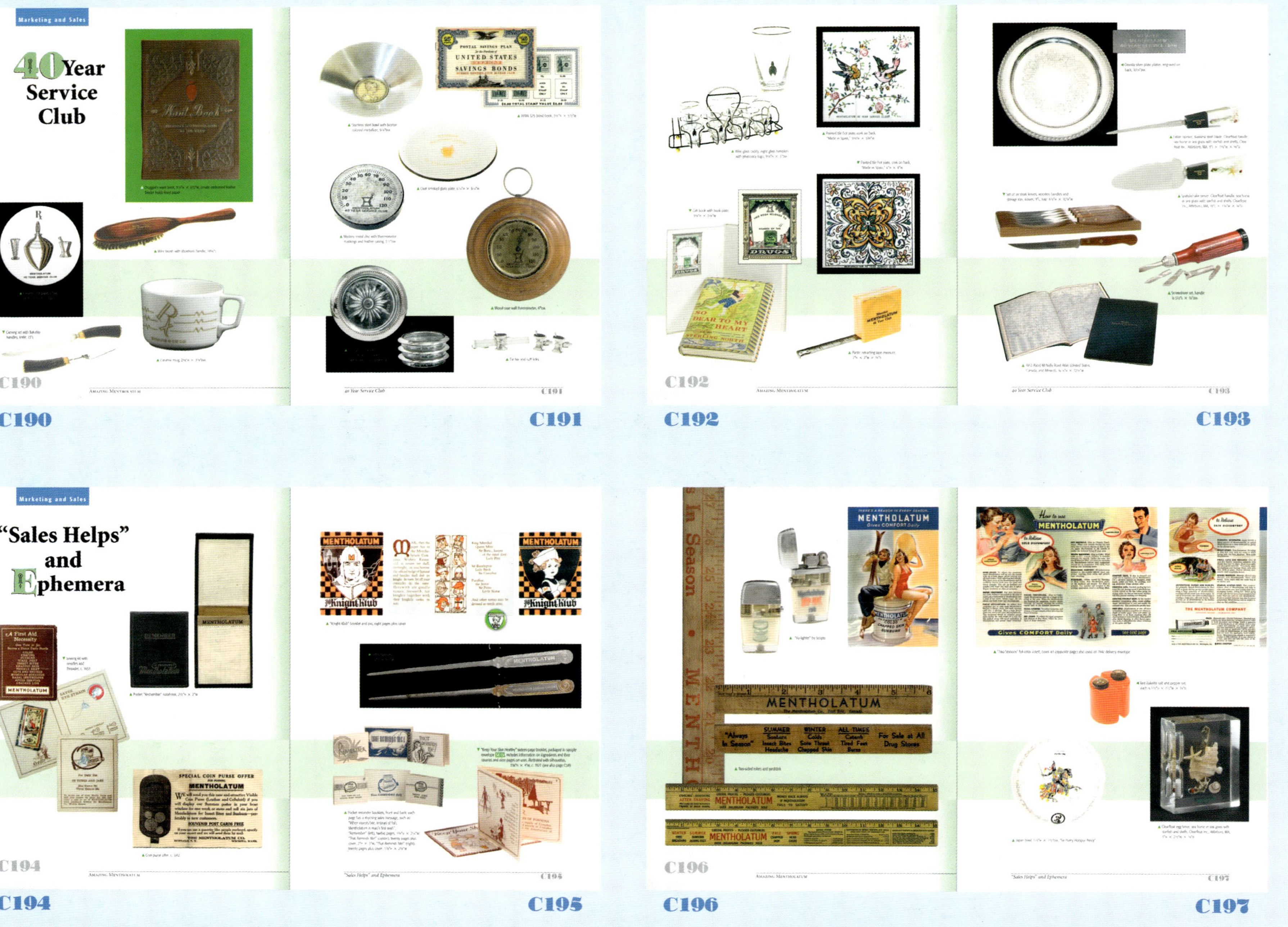
Marketing and Sales
40 Year Service Club
C190
C191
C192
C193
Marketing and Sales
"Sales Helps" and Ephemera
C194
C195
C196
C197